Body Fat Distribution & Health

Moderate amounts of body fat do not compromise health. However, excess fat above the hips carries a far greater health risk than fat on or below the hips - better to be a 'pear-shape' than an 'apple-shape'.

Abdominal obesity greatly increases the risk of developing diabetes, heart disease, high blood fats, hypertension, stroke, sleep apnea, arthritis and some cancers. So-called **'cellulite'** carries no extra health risk.

Waist Circumference directly reflects the increased health risk of abdominal obesity. Waist size associated with a high health risk:
Men ~ Over 40 inches **Women** ~ Over 35 inches

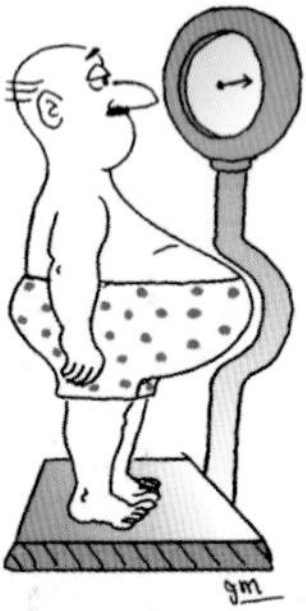

Abdominal obesity greatly increases the risk of ill-health and earlier death.

Body Mass Index (BMI)

BMI is a general (but not specific) indicator of body fatness. Although BMI alone is not diagnostic, the higher the BMI, the greater the health risk of developing diabetes, high blood pressure and heart disease. BMI does not apply to heavily muscled persons. BMI is used in a different way for children.

Check Your BMI: Find your height (no shoes) - look across the row to the weight nearest your own. Then track down to BMI.

Ht	WEIGHT (LBS) ~ ADULTS													
5'1"	100	106	111	116	122	127	132	137	143	148	153	158	185	211
5'2"	104	109	115	120	126	131	136	142	147	153	158	164	191	218
5'3"	107	113	118	124	130	135	141	146	152	158	163	169	197	225
5'4"	110	116	122	128	134	140	145	151	157	163	169	174	204	232
5'5"	114	120	126	132	138	144	150	156	162	168	174	180	210	240
5'6"	118	124	130	136	142	148	155	161	167	173	179	186	216	247
5'7"	121	127	134	140	146	153	159	166	172	178	185	191	223	255
5'8"	125	131	138	144	151	158	164	171	177	184	190	197	230	262
5'9"	128	135	142	149	155	162	169	176	182	189	196	206	236	270
5'10"	132	139	146	153	160	167	174	181	188	195	202	207	243	278
5'11"	136	143	150	157	165	172	179	186	193	200	208	215	250	286
6'0"	140	147	154	162	169	177	184	191	199	206	213	221	258	294
6'1"	144	151	159	166	174	182	189	197	204	212	219	227	265	302
6'2"	148	155	163	171	179	186	194	202	210	218	225	233	272	311
6'3"	152	160	168	176	184	192	200	208	216	224	232	240	279	319
6'4"	156	164	172	180	189	197	205	213	221	230	238	246	287	328
BMI	**19**	**20**	**21**	**22**	**23**	**24**	**25**	**26**	**27**	**28**	**29**	**30**	**35**	**40**

BMI Classification:

BMI Below 19
Underweight

BMI 19-24.9
Healthy Weight (Low Health Risk)

BMI 25-29.9
Overweight (Moderate Health Risk)

BMI 30-40
Obese (High Health Risk)

BMI Over 40
Morbid Obesity (Very High Risk)

Interactive BMI Calculator
www.calorieking.com

Calories & Weight Loss

Calories in Food

Calories in food are derived from protein, fat and carbohydrate. Alcohol also provides calories. Vitamins, minerals and water provide no calories.

Calorie Values Per Gram

Fat/Oil	~ 9 Calories
Carbohydrate	~ 4 Calories
Protein	~ 4 Calories
Alcohol	~ 7 Calories

Note that fats have over double the calories of protein and carbohydrate. The higher the fat content of food, the higher the calories.

Sample Calculation

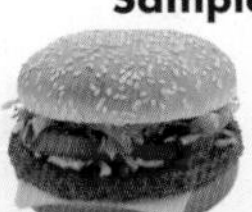

QUARTER POUNDER® WITH CHEESE has 530 calories derived from:

30g Fat (x 9 cals/gram)	= 270
38g Carbohyd.(x 4 cals/gram)	= 152
27g Protein (x 4 cals/gram)	= 108
Total Calories	= 530

Calorie Levels for Weight Loss

Start with a calorie-controlled diet that allows a moderate weight loss of ½ - 1 pound per week. Weight loss is usually much greater in the first few weeks due to extra fluid losses.

Note: It is better to increase exercise rather than lessen food calories too drastically.

Suggested Calories for Weight Loss

Women:	Non-active	1000 - 1200
	Active	1200 - 1500
Men:	Non-active	1200 - 1500
	Active	1500 - 1800
Teenagers:		1200 - 1800

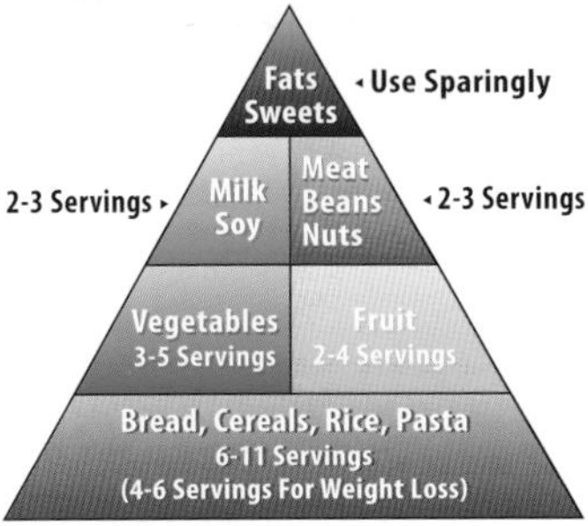

The Food Guide Pyramid emphasizes eating a wide variety of foods from the 5 major food groups. For weight loss, make low-fat choices and eat the lower number of servings.

Examples of Serving Size

Bread & Cereal Group:

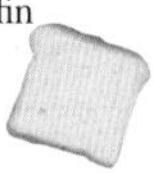

- 1 slice bread
- ½ bun, small bagel or English muffin
- 4 small crackers or 1 tortilla
- 1 oz ready-to-eat cereal
- ½ cup cooked cereal, rice or pasta

Fruit Group:

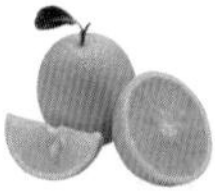

- 1 medium apple, orange, banana
- ½ cup canned fruit
- ¼ cup dried fruit
- ¾ cup fruit juice
- ¼ medium avocado

Vegetable Group:

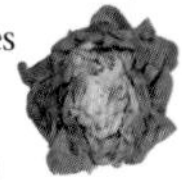

- 1 cup raw leafy vegetables
- 1½ cups raw chopped vegetables
- ½ cup cooked vegetables
- ½ - ¾ cup vegetable juice

Meat & Alternatives Group:

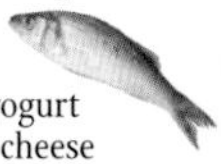

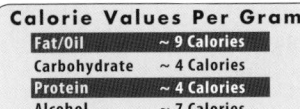

- 2-3 oz (cooked) lean meat/poultry/fish
- 2 eggs **or** 7 oz tofu **or** ¼ cup nuts
- 1 cup (cooked) dried beans **or** chickpeas
- 4 Tbsp peanut butter

Milk & Alternatives Group:

- 1 cup (8 fl.oz) milk, soy drink, yogurt
- 1½ oz cheese or ½ cup cottage cheese

Portion Size Counts!

Food portion size is critical to controlling calorie intake for weight control.

Super-sized food servings have become more common when eating out and in the home. This can mean a day's worth of calories being consumed in one meal; or a snack being equivalent to a full meal.

It is easy to underestimate portion size of foods and drinks, and unwittingly consume excess calories – even if the fat content is low or even zero!

To more accurately estimate portion size of different foods, weigh and measure your food with food scales, measuring spoons and cups. Better control of calories will result.

For a visual idea of portion sizes, visit www.CalorieKing.com. See examples (fries and cola) on this page.

Allow for Extra Calories in Packaged Food

The actual weight of packaged foods is usually 5-10% more than the label net weight (the minimum legal weight) - and in some cases up to 50% more. However, manufacturers calculate the calories based on the net weight. For actual calories, weigh the product and calculate the extra calories. **For extra details see www.CalorieKing.com**

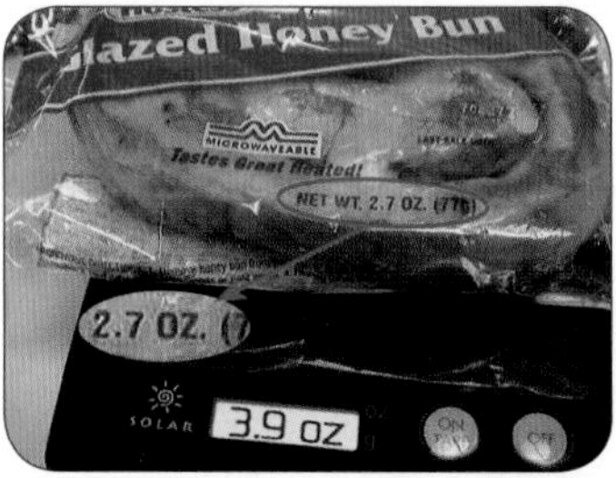

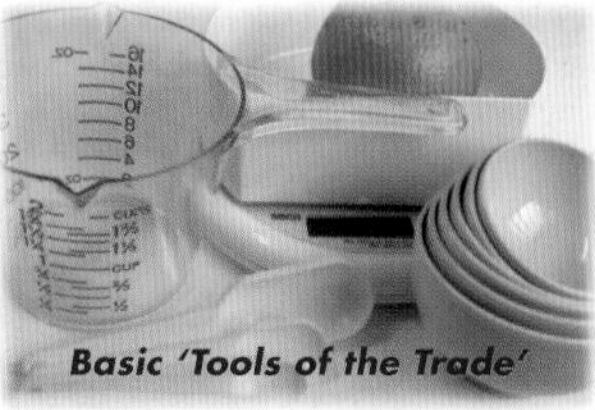

Basic 'Tools of the Trade'

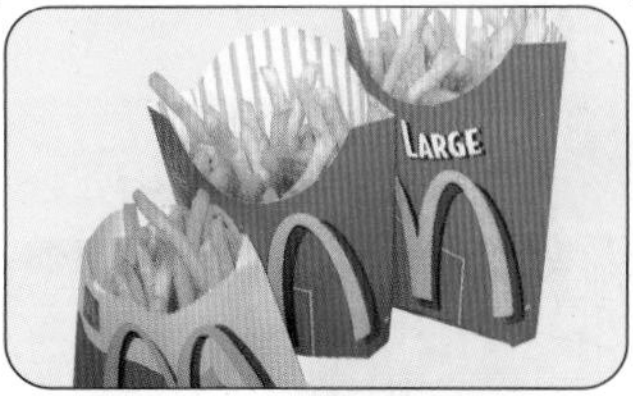

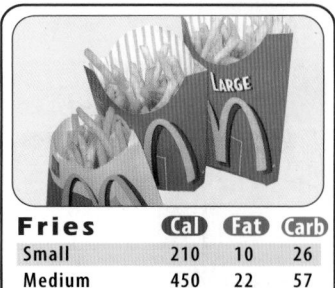

Fries	Cal	Fat	Carb
Small	210	10	26
Medium	450	22	57
Large	540	26	68

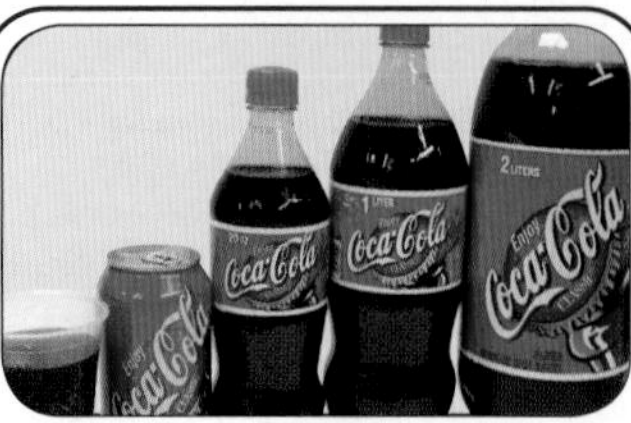

Cola	Cal	Fat	Carb
8 fl.oz Cup	100	0	25
12 fl.oz Can	150	0	37
20 fl.oz Bottle	250	0	63
1 Liter Bottle	400	0	100
2 Liter Bottle	800	0	200

Recommended Fat Intake

Americans consume too much fat with many getting over 40% of total calories from fat – either as fat or oil, or as fat in foods and drinks. A range of 20-30% is healthier.

Fat Intake - Healthy Ranges

Children	~	30-60g
Teenagers (Active)	~	40-80g
Women	~	30-60g
Men: Active	~	40-80g
Heavy Activity/Athlete	~	80-120g

MAXIMUM DESIRABLE FAT INTAKE (Daily)

Calories	Fat	% Fat Cals
1200 cals	30g fat	23%
1500 cals	40g fat	24%
1800 cals	50g fat	25%
2000 cals	60g fat	27%
2200 cals	70g fat	28%
2500 cals	80g fat	29%
3000 cals	100g fat	30%
4000 cals	135g fat	30%

Percentage Fat Calories Formula:

$$\frac{\text{Grams of Fat Per Serving x (900)}}{\text{Total Calories Per Serving}}$$

Fat Percent Content

(Grams of fat per 100 grams of food)

Don't be fooled by promotion of foods claiming to have a low percentage of fat. **It's serving size and total grams of fat that count.**

For example, whole milk with 3.5% fat sounds low (3.5g fat/100ml) but an 8 fl.oz cup contains 8g fat; and 2 cups contain 16g fat.

Ice cream with 10% fat seems high, yet a regular scoop (3 fl.oz) has only 5g fat.

(Low-fat ice cream has less than 2g fat/serve.)

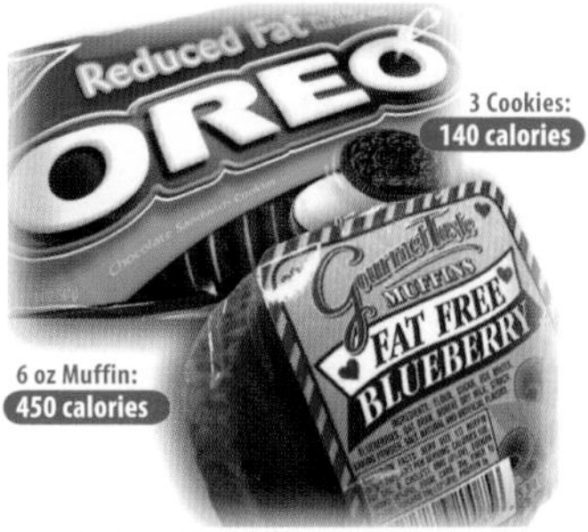

Reduced fat & fat-free foods are not necessarily low calorie. Portion size is still important.

It is a mistake to think that eating low-fat or fat-free foods allows you to eat double the quantity. You can end up with even more calories than when you eat smaller amounts of regular fat products.

Also fat-free but high in calories are soda drinks, fruit juices, beer, alcoholic spirits, sugar and sugar candy. Bread, rice and pasta also have negligible fat.

Total Calories Count!

Ultimately, **it is food portion size and total calories that count** whether from fat, carbohydrate or protein. Remember, cows get fat on grass!

FOOD LABEL MEANINGS

FDA Nutrition Claim Definitions

(All are on a Per Serving Basis)

Low Calorie: 40 Calories or less

Light or Lite: One third fewer calories or, 50% or less fat than regular product

Fat-Free: Less than half a gram of fat

Low-Fat: 3 grams or less of fat

Reduced Fat: 25% less fat than regular product

Fewer or Less Calories: At least 25% fewer calories than regular product

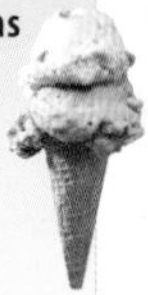

Meats, Poultry, Fish

- Choose **lean cuts** of meat with little marbling. **Trim all visible fat** from meat and remove the skin from poultry. Removal of fat after cooking, is okay (to prevent dryness). Choose 'extra lean' ground beef.
- **Avoid high-fat meat products** such as salami, bacon, sausage and franks.
- **Broil or bake. Avoid frying in oil.** Allow casseroles to cool and skim off surface fat.
- **Avoid fried fish,** frozen fish in batter and canned fish in oil.

Fats & Oils

- **Use minimal amounts** of all types of fat and oil. All are high in calories.
- **Choose** 'light' and 'reduced fat' spreads but still use sparingly.
- Use minimal amounts of oil when stir-frying. Use no-stick sprays like Pam.

Salad Dressings & Sauces

- **Avoid regular mayonnaise and oil dressings.** Choose 'light', 'reduced fat' or 'fat-free' brands.
- **Choose** low-fat or fat-free sauces (mainly tomato-based). Avoid 'pesto', 'alfredo', 'cheese' and 'creamy' sauces.

Milk, Cheese

- **Choose** low-fat or nonfat milks and yogurts. **Avoid** full-cream milk, cream, Half & Half.
- **Cheese:** Choose fat-free, low-fat and fat-reduced (e.g. cottage, part-skim ricotta). Cheese substitutes can still be high in fat.

Snacks, Cookies, Candy

- **Avoid** high-fat snacks such as potato chips, corn/tortilla chips, cheesy balls, buttered popcorn, chocolate and carob bars.

Desserts/Sweets

- **Avoid high-fat desserts,** such as fruit pies, pastries, cheesecake, cheese board.
- **Choose** fresh fruits, fresh fruit salad, canned fruit in water pack, low-fat ice cream. Use low-fat yogurt in place of cream.

Fast-Foods & Take-Out

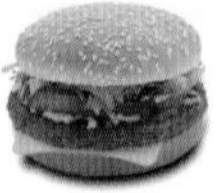

Check the Fast-Foods Section of this book for actual fat and calorie counts.

- **Avoid deep-fried chicken,** french fries; onion rings
- **Pizzas:** Avoid sausage/pepperoni. Choose vegetarian topping and modest quantity of cheese. Eat a moderate serving. Eat extra salad and fresh fruit.
- **Hamburgers:** Choose medium size, lower fat burgers. Avoid bacon. Have a side salad (with fat-free dressing).
- **Delis:** Choose sandwiches/bread rolls, pitas with low-fat fillings and plain salad. Limit meat/cheese to small portions.
- **Coffees:** Avoid large sizes of latte and frappuccino. Request nonfat milk and no whipped cream. Avoid cookies.

Extra Information: www.CalorieKing.com

FRYING ADDS FAT!

The greater the surface area of potato exposed to fat or oil, the higher the fat content.

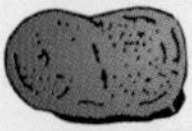

Whole Potato (3 oz)
0g Fat, 65 Cals

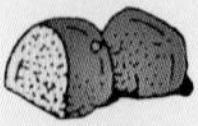

Roast Potato (3 oz)
5g Fat, 155 Cals

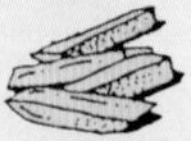

Fries (Large cut, 3 oz)
12g Fat, 220 Cals

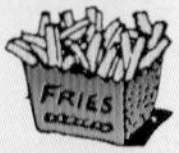

Fries (Small, 3 oz)
15g Fat, 265 Cals

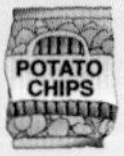

Potato Chips (3 oz)
30g Fat, 450 Cals

Carbohydrates ~ Friend or Foe?

Naturally Friendly Carbs

- **Carbohydrate foods in their more natural forms** (not overly processed) are essential to good health. They are the main source of fuel for the body, and also provide important vitamins, minerals, antioxidants and fiber – all of which help protect against heart disease, diabetes, hypertension, constipation-related ailments and many other diseases.
- Carbohydrates even stimulate production of serotonin, the 'feel good' brain chemical that helps control appetite and overeating. Too little serotonin can lead to mood swings and depression.

Carbohydrates are found in different forms in food as:

- Sugars in fruit, sugar cane, milk
- Starches in whole grains, legumes, nuts, seeds and vegetables
- Dietary fiber – (See Fiber Guide ~ Page 282)

Glycemic Index & Diabetes ~ Page 21

RECOMMENDED CARBOHYDRATE INTAKE

Calories (Daily)	Carbohydrate (Grams)	Percent Carbohydrate Calories
1200 cals	120g	40%
1500 cals	170g	45%
1800 cals	210g	47%
2000 cals	250g	50%
2500 cals	345g	55%
3000 cals	450g	60%

How Much Do We Need?

- As shown in the chart, well-balanced diets above 2000 calories contain 50-60% of total calories from carbohydrate.
- At lower calorie levels used for weight control (1200-1500 calories), carbohydrates account for as little as 40% of total calories. This is because protein calories have nutritional priority.

Low carb diets only work if total calories are reduced.

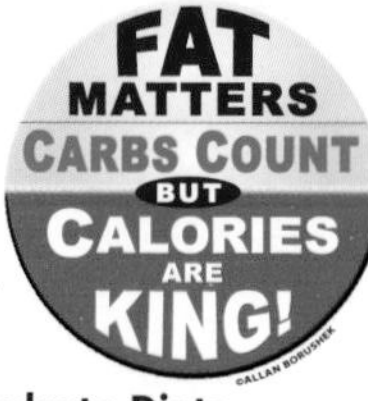

Low Carbohydrate Diets

- Popular low carbohydrate diets are extreme in their recommendations to initially cut carb intake to as little as 20 grams per day – the amount in 1 thick slice of bread, or 1 medium apple, or 1 small potato.

  This greatly increases the risk of nutritional deficiencies and compromises health, particularly if fat intake is excessive through fatty meats, high-fat dairy products, and fried foods.
- While overweight Americans do need to reduce carbohydrate intake, it should be done **sensibly as part of reducing portion size and total calories.**
- Simply eating 'low carb' food products without regard to portion size, calories or fats, will do little to promote weight loss or good health.
- **Low carb diets (and indeed any diet) only work if total calories are reduced.**
- Refined sugars should be one of the first targets in moderating carb intake.

Extra Info ~ www.CalorieKing.com

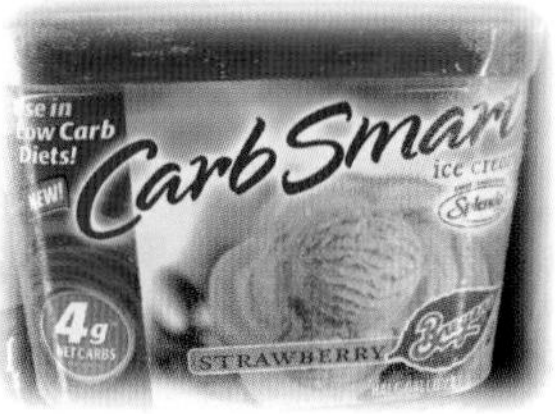

Low carbohydrate products may still be high in calories and fat.

- Many overweight, inactive people consume over 500 calories of refined sugars per day either self-added or as part of food products. This is equivalent to over 30 level teaspoons - a significant amount in weight control terms. Halving this amount would be reasonable and worthwhile.

  Note: Naturally occurring sugars in fruits, vegetables and milk are fine when consumed in normal recommended amounts. These foods are also rich in other nutrients.

  Refined sugar is referred to as having 'empty calories' because it supplies calories but negligible nutrients and no fiber.
- **Most sugar in our diet is 'hidden'** in processed foods such as soft drinks, fruit drinks, candy, cookies, cake, jam, sauces, ice cream, desserts, canned foods, and breakfast cereals.

  Certainly enjoy moderate quantities of these foods, but for serious weight control, look for 'low calorie', 'diet' or 'sugar-free'.

  However, be careful not to substitute sugar-rich foods with high-fat foods which might boost calories even more!
- Be aware that sugar comes in different forms such as sucrose, glucose, fructose, malt, high-fructose corn syrup, molasses, honey and maple syrup. Check the label.
- **Sugar alcohols such as sorbitol,** mannitol and maltitol are carb-based and have ½ - ¾ the calories of regular sugar. While not counted as sugar on food labels, they do add to the carb count. Excess amounts can cause bloating, gas and diarrhea.
- **Sugar-free sweeteners** such as *Equal, DiabetiSweet, NutraSweet, Splenda, Sweet'n Low* and *Stevia* make it easy to reduce sugar in drinks and recipes. Use only in moderation.

  Note: Most recipes can be adapted to contain less sugar with little effect on taste or quality.

Extra Info ~ www.CalorieKing.com

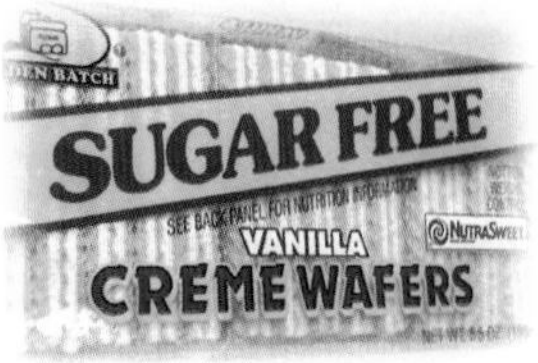

Sugar-free snacks and foods may be higher in fat and calories than the regular product.

Example ~ Creme Wafers (3):
Regular ~ 115 cals, 6g fat
Sugar-Free ~ 160 cals, 10g fat

SUGAR CONTENT OF SOME COMMON FOODS

	Teaspoons of Sugar
Coca Cola or *Pepsi*, 12 fl.oz	10
20 fl.oz size	17
Iced Tea, sweetened, 12 fl.oz	8
Chocolate Milk, 12 fl.oz	6
Honey Smacks Cereal, 1 oz	4
Popcorn, caramel, 1 cup	3.5
Chocolate Bar, 1.5 oz	6
M&M's 1.7 oz pkg	7
Muffin, large, 4 oz	6
Choc Chip Cookie, 1 oz	2
Donut, iced	6
Apple Pie, 1 piece	7
Jell-O, ½ cup	4.5
Jam, 1 Tbsp, 20g	2.5
Syrup, maple, 1 Tbsp	3

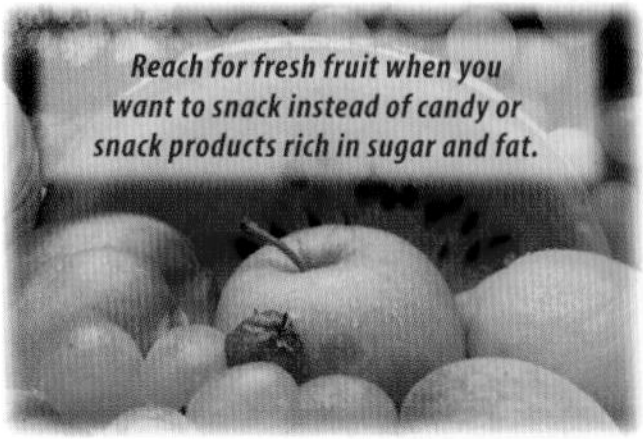
Reach for fresh fruit when you want to snack instead of candy or snack products rich in sugar and fat.

Tips For Overweight Kids & Parents!

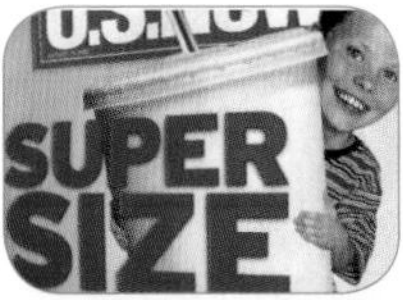

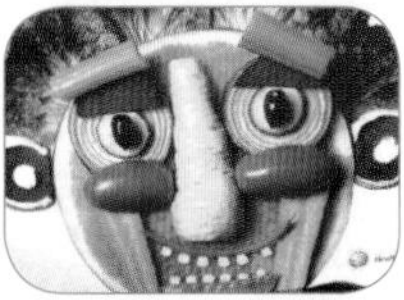

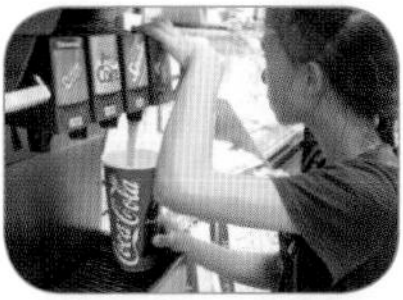

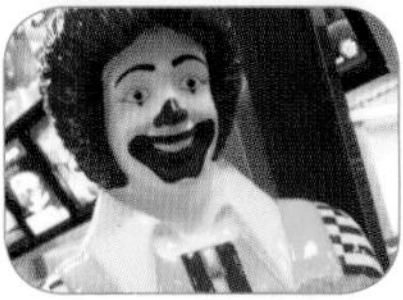

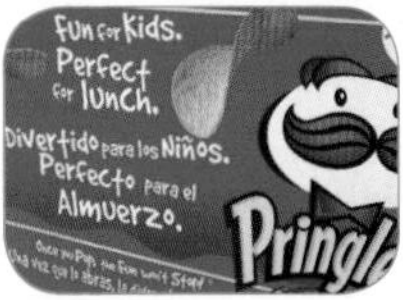

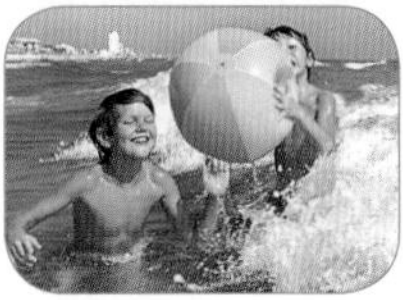

The XL Generation

Some 15% of American kids and adolescents are overweight; and childhood obesity has doubled over the last 20 years. Diabetes, high blood pressure and high cholesterol are major problem areas for overweight children and adolescents, as are depression, low self-esteem, sleep apnea and bone joint problems.

To address this problem, cooperation is required between kids, parents, schools and government. Weight control is a family and community affair.

Some simple tips to get started:

» Watch Soda Intake!

Limit soda and sugary drinks to one serving on the weekends. Soda should not be an everyday beverage. Try water instead. When at fast-food restaurants or using a soda fountain, choose small servings with ice or choose diet soda instead. Schools should provide water and restrict access to soda. Parents need to supervise kids at the soda fountain!

» Cut back on Fast-Foods and Eating Out

Many more calories are consumed when you eat out. Healthy meals prepared at home are best for the whole family.

» Say "No" to Super-Sizing!

Portion sizes are on the increase, and for just a few cents, meals can be upsized - with loads more calories. Choose sensible portion sizes when dining out and at home. Use smaller plates and choose smaller packages.

» Limit Between-Meal Snacking

Watch out for high-fat and high-calorie snacks – they can have more calories than a meal. Keep your eye on portion sizes and limit foods like chips and candy to parties and special occasions. Choose fresh fruit and vegetables instead.

» Get Moving ~ Watch Less TV!

Kids need at least 60 minutes of physical activity every day. Limit time spent in sedentary activities (such as playing computer games or watching TV to just one hour per day.) Also limit the accompanying snacks! Include exercise in family activities.

Note: When kids watch TV in a motionless trance, they burn even less calories than if simply sitting, reading or talking.

For extra information and tips see www.CalorieKing.com

Sample Diet Plan - 1300 Calories

For Overweight Persons. Please Check With Your Doctor.
(Menu contains approximately 30-35 Grams Fat)

Breakfast (approx. 250 cal)

	1 Small Fruit or 1/2 oz Dried Fruit
Plus	Cereal: 1 1/2 oz Dry (high fiber)
	or 1 cup cooked Oatmeal
Plus	Milk (from daily allowance)

Daily Milk Allowance (160 calories)
2 cups Skim Milk or 1 1/2 cups Low-fat (1%) Milk
or equivalent Soy Drink, Yogurt, Cheese, Tofu

Fat Allowance (140 calories; 15g Fat)
4 tsp Fat or 6-8 tsp Diet Margarine or 3 tsp Oil
or 1 1/2 Tbsp Mayonnaise or 1/2 medium Avocado
or 1 1/2 Tbsp Peanut Butter or 30g Nuts/Seeds

Breakfast ~ Choice 2

	1 Small Fruit
Plus	1 Egg (no added fat)
	or 3/4 oz Cheese
	or 2 oz Cottage Cheese
	or 1 oz Lean Bacon
Plus	1 Toast or 1/2 Muffin (English)

Lunch (approx. 440 calories)

	2 slices Bread (2 oz) or 1 medium Roll or Bagel
	or 4 Crispbreads/Crackers or 6" Pita
Plus	2 oz lean Meat, Chicken or Turkey
	or 3 1/2 oz Tuna (in water) or 2 1/2 oz Salmon
	or 1 oz Cheese or 1/2 cup (4 oz) Cottage Cheese
	or 1/2 cup (4 oz) Ricotta Cheese (low-fat)
	or 1/2 cup (4 oz) Fruit Yogurt (low-fat)
	or 1/2 cup (4 oz) Bean Salad
Plus	Large Salad (Oil-free dressing)
Plus	1 small Fruit or 1/2 oz Dried Fruit

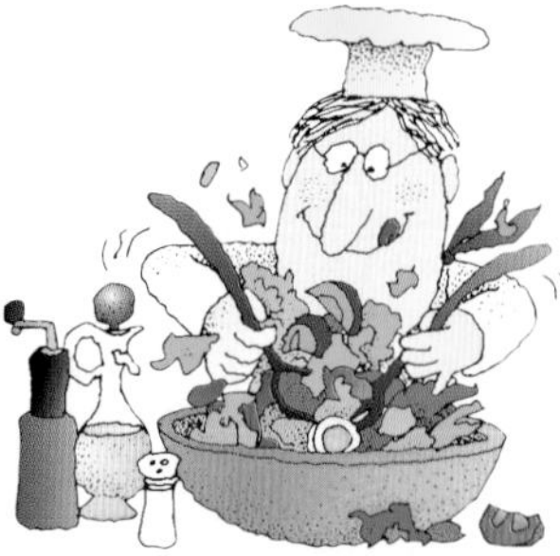

Dinner (approx. 360 calories)

	Soup (fat-free)
Plus	3 oz lean Meat (cooked weight)
	or 4 oz Chicken Breast (no skin)
	or 3 oz Chicken Thigh/Leg (no skin)
	or 5 oz Fish (grilled, no fat)
	or 3/4 cup (6 oz) Beans (Soy, Kidney, Pinto etc)/Lentils
	or Low-fat Entree (e.g. Lean Cuisine) or Recipe Dish
Plus	1 small Potato or 1/2 cup Rice/Pasta or 1 slice Bread
Plus	2-3 servings Vegetables/Salad
Plus	1 small Fruit + Diet Gelatin Dessert

Between Meals

Water, Coffee, Tea, Diet drinks,
Fruit from main meals; Raw vegetable pieces, Milk from Allowance

Note: Take a multivitamin/mineral supplement daily while dieting.

Exercise & Weight Control

- **People who exercise regularly lose more weight** and keep it off longer than non-exercisers.
- Exercise also improves general health and well-being. **Mood, confidence and self-esteem are** enhanced by a sense of control and accomplishment.
- **Exercise increases the metabolic rate** of the body even for hours after exercise – a good way to 'wake up' a sluggish metabolism and burn extra fat.

  Exercise compensates for any decrease in metabolic rate with increasing age and also in some heavy smokers who stop smoking.
- **Strength training** further builds muscle and aids body reshaping. You can also eat more food!

Note: It is muscle which burns calories. Each extra pound of muscle burns an extra 100 calories daily – even while you sleep! Weight from exercised muscles is okay. It is surplus fat that is potentially harmful.

- **Avoid injury** by beginning with walking, low impact aerobics, or weight-supported exercise (e.g. swimming, cycling). Avoid competitive sports.
- **How Much?** Start with 10 - 20 minutes/day and progress to 30-45 minutes/day – even if broken into 5-10 minute lots. It all adds up! **Aim to achieve 250-500 calories of exercise daily.**

  Also walk up stairs instead of using elevators. Take a brisk walk at lunch. Use an exercise bike, treadmill or stair machine while watching TV.
- **How Often?** While aerobic fitness requires only 3 - 4 sessions weekly, **weight control is a daily event which requires daily exercise.**

TV CAN BE FATTENING!

Many adults and children watch over 20 hours of television per week (plus computer hours). At the same time, high-calorie snacks and drinks are consumed – potent contributors to obesity.

Are you a TV couch potato? Limit your TV hours and plan healthy physical activities. At least use an exercise bike or treadmill while watching TV!

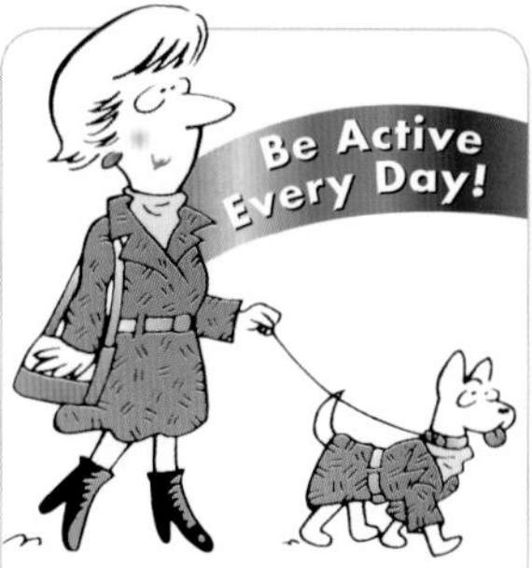

Brisk walking each day is a safe and effective way to keep trim and fit. Try it - you'll like it!

Strength-training with light weights helps to retain or rebuild muscle tissue. It enhances weight control.

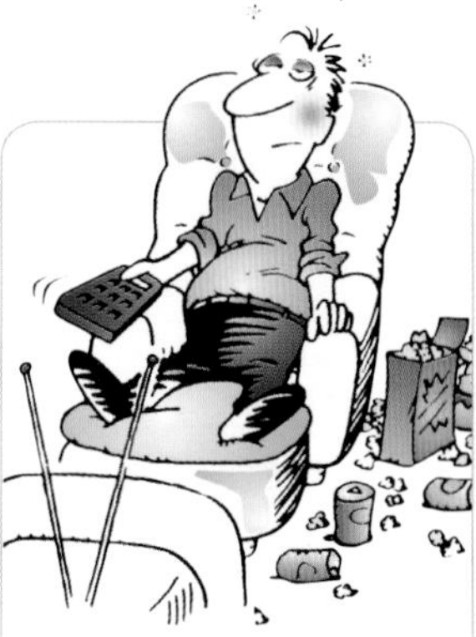

Middle-age spread has little to do with getting older. Too little exercise is the main culprit.

Daily exercise and sensible eating can minimize middle-age spread.

Calories Used in Exercise

LIGHT
4 Calories/Minute

- Walking, slow
- Cycling, light
- Gardening light
- Golf, social
- Tennis, doubles
- Housework, cleaning
- Calisthenics, Yoga
- Bowling
- Ping-pong, social
- Ice Skating
- Aquarobics, light
- Skate Boarding
- Line/Square Dancing

MODERATE
7 Calories/Minute

- Walking, brisk
- Cycling, moderate
- Swimming, crawl
- Weight-training, light
- Tennis, moderate
- Racquetball, beginners
- Aerobics, light
- Football, Grid Iron
- Basketball, Baseball
- Walking Downstairs
- Snow Skiing (downhill)
- Shovelling snow
- Dancing (ballroom)

HEAVY
10 Calories/Minute

- Walking (power), Jogging
- Cycling (vigorous), Spinning
- Swimming, strenuous
- Weight-training, heavy
- Wrestling/Judo, advanced
- Racquetball, advanced
- Tae Bo, Kick Boxing
- Football, training
- Basketball (Pro)
- Climbing Stairs
- Skipping Rope
- Skiing (cross country)
- Aquarobics, advanced
- Dancing (strenuous), Zumba

Note: Only those sports or activities that are sustained over a period of time (e.g running) qualify for heavy exercise. Stop-start sports such as tennis are considered 'moderate'.

10,000 STEPS PER DAY

PEDOMETERS

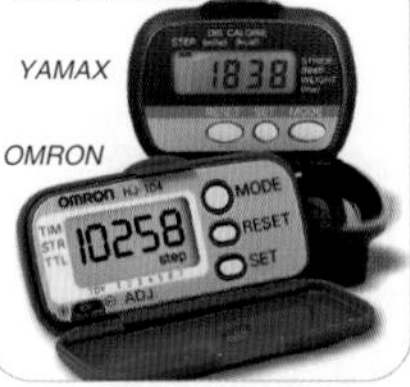

A pedometer can motivate you to be more active every day.

Different models count steps, miles and even calories used. It clips to your belt or waist band and registers each step.

Aim for 8,000 - 10,000 steps per day, instead of an average of only 3,000 - 4,000 steps.

Ordering Details ~ Page 303

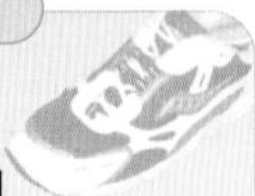

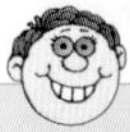

WALKING PROGRAM

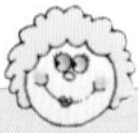

Weeks	Distance To Walk	Time Taken	Calories Used (140lb Person)
Weeks 1-2	1 mile	20 mins	140 calories
Weeks 3-5	1.5 miles	28 mins	200 calories
Weeks 6-8	2 miles	35 mins	250 calories
Weeks 9-10	2.5 miles	45 mins	310 calories
Weeks 11+	3.5 miles	60 mins	420 calories

Reshaping Eating Behaviors

- Eating is a behavior that is largely controlled by people with whom we live or socialize, places in which we carry out our lives, and our emotions. Become aware of those situations that commonly lead to extra food being eaten.
- We may also be unaware of 'bad' eating habits that can lead to excess calorie intake; e.g. eating quickly, large mouthfuls, eating when tense or bored, finishing a large serving of food when not hungry.

Tips to help uncover and correct those 'bad' eating habits:

- **Don't eat while engaged in other activities;** for example, watching TV, reading. Eat only at the table, not at the fridge or while standing.
- **Don't eat quickly.** Chewing slowly allows time to register a feeling of fullness. Don't use fingers, only utensils. Cut food into smaller pieces. Don't load your fork until the previous mouthful is finished.
- **Don't purchase problem high calorie foods.** Shop from a set list to prevent impulse buying. Avoid shopping with children.
- **Buy snack foods** in the smallest package. The larger the serving size or package, the more you are likely to eat or drink.
- **Plan meals in advance. Stick to a set menu.**
- **Plan a strategy to avoid uncontrolled eating** and drinking at social events, or when your emotions urge you to binge.

  Rehearse repeatedly in your mind exactly what you will do in such situations. Remind yourself several times each day that you are in charge of your actions and that you can be strong-willed. Seek counseling or coaching on various strategies.
- **Promise yourself** that when you feel the urge to snack, you will engage in some activity that will distract you away from food (e.g. go for a walk, brush your teeth, phone a friend.)

  If you eat out of boredom, find some new hobby or interest that gets you out of the house. Even enroll in an adult education class.

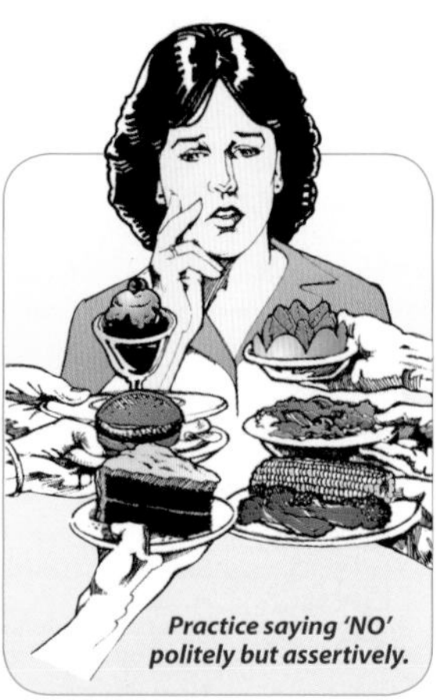

Practice saying 'NO' politely but assertively.

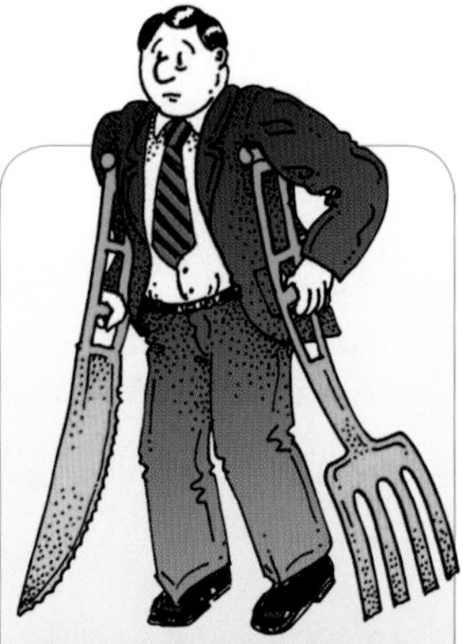

Do you use food as an emotional crutch? If so, professional counseling may be helpful.

The food diary is the most powerful proven aid for dieters. Persons who keep a food and exercise diary not only lose more weight they also keep it off. Here are some of the reasons:

- Recording your eating and exercise habits jolts you into realizing just what you do eat and drink each day; and also whether you exercise sufficiently.
- **Helps you identify problem foods** and drinks with excessive calories and fat.
- **Helps identify moods**, situations and events that lead to excessive eating of unwanted calories. You can then plan to overcome or avoid them.
- **Prevents 'calorie amnesia'**, the forgetfulness that leads to rebound weight gain after successful weight loss. Recording puts you back on the right track.
- **Helps you develop greater self-discipline.** You will think twice about overindulging if you have to record it - especially if someone checks your diary regularly. It certainly keeps you honest!
- **Motivates you** to carefully plan your meals and to exercise each day.
- **Serves as a check system** for your doctor, dietitian or counselor to assess your progress and make recommendations.

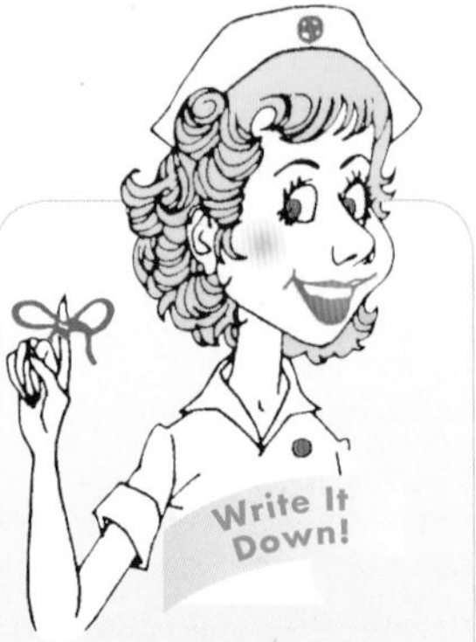

"Keeping a diary gives me feedback on exactly what I eat and drink each day.

It helps prevent 'calorie amnesia' and reminds me to exercise each day.

It's a must for successful weight control!"

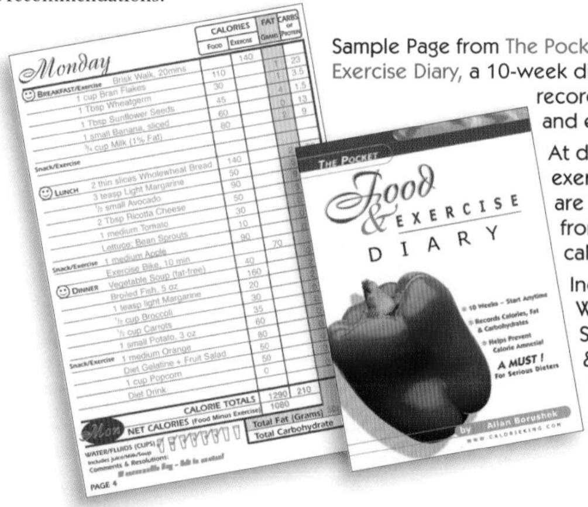

Sample Page from The Pocket Food & Exercise Diary, a 10-week diary to record food and exercise.

At day's end, exercise calories are deducted from food calories.

Includes Weekly Summary Page & Progress Checklist.

EXTRA DETAILS

~ SEE PAGE 302

What is Diabetes?

Diabetes is a disorder in which the body cannot make proper use of carbohydrates (sugar and starches).

- After digestion, sugar and starches are changed into **glucose** – the simplest form of sugar vital for body energy and growth.
- **Insulin** is the hormone which acts like a key that opens the door to body cells and allows glucose to enter.
- **Without sufficient insulin,** unused glucose builds up in the blood and passes into the urine. This produces symptoms of frequent urination, continual thirst and tiredness.
- **Untreated diabetes** increases the risk of damage to nerves and blood vessels. This, in turn, increases the risk of heart disease, stroke, blindness, kidney damage, foot ulcers and gangrene (with amputation), impotence and other complications.

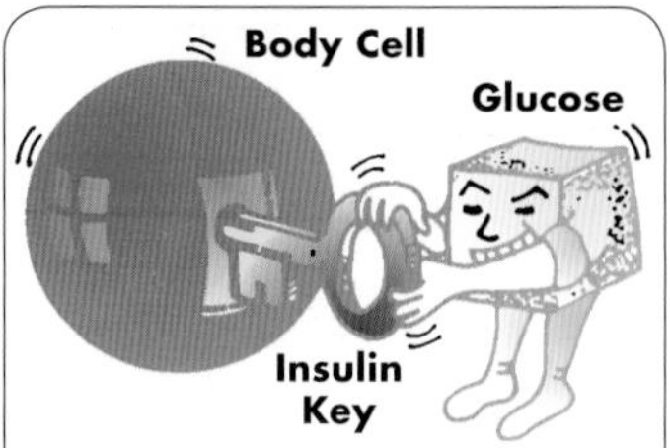

*Insulin acts like a key.
It opens the door to body cells and allows glucose to enter.*

People with Type-1 diabetes and some with Type-2 have too few or no keys and require insulin injections.

Others (most Type -2) have ample keys but 'misshapen' key holes (insulin resistant) – particularly if obese and inactive.

TYPE-1 DIABETES

Insulin-Dependent Diabetes

- Occurs in 10% of diabetes cases
- Usually in children and young adults
- Pancreas gland produces little or no insulin. Daily insulin injections are necessary, plus:
- Regular meals with even carbohydrate distribution to match insulin dosage. Regular exercise and weight control are also important.

WARNING SIGNALS

- Frequent urination
- Continual thirst
- Rapid weight loss
- Unusual hunger
- Extreme weakness/fatigue
- Nausea, vomiting, irritability

TYPE-2 DIABETES

Non-Insulin Dependent

- Occurs in 90% of diabetes cases
- Occurs mainly in adults - particularly in overweight and inactive persons
- Insulin is produced but body cells resist its action and glucose cannot enter cells.
- Usually treated with diet and exercise. Sometimes requires medication (tablets or insulin injections).

WARNING SIGNALS

- Any Type-1 symptom
- Blurred vision
- Excessive itching
- Skin infections with slow healing
- Tingling/numbness in feet

GESTATIONAL DIABETES • Occurs during pregnancy • Usually disappears on the baby's birth • Over 50% of these mothers develop diabetes within the next 20 years. • Requires weight control, a healthy lifestyle and regular medical checks.

Prediabetes - An Early Warning!

- Prediabetes means you don't have diabetes now but are likely to develop it in the future - if serious preventive action is not taken now! Your risk for heart disease and stroke is also increased by 50%.
- You are prediabetic if your blood sugar level is between 100 and 125 mg/dL (after an overnight fast).

  These levels are higher than normal but not high enough to be diabetes.
- Risk factors for prediabetes include being overweight or obese, a family history of diabetes, high blood lipids, hypertension, and a history of gestational diabetes (during pregnancy).
- Most people with prediabetes can prevent full-blown diabetes (usually Type 2) by adopting a healthier lifestyle. This includes **losing weight if overweight, and exercising for 30 minutes at least 5 days a week.**
- Your doctor and dietitian can plan a preventive lifestyle program for you.

NEW BLOOD SUGAR CLASSIFICATION FOR DIABETES

(American Diabetes Association, 2003)

NORMAL:
Below 100 mg/dL

PREDIABETES:
100-125 mg/dL

DIABETES:
Over 125 mg/dL

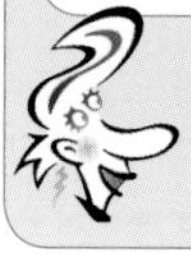

Everyone 45 and over should have a blood glucose test every 3 years.

Importance of Weight Control

- **Type-2 diabetes** occurs 2-3 times more often in overweight persons – particularly if inactive.
- Such persons do not usually lack insulin. Rather, their insulin is less effective. As obesity develops, muscle and other body cells may resist insulin in varying degrees. The resultant build-up of blood glucose may lead to diabetic symptoms.
- **Weight loss alone** often corrects this condition in Type-2 diabetes. If overweight, try a moderate diet of 1200-1500 calories **plus daily exercise.**

  Within several weeks, body cells can lose their resistance and become sensitive once again to the effects of insulin. Insulin and blood glucose levels may normalize, and symptoms may disappear.

  Further, the need for oral antidiabetic drugs might be prevented or much lessened in dosage. **So, give diet and exercise a fair chance** – and maintain them to keep symptoms under control.

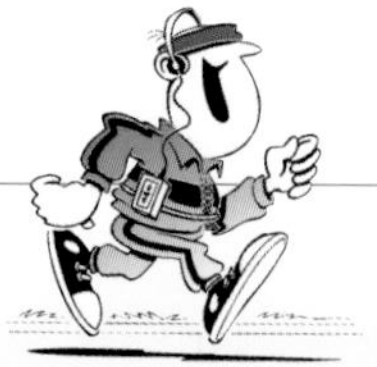

Get Moving! Everyday, do at least 30 minutes of moderate intensity exercise. It's the key to improving insulin sensitivity.

Add strength-training 3-4 times a week to double the benefits.

Managing Diabetes

Don't battle diabetes alone. Establish a partnership with your doctor, dietitian, certified diabetes educator and pharmacist. **Extra Support:** • *American Diabetes Association* • *American Diabetes Educators Association* • *National Diabetes Education Program*

Hints to keep blood glucose within safe limits:

- **Control your diet.** Know what and when you will eat. Seek referral to a dietitian for expert advice.
- **Exercise regularly.** It assists weight control and can improve sensitivity of body cells to insulin. Plan exercise into your daily routine.
- **Monitor your blood glucose** at home and work – ideally with a portable blood glucose meter. It will help you become familiar with your blood glucose patterns, and the effects of diet, exercise and medication. Insulin pumps can also help control blood glucose levels around the clock.
- **Don't skip prescribed insulin or oral medication.** If on insulin, know what action to take if hypoglycemia (low blood glucose) occurs. Also educate your family and friends.

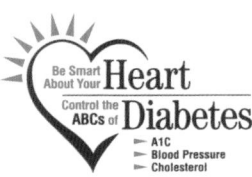

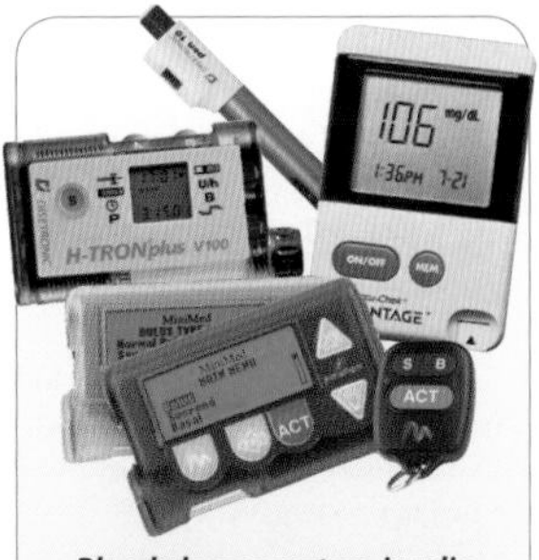

Blood glucose meters, insulin pumps and pens can greatly improve control of diabetes and lifestyle choices.

Be Heart Smart ~ Know Your ABC's

If you have diabetes, you are at high risk for heart attack and stroke. Heart disease is more likely to strike you – and at an early age – than someone without diabetes.

But you can fight back. Be smart about your heart. **Take control of the ABC's of diabetes** and live a long and healthy live. Talk to your health care provider about your ABC targets.

Be Smart About Your Heart
Control the ABCs of Diabetes
- A1C
- Blood Pressure
- Cholesterol

National Diabetes Education Program

A is for A1C

The A1C (A-one-C) test – short for hemoglobin A1C – measures your average blood glucose (sugar) over the last 3 months. **Suggested target: below 7**

B is for Blood Pressure

High blood pressure makes your heart work too hard. **Suggested target: below 120/80**

C is for Cholesterol

Bad cholesterol, or LDL, builds up and clogs your arteries. **Suggested target: below 100**

A1C Values	AVERAGE DAILY BLOOD GLUCOSE
6%	120 mg/dL Excellent Control
8%	180 mg/dL Needs Treatment Change
10%	240 mg/dL Poor Control
13%	330 mg/dL Seriously Out of Control

Guidelines for choosing a healthy diet apply equally to people with or without diabetes. Eating a wide variety of foods that are mainly low in fat and refined sugars, and high in fiber, is recommended.

However, actual food quantities, as well as when you eat, will also influence control of blood glucose. Your dietitian will individualize a diet plan to suit your food preferences, lifestyle and medical status. Here are a few hints:

- **Maintain a healthy weight.** If overweight, even a modest weight loss plus daily exercise can help to normalize blood glucose in Type-2 diabetes.
- **Don't skip meals.** If you take insulin or an oral hypoglycemic agent, regular meals are important.
- **If on insulin,** eat meals at the same time each day. Eat a similar amount of food at each meal. Even distribution of carbohydrate over the day will make best use of the available insulin and prevent wide variations in blood glucose levels.

  Note: Take your rapid-acting insulin no more than 15 minutes before eating. Regular and combination insulins are best taken with about 30 minutes between insulin injection and breakfast.
- **Choose wholegrain breads, cereals and pasta.** Eat fresh fruits, vegetables and legumes. These foods contain more fiber and slow the release of glucose into your blood after a meal.
- **Limit foods high in saturated fat and cholesterol.** Enjoy fish, soy foods, and other foods rich in omega-3 fats. **Extra Notes** ~ *See Fats & Cholesterol Guide, Page 271*
- **Avoid sugars and foods high in added sugar** particularly if overweight. Small amounts of sugar as part of a meal may occasionally be okay. Check with your dietitian. Use *Equal, Splenda* and *NutraSweet* – sweetened foods and drinks.
  Extra Notes ~ *See Page 9*
- **Foods (and supplements) rich in antioxidant vitamins C, E and beta-carotene,** as well as omega-3 fats, magnesium, zinc and chromium may help prevent long-term complications of diabetes (such as damage to small blood vessels and nerves). Be sure to check with your doctor.

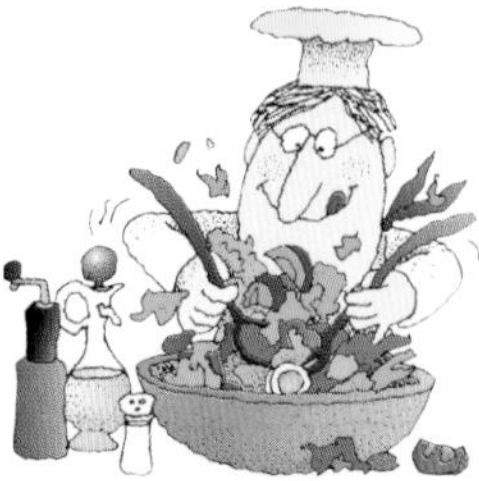

Eat a well-balanced diet, high in fiber-containing foods and low in saturated fat.

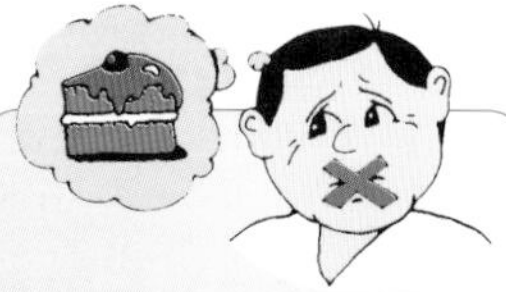

Modest weight loss and daily exercise can greatly improve control of Type-2 diabetes.

Excess Alcohol
contributes to obesity, diabetes, and high blood pressure.

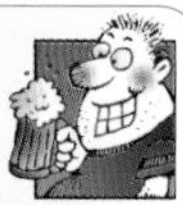

The risk of hypoglycemia (low blood sugar) and drug interactions with alcohol is also increased.

Diabetes & Carbohydrate Distribution

- **For people with diabetes,** regular meals with even distribution of carbohydrate over the day are important for good control of blood sugar levels.
- **Smaller amounts of food** eaten more frequently result in steadier, more even blood glucose levels. (Be sure to control your weight.) Recommended daily eating patterns for good blood glucose control:

1. **Three Meals & Three Snacks** ~ Best for persons on insulin (Type-1 diabetes) with normal blood glucose variations.
2. **Three Meals** ~ Best for Type-2 diabetes (especially if overweight).

Note: If blood sugar levels show excessive variations see your doctor and dietitian.

- **Your doctor or dietitian** will select the level of calories and carbohydrate most appropriate to your weight, medication and activity. (Regular blood glucose checks will provide feedback on the level of control.)
- **Amounts of carbohydrate** in the guide below provide an average of 50% of total calories. **A rough rule of thumb is:** 13 grams of carbohydrate per 100 calories.

At calorie levels above 2000, carbohydrates approach 50-60% of total calories.

At lower calorie levels used for weight loss (1200-1500 calories), carbohydrates account for as little as 40% of total calories. This is because protein has nutritional priority.

These carbohydrate quantities (and percentages) apply equally to persons with or without diabetes.

IDEAL CARBOHYDRATE DISTRIBUTION For Type-1 Diabetes (Insulin Dependent)

3 MEALS & 3 SNACKS

Balanced Blood Sugar Levels

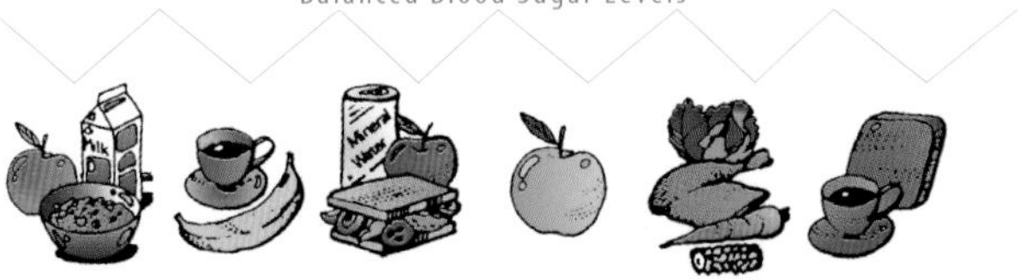

GUIDE TO CARBOHYDRATE DISTRIBUTION

Daily Total Calories		Daily Total Carbohydrate	Percent Carbohyd. Cals	Each Main Meal (3)	Between Meals (3)
1200 Cals	~	120g	40%	30g	10g
1500 Cals	~	170g	45%	40g	15g
2000 Cals	~	250g	50%	60g	25g
2500 Cals	~	345g	55%	70g	45g
3000 Cals	~	450g	60%	90g	60g

Note: Check with your dietitian as to the best eating plan for you.

Carbohydrate Type Affects Blood Glucose

The various forms of carbohydrate affect blood glucose levels in different ways. It is difficult to predict the effect of particular foods, sugars or meals, simply by their carbohydrate content.

Thus the same amount of carbohydrate from different foods may affect blood sugar levels very differently. Many factors affect the rate of digestion and absorption – particularly the type of sugar, starch and fiber; the degree of processing and cooking (which increases digestion rate); and the amount of protein and fat (which slows stomach emptying and digestion).

Glycemic Index (GI)

The GI is a method of ranking carbohydrate foods on a scale (0-100) according to how they affect blood glucose levels. (See next column). The higher the GI value, the greater the food's ability to rapidly raise blood glucose levels and the more insulin needed by the body (not desirable).

Eating low GI foods leads to better control of blood glucose and insulin levels (which in turn lowers the risk of damage to blood vessels and nerves). The slower digestion of low GI foods also helps to delay hunger pangs, and benefit weight control.

Of course, choosing low GI foods is not a licence to eat unlimited amounts – **calorie restriction and portion control for weight control is of prime importance.**

Extra Notes: * GI is not meant to be used in isolation without regard to portion size, and other dietary recommendations for healthy eating. Foods are not good or bad on the basis of their GI.

* The GI concept is yet to be adopted by the American Diabetes Assoc. and American Dietetic Assoc. There are other important aspects to consider for wise use of GI, including GL (Glycemic Load).

Extra Information ~ www.calorieking.com

LOWER GLYCEMIC FOODS

Slower Acting Carbohydrates

These foods are more slowly digested and absorbed. They help maintain more even blood glucose levels, as long as excessive amounts are not eaten. Use these foods regularly but still limit portion size for weight control.

Examples:

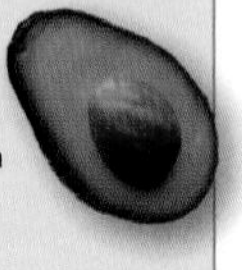

- Dried beans, peas, lentils
- Nuts and seeds
- Wholegrain breads and pita
- Bran cereals, oats
- Barley, buckwheat, bulgur
- Spaghetti, pasta, Basmati Rice
- Fresh fruit: apples, avocados, bananas (firm), cherries, grapefruit, grapes, olives, oranges, peaches, pears, plums. Fresh juices.
- Vegetables: sweet potatoes, yam
- Milk, yoghurt, soy drinks
- Sugar alcohols (Sorbitol, Maltitol)

HIGHER GLYCEMIC FOODS

Quicker Acting Carbohydrates

These foods more rapidly raise blood glucose levels. Eat only in moderation.

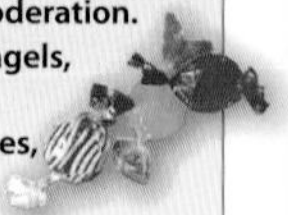

- White bread, rice cakes, bagels, croissants, doughnuts
- Low fiber cereals: Cornflakes, *Rice Krispies, Froot Loops*
- White potatoes, white rice, corn
- Watermelon, ripe bananas, cantaloupe, pineapple
- Soda, sugar-sweetened sports/energy drinks
- Sugar, Sugar Candy
- Ice Cream (low-fat), Frozen Yogurt

EXTRA INFORMATION

- **Book:** The New Glucose Revolution by Jennie Brand-Miller
- **www.glycemicindex.com**
- **www.CalorieKing.com**

Unexplained Weight Gains

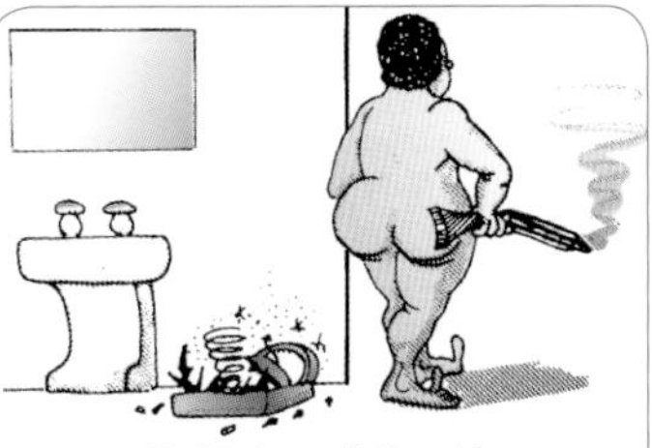

Scales do not distinguish between fat, muscle and fluids.

» Body Fluid Changes

Body weight fluctuates from day to day. This is mainly due to changes in body fluids which make up around 70% of total body weight. It can be affected by changes in hormone levels, dietary factors such as salt and carbohydrate, and even exercise.

Weight change over several weeks is more likely to reflect changes in levels of fat and muscle rather than fluid. Unfortunately, the scales do not distinguish between weight changes due to water, fat or muscle. This is why **we shouldn't allow every fluctuation in weight to rule our lives.**

To limit fluid retention, avoid salty foods and go easy on the salt shaker. Eating sufficient fruit and vegetables supplies extra potassium which counteracts sodium and encourages fluid loss. However, **do not limit water intake.** Be sure to drink at least 6-8 glasses of water or other fluids per day.

When dining out, be aware that the extra pound or two that might show on the scales the next morning is not the result of a small dietary indiscretion. It is more likely due to fluid retention resulting from more highly seasoned and salty food.

Monthly hormonal changes in women can also account for a build-up of fluids of several pounds prior to menstruation.

» Menopausal Weight Gains

Most women gain an average of 4-5 pounds in the years leading up to menopause – usually in their middle to late 40's. This can occur even when exercise and eating habits have not changed significantly.

With hormonal changes occurring at that time, body fat also tends to be redistributed from thighs, buttocks and hips to the breast and stomach areas (a greater health risk).

Be sure to eat wisely and continue daily physical activity including strength-training to maintain or build muscles – and to boost metabolism and self-esteem.

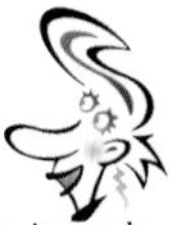

» Underactive Thyroid

Thyroid hormone is made by the thyroid gland in the neck.

When insufficient thyroid hormone is made, metabolism and body processes slow down and weight gain can occur.

Symptoms of hypothyroidism can be subtle and easily overlooked as signs of normal aging. **Early symptoms** may include fatigue, muscle weakness, sluggishness, a swollen tongue that you keep biting, and a puffy face.

As metabolism continues to slow, further **signs can include** chronically cold hands and feet, slow reflexes, constipation, dry skin and coarse hair, brittle nails, heavy menstrual periods, slower pulse, and a husky voice.

Depression-like symptoms may also develop such as forgetfulness, loss of interest, mood swings and irritability.

Weight gains of as much as 10-20 pounds (mainly fluid) can occur, as well as a raised **blood cholesterol level.**

The condition is more common in women, especially following pregnancy, around menopause, or after age 60.

A simple blood test through your doctor can detect hypothyroidism. It is easily treated in most cases with thyroid hormone pills.

Adults 35 and older should have a TSH (thyroid stimulating hormone) test every 5 years. Testing when pregnant is also wise.

Notes, Abbreviations, Measures

» **Calorie and fat values have been rounded off.**
Calories ~ to the nearest 5 or 10 calories.
Fat ~ to nearest half gram. **Note:** Trace amounts of fat (less than 0.3 grams) have been treated as zero.

» **Carbohydrate figures** in this book are for total carbohydrate, and not **Net Carbs** (which deducts fiber, polydextrose and sugar alcohols from total carbs).

» Because manufacturer's figures on labels are rounded off, figures in this book may differ slightly from the label. Serving sizes may also vary.

» Food product formulations change occasionally, and hence the need to regularly update this type of publication. Many products also come and go. Check the food label for any changes.

» **Seek Professional Advice:** This book is intended for educational purposes only. It is not a substitute for professional advice.

» **Feedback Welcome:** Please contact the author directly with your queries, and suggestions for foods to be included in future editions.

Write to: Allan Borushek (Dietitian)
1001 West 17th Street, Costa Mesa CA 92627
Email: allan@calorieking.com

» **Food Product Updates:** Check the author's website.

www.CalorieKing.com

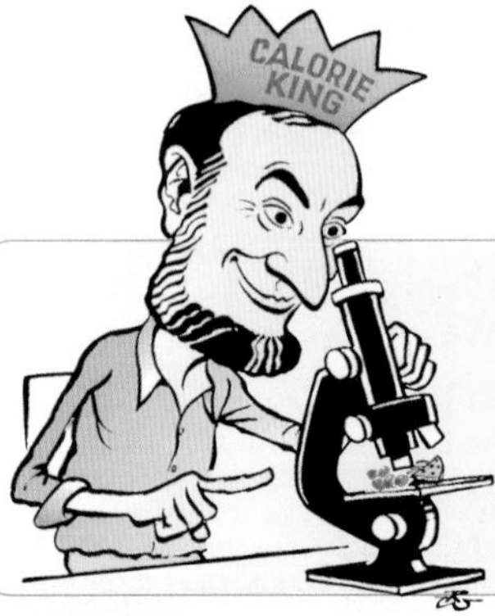

C ~ **Calories**
F ~ **Fat (grams)**
Cb ~ **Carbohydrate (grams)**

Abbreviations

tsp = teaspoon
Tbsp or T = Tablespoon
oz = ounce(s)
c = cup
fl.oz = fluid ounce(s)
g = gram(s)
avg = average
pkg = package

Volume Measures

(All measures are level)

3 tsp = 1 Tbsp
2 Tbsp = 1 fl.oz
½ cup = 4 fl.oz
1 cup = 8 fl.oz
2 cups = 1 Pint
2 Pints = 1 Quart

Note: 8 oz weight is not the same as 8 fl oz volume (space occupied). Dense foods weigh more per set volume. Examples:

1 cup popcorn weighs ½ oz
1 cup milk weighs 8½ oz
1 cup pudding weighs 10 oz

Metric Conversion

½ oz = 14 grams
1 oz = 28.4 grams
2 oz = 57 grams
3½ oz = 100 grams
1 fl.oz = 30 mls
1 cup (8 fl.oz) = 240 mls
33 fl.oz = 1 liter (volume)

SOURCES OF INFORMATION

- U.S. Dept. of Agriculture
- Food Manufacturers
- Food Industry Boards & Councils
- Independent laboratory analysis
- Scientific publications
- Overseas food composition tables
- Author extrapolations

Quick Guide

	C	F	Cb
Cow Milk ~ *Average All Brands*			
Whole (3.5% fat):			
2 Tbsp, 1 fl.oz	**20**	1	1.5
1 Glass, 6 fl.oz	**110**	6	8.5
1 Cup, 8 fl.oz	**150**	8	12
1 Pint, 16 fl.oz	**300**	16	23
1 Quart, 946 ml	**600**	32	46
Reduced-Fat (2% fat):			
2 Tbsp, 1 fl.oz	**15**	0.5	1.5
1 Glass, 6 fl.oz	**90**	4	8.5
1 Cup, 8 fl.oz	**130**	5	13
1 Pint, 16 fl.oz	**260**	10	26
1 Quart, 946 ml	**520**	20	52
Light/Low-Fat (1% fat):			
2 Tbsp, 1 fl.oz	**12**	0.3	1.5
1 Glass, 6 fl.oz	**75**	2	8.5
1 Cup, 8 fl.oz	**120**	2.5	14
1 Pint, 16 fl.oz	**240**	5	28
1 Quart, 946 ml	**480**	10	56
Light/Low-Fat (½ % fat):			
2 Tbsp, 1 fl.oz	**12**	0.1	1.6
Fat Free/Skim:			
2 Tbsp, 1 fl.oz	**10**	0	1.5
1 Cup, 8 fl.oz	**90**	0.5	13
1 Pint, 16 fl.oz	**180**	1	26
w. Replace (Oatrim Fiber): 1 cup	**85**	0	12
Protein-Fortified:			
2% fat, 1 cup	**140**	5	14
1% fat, 1 cup	**120**	3	14
Skim, 1 cup	**100**	0.5	14
Acidophilus: Average All Brands			
Reduced Fat (2%), 1 cup	**130**	5	13
Low-Fat (1%), 1 cup	**100**	2	13
Buttermilk: Average All Brands			
Reduced-Fat (2%), 1 cup	**120**	5	10
Low-Fat (1%): 1 cup	**100**	2.5	12
Lactose-Reduced:			
Reduced-Fat: *Lactaid,* 1 cup	**130**	5	12
Dairy Ease 100, 1 cup	**130**	5	12
Low-Fat: *Lactaid,* 1 cup	**110**	2.5	13
Fat-Free: *Lactaid/Lucerne,* 1 cup	**80**	0	13
Lactaid with Soy Protein	**110**	0	13
Lower Carb Dairy Drinks: *Per 8 fl.oz Cup*			
Carb Countdown (Hood): Regular	**130**	8	3
2% Reduced-Fat, 1 cup	**100**	4.5	3
Fat-Free, 1 cup	**70**	0	3
LeCarb: 2% Low-Fat Dairy, 1 cup	**105**	4.5	4
Homogenized Dairy	**140**	9	4

Soy/Non-Dairy Drinks

~ *See Page 27*

Goat/Sheep Milk, Kefir

	C	F	Cb
Goat's Milk (Meyenberg):			
Whole, 1 cup, 8 fl.oz	**140**	7	11
Light/Low-Fat (1%), 8 fl.oz	**90**	2.5	9
Evaporated, reconst., 8 fl.oz	**145**	8	11
Kefir: *Steve's Kefir Peach*, 1 cup	**220**	9	25
Nancy's, fruit flavors, avg, 1 cup	**200**	8	25
Sheep's Milk: Whole, 1 cup	**265**	17	13

Canned & Dried Milk

	C	F	Cb
Condensed: Reg. 2 Tbsp, 1 fl.oz	**130**	3	22
Low-Fat *(Eagle)*, 2 Tbsp	**120**	1.5	23
Fat-Free *(Eagle)*, 2 Tbsp	**110**	0	24
Evaporated: Whole, 2 Tbsp	**40**	3	3
Whole, ½ cup	**170**	10	13
Low-Fat *(Carnation)*, 2 Tbsp, 1 oz	**25**	0.5	3
½ cup, 4 fl.oz	**115**	2.5	14
Fat-Free, 2 Tbsp, 1 oz	**25**	0	4
Dried: Whole, ¼ cup, 1 oz	**150**	8	11
Skim/Non-Fat, ⅓ cup	**80**	0	12
Made-up, 1 cup, 8 fl.oz	**80**	0	12
Buttermilk sweetcream, 1 oz	**110**	2	3
Non-Fat, 1 Tbsp	**25**	0	3

Whey Drink

	C	F	Cb
Acid: Dry, 1 Tbsp, 3g	**10**	0	2
Fluid, 1 cup, 8 fl.oz	**60**	0	13
Sweet: Dry, 1 Tbsp, 8g	**25**	0	6
Fluid, 1 cup, 8 fl.oz	**65**	1	13
Nutri Mil: Orig./Low-Fat 8 fl.oz	**80**	3	11
Chocolate, 8 fl.oz	**110**	3	19
Fat-Free (Calcium Enriched)	**60**	0	11

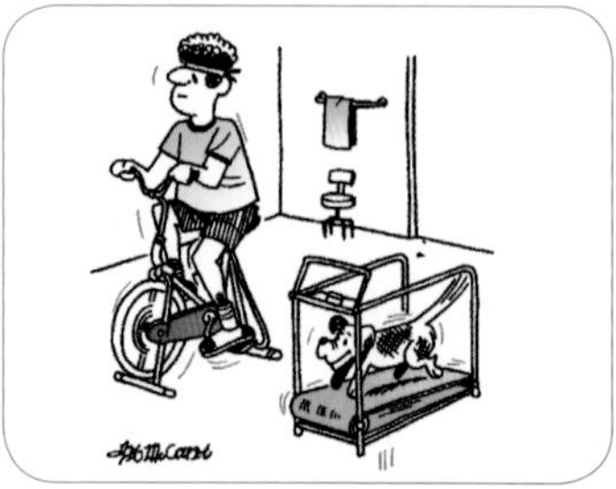

Flavored Milk Drinks

Quick Guide

Chocolate Milk	C	F	Cb
Average All Brands: *Per Cup (8 fl.oz)*			
Whole Milk (3.3%): 1 cup	**225**	9	26
1 Pint	**450**	18	52
Reduced-Fat (2%), 1 cup	**190**	5	26
Low-Fat (1%), 1 cup	**160**	3	26

Brands ~ Flavored Milk

Ready-To-Drink: *Per 8 fl.oz Cup Unless Indicated*	C	F	Cb
Albertson's, low-fat, 1 cup	**170**	2.5	30
Bodywise, non-fat, 1 cup	**180**	0	35
Borden Dutch Choc., 1 cup	**220**	8	28
Bosco, 1 cup	**230**	8	33
Brown Cow Farm, 1 cup	**250**	8	39
Carb Countdown (2%), Choc	**100**	4.5	3
Deans'Chug': Regular	**220**	9	26
Low-Fat, 1 cup	**160**	2.5	27
Dominick's Low-Fat, 1 cup	**170**	2.5	28
Golden Guernsey, 1 cup	**130**	2.5	15
Grocers Pride Choc D'Lite, 1 cup	**120**	3	22
Hershey's: Fat-Free Chocolate	**165**	0	30
Reduced-Fat Chocolate/Strawb.	**200**	5	31
White Chocolate	**130**	5	12
MilkShake, avg, 8 fl.oz	**285**	8	44
Hood: Low-fat (1%), Chocolate	**150**	2	27
Carb Countdown 2% Reduced-Fat	**100**	4.5	3
Horizon Organic	**160**	2.5	27
Knudsen	**200**	3	32
Kroger (3.25% milk)	**220**	9	28
Lactaid (1%)	**160**	3	26
Land O'Lakes, low-fat (0.5%)	**150**	1.5	35
Meadow Gold (3.5%)	**230**	8	31
Nesquik: 16 fl.oz bottle	**460**	16	64
Banana, 16 fl.oz	**385**	10	40
Choc., Fat Free, 16 fl.oz bottle	**320**	0	64
Double Choc., 16 fl.oz bottle	**395**	10	60
Very Vanilla, 16 fl.oz	**370**	10	60
Oak Farms, 1 cup	**210**	8	26
Parmalat (2%)	**180**	5	28
Ralph's	**240**	3	34
Sobe Love Bus Chocolate, 8 fl.oz	**140**	1	28
Viva, Low-Fat	**130**	2.5	26
Yoo Hoo Choc Drink, 8 fl.oz	**130**	1	29

Bottled Coffee

See Coffee Section: *Page 164*

Shakes & Smoothies

Smoothies	C	F	Cb
Made Up Ready-To-Drink (8 fl. oz Milk/Soy + Fruit): *Per 12 fl.oz*			
Average all types w. Whole Milk	**300**	8	50
+ Icecream, 1 scoop	**400**	13	62
with Non-Fat Milk	**240**	0	50
Freshens; Jamba Juice; TCBY: *See Fast-Foods Section*			
Shakes			
Regular: Chocolate, 10 fl.oz	**360**	11	58
Vanilla/Strawberry, 10 fl.oz	**320**	9	53
Carb Options, 11.3 fl.oz can	**185**	9	6
Burger King; McDonald's: *See Fast-Foods*			

Cocoa-Chocolate Mixes

Add extra cals/fat/carbohydrate for milk	C	F	Cb
Alba '66 Milk Choc, 1 pkg	**60**	0	14
Carnation Breakfast Drinks: *See Page 158*			
Hershey's, 1 Tbsp	**20**	0.5	3
Horlicks, Malt Extract, 1 oz	**20**	0	3
Land O' Lakes: *Per 1¼ oz Pkg*			
Choc.Mint/Raspb./Supreme	**160**	5	25
Nescafe Frothe, 3 T., makes 8 fl.oz	**15**	0.5	2.5
Nestle: French Vanilla, 1 envelope	**120**	3	22
Hot Cocoa, 2 Tbsp	**85**	2.5	15
Fat-Free Hot Cocoa, 2Tbsp	**25**	0	4
w. Marshmallows, 1 envelope	**35**	0	8
Nesquik Powder *(Nestle): Per 2 Tbsp*			
Choc.; Dble Choc; Strawberry	**90**	0.5	19
Chocolate, No Added Sugar	**40**	1	7
Ghirardelli: *Per 2 Heaping Teaspoons*			
Choc. Mocha/Hazelnut/Dble Choc	**80**	1.5	21
Pralines & Creme, 2 Tbsp	**90**	0	23
Ovaltine Cocoa Mixes, 4 tsp	**80**	0	20
Swiss Miss: Cocoa Mixes,			
Milk Chocolate, 1 oz pkt	**110**	1.5	22
w. Marshmallows, 1.2 oz pkg	**140**	3	22
Choc. Sensation, 1.25 oz pkg	**150**	4	27
Lite, 1 pkg	**70**	0	18
Diet Cocoa Mix, 1 pkg	**25**	0	4
Hot Cocoa Sugar Free, 1 pkg	**60**	0	10
Fat-Free, 0.53 oz	**50**	0	9
Vending Machine, 1.34 oz pkg	**145**	2	24
Weight Watchers: Hot Cocoa Mix	**70**	0	10

Soy ~ Ready-To-Drink

Per 1 Cup Serving (8 fl.oz)	C	F	Cb
Cereal Match, 1 cup	100	3	17
Eden Blend, 1 cup	125	3	18
Edensoy: Extra Original	130	4	13
Unsweetened	120	6	5
Extra, Vanilla	150	3	23
Carob	170	4	27
Chocolate	175	4	28
Light: Original	100	2	14
Vanilla	120	2	20
8th Continent: Original, Low-Fat	80	3	8
Original, Light	50	1.5	2
Chocolate: Low-Fat	140	3	23
Light	90	1.5	13
Vanilla: Low-Fat	90	3	11
Light	60	1	5
Hain Soy Supreme: Original	80	3	9
Vanilla, 1 cup	100	3	12
Hansen's Soy Smoothies: *See Page 153, 158*			
Harmony Farms: Regular	80	1.5	10
Enriched; Vanilla	80	1.5	10
Health Source: All flavors	150	1.5	23
Health Source Plus	160	1	17
Soy Protein Shake	100	1	4
It's Soy Delicious: Vanilla	110	1	22
Awesome; Chocolate	120	2	22
Lifeway, Soy Treat, Apple; Caramel	160	4	23
Naked Juice: *See Page 155*			
Odwalla Future Shake: Chocolate	160	3	27
Vanilla al'monde	190	6	24
Pacific: Select Plain, Low -Fat	70	2.5	9
Select Vanilla, Low-Fat	80	2.5	11
Organic, Original Unsweetened	90	4.5	4
Ultra (Extra Protein/Calcium): Plain	120	4	12
Vanilla	130	4	14
PowerDream: Mango Passion	320	5	65
Java Jolt, Chai, Vanilla Blast	250	5	42
X-treme Chocolate	260	5	48
Silk *(White Wave):* Plain, regular	95	4	8
Plain, unsweetened	90	4	5
Chai, 1 cup	140	4	19
Chocolate, 1 cup	140	3.5	23
Coffee Soylatte, 1 cup	150	3.5	25
Enhanced, 1 cup	110	5	8
Mocha, 1 cup	140	3.5	22
Spice Soylatte, 11 oz bottle	190	5	27
Vanilla	100	3.5	10
Silk Creamer, 1 Tbsp	15	1	1
Slim-Fast: w. Soy Protein,			
Orange Pinepple Shake, 1 can	220	1	46

	C	F	Cb
SoyDream: Orig./Enriched 8 fl.oz	130	4	17
Carob/Chocolate Enriched	210	3.5	37
Vanilla; Vanilla Enriched	150	4	22
Soy Fusion: Berry, 1 cup	120	1.5	24
Soy Nice: *Per 1 Cup (8 fl.oz)*			
Natural, 8 fl.oz	70	3.5	2
Original	80	3	6
Chocolate, 1 cup	110	3	17
Vanilla	100	3	11
SunSoy: Chocolate, 1 cup	150	3.5	26
Creamy Original, 1 cup	100	4	8
Vanilla, 1 cup	100	3.5	12
Vitasoy: Refrigerated, Creamy Orig.	100	4	9
Rich Chocolate	160	4	24
Smooth Vanilla	110	4	12
Long Life: Creamy Original	110	4	11
Classic Original	120	4.5	11
Green Tea Soy Drink	120	4	13
Rich Chocolate	160	4	24
Unsweetened Original	80	4	5
Vanilla Delight	120	4	13
Light: Original	60	2	7
Chocolate	110	2	17
Vanilla Soy Drink	70	2	10
WestSoy: *Plus,* Plain, 8 fl.oz	130	3	17
Plus, Vanilla	130	3	19
100% Organic: Original (2% fat)	130	3.5	18
Unsweetened, Plain	90	4.5	5
Unsweetened, Vanilla	100	4.5	5
Nonfat: Plain, 8 fl.oz	70	0	10
Vanilla	80	0	14
Lite: Plain, 1 cup, 8 fl.oz	90	1.5	15
Chocolate	130	1.5	25
Vanilla	110	1.5	19
Low-fat: Plain	90	1.5	14
Chocolate	140	3	24
Strawberry	160	3	25
Vanilla	120	1.5	21
Soy Slender, avg., all flavors	70	3	5
Chai, Original, 8 fl.oz	130	3	25
Smoothies, all flavors, 8 fl.oz	140	1.5	28
Soy Shakes, Choc; Vanilla	170	3.5	30
Vigor Aid: Vanilla	230	5	37
Chocolate	260	5	42
Juice Bar, average all flavors	120	1.5	24
Vitamite 100: 1 cup, 8 fl.oz	110	5	14
Wild Oats: Original, 1 cup, 8 fl.oz	100	3.5	12
Wildwood: Organic Chocolate	135	3.5	19
Original; Vanilla, 8 fl.oz	105	3	14
Smoothies, 10 fl.oz bottle	130	3.5	18
Zen Soy: Plain, 8 fl.oz	95	3.5	9
Chocolate	170	4	27
Cappuccino	150	3.5	22
Vanilla	115	3.5	14

Soy Powder Mix

	C	F	Cb
1 oz (¼ cup) mix makes 1 Cup (8 fl.oz)			
Soy Protein Isolate, 1 oz dry	95	1	0
Better Than Milk: Original, 1 oz	100	2.5	16
Light, 1 oz	80	0.5	13
Joy Soy: Extra (Carob/Van.), 2 T.	80	3	11
Revival Soy Shakes: *Per Packet*			
Plain; Chocolate Daydream	110	1.5	2
Flavors, average: with Fructose	225	2	33
Unsweetened or Splenda	130	2	4
Soyagen: Reg./No Sugar, 1 oz dry	130	6	12
Carob, 1 oz dry	130	6	13
Soy Quik *(Ener-g)*, 1 oz dry	100	4.5	8

Rice & Cereal Drinks

	C	F	Cb
Almond Breeze: Original, 8 fl.oz	60	2.5	8
Chocolate, 8 fl.oz	110	3	22
Vanilla, 8 fl.oz	90	2.5	16
Amazake, Almond Light, 8 fl.oz	110	2	20
Horchata: Don José, 8 fl.oz	140	4	25
Kerns, Aguas Frescas, 8 fl.oz	140	3	26
Eden Blend, Rice & Soy, 1 cup	120	3	18
Hain Rice Supreme: Low-Fat Orig.	100	3	16
Low-Fat Cinnamon, 8 fl.oz	130	3	22
Pacific: Multigrain, 8 fl.oz	160	2	30
Organic Oat: Original, 1 cup	130	2.5	24
Vanilla, 1 cup, 8 fl.oz	130	2.5	24
Almond: Original, 1 cup	80	2.5	11
Vanilla, 1 cup, 8 fl.oz	100	2.5	15
Hazelnut: Original, 1 cup	110	3.5	18
Pacific Rice: Low-Fat,			
Plain/Vanilla, 1 cup	130	2	27
Rice Dream: Carob, 1 cup	150	2.5	32
Chocolate; Enriched, 1 cup	170	3	36
Vanilla/Vanilla Enriched, 1 cup	130	2	28
Original/Original Enriched, 1 cup	120	2	25
Westbrae Rice, Plain/Van., 8 fl.oz	110	2.5	20
Wild Oats: Vanilla, 1 cup, 8 fl.oz	120	2	26
Original, 1 cup, 8 fl.oz	100	2	20

Rice/Nut Drink Mixes

	C	F	Cb
Better Than Milk: Light, 19g	70	0.5	14
Original, 23g	100	2.5	16
Nut Quik, 2 Tbsp powder, 18g	110	9	3
Rice Moo, 2 Tbsp powder, 19g	72	0	17
Solait, 3 Tbsp powder, 22g	80	1.5	13
Sun's Up, 2 scoops, 40g powder	160	2	36

Quick Guide

	C	F	Cb
Yogurt			
Average All Brands: *Per 8 oz Cup*			
Plain Yogurt: Whole, 8 oz	180	7	11
Low-Fat	140	4	16
Non-Fat	110	0	18
Fruit Flavored: Whole, 8 oz	250	6	38
Low-Fat	230	3	32
Non-Fat, regular	150	0	32
Non-Fat, no sugar added	120	0	32
Goat's Milk Yogurt ~ *Same as Regular Yogurt*			

Yogurt ~ Brands

	C	F	Cb
Alex Rod: Fat-Free, all flav., 8 oz	70	0	12
Albertson's (Low-Fat):			
Swiss, avg. all flavors, 8 oz	280	2.5	54
Fruit on the Bottom (low-fat):			
Average all flavors, 8 oz	260	2.5	49
Alta Dena: *Per Cup (8 oz)*			
Low Fat: Average all flavors	220	2	41
Non-Fat: Fruit Flavors, average	190	0	38
Plain	110	0	16
Vanilla	160	0	30
America's Choice: Swiss Style	210	2.5	41
Non-Fat, all flavors, 8 oz	100	0	15
Berkeley Farms: Non-Fat, avg.	100	0	16
Low-Fat: Boysenberry/Cherry	230	2.5	46
Raspberry	220	2.5	43
Strawberry, Lemon, Vanilla	270	2.5	52
Blue Bunny: Lite85, 6 oz	80	0	14
Low-Fat, average all flavors, 6 oz	85	3	5
Swirl'n Magic, Strawb. & Cherry, 4 oz	75	1	12
Yo-Pals, Strawb. & Banana, 4 oz	125	3	19
Breyers: Light (Fat-Free), 8 oz	120	0	22
Fruit On The Bottom, 8 oz	240	2	46
Creme Savers, all flavors, 8 oz	240	3	45
Smooth & Creamy, avg., 8 oz	240	2	48
Brown Cow: *Per 8 oz*			
Cream Top: Plain	170	10	12
Chocolate	250	8	39
Creamy Coffee, Vanilla	210	9	25
Fruit Flavors, average	230	8	35
Low-Fat: Plain	130	3	18
Flavors, average	220	3	41
Non-Fat: Plain	115	0	17
Fruit Flavors, average	190	0	39
Cabot: Plain, 8 oz	140	4	16
Flavors, 8 oz	220	3	42
Cascade Fresh: Low-Fat, 6 oz	140	2	23
Fat-Free, all flavors, 6 oz ctn	110	0	20
Whole Milk, 8 oz	170	8	12

Yogurt ~ Brands (Cont)

	C	F	Cb
Carb Countdown (Hood)			
Average all flavors, 6 oz	80	1.5	4
Colombo			
Light, all flavors, 8 oz	110	0	20
Classic, avg. all types, 8 oz	220	3	41
Fat-Free, Plain, 8 oz	110	0	16
Continental: Non-Fat, 8 oz ctn			
Fruit on the Bottom, 8 oz	190	0	38
Vanilla	190	0	38
Crowley: Low-Fat Blueberry, 8 oz	240	2.5	48
Dannon: Plain (Natural), 8 oz	170	8	14
Danimals: Super Creamy, 4 oz	120	1	18
Squeezable, 2 oz	140	5	20
Drinkable, 3.3 fl.oz	120	0	22
Fruit Blends: Blueberry, 6 oz	170	1.5	33
Creamy, avg., 6 oz	170	2	32
Strawberry Blueberry, 4 oz	110	1	21
Fruit on the Bottom, 6 oz ctn	160	1.5	29
Frusion Smoothie, 10 fl.oz bottle	280	3.5	53
la Creme: Avg. all flavors, 4 oz	150	5	21
Mousse, all flavors 2.6 oz	120	5	15
Light 'n Fit (0% Fat): Avg., 6 oz	95	0	16
Carb Control, 4 oz	60	3	3
Creamy, avg. all flavors, 6 oz	100	0	17
Smoothie, 7 fl.oz bottle	80	0	15
Natural, avg. all flavors, 6 oz	160	2.5	22
Sprinkl'ins, all flavors, 4.1 oz ctn	120	1.5	22
Whipped, avg. all flavors, 4.6 oz	160	3	28
Dominick's: Low-Fat, 8 oz	230	2	40
Fruit on the Bottom, avg, 8 oz	230	2	40
Fat-Free 80 Calories, 8 oz	80	0	13
Plain: Low-Fat, 8 oz	130	2.5	15
Non-Fat, 8 oz	120	0	17
Friendship: Regular type, 6 oz	190	5	31
Grocer's Pride: Low-Fat, 4.4 oz	140	1.5	28
Hood: Fat Free, Plain, 8 oz	130	0	18
Flavors, average, 8 oz	190	0	40
Horizon Organic			
Whole Milk, Plain Vanilla, 8 oz	220	6	32
Low-Fat: Blended, 6 oz cup	165	2	30
Tubes (1)	65	1	12
Fat-Free, all varieties, 6 oz	132	0	26
32 oz Carton, Plain, 8 oz	110	0	15
Yo Yo's, 4 oz	105	1	20
Jerseymaid (Vons)			
Fruit on the Bottom, 8 oz	240	2.5	46
Prestirred (low-fat), average	240	2.5	46
Plain, low-fat, 8 oz	140	3.5	18

	C	F	Cb
Jell-O: Spaceship, 4 oz	110	1	22
Hellios: Kefir Organic, 1 cup	120	5	13
Jewel: Low-Fat, average, 8 oz	250	2.5	48
Kemps: 100 Calories Nonfat, 5 oz	100	0	22
Classic Low-Fat, 6 oz	160	1.5	30
Free Non-Fat, 6 oz	90	0	22
Knudsen: 70 Calories, 6 oz	70	0	11
Free, average, 6 oz	170	0	33
Kroger: *Per 8 oz Ctn*			
Lite (Non-Fat) avg. all flavors	100	0	16
Low-fat: Plain, 8 oz	120	0	17
Flavors, average, 8 oz	250	2.5	47
Fruit on the Bottom, 8 oz	225	3	41
Lactaid: Low-Fat Vanilla, 8 oz	240	2.5	45
La Yogurt: Light, avg., 6 oz	90	0	17
Custard Classics, avg., 6 oz	170	2	32
French Style, avg., 6 oz	160	2	32
Fruit on the Bottom, avg., 8 oz	235	2.5	45
Latin Style, avg., 6 oz	180	2	33
LeCarb: YoCarb Plain, 4 oz	55	2.5	3
YoCarb Flavors, 4 oz	45	1	4
Light n' Lively			
Free 50 Calories, 4 oz	50	0	8
Free 70 Calories, 6 oz	70	0	11
Free (Regular): Vanilla, 6 oz	160	0	32
Fruit Flavors, average, 6 oz	180	0	36
Kidpack/Multipack, avg 4.4 oz	140	1	28
Lucerne			
Low-Fat: Plain, 8 oz	150	3.5	18
Fruit flavors, average, 8 oz	240	2.5	47
Vanilla	230	2.5	43
Fat-Free: Plain, 8 oz	130	0	19
Light Fat-Free, fruit, 8 oz	120	0	22
YoCups, avg all flavors, 4 oz	130	1	27
Yo On The Go, 2.25 oz tube	80	2	13
Meadow Gold: Plain, 8 oz	160	5	16
Flavors, average, 8 oz	250	4	42
Mountain High			
Original Style, plain, 8 oz	190	8	18
European Delight, all flavors, 4 oz	115	2	20
Naturally Nutritious, all flavors, 4 oz	95	0.5	18
Low-Fat: Plain, 8 oz	150	2	22
Classic, 8 oz	150	1	29
Fat-Free: Plain, 8 oz	120	0	19
Natural, 8 oz	165	0	33
Mystic Lake Dairy (Goat Milk Yogurt)			
Plain, 1 cup, 8 oz	120	6	9

Brands (Cont)

	C	F	Cb
Nancy's: *Per 8 oz Serving*			
Whole Milk: Honey, plain, 8 fl.oz	**180**	8	17
w. Fruit Cup, avg, 9.5 oz	**230**	8	29
Low Fat: Plain/Lemon/Vanilla, avg	**140**	3	16
Other flavors, average	**180**	3	28
Nonfat: Plain, 8 oz	**120**	0	17
Maple, Vanilla (8 oz ctn)	**160**	0	27
w. Fruit Cup, avg, 9.5 oz	**165**	0	29
Vanilla (32 oz ctn), swtn'd, 8 oz	**220**	0	40
Soy Cultured: (6 oz ctn): Plain	**145**	3	25
Berry flavors, average	**150**	3.5	24
Vanilla	**120**	3	19
Kiwi-Lime; Mango, average	**170**	3	33
Old Home: 100 Cal., Non-Fat, 6 oz	**100**	0	20
Velvet Delight, average, 6 oz	**240**	7	39
Pavel's: Original Russian, 8 oz	**140**	8	10
Low-Fat Vanilla, 8 oz	**120**	4	12
Non-Fat Russian, 8 oz	**110**	0	15
Mountain Dairy, 6 oz	**150**	1.5	27
Publix: Fat-Free, Plain, 8 oz	**140**	0	23
Swiss Style (low-fat), 8 oz	**240**	2.5	41
Redwood Hill Farm (Goat Milk Yogurt)			
Vanilla; Fruit flavors, avg., 8 oz	**180**	5	28
Plain, 8 oz	**125**	6	10
Silk (Soy): Plain, 1 cup, 8 oz	**135**	3	22
Vanilla, 6 oz ctn	**170**	3	30
Other flavors, average, 6 oz	**170**	2	31
Sky Hill Napa Valley, Plain, 8 oz	**130**	8	8
Snackwell's, Non-Fat, 6 oz	**160**	0	36
Stater Bros: Non-Fat, avg, 8 oz	**130**	0	16
Stonyfield Farm (Organic)			
All Natural Fat-Free: Plain, 6 oz	**90**	0	14
Chocolate Underground, 6 oz	**185**	0	39
Other varieties, 6 oz	**130**	0	26
Low-Fat: Caramel	**190**	1.5	38
Plain	**95**	1.5	13
Other varieties, average	**140**	1.5	25
Whole Milk Yogurt:			
French Vanilla; Mocca-ccino, 6 oz	**185**	6	27
Vanilla Truffle, 6 oz	**235**	5	41
Other varieties, avg.	**170**	6	24
Moo-La-La, flavors, avg., 4 oz	**160**	5	25
Moove Over Carbs, 16 oz	**70**	3	14
O'Soy: Choc.; Vanilla, avg., 6 oz	**160**	2	27
Fruit on Bottom, average, 6 oz	**180**	2	33
Smoothies: Peach, 10 oz	**265**	3	49
Other varieties, 10 oz	**250**	3	46
Squeezers, all flavors, 57g	**60**	1	11
Yo Self, Low-Fat, average, 4 oz	**110**	1	21
Stop & Shop, Blended Lite, 8 oz	**120**	0	20
"TCBY" Fat-Free (Fantasies):			
Banana Creme Pie, 6 oz	**110**	0	18
White Chocolate, 6 oz	**90**	0	12
Trader Joe's			
Low-Fat, average, 8 oz	**230**	2.5	44
Non-Fat: Regular 8 oz	**190**	0	40
French Village, Vanilla, 8 oz	**170**	0	32
Organic Vanilla, 8 oz	**160**	0	27
Organic Low-Fat, average, 6 oz	**150**	2.5	24
Cultured Soy, all varieties, 6 oz	**140**	2.5	28
Wallaby (Organic), avg., 6 oz	**150**	2.5	24
Wildwood: Soyogurt Plain, 6 oz	**105**	5	6
Other varieties, avg., 6 oz	**130**	3.5	20
WholeSoy: Plain, 6 oz ctn	**140**	2.5	24
Other flavors, avg, 6 oz ctn	**150**	2.5	27
YoFarm, all flavors, avg, 8 oz	**220**	6	37
YoCrunch: *Low-fat w. Toppings, 6.5 oz Cup*			
Oreo Cookies	**190**	4	35
Peach/Strawb./Rasp. w. Granola	**220**	2	46
Average other varieties	**240**	6	41
Yoplait: Fruit Flavors, 6 oz	**165**	1.5	33
Coconut Cream Pie, 6 oz	**185**	3	34
Lemon Burst, 6 oz	**180**	1.5	36
Pina Colada, 6 oz	**170**	2	33
Light (Fat-Free): Fruit, 6 oz	**95**	0	19
Indulgent flavors, 6 oz	**105**	0	20
Custard Style, all flavors, 6 oz	**190**	3.5	32
Go-Gurt, 2.25 oz tube	**80**	2	13
Grande: Avg. all flavors, 8 oz	**250**	2.5	48
99% Fat-Free Plain, 8 oz	**135**	0	19
Trix, avg., all flavors, 4 oz	**120**	1.5	23
Ultra Creme, 6 oz	**85**	2.5	8
Whips!, 4 oz ctn	**145**	2.5	25
Yumsters, 4 oz	**120**	2	21

Yogurt Drinks & Probiotics

	C	F	Cb
Actimel *(Dannon)* Probiotic, 3.3 fl.oz	**95**	2	16
Alta Dena, Drinkables, 1 cup	**220**	0	46
Carb Countdown, 10 fl.oz	**100**	3	4
Carbolite, 8 fl.oz	**85**	2	8
Creme Savers *(Breyers),* 10 oz	**190**	3	32
Dannon: Danimals, 3.4 fl.oz bottle	**90**	1.5	16
DanActive, 3.4 fl.oz	**95**	1.5	18
Glen Oaks, all flavors, avg, 1 cup	**250**	4	46
Nouriche: Regular, 11 fl.oz	**280**	0	60
Light, 11 fl.oz	**170**	0	33
Stonyfield Farm, 10 fl.oz	**250**	3	48
WholeSoy, 12 fl.oz bottle	**210**	3	35
Yo Soy, 8 fl.oz	**80**	4	4
Yonique: Pina Colada, 6 fl.oz	**190**	4	30
Peach; Banana; Guava, 6 fl.oz	**170**	2	30

Quick Guide

Ice Cream

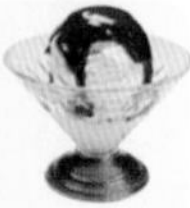

Vanilla: *Average All Brands*

Other flavors ~ See Brand Listings.

	C	F	Cb
Regular Ice Cream (10% fat):			
(Examples: *Borden/Hood*)			
3 fl.oz scoop	**100**	5	12
½ cup, 4 fl.oz	**130**	7	16
1 Pint, 16 fl.oz	**520**	28	62
½ Gallon (4 Pints)	**2100**	112	248
Rich (16% fat):			
3 fl.oz scoop	**130**	8	12
½ cup, 4 fl.oz	**170**	10	17
1 Pint	**690**	40	68
Super-Rich (20% fat): *(Haagen-Dazs/Ben & Jerry's)*			
3 fl.oz scoop	**200**	14	16
½ cup, 4 fl.oz	**270**	18	21
1 Pint	**1100**	72	84
Reduced-Fat/Light (6% fat):			
(Breyer's Light/Hood Light)			
3 fl.oz scoop	**100**	3	14
½ cup, 4 fl.oz	**140**	4	18
1 Pint	**560**	16	72
Low-Fat (less than 4% fat):			
(Healthy Choice/Weight Watchers/Snackwell's)			
3 fl.oz scoop	**90**	2	17
½ cup, 4 fl.oz	**120**	2.5	22
1 Pint	**480**	10	88
Fat-Free: *(Baskin-Robbins FF/Borden FF/ Breyers FF/Dreyers FF/Hood FF)*			
3 fl.oz scoop	**75**	0	17
½ cup, 4 fl.oz	**100**	0	22
1 Pint	**400**	0	88
Soft Serve: Regular, ½ cup	**140**	5	20
1 cup	**280**	10	40
Non-Fat, ½ cup	**90**	0	23
1 cup	**180**	0	46

Quick Guide

Frozen Yogurt

Average All Brands

	C	F	Cb
Hard: Low-Fat, ½ cup	**140**	3	26
Non-Fat, ½ cup	**110**	0	29
Soft: Low-Fat, ½ cup	**120**	2.5	28
Non-Fat, ½ cup	**100**	0	30

Brands: *See Ice Cream & Ices Section*

Quick Guide

Gelato/Ices

	C	F	Cb
Gelato: *Per ½ Cup*			
Milk base: Vanilla	**200**	15	18
Choc. Hazelnut	**370**	29	26
Water base: ½ cup	**100**	0	25
Ice (Milk base): Average all flavors			
Hard (4% fat), ½ cup	**100**	3	15
Soft Serve (3% fat), ½ cup	**110**	2	19
Shaved Ice: Average, 12 fl. oz	**160**	0	40
Sherbet: Average, ½ cup	**120**	2	28
Sorbet: Fruit (no fat), ½ cup	**120**	0	30
Fruit Ice Pops	**80**	0	20

Tofu Frozen Desserts: *See Page 35*

Sundaes

	C	F	Cb
Denny's: **Sundaes,**			
Single Scoop, no topping	**195**	14	14
Double Scoop, no topping	**385**	27	29
Banana Split	**930**	43	121
Toppings: Blueberry, 2 oz	**105**	0	26
Chocolate, 2 oz	**340**	25	27
Fudge, 2 oz	**215**	10	30
Strawberry, 2 oz	**115**	1	26
McDonald's: **Sundaes,**			
Hot Fudge Sundae, 6.3 oz	**350**	12	52
Strawberry Sundae	**290**	7	50
Toppings: Nut/Sundae, ¼ oz	**50**	3.5	2

Ice Cream Bars & Pops

See Pages 36-38

Ice Cream, Cones & Cups

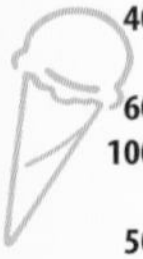

Average All Brands	C	F	Cb
Wafer Cone/Cup, average	**20**	0	4
Sugar Cone, average	**40**	0	9
Waffle Cone:			
Small	**60**	0	11
Large	**100**	1	22
Brands:			
Oreo Chocolate Cone	**50**	1	10
Comet Sugar Cone	**50**	0	11
Keebler Sugar Cone	**45**	0	11

Brands	C	F	Cb
Aspen: Ice Cream, ½ cup	170	0	4
Wow Cow Frozen Yogurt, ½ cup	40	0	8
Atkins: *Per ½ Cup*			
Endulge, average all flavors	130	11	6
Baskin-Robbins: *See Fast-Foods Section*			
Ben & Jerry's: *Per ½ Cup*			
Carb Karma: Chocolate	170	12	11
Half Baked	210	13	18
Vanilla Swiss Almond	205	15	13
Light: Chocolate Chip Cookie Dough	200	6	33
Chocolate Mint & Cookies	205	8	28
Vanilla	155	7	19
No Sugar Added: Strawberry	160	9	18
New York Super Fudge,	250	18	18
Original: Brownie Batter	310	18	32
Butter Pecan	285	21	20
Cherry Garcia	255	15	26
Chocolate	260	16	25
Chocolate Chip Cookie Dough	280	15	32
Chocolate Fudge Brownie	265	13	32
Chubby Hubby	345	21	32
Chunky Monkey	305	19	30
Coffee	235	15	21
Coffee Heath Bar Crunch	295	18	29
Di's Candy Drawer	310	18	32
Everything But The...	310	19	30
Fudge Central	300	18	31
Half Baked	275	13	34
Karamel Sutra; One Sweet Whirled	285	15	33
Mint Chocolate Cookie	265	16	26
New York Super Fudge Chunk	320	20	30
Oatmeal Cookie Chunk	290	16	32
Peanut Butter Cup	380	26	29
Phish Food	285	13	38
Pistachio Pistachio	280	19	21
Primary Berry Graham	265	15	29
Strawberry	245	14	26
Uncanny Cashew	295	19	27
Vanilla	245	16	21
Vanilla Heath Bar Crunch	305	19	29
Vanilla Swiss Almond	285	19	24
Frozen Yogurt: *Per ½ Cup*			
Cherry Garcia Yogurt	170	3	32
Choc. Fudge Brownie Yogurt	190	2.5	36
Half Baked Yogurt	195	3	37
Phish Food Yogurt	230	5	42
Sorbet: Average all flavors	120	0	30
Bars/Pops: *See Page 36*			

Blue Bunny	C	F	Cb
Fat-Free, No Added Sugar: *Per ½ Cup*			
Brownie Sundae; Burgundy Cherry	105	0	23
Caramel Toffee Crunch	110	0	24
Average other flavors	90	0	20
Reduced-Fat, No Added Sugar: *Per ½ Cup*			
Banana Split; Butter Pecan, avg.	135	6	18
Exquisite Mint; Tin Roof, avg.	145	6	20
Rocky Road; Turtle Sundae	155	7	20
Other flavors, avg.	120	5	16
Hi Lite: Butter Pecan	120	4.5	17
Caramel Pecan; Fudge Nut	130	4	21
Cookies & Cream; Vanilla	130	3.5	21
Other varieties, avg.	110	2.5	17
Carb Freedom: Vanilla Bean	100	6	10
Mint Chip; Butter Pecan	110	8	11
Choc. Almond Fudge	120	8	13
Double Strawberry	100	6	13
Frozen Yogurt, 6 fl.oz	75	0	13
Bars/Pops: *See Page 36*			
Bon Bon's *(Nestle)*: Milk Choc. (8)	330	23	27
Dark Chocolate, (8)	310	21	26
Bresler's: *Per ½ Cup*			
All Flavors Ice Cream: average	230	12	23
Royal Cremes, average	260	16	24
Royal Lites, average	220	0	49
Breyers: *Per ½ Cup*			
CarbSmart: Chocolate Almond	160	12	10
Chocolate Caramel	120	4	18
Strawberry; Vanilla	150	9	10
Other varieties, avg.	155	12	10
98% Fat-Free, average	105	1.5	20
All Natural: Banana Fudge Chunk	175	9	21
Butter Almond/Pecan	160	10	14
Caramel Praline Crunch; Heath	175	9	22
Chocolate Chip Cookie Dough	175	9	20
French Vanilla; Coffee; Cherry	145	8	15
Fruit Sherbet	120	1.5	26
Mocha Almond Fudge	170	9	18
Lactose Free; Peach; Strawb.	125	7	14
Peanut Butter & Fudge	175	10	17
Rocky Road	165	8	20
Take Two: Vanilla & Chocolate	150	8	16
Vanilla & Orange Sherbert	135	4.5	21
Vanilla & Choc. & Strawberry	140	8	15
Vanilla Fudge Brownie; Almond	170	9	19
Other varieties, avg.	155	8	16
Light: French Vanilla	120	4	18
French Chocolate	140	5	20
Vanilla	105	3	17
Other varieties, avg.	140	5	20

Brands (Cont)

	C	F	Cb
Breyers (Cont): *Per ½ Cup*			
No Sugar Added: Butter Pecan	135	7	15
Chocolate Caramel	160	4	18
Other varieties, avg.	115	4	14
Premium Edition: Turtle Sundae	190	11	20
Caramel Toffee Crunch; Reese's	180	9	22
Deep Chocolate Fudge	205	12	21
Ice Cream Cake, 1/13 cake, avg	185	10	21
Frozen Yogurt: *Per ½ Cup*			
98% Fat-Free: Fudge Brownie	105	1.5	20
Other varieties, average	120	1.5	23
All Natural: Average	140	4.5	22
No Sugar Added Vanilla Yogurt	120	4.5	13
Brigham's: *Per ½ Cup*			
Ice Cream: Big Dig	215	12	24
Chocolate/Chip; Vanilla	205	13	19
Chocolate Chip Cookie Dough	225	13	24
Mississippi Mud; Mocha Almond	220	14	20
Raspberry Lime Rickey Sherbert	130	2	27
Bruster's: Ice Cream, ½ cup	160	8	20
Frozen Yogurt, ½ cup	110	3	17
Fat-Free Ice Cream, ½ cup	110	0	23
Reduced-Carb Ice Cream, ½ cup	135	7.5	27
Carb Promise: *Per ½ Cup*			
Butter Pecan	150	11	10
Chocolate Peanut Butter Cup	170	12	12
Cow Tracks	150	8	18
Toffee Fudge Chunk	140	9	12
Vanilla	125	8	10
Vanilla Fudge Nut Sundae	165	11	14
CarbSmart: *See Breyers*			
Carvel Ice Cream: *See Fast-Foods Section*			
Coldstone Creamery: *See Fast-Foods Section*			
Colombo: *Per ½ Cup*			
Frozen, Soft Serve: Non-Fat var.	100	0	22
Slender Sensations varieties	60	0	11
Low-Fat: Old Worlde; Cookies	120	2.5	20
Sorbet: Vanilla	140	0	29
Other flavors	95	0	24
Costco: Frozen Yogurt, ½ cup	95	0	20
CremaLita (Soft Serve)			

Calories will vary with density (air in product) and serving size. Best to weigh product and calculate on 25 cals per 1 oz weight.

	C	F	Cb
Vanilla: Small (4 fl.oz cup),			
If 2½ oz weight	60	0	14
If 4 oz weight*	100	0.5	23
If 6 oz weight*	150	1	35
(*) Most common weights			
Medium (8 fl.oz cup), 11 oz wt	275	1.5	63
Chocolate: Small, 6 oz weight	160	1	36

	C	F	Cb
Dairy Queen/Brazier: *See Fast-Foods Section*			
Dannon Frozen Yogurt: *Per ½ Cup (4 fl.oz)*			
Light Soft, all flavors, average	90	1	21
Light 'N Crunchy, all flavors, avg.	110	1	23
Pure Indulgence, all flavors, avg.	150	3	25
Dolewhip (Soft Serve): *Per ½ Cup (4 fl.oz)*			
Chocolate; Vanilla	100	3	18
Fruit flavors, average	80	0.5	16
Dreyers: *Per ½ Cup*			
Fat-Free Ice Cream: Avg. all flav.	100	0	20
Carb Benefit, average	170	12	13
Grand: Almond Praline	170	8	21
Chocolate; Coffee, avg.	150	8	16
Fudge Tracks; Peanut Butter Cup	185	11	18
Grovestand Peach	120	5	17
Neapolitan	135	7	16
Nestle Drumstick Sundae Cone	180	10	19
Real Strawberry	125	6	16
Toasted Almond	155	9	15
Vanilla; Americans Vanilla	155	10	14
Vanilla Bean/Chocolate	140	8	15
Other flavors, avg.	165	9	18
Grand Light Ice Cream: Vanilla	105	3.5	15
Average other flavors	115	4	17
Homemade: Chocolate	150	7	19
Grovestand Peach	120	5	17
Mint Choc. Chunk; Van. Custard	160	8	18
Old Fashioned Butter Pecan	150	9	15
Strawberries and Cream	130	6	17
Vanilla	135	7	15
Frozen Yogurt: Vanilla; Raspb.	100	2.5	17
Other flavors, avg., ½ cup	120	3.5	19
Fat-Free, average all flavors	90	0	20
Sherbet, avg. all flavors	130	2	30

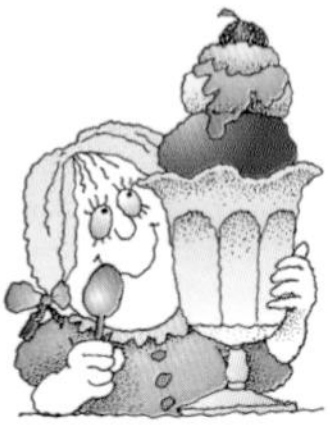

Brands (Cont)

	C	F	Cb
Edys: *Per ½ Cup*			
Banana Split; Choc. Fudge Mousse	160	8	19
Cherry Choc; Van./Choc.; Espresso	150	8	17
Choc. Fudge Sundae; Dble Fudge	170	9	19
Ice Cream Sandwich	150	7	19
Grand Light: Vanilla	100	3	15
Butter Pecan; Choc. Almond	120	5	16
Chiquita 'N Chocolate	110	5	13
Choc. Fudge Mousse	110	3	17
Cookie Dough; P'nut Butter Cups	130	5	18
Cookies 'n Cream; Rocky Road	120	4	18
French Silk	130	4.5	19
Fat-Free: Average all flavors	115	0	25
Eskimo Pie: *Per ½ Cup*			
Reduced-Fat: Butter Pecan	140	7	16
Choc. Marshmallow	130	4	23
Neopolitan; Vanilla	110	4	18
Other flavors, avg.	120	4	19
Bars: *See Page 37*			
Friendly's			
Ice Cream: Chocolate Almd Chip	170	10	18
Forbidden Chocolate	150	9	14
Fudge Nut Brownie	200	11	23
Vanilla Choc. Strawb.; Vanilla	150	8	16
Vienna Mocha Chunk	180	11	19
Frozen Yogurt: *Per ½ Cup*			
Regular flavors, average	150	4	24
Low-Fat flavors, average	120	3	20
Sundaes: *Per 3 Scoops*			
Apple Pie	700	30	98
Candy Shop Satisfaction Snickers	810	35	100
Dble Deluxe Caramel Fudge Blast	700	30	98
Cyclones: *Per 12 fl.oz*			
Fudge Brownie	790	25	127
Reese's Peanut Cup	880	43	100
Frostline (Soft Serve): Chocolate	90	2	20
Vanilla, ½ cup	90	3	18
Frusen Gladje: *Per ½ Cup*			
Butter Pecan	280	21	16
Chocolate	240	17	17
Strawberry	230	15	20
Swiss Choc. Candy Almond	270	19	18
Vanilla	230	17	16
Vanilla Swiss Almond	270	19	18
Other flavors, average	275	18	22

	C	F	Cb
Gelatida: *Per ½ Cup*			
Almond Biscotti	150	3	26
Amaretto Chocolate	150	4.5	23
Average other flavors	130	2	22
Godiva: *Per ½ Cup*			
Belgian Dark Chocolate	280	17	26
Choc Hazelnut Truffle	350	23	31
Choc Raspberry Truffle; Vanilla	290	16	33
Chocolate Cheesecake	310	17	36
Chocolate w. Chocolate Hearts	330	20	32
Classic Milk Chocolate	290	18	28
Pecan Caramel Truffle	320	19	32
White Choc. Raspberry	260	12	32
Good Humor: *Per ½ Cup*			
Light: Choc. Chip, Toffee Bar Crunch	130	4	20
Cookies n' Crm; Praline Alm. Crnch	130	3	21
Other varieties, avg.	110	3	19
Haagen-Dazs			
Ice Cream, Sorbet, Frozen Yogurt: *See Fast-Foods Section*			
Bars: *See Page 37*			
Healthy Choice: *Per ½ Cup*			
Brownie Bliss	125	2	25
Cookies 'N Cream	130	2	24
Double Karma; Happy Together	140	2	29
Jumpin' Java	130	2	25
Peanut Butter Cup	110	2	19
Praline & Caramel; Rocky Road	130	2	25
Vanilla; Mint Choc Chip	100	2	18
Other flavors, average	120	2	18
Low-Fat, No Sugar Added: Vanilla	90	2	18
Coffee Almond Fudge	110	2	20
Chocolate Fudge Brownie	115	2	20
Mint Chocolate Chip	100	2	18
Hood: *Per ½ Cup*			
Regular Ice Cream: Avg. all flavors	150	8	17
Light Ice Cream: Creamy Vanilla	110	3.5	18
Raspb. Swirl; Heavenly Hash, avg	130	3.5	22
Other flavors, average	140	5	22
No Sugar Added, Low-Fat Ice Cream:			
Vanilla Dream; Classic Trio	100	1.5	19
Choc Frenzy	120	2.5	19
Chocolate Chip	155	2.5	30
Fat-Free Ice Cream: Avg. all flavors	100	0	23
Frozen Yogurt: Avg. all flavors	150	8	17
Non-Fat: Strawb., Old Fashion. Van.	110	0	24
Other flavors, average	120	0	27
Bars: *See Page 37*			
I Can't Believe It's Yogurt: *See Fast-Foods Section*			

Brands (Cont)

	C	F	Cb
Jerseymaid (Vons): *Per ½ Cup*			
After Dinner Mint; Cookies & Crm	**170**	9	19
Choc Chip; Mint Choc Chip	**160**	9	17
Heavenly Hash; Nut Chunky Choc.	**170**	8	22
Mocha Almd Fudge; Rocky Road	**160**	7	20
Neopolitan; Vanilla	**140**	7	16
Strawberry	**140**	6	18
Kilwin's: *Per ½ Cup*			
Butter Pecan	**190**	13	16
Butter Pecan Yogurt	**130**	6	17
Chocolate	**170**	10	17
Average other flavors	**190**	10	20
Fat-Free Ice Cream, avg. all flavors	**100**	0	23
Topping: Caramel	**160**	4.5	31
Fudge	**110**	6	28
LeCarba: *Per ½ Cup*			
Chocolate Almond	**120**	9	6
Lemon	**90**	6	6
Other flavors	**100**	7	6
Luigi's Real Italian Ice: *Per Cup (6 fl.oz)*			
Chocolate	**160**	0	40
Other flavors	**125**	0	31
Swirl, all flavors	**155**	0	39
Rice Dream *(Non-Dairy): Per ½ Cup*			
Vanilla Carob/Choc/Cappuccino	**150**	6	23
Other varieties	**170**	8	26
Sealtest: *Per ½ Cup*			
Butter Pecan	**160**	9	16
Choc. Chip Cookie Dough	**160**	8	20
Fudge Royal; Heavenly Hash	**150**	7	20
Vanilla/Choc. Strawberry	**140**	7	16
Snackwell's: *Per ½ Cup*			
Brownie; Rocky Road; Praline	**140**	2	28
Vanilla	**100**	2	18
Soy Delicious (Organic): *Per ½ Cup*			
Novelties: Twisted Van. Orange	**120**	2	24
Mocha Fudge	**150**	3.5	27
Other flavors, avg	**145**	5	23
Fruit Pints: Almond Pecan	**160**	6	24
Choc Almond/P'Nut Butter	**155**	5	25
Other flavors, average	**130**	3	25
Purely Decadent: Zig Zag; Banana	**255**	13	32
Other flavors, average	**215**	9	32
Sweet Nothings, avg.	**115**	0	29
Soy Dream (Non-Dairy): *Per ½ Cup*			
Butter Pecan	**160**	10	17
Chocolate Fudge Brownie	**150**	8	20
Mint Chocolate Chip	**150**	9	19
Average other flavors	**140**	6	20

	C	F	Cb
Starbucks: *Per ½ Cup*			
Caramel Cappuccino	**240**	12	30
Classic Coffee; Italian Roast	**230**	12	26
Coffee Almond Fudge; Java Chip	**250**	13	29
Mud Pie	**240**	11	32
White Chocolate Latte	**280**	15	31
Low-Fat: Mocha Mambo; Latte	**170**	3	30
Bars: *See Page 38*			
Stonyfield Farm (Organic): *Per ½ Cup*			
Ice Cream: Chocolate	**260**	18	22
Vanilla	**255**	18	20
Other flavors, average	**260**	16	26
Frozen Yogurt:			
Non-Fat: Vanilla Fudge Swirl	**110**	0	23
Other varieties	**90**	0	19
Low-Fat: Creme Caramel	**120**	1.5	23
Choc Mint; Mocha Almd, avg.	**130**	3	22
Sweet Nothings *(Non-Dairy/Fat-Free)*			
Average all flavors, ½ cup, 3 oz	**120**	0	28
TCBY: *Per ½ Cup*			
Frozen Yogurt: Non-Fat, all flavors	**110**	0	23
96% Fat-Free, all flavors	**140**	3	23
No Sugar Added, all flavors	**90**	0	20
Hand-Dipped Icecrm: Butter Pecan	**260**	20	17
Chewy Chocolate Fudge	**270**	16	27
Chocolate Chocolate; Pralines	**215**	13	21
Choc. Chunk Cookie Dough	**210**	14	18
Lemon Meringue Pie	**235**	12	29
Oatmeal Raisin	**220**	12	25
Vanilla Bean	**195**	13	17
Very Berry Strawberry	**185**	11	19
White Macadamia; Mint Choc.	**250**	16	23
Sorbet, ½ cup	**95**	0	24
Tasti D-Lite (Soft Serve)			
Calories will vary with density (air in product) and serving size. Best to weigh product and calculate on 25 cals per 1 oz weight.			
Vanilla: Small (4 fl.oz cup), 6 oz wt	**180**	4	35
Medium (8 fl.oz cup), 11 oz wt	**330**	7	64
Tofutti Non-Dairy Dessert: *Per ½ Cup*			
Low-Fat Supreme: Average	**110**	2	25
Too Toos: Vanilla S'wich	**215**	10	28
Van. Choc. Swirl/Chip S'wich	**230**	11	30
Premium: Vanilla	**190**	11	20
Better Pecan; Alm. Bark	**220**	13	22
Choc. Cookie Crunch	**210**	11	26
Chocolate Supreme	**180**	11	18
Van. Fudge; Wildberry	**190**	9	24
Cutie Pies: Average, 67g bar	**250**	19	18
Teddy Fudge, 52g bar	**70**	1	19

Brands (Cont)

	C	F	Cb
Turkey Hill: *Per ½ Cup*			
Black Cherry	140	7	18
Butter Pecan	170	11	16
Choco. Mint Chip, Cookies 'n Crm	160	10	17
Rocky Road	170	8	23
Other flavors, average	140	8	16
Lite: Choco Mint Chip	140	5	19
Cookies 'n Cream	130	5	21
Vanilla & Choc., Van. Bean	110	3	18
Weight Watchers: *Per ½ Cup*			
Cookie Dough Craze	140	3.5	24
Oh! So Very Vanilla	120	2.5	20
Triple Chocolate Tornado	150	3.5	26
Other varieties, avg.	140	3	24
Smart Ones Bars: *See Page 38*			
WholeSoy Glace: *Per ½ Cup (70g)*			
Mocha Fudge	130	4	21
Swiss Chocolate	180	9	21
Strawberry	150	6	20
Vanilla Bean	190	9	25

Bars & Pops

	C	F	Cb
Per Bar/Serving			
Baby Ruth *(Nestlé)*	180	12	15
Barg's Root Beer & Ice Cream Float, 4 oz cup	120	3	22
Baskin Robbins: Tiny Toons	140	17	20
Cappuccino Blast, average	120	4	20
Sundae Bar, Pralines 'n Cream	280	17	28
Ben & Jerry's: 'Wich Cookie S'wich	340	17	44
Peace Pops: Cherry Garcia (1)	280	18	29
Cookie Dough (1)	380	22	41
One Sweet Whirled (1)	270	16	28
Vanilla (1)	300	20	26
Vanilla w. Heath Toffee (1)	320	21	30
Big Bear: *See Klondike*			
Big Ed's Super Saucer, 10 fl.oz	420	28	32
Blue Bunny: Ice Pops, avg.	40	0	10
Bomb Pops, avg.	45	0	10
Chocolate Cup, 1.7 oz	100	5	12
Fudge Bar, 2.7 oz	110	1.5	21
Health Smart, 2.2 oz	70	0	17
Sweet Freedom S'wich, avg.	160	2	32
Vanilla Nutty Cone, 3 oz	245	10	34
Carb Freedom: Vanilla Bar	140	12	11
Almond Bar	160	13	11
Fudge Bar	90	4	12
Bon Bons *(Nestlé):* Milk Choc., (8)	330	23	27
Dark Chocolate, 8 pces	310	21	26

Bars & Pops (Cont)

	C	F	Cb
Per Bar/Serving			
Borden: Sundae Cone	210	10	27
Twin Pops	60	0	14
Bounty, all varieties	70	5	7
Breyers: Lemonade Ice Cup	295	0	74
Ice Cream Cups, 4 fl.oz	155	9	19
All Natural Fruit Bars: Strawb.	120	0	30
Other varieties, 50ml	50	0	13
Fruit Bars, N.A.S., 50ml	35	0	8.5
Fruit Juice Bar, 3.75 fl.oz	120	0	30
Fruit Swirls, 4 fl.oz	165	9	19
Hershey's Almond Bar, 4 fl.oz	265	19	20
Tropical Fruit Bar, 2.75 fl.oz	80	0	20
Butterfinger Bar, 2.5 oz	190	13	16
CarbSmart: *See Klondike*			
Carnation: Orange Sherbet, 3 oz	90	1	19
Ice Cream Cup: Choc., 3 fl.oz	140	8	16
Strawb., Vanilla, 3 fl.oz	100	6	12
Choc./Vanilla Malt, 12 oz	270	6	48
Sundae Cup, all types, 5 fl.oz	210	9	30
Chipwich Jr: Choc. Chip S'wich	240	10	35
Chiquita: Swirls, all flavors	80	3	12
Cool Creations: Mini Sandwich	110	5	16
Cookies & Cream Sandwich	240	11	34
Pops, all types, 2 oz	60	0	14
Mickey Mouse: 2.5 oz Bar	120	8	10
Creamsicle: Sugar-free pops	25	0	15
Orange, 2.8 fl.oz	110	3	20
Crunch *(Nestlé)*: King, 4 oz	270	19	21
Reduced-Fat, 2.5 oz	130	7	14
Regular Ice Cream Bar, 3 oz	200	14	16
Crystal Light: Cool 'n Creamy	50	2	7
Dole: Fruit 'N Juice Bars, 2.5 fl.oz	70	0	18
Fruit Juice Variety Pack, all flavors (1)	45	0	11
No Sugar Added varieties	30	0	7
Dove Bar: Almond	340	22	30
Bite Size, 5 pces, average	350	22	36
Caramel Pecan	350	35	35
Mocha Cashew; Van. Milk Choc.	260	17	25
Peppermint	390	17	31
Vanilla Dark Choc; Cookie	340	21	35
Dreyers: Ice Cream Bars, average	250	17	22
Fruit Bars: Coconut	125	3	21
Grape; Cherry; Tropical	70	0	17
Sundae Cone, 4 fl.oz	240	11	31
Whole Fruit Bars, 1.75 fl.oz	30	0	8
Drumstick *(Nestlé)*: Chocolate	320	17	36
Choc. Dipped	320	16	40
Original Vanilla	340	19	35
Vanilla Caramel/Fudge	360	20	39

Bars & Pops (Cont)

Per Bar/Serving	C	F	Cb
Eskimo Pie: Arctic Madness, 2.5 oz	230	15	23
Bars: Milk/Dark Choc, 50g	160	11	15
Fudge Bar, 55g	60	1	11
Reduced-Fat varieties	120	8	13
Crispy Bar, 47g	130	8	13
Pecan, 51g	190	15	12
Big Bar, 99g	300	20	26
Ice Cream Sandwich, 65 g	160	4	27
Cones, 74g	210	12	24
No Sugar Added: Bar, 49g	120	8	13
Pudding Bar, 59g	90	1.5	16
Flintstones: Push Up Sherbet	100	2	20
Push Up Pebbles, 2.75 oz	120	6	15
Cool Cream, 2.75 oz	90	2	18
Frosty Dreams *(Nestlé)*	100	2	19
Frosty Pops *(Nestlé)*	40	0	11
FrozFruit: Peach Boost Bar	70	0	17
Banana; Strawb. Crm Bar, avg.	155	8	21
Fruit Bars: Mango	105	0	26
Other varieties, avg.	80	0	20
Fruit A Freeze: Coconut	130	5	20
Lime	65	0	16
Banana; Strawberry	90	1.5	19
Dark Choc-Dipped Strawberry	90	3.5	14
Fudge Bar *(Nestlé)*	110	1	23
Fudgesicle: Fudge Bar (1)	45	0.5	9
Fat-Free (1)	60	0	13
Fudgetastics Sticks Sundae	220	15	37
Godiva Pecan Caramel Bar	380	23	39
Good Humor: Bubble Play	105	0	26
Candy Center Crunch	315	23	24
Chocolate Eclair	225	11	30
Great White	70	0	18
Hyper Stripe	80	0	19
Number 1	200	11	21
Premium Vanilla	260	17	23
Reese's Peanut Butter Cup	315	21	27
Strawb. Shortcake; Tstd Almd	230	10	35
Cones: Giant King	395	21	44
King	255	13	30
Premium Sundae	265	15	29
Strawberry Shortcake	235	10	34
Sundae Twist	165	2.5	33
Sandwiches: Premium Vanilla	190	7	29
Giant Mississippi Mud	300	14	37
Giant Neapolitan/Vanilla	260	10	37
Premium Cookie	295	13	41

Per Bar/Serving	C	F	Cb
Haagen-Dazs: Vanilla & Almonds	215	12	22
Chocolate & Dark Chocolate	290	20	23
Chocolate Fudge & Almonds	325	23	25
Chocolate Sorbet Bar	85	0	20
Coffee & Almd; Cookies & Crm	310	12	23
Dulce De Leche (Caramel)	300	19	28
Raspb. Sorbet & Van. Yogurt	90	0	21
Strawberry Cheesecake	360	25	30
Vanilla Caramel & Pecans	360	26	27
Vanilla & Dark/Milk Chocolate	280	20	22
Health Smart *(Blue Bunny)*, avg.	80	0	18
Healthy Choice: Fudge Bar	75	1	13
Caramel Swirl Sandwich	145	3	27
Fudge Swirl Sandwich	145	3	27
Strawberry & Cream	80	1.5	13
Vanilla Sandwich	130	3	24
Hood: Chocolate Eclair, 1 bar	150	10	14
Fudge Bar: Chocolate	95	0.5	21
No Added Sugar	60	1.5	9
Dipped Delights	130	8	14
Java Smoothie	95	2.5	17
Hoodsie/Mint Sandwich	105	4	15
Light Sandwich	160	3.5	29
Hoodsie Cup Van./Choc.	100	5	12
Orange Cream Bar	90	1.5	18
Rockets, each	120	5	18
Vanilla Bar	160	12	11
Ice Cream Sandwich *(Nestle)*	170	6	26
Jell-O: Pop Bars	31	0	7
Jigglers, all varieties, 6 oz	215	1.5	50
Pudding Bars	80	2	13
Klondike: Choco Taco, 4 fl.oz	300	16	35
Dark Chocolate Crunch, 2.5 fl.oz	140	8	15
Heath, 5 fl.oz	295	20	26
Krunch, 5 fl.oz	280	19	25
Mini's Vanilla Ice Cream, 3 fl.oz	170	11	15
Movie Bites, 4.5 fl.oz	320	22	26
No Sugar Added Red. Fat, 4 fl.oz	180	9	21
Oreo, 3 fl.oz	160	10	17
Original, 5 fl.oz	280	19	24
Planters Caramel & Peanut	310	20	28
Reese's Peanut Butter, 2.9 fl.oz	220	15	20
Slim-a-Bear, 5 fl.oz	270	15	31
CarbSmart: Fudge Bar	105	7	9
Ice Cream Bar	180	15	9
Sandwich	115	4.5	10
Ice Cream Cone	210	16	14
Cones: Big Bear Sundae Cone	315	17	36
Big Bear Vanilla Sundae Cone	300	17	31
Oreo Cone	250	12	32
w. Oreo Cookies	230	9	34

Bars & Pops (Cont)

Per Bar/Serving	C	F	Cb
Klondike (Cont): Cup, 6 fl.oz	280	17	26
Sandwich: Big Bear	190	7	28
Giant Cookie w. Hershey's	470	20	66
w. Oreo Cookies	230	9	34
Kool-Aid Pops	40	0	10
Krispy Frostick	150	10	13
Juice Flavored Sticks	50	0	13
M&Ms Cookie Ice Cream S'wich	220	11	29
Mars Almond Bar	210	14	20
Matterhorn Cone, 10 fl.oz	510	38	19
Milky Way: Choc, Reduced-Fat	140	7	19
Caramel Swirl, 1 bar	180	10	21
Snack Bar, Vanilla/Chocolate	70	4	9
Minute Maid Fruit Juice Pops	60	0	15
Nestlé: Push Up Pop	90	1.5	19
Crunch: 3 oz bar	215	15	18
Multipack, 2.5 oz bar	150	8	18
Drumstick: S'Mores, 4.3 fl.oz	310	18	34
Strawberry Cheesecake	260	12	35
Original, 4.6 fl.oz	280	13	36
Fruit 'N Juice Lemonade	70	0	17
Ice Pops: Bubble Gumstix	90	0	23
Fudge Itzakadoozie	130	2	26
Juicy Juice Pops	30	0	8
Nesquik Pops, Chocolate	115	6	13
Push-Up Sherbet Treats	80	1	18
Push-Up Sundae	95	1.5	20
Oreo: Big Stuf, 1 sandwich	240	10	33
Cookies n' Cream, 1 bar, 59g	180	12	18
Pathmark Vanilla w. choc. coat.	150	10	14
Polar Bar: Vanilla w. choc. coat.	240	18	15
Choc. Chip Cookie Dough	450	28	48
Pops (water/juice), average	60	0	14
Popsicles: Big Stick Ice Pops	70	0	17
Creamsicle Pop	70	2	13
Crispy Cones, 2.5 fl.oz	150	7	20
Fudgesicle Fudge Pop	90	1.5	16
Firecracker Super Hero; Fruit Shot	40	0	10
Minis Ice Cream Pop	190	13	18
Rainbow Floats, 1.75 fl.oz	60	1.5	11
Sponge Bob Squarepants Pop Up	90	1.5	17
Scribblers Ice Cream: 2 pces	130	7	15
Juice Pops, 2 pces	60	0	16
Ice Pops: 1 pce	45	0	11
Sugar-Free, 1 pce, 1.9 oz	15	0	3
Reese's: Peanut Butter Ice Cream	160	11	22

Per Bar/Serving	C	F	Cb
Rice Dream: Pies, all flavors	320	18	40
Bars: Strawberry	250	13	31
Chocolate, Vanilla	270	15	32
Choc/Vanilla Nutty	270	18	23
Safeway Select Coffee Almd Bar	270	17	26
Silhouette *(The Skinny Cow)*			
Cookies 'N Cream Bar	120	1.5	23
Fat-Free Fudge Bar	90	0	19
Sandwich, Low-Fat, avg. all flav.	140	2.5	23
Sundae Cups: Chocolate	130	1	29
Vanilla Strawberry	120	0	27
Van. w. Choc. Fudge Topping	130	0.5	29
Slim-Fast: Fudge Bar	110	1.5	22
Ice Cream Sandwich: Vanilla	130	1	27
Chocolate	130	1.5	27
Smart Ones *(Weight Watchers)*:			
Chocolate Mousse; Orange	40	1	9
Chocolate Treat	100	0.5	20
English Toffee Crunch	110	6	12
Giant Fudge Bar, 76g	80	0	20
Mocha Java	80	1.5	15
Vanilla Low-Fat Sandwich	150	3	28
Snackwell: Ice Cream Sandwich	90	1.5	18
Yogurt Bars, 1 bar, 80g	120	2	22
Snickers: Ice Cream Bar	180	11	18
Pralines n' Creme	220	13	22
Ice Cream Bar (The Big One)	250	15	25
Snack, 4 bars	390	25	38
Soy Delicious: Li'l Buddies S'wich	165	4.5	28
Soy Dream (Non-Dairy):			
Dreamwich Vanilla	130	6	15
Heavenly Pies: Mocha; Vanilla	290	14	40
Lil' Dreamers: Choc; Vanilla	60	3	7
Rocket Bars: Choc; Vanilla	220	12	29
Starbuck's Frappuccino Bars, avg.	130	2	25
Starburst Juice Bars	20	0	5
Super Sundae Bar, 86g	310	20	26
3 Musketeers: 2 fl.oz bars	170	10	21
Snack Bars, regular	60	4	16
Tandem *(Nestlé)* Sandwich	380	21	39
Twin Pop *(Nestlé)*	60	0	14
Twix Bar	180	10	19
Vitari Soft Serve, 4 fl.oz, average	80	0	20
Welch's: Fruit Juice Bars, 92g	80	0	19
Tropical Coolers, 92 bar	45	0	11
No Sugar Added, 1 bar	25	0	6
Fruit Smoothie, 1 ctn	240	0	59

Quick Guide

Cream

Average All Brands	C	F	Cb
Half & Half Cream: 1 Tbsp, 0.5 oz	20	2	0.5
2 Tbsp, 1 oz	40	4	1
Light, coffee/table (20% fat): 1 T.	30	3	0.5
2 Tbsp, 1 oz	60	6	1
Medium (25% fat), 2 Tbsp, 1 oz	40	4	0.5
Sour Cream:			
Regular, 1 Tbsp, 0.5 oz	30	3	0.5
1 cup, 8 oz	490	48	8
Low-fat/Light, 1 Tbsp, 0.5 oz	20	2	1.5
2 Tbsp, 1 oz	40	2.5	2
Half & Half, 1 Tbsp, 0.5 oz	20	2.5	0.5
Fat-Free, 2 Tbsp, 1 oz	20	0	3
Fat Free: *(HeluvaGood),* 2 Tbsp	20	0	6
(Kroger), 2 Tbsp, 1 oz	25	0	5
(Naturally Yours; Oak Farm), 2 T.	20	0	3
(Knudsen), 2 Tbsp, 1 oz	35	0	6
Sour Cream Substitute:			
(Albertson's/ IMO), 2 T., 1 oz	60	5	2
(Tofutti) Sour Supreme, 1 oz	50	5	1
Whipping Cream:			
Heavy (37% fat):			
1 Tbsp fluid/2 Tbsp whipped	50	5	1
¼ cup whipped	100	11	2
½ cup fluid/1 cup whipped	400	44	8
Light (30% fat):			
1 Tbsp fluid/2 Tbsp whipped	45	4,5	0.5
½ cup fluid/1 cup whipped	350	37	4

Coconut Cream/Milk

	C	F	Cb
Coconut Cream (Canned),			
Plain/unsweetened, 2 Tbsp, 1 oz	70	6	4
½ cup, 4 oz	280	24	16
Sweetened: Coco Lopez, 1 oz	120	5	20
½ cup, 4 oz	480	20	80
Coconut Milk (Canned):			
Natural Value: Reg., ¼ c., 2 fl.oz	90	9	1
Lite, ¼ cup, 2 fl.oz	55	5	1
Thai Kitchen: Reg., ¼ c., 2 fl.oz	125	7	3
Lite, ¼ cup, 2 fl.oz	50	3	2
Premium, 2 fl.oz	125	12	3
Coconut Water (Center), 1 cup	45	0.5	9

Whipped Toppings

Average All Brands	C	F	Cb
Cream (Pressurized): 2 Tbsp	20	2	1
¼ cup	45	4	2
½ cup	90	8	4
Cream Toppings: *(Jewel)* Lite, 2 T.	20	1	2
Cool Whip: Extra Creamy, 2 T.	25	1.5	2
Lite, 2 Tbsp, 9g	20	1	2
Free, 2 Tbsp, 9g	15	0	3
Non-Dairy, 2 Tbsp	22	2	2
Kraft: Whipped, 2 Tbsp	20	2	1
Real Cream, 2 Tbsp	20	2	1
Reddi-Wip: Original, 2 T., 8g	10	1	0.5
Original Light, 2 Tbsp	15	1	2
Non-Dairy, 2 Tbsp, 8g	20	1.5	2
Extra Creamy, 2 Tbsp, 8g	15	1.5	0.5
Fat-Free, 2 Tbsp, 8g	10	0	2

Non-Dairy Coffee Creamers

	C	F	Cb
Powder: **Coffee-Mate/Cremora/N-Rich**			
Regular, 1 tsp	20	2	1
1 heaping tsp	25	2	2
Fat-Free, 1 tsp	10	0	2
Lite, 1 tsp	10	0.5	2
Flavors: 1⅓ Tbsp	60	3	9
Fat-Free: Average, 1⅓ Tbsp	50	0	11
Liquid/Refrigerated: *Per Tablespoon*			
Coffee-Mate Non-Dairy Creamer:			
Plain: Regular/Plain, 1 Tbsp	20	1	2
Fat-Free, 1 Tbsp	10	0	2
Lite, 1 Tbsp	10	0.5	1
Flavors: All flavors, 1 Tbsp	40	2	5
Fat-Free, all flavors, 1 Tbsp	25	0	5
Crème de la Soy *(Westsoy):*			
Original, 1 Tbsp	20	1.5	2
Amaretto; French Vanilla, 1 T.	25	1	4
Hood (Non-Dairy), 1 Tbsp	25	1.5	2
International Delight: 1 Tbsp	35	1.5	6
Fat-Free flavors, 1 Tbsp	30	0	7
Mocha Mix: Original, 1 Tbsp	20	1.5	1
Fat-Free, 1 Tbsp	10	0	1
Lite, 1 Tbsp	10	0.5	1
Morningstar, 1 Tbsp	40	1.5	7
Rich's Coffee Rich: Regular, 1 T.	25	1	2
Light	15	0.5	0.5
Rich's Farm Rich: Regular, 1 Tbsp	20	1	2
Light/Fat-Free	10	0	0.5
Silk *(White Wave)* Creamer, 1Tbsp	15	1	1
French Vanilla, 1 Tbsp	20	1	3

Fats, Spreads & Oils

Quick Guide

Butter & Margarine	C	F	Cb
Average All Brands			
Regular: 1 tsp (5g)	35	4	0
1 Pat (5g)	35	4	0
1 Tbsp, approx. ½ oz	100	11	0
2 Tbsp, 1 oz	205	23	0
1 Stick, ½ cup, 4 oz	810	92	0
1 Pound, 2 cups, 16 oz	3240	368	0
Light (Regular) 40% Fat:			
1 tsp, 5g	17	2	0
1 Tbsp, ½ oz	50	6	0
2 Tbsp, 1 oz	100	11	0
Whipped Butter (Regular):			
1 tsp (4 g)	27	3	0
1 Tbsp (10g)	70	7.5	0
1 Stick, ½ cup, 2 ⅔ oz	570	60	0
Whipped Light Butter 40% Fat:			
1 tsp, 5g	10	1	0
1 Tbsp, 9g	35	3.5	0
2 Tbsp, 18g	70	7	0
Unsalted: Same as Regular			

Clarified Butter

	C	F	Cb
100% Fat: 1 Tbsp, ½ oz	130	15	0
2 Tbsp, 1 oz	260	30	0

Flavored Butter/Spread

Average All Brands	C	F	Cb
Honey Butter (60% Fat):			
1 Tbsp, ½ oz	90	7	4
Downey's, 1 Tbsp, ½ oz	60	1	11
Garlic Butter (80% Fat):			
1 Tbsp, ½ oz	100	11	0
Macadamia Butter *(Atkins)*, 1 T.	125	12	2.5
Sweet Cream Butter:			
Regular, 1 Tbsp	100	11	0
Stick (70% Fat), 1 Tbsp	90	10	0
Tub (60% Fat), 1 Tbsp	80	9	0

Other Spreads & Fats

	C	F	Cb
Copha, Dripping, Lard, Suet, Shortening:			
1 Tbsp, ½ oz	120	13	0
Chicken, Duck, Goose Fat:			
1 Tbsp, ½ oz	115	13	0

Light & Reduced Fat Spreads

Per 1 Tbsp, ½ oz (Unless Stated)	C	F	Cb
Benecol: Spread, 1 Tbsp, 14g	80	9	0
Light, Spread, 1 Tbsp, 14g	45	5	0
Blue Bonnet, Homestyle (48% Veg Oil)	60	7	0
Breakstone's, Whipped Butter	60	7	0
Brummel & Brown, Spread	45	5	0
Chiffon, Whipped, 1 Tbsp	70	7	0
Country Crock *(Shedd's):* Regular	60	7	0
Light; Calcium & Vitamins	50	5	0
Country's Delight (70% Veg.)	90	10	0
Country Morning, Light	50	6	0
Downey's, Honey Butter	60	1	0
Dutch Farms, 52% Veg. Spread	70	7	0
Fleischmann's: Soft Spread	80	9	0
Original Stick	100	11	0
Light Spread	40	4.5	0
'I Can't Believe It's Not Butter': Reg.	90	10	0
Light; Sweet Cream	50	6	0
Imperial, Diet, 1 Tbsp	50	6	0
Jewel: Soft Spread	60	7	0
Unbelievably Butter	90	9	0
Kraft, 'Touch of Butter' (bowl)	50	6	0
Land O'Lakes: Fresh Buttery Taste	80	8	0
Honey Butter	90	7	4
Light Butter Whipped	35	3.5	0
Light Butter	50	6	0
Mazola, Diet	50	6	0
Mother's, Mrs Filbert's, 1 Tbsp	70	8	0
Miracle: Soft	60	7	0
Stick	70	7	0
Nucoa, HeartBeat Margarine	25	3	0
Olivio, Vegetable Spread	80	8	0
Parkay: Squeeze, 1 Tbsp	80	9	0
Stick, ⅓ Less Fat	70	7	0
Tub, 1 Tbsp	60	7	0
Tub, Light/Soft Diet	50	6	0
Whipped	70	7	0
Promise: Regular	90	10	0
Extra Light	50	6	0
Buttery Light	45	5	0
Ultra, w. Canola Oil	35	4	0
Smart Balance: Regular, 1 Tbsp	80	9	0
Light, 1 Tbsp	45	5	0
Smart Beat, Fat-Free	10	0	3
Take Control: Regular Spread	80	8	0
Light Spread	45	5	0
Weight Watcher's, Light	45	4	2

Butter Substitutes

	C	F	Cb
Bake It Perfect (Fat-Free Spread), 1 T.	5	0	0
Best O'Butter, ½ tsp	4	0	0
Butter Buds, 1 serving, ½ tsp	4	0	0
Butterlike Saute Butter, 1 Tbsp	35	2	0
Butter Sprinkles *(Watkins)*, 1 tsp	5	0	0
Earth Balance, Non GMO, 1 tsp	35	3.5	0
Molly McButter, ½ tsp	5	0	0
Mrs Bateman's Baking Butter, 1 T.	35	1	0
Natural Touch Soy, 1 Tbsp	85	5.5	5

Spreads Comparison

	C	F	Cb
Mayonnaise: Regular, 1 Tbsp	100	11	0
Light, average, 1 Tbsp	50	5	1
Fat-Free, 1 T.	10	0	3
Miracle Whip *(Kraft)*:			
Regular, 1 Tbsp	70	7	2
Light, 1 Tbsp	40	3	3
Free, 1 Tbsp	15	0	3
SmartBeat Dressing: 1 Tbsp	10	0	3

Extra Listings for Mayonnaise & Dressings
~ See Page 89 ~

	C	F	Cb
Avocado, mashed, 1 Tbsp	25	2.5	2
Peanut Butter, 1 Tbsp	100	8	3.5
Nutella, 1 Tbsp	100	5.5	12

"I push myself away from the table but my wife's good cooking pulls me right back."

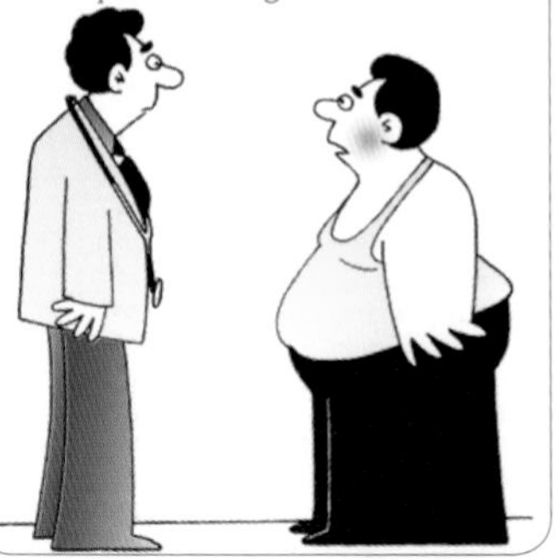

Animal Fats/Lards

	C	F	Cb
Average All Types			
Beef Tallow/Drippings, Lard (Pork), Chicken, Duck, Goose, Turkey.			
1 Tbsp (13g)	115	13	0
2¼ Tbsp, 1 oz	255	28	0
1 cup, 7¼ oz	1850	205	0
½ pound, 8 oz	2040	227	0
Ghee/Butter Oil: 1 Tbsp, 13g	110	13	0
2¼ Tbsp, 1 oz	250	28	0

Vegetable Shortening

	C	F	Cb
Average All Types (example, Crisco)			
1 Tbsp, 0.44 oz	113	13	0
2¼ Tbsp, 1 oz	250	28	0
1 cup, 7¼ oz	1810	205	0

Vegetable Oils

Includes almond, avocado, canola, corn, coconut, flaxseed, grapeseed, linseed, mustard, olive, palm, peanut, rice-bran, safflower, sesame, sunflower, soybean, wheatgerm. Note: Oil is 100% fat.

	C	F	Cb
1 tsp, 5g	45	5	0
1 Tbsp, ½ oz	120	14	0
2 Tbsp, 1 oz	250	28	0
1 cup, 7¾ oz	1930	205	0

Fish Oils

Average All Types (Includes cod liver, herring, salmon, sardine):

	C	F	Cb
1 Tbsp, ½ oz	125	14	0

Cooking Sprays/Squeezes

	C	F	Cb
Cooking Sprays *(Pam, Mazola, I Can't Believe It's Not Butter, Weight Watchers, Wesson)*:			
Per serving	2	0	0
1-3 second spray	6	1	0
I Can't Believe It's Not Butter	0	0	0
Parkay Buttery Spray	0	0	0
Squeeze (Parkay), 1 Tbsp, 0.5 oz	70	8	0

Olestra (Olean)

	C	F	Cb
Olestra *(Olean)*	0	0	0

Olean *is Proctor & Gamble's* brand name for olestra – a no-calorie cooking oil that gives snacks (like potato chips, tortilla chips and crackers) taste and texture without adding fat or calories.

Quick Guide

	C	F	Cb
Firm/Hard Cheeses			
(American, Cheddar, Colby, Coon, Swiss)			
Regular Cheese:			
1 oz slice/piece	110	9	0.5
8 oz package	880	72	4
16 oz (1lb) package	1760	144	8
Cubes: 1" cube, ¾ oz	55	5	0.5
1¼" cube, 1 oz slice	110	9	0.5
Diced: 1 cup, 4½ oz	500	40	2
Grated: 1 Tbsp, ¼ oz	27	2	0
Shredded:			
¼ cup, 1 oz	110	9	0.5
1 cup, 4 oz	440	36	4
Sliced: 1 thin (3½" sq.), ¾ oz	85	7	0.5
Rectangular (7"x 4"x ⅛"), 1½ oz	165	14	1
Round (3¼" diam. x ⅛"), ¾ oz	85	7	0.5
Semi-circular, 1¼ oz			
(5½" long, 3½" radius, ⅛" thick)	140	11	0.5
Light: Average All Brands, 1 oz	80	5	0.5
Fat-Free: Average All Brands, 1 oz	50	0	2
Low-Fat: Average All Brands, 1 oz	50	1.5	1

Cheese

	C	F	Cb
Per 1 oz Unless Indicated			
American:			
Regular, 1 slice, 1 oz	110	9	1
Kraft 0.7 oz slice	60	4	1
Grated, 1 Tbsp, ¼ oz	23	2	0
Light: *Borden,* 1 oz	70	4	0.5
Land O'Lakes, 1 oz	70	5	0.5
Smart Beat, 0.6 oz slice	35	2	0
Kraft, (2% Milk), 0.7 oz slice	45	3	1
Fat-Free: *Kraft,* 0.75 oz slice	30	0	2
Alpine Lace, 1 oz	45	0	2
HealthyChoice, Singles, 0.7 pce	75	6	0
Weight Watchers, ¾ oz	30	0	3
Babybel *(Laughing Cow),* 1 oz	90	7	0
Swiss Light Creamy, 21g pce	70	2	10
Bonbel *(Laughing Cow),* 1 pce	75	6	0
Swiss Light Creamy, 21g pce	70	2	10
Brick, 1 oz	100	8	0
Brie, 1 oz	95	8	1
Camembert, 1 oz	90	7	1
Caraway, 1 oz	105	8	1

	C	F	Cb
Cheddar: (Also see 'Quick Guide')			
Regular, 1 oz	110	9	0.5
Reduced-Fat/Light, 1 oz	80	5	0.5
Cabot Vermont, 50% Light	70	4.5	1
Weight Watchers, 1 oz	80	5	1
Fat-Free: *Alpine Lace,* 1 oz	45	0	2
Weight Watchers, 1 sl., ¾ oz	30	0	3
Cheese Balls *(Kaukauna),* 1 oz	100	7	0.5
Cheese Nut, average, 1 oz	100	7	2
Cheese Logs, average, 1 oz	100	7	0.5
Cheshire, 1 oz	110	9	1.5
Colby: Regular, 1 oz	110	9	0.5
Reduced-Fat *(Alpine Lace),* 1 oz	80	5	1
Colby-Jack, 1 oz	110	9	0.5
Cottage Cheese: *Average All Brands*			
Creamed (4% milk fat): 2 Tbsp, 1 oz	30	1	1
½ cup, 4 oz	120	5	4
w. fruit, ½ cup, 4 oz	130	4	15
Reduced-Fat (2%), 2 T., 1 oz	25	0.5	1
½ cup, 4 oz	100	2	4
Low-Fat (1%), 2 Tbsp, 1 oz	20	.5	1
½ cup, 4 oz	80	1	3
Fat-Free/Non-Fat, 2 Tbsp, 1 oz	20	0	1
½ cup, 4 oz	80	0	3
Borden Dry Curd (0.5%), ½ c., 4 oz	80	0	0
Friendship: Low-Fat P'apple, 4 oz	120	1	17
Non-Fat Plus Peach, ½ c., 4 oz	110	0	15
Pot Style, ½ cup, 4 oz	90	3	3
w. Pineapple, 4 oz	140	4	16
Hood Fruit Stirs, avg, 110g ctn	200	2.5	24
Knudsen: 1.5% Fruit, 4 oz	110	2	12
Free: Non-Fat, ½ cup, 4.3 oz	80	0	7
Low-Fat, 4 oz	85	2	4
Cottage Doubles, avg, 5.5 oz ctn	150	2.5	18
4% Milk-Fat, ½ cup, 4.3 oz	120	5	5
Light N' Lively: Garden Salad, 4 oz	90	2	5
Peach and Pineapple,			
½ cup, 4.3 oz	120	1	14
Cream Cheese: *See Page 45*			
Dorman's Castello, 1 oz	135	12	1
Edam, Regular, 1 oz	100	8	0
Farmer *(Friendship),* 2 Tbsp, 1 oz	50	3	0
Feta: Regular, Frigo, 1 oz	100	8	1
Crumbled, ½ cup, 2½ oz	190	15	2.5
Reduced-Fat *(Alpine Lace)*	60	4	1
Fontina *(Sargento/Classica),* 1 oz	110	9	0.5
Gjetost (Goat's Milk, fresh), 1 oz	85	7	0.5
Sargento, 1 oz	130	8	12
Goat's Milk: Soft: *Chevre,* 1 oz	70	6	0.5
Chavril, 3 Tbsp, 1 oz	60	4.5	0.5

Goat's Milk Cheese (Cont)	C	F	Cb
Semi-Soft: 1 oz	100	8.5	1
Hard: *Sargento*, 1 oz	130	10	0.5
Gorgonzola, 1 oz	110	9	0.5
Galbani Dolcelatte, 1 oz	95	8	1
Gouda, 1 oz	100	8	0.5
Gruyere, 1 oz	115	9	0
Havarti, 1 oz	120	11	0
Italian *(Classica Italiano)*, 1 oz	110	10	1
Jarlsberg, 1 oz	100	7	1
Jarlsberg Lite shredded, 1 oz	70	4	1
Kefir, 2 Tbsp, 1 oz	60	4	1
Limburger, 1 oz	90	8	0
Mascarpone, 1 oz	130	13	1
Mexican (*Sargento* Recipe Blend),			
Shredded, ¼ cup, 1 oz	110	9	0.5
Monterey, 1 oz	105	8.5	0
Monterey Jack: Regular, 1 oz	110	9	0
Light Naturals (Kraft), 1 oz	80	5	0
Alpine Lace, Monti-Jack Lo, 1 oz	80	5	0
Weight Watchers, 1 oz	90	6	1
Mozzarella:			
Regular: *Kraft/Dorman's*, 1 oz	90	7	0.5
Land O'Lakes/Polly-O, 1 oz	80	6	0.5
Shredded, ¼ cup, 1 oz	80	6	0.5
Light: *Polly-O Lite*, 1 oz	60	2.5	0.5
Kraft Light Naturals, 1 oz	80	5	0.5
Sorrento Lite, 1 oz	60	3	0.5
Part Skim *(Alpine Lace)*, 1 oz	70	5	0.5
Polly-O, 1 oz	90	6	0.5
Fat-Free: *Healthy Choice*, ¼ c.,1oz	45	0	1
Polly-O, 1 oz	35	0	1
Kraft, shredded, ¼ cup, 1 oz	50	0	2
Muenster: Regular, 1 oz	110	9	0
Reduced-Fat *(Dorman's)*, 1 oz	80	5	0
Myzithra, 1 oz	115	9	1
Neufchatel: *Dominick's*, 1 oz	70	6	2
Philadelphia, 1 oz	70	6	0.5
Flavored: Fruit/Herbs	80	7	1
Chocolate *(Hickory Farms)*, 1 oz	110	8	1
Parmesan: Fresh/Block, 1 oz	110	7	1
Shredded/Grated, 1 Tbsp	22	1.5	0
Grated (Packaged): 1 Tbsp	26	2	0
1 oz quantity	130	9	1
½ cup, 1¾ oz	230	16	2
w. Romano *(Frigo)*, grated, 1 oz	130	9	1

Note: Packaged grated and shredded Parmesan have more calories (per unit weight) than block Parmesan due to a lower moisture content.

Pizza Cheese, shredded:	C	F	Cb
Regular *(Frigo)* ¼ cup, 1 oz	90	7	1
Low-Fat *(Frigo)*, 1 oz	65	3	1
Port Du Salut, 1 oz	100	8	0.5
Port Wine *(Hickory Farms)*, 1 oz	100	7	2.5
Pot *(Sargento)*, 1 oz	25	0	1
Provolone: Regular, 1 oz	100	8	1
Reduced-Fat, *Alpine Lace*, 1 oz	70	5	1
Pub *(Hickory Farms)*, 1 oz	95	7	1
Quark: 40% fat, 1 oz	47	3	1
20% fat, 1 oz	32	1.5	1
Skim/Non-Fat, 1 oz	22	0	1.5
Queso: Anego/Asadero/Blanco	105	9	1
Queso Chichuahua/De Papa	110	9	2
Ricotta Cheese:			
Whole Milk, 2 Tbsp, 1 oz	50	3.5	1
½ cup, 4½ oz	225	16	4.5
Part Skim, 2 Tbsp, 1 oz	40	2.5	1
½ cup, 4½ oz	180	12	4.5
Light/Low-Fat, 2 Tbsp, 1 oz	25	1	1
½ cup, 4½ oz	100	2.5	5
Fat-Free, ½ cup, 4½ oz	100	0	4
Knudsen 'On The Go': Low-Fat, 4 oz	90	2	4
Free (Non-Fat), 4 oz container	80	0	6
Baked Ricotta, 2 oz portion	130	9	3
Romano: Block/Loaf, 1 oz	110	8	1
Grated (Pkg), 1 oz	120	9	1
1 Tbsp	26	2	0.5
Roquefort, 1 oz	105	9	0.5
Slim Jack *(Dorman's)*, 1 oz	90	7	1
Sheep's Milk *(Hollow Rd Farm)*	45	3	1
Smoked: *Sargents*, Smokestick	100	7	1
Hickory Farm, Smoky Lyte, 1 oz	80	6	1
Stilton, 1 oz	118	10	1
String *(Frigo/Kraft/Sargento)*, 1 oz	80	5	1
Light String-Ums, 1 stick	60	2.5	0.5
String Lite *(Frigo)*, 1 oz	60	2	1
Mootown Light *(Sargento)*, 1 stick	50	2.5	0.5
Swiss: Regular, 1 oz	110	9	1
Reduced-Fat: *Alpine Lace*, 1 oz	90	6	1
Dorman's/Kraft Light Naturals	90	5	1
Weight Watchers, ¾ oz slice	30	0	2
Taco Cheese, shredded, ¼ cup	110	9	1
Tilsit *(Sargents)*, 1 oz	100	7	0.5
Tybo *(Dorman's/Sargents)*, 1 oz	100	7	0.5
Vermont *(Churny)*, 1 oz	100	9	1
Wensleydale, 1 oz	108	9	0
Whey Cheese, 1 oz	125	8	9

Cheese Products

	C	F	Cb
Cheese Food:			
Average all flavors: ¾ oz slice	**70**	5	1.5
1 oz slice	**90**	6	2
Alouette: Fr. Onion/Garl.,2 T., 0.8oz	**70**	7	1
Light Garlic, 2 Tbsp, 0.8 oz	**50**	4	1
Cracker Barrel, Cheddar, 1.1 oz	**100**	8	4
Delico: Alouette Cajun, 2 T., 0.8 oz	**70**	7	1
Garden Vegetable, 2 T., 0.8 oz	**60**	6	1
Handi-Snacks:			
Cheez'n Breadsticks, 1 pkg	**130**	7	11
Cheez'n Pretzels, 1 oz pkg	**110**	6	11
Cheez'n Crackers, 1.1 oz pkg	**130**	8	10
Mozzarella Stringchse Stick, each	**80**	6	0.5
Healthy Choice, Amer. Singles, 1 sl.	**30**	0	2
Heluva Good Cheese:			
American, 1 slice	**45**	5	2
Cheddar w. H/radish, 2 Tbsp, 1oz	**90**	7	3
Jalapeno, avg., all brands, 1 oz	**90**	7	2
Kraft: American grated, 1T., 0.2 oz	**25**	2	1
Singles, 1 slice, ¾ oz	**70**	6	1
Free Singles, 1 slice, 0.7 oz	**40**	3	3
Pimento Spread, 2 Tbsp, 1.1 oz	**80**	6	3
Velveeta (Process Cheese Spread)			
Regular, ⅜" slice, 1 oz	**100**	6	3
Light, ⅜" slice, 1 oz	**60**	3	3
Rip-Ums, 1 strip, 0.75 oz	**80**	7	0.5
String-Ums (Lite), 1 stick	**60**	2.5	0.5
Lifeway Farmers Cheese, 2 oz	**75**	5	2.5
Precious String Chse Stuffsters, 1 oz	**70**	4.5	1
Roka Blue, 2 Tbsp, 1.1 oz	**80**	7	2
Rondele: Soft Spread., 2 T., 1 oz	**100**	9	1
Light, 2 Tbsp, 0.9 oz	**60**	4	2
SmartBalance Crmy Cheddar, 1 sl.	**40**	2	2
Spreadery: Vermont, 2 Tbsp, 1 oz	**80**	5	3
Neufchatel, all flavors, 2 T, 1 oz	**80**	7	1
Velveeta: Cheese, 1 slice, 1 oz	**100**	6	3
Light, 1 oz	**60**	3	3
Shredded, ¼ cup, 1.3 oz	**130**	9	3
WisPride: Hickory Smoked Cup;			
Port Wine Ball/Cup, 2 T., 1.1 oz	**100**	7	4
Light, 2 Tbsp., 1.1 oz	**80**	3	5

Cheese Whiz (Sauce)

	C	F	Cb
Regular, 2 Tbsp, 33g	**90**	7	2
Light, 2 Tbsp, 33g	**80**	3	6
Squeezable, 2 Tbsp, 33g	**80**	6	2

Cheese Substitutes

	C	F	Cb
Per 1 oz Unless Indicated			
Almond Rella *(Nu Soya):*			
Cheddar; Garlic & Herb, 1 oz	**70**	3.5	3
Borden, Taco-Mate, 1 oz	**100**	7	2
Delicia American Colby	**80**	6	1
Dorman's Lo Chol	**100**	7	1
Formagg: Cheddar, 1 slice, 0.7 oz	**60**	4	0.5
American Wh./Yellow, 1 sl. 0.7oz	**60**	4	0.5
Mozzarella (Old World), 1 oz	**60**	3	1
Parmesan Grated, 1 Tbsp, ¼ oz	**20**	1.5	1.5
Provolone (Vintage), 1 oz	**60**	3	1
Swiss White, 1 slice, 0.7 oz	**60**	4	0.5
Frigo Cheddar; Mozzarella, 1 oz	**90**	7	1
Georgio's: Imitation Cheddar;			
Mozzarella., shredded, ¼ c., 1 oz	**90**	7	1
Golden Image: American, 0.7 oz			
Mild Cheddar, 1 slice, 0.7 oz	**70**	5	1
Harvest Moon: *Per ¼ Cup, 1.3 oz*			
Shredded: American; Cheddar	**120**	9	3
Mozzarella	**110**	9	3
Nu Tofu: Mozzarella, 1 oz	**70**	4	2
Fat-Free: Mozz./Ched./Jack, 1 oz	**40**	0	2
Sargento Classic Supreme:			
Cheddar, shredded, 1 oz	**90**	6	2
Mozzarella, shrd, ¼ cup	**80**	6	0.5
Smart Beat, Fat-Free, 0.6 oz sl.	**35**	0	3
Soya Kaas: Regular, 1 oz	**70**	5	1
Fat-Free, all varieties, 1 oz	**40**	2	1
Soyco: Almond/Oat/Rice Slices,			
1 slice, 0.7 oz	**40**	2	1
Veggy Singles, 1 slice, 0.7 oz	**40**	2	1
Grated Parmesan, 2 tsp, 5g	**15**	0.5	0
Tofum Rella, avg. all varieties, 1 oz	**80**	5	3
Tofutti Better Than Cream Cheese	**80**	8	1
Weight Watchers: Fat-Free Slices,			
All varieties, ¾ oz slice	**30**	0	3
Grated Italian Topping, 1 Tbsp	**20**	0	2
White Wave: Soy A Melt,			
Cheddar/Mozz./Mont. Jack, 1 oz	**80**	5	1
Fat-Free, 1 oz	**40**	0	3
Singles: Amer./Mozzarella, ¾ oz	**60**	4	1
Yves, Good Slice, ¾ oz slice, avg.	**35**	2	1

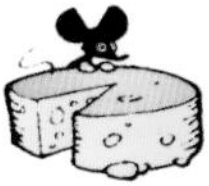

Cream Cheese

Cream Cheese	C	F	Cb
Regular/Soft: 2 Tbsp, 1 oz	100	10	1
3 oz pkg	300	30	2
w. Chives/Herbs/Pimento, 1 oz	90	9	0.5
w. Fruit/Strawb./P'apple, 1 oz	90	8	5
Lox, 1 oz	90	9	0.5
Philadelphia *(Kraft): Per 2 Tbsp*			
Original, 1 oz	100	10	1
⅓ Less Fat, 1 oz	70	6	1
Light: Plain, 1 oz	60	4.5	2
Strawberry, 0.7 oz	70	7	1
Fat-Free, 1 oz	25	0	2
Flavored: Blueberry/Raspberry, 1 oz	95	8	5
Strawberry, 1 oz	90	8	4
Garden Vegetable, 1 oz	95	9	2
Snacks: Bars, avg, all types (1)	180	11	20
Snack Bites (1) 1 oz	130	7	15
Bagel & Crm Chse To Go, 3.2 oz	240	9	36
Whipped: Regular, 2 Tbsp, 0.7 oz	60	6	1
Mixed Berry, 2 Tbsp, 0.7 oz	70	6	3
Alpine Lace, Fat-Free, 2 T., 1 oz	30	0	1
Weight Watchers, 2 Tbsp, 1 oz	40	2.5	1

Dips/Spreads ~ *Per 2 Tbsp (1 oz)*

Dips/Spreads	C	F	Cb
Avocado/Guacamole	50	4	4
Baba Ghannoush *(Eggplant/Sesame)*	70	6	2
French Onion Dip, avg. all brands	60	6	3
Guacamole, 2 Tbsp, 1 oz	50	4	4
Hummus: 2 Tbsp, 1 oz	50	1	5
½ cup, 4.5 oz	220	4.5	23
Tzatziki *(Cucumber/Yogurt Dip)*	40	3	1
Best Foods			
Dippin' Sauce: *Per 2 Tbsp*			
Honey Mustard Madness	60	2	10
Rockin' Ranch	90	6	8
Totally BBQ	110	12	1
Birdseye No-Fat Veggie Dip, 1.1 oz	25	0	5
Breakstone's Sour Cream, all flav.	50	4	4
Chalco: Quéso Quesadilla; Cotija	120	10	0
Fresco, 2 Tbsp, 1 oz	70	8	0
Cheese Fondue, ½ cup, 4 oz	210	14	4
Chi-Chi's: Con Quéso, 2 Tbsp	90	7	4
Hot/Medium/Mild/Acante, 2 T.	10	0	2
Cool Cuts: Carrot & Ranch	60	4	5
Celery & Peanut Butter	170	14	9
Frito Lay: Chili Cheese; Jalapeno	50	3	3
French Onion	60	5	4
Bean/Jalapeno Bean	40	1	6
Guiltless Gourmet: Nacho Dip	25	0	5
Other varieties	30	0	5
Heluva Good *Cheese:* Chse 'N Salsa	80	3	3
Clam/French Onion	50	5	2
Bacon/Homestyle/Ranch	60	5	2
Light Fr. Onion/Jalapeno Cheddar	40	2	3
Hy-Top Pimiento, 1 oz	90	8	3

Dips/Spreads (Cont)

Dips/Spreads (Cont)	C	F	Cb
Per 2 Tbsp (1 oz)			
Kaukauna Nacho Cheese	90	7	4
Knudsen Nacho Cheese	60	4	3
Sour Cream Bacon & Onion	60	5	2
Sour Cream French Onion	50	4	2
Kroger The Big Dipper; all flavors	60	5	2
Kraft: Average all flavors, 2 Tbsp	60	5	4
Philly flavors:			
Bacon & Cheddar	60	5	3
Average other flavors	55	4.5	3
Fat-Free: Strawberry	25	0	2
Garden Veges	30	0	2
Lay's Low-Fat Sr. Cream, Onion	40	1	0
Louise's: (Fat-Free) Honey Mustard	40	0	0
Sour Cream & Onion/White Chse	25	0	0
Luisa's Fiesta Dip, 2 Tbsp	35	2	3
Marie's: Reg, all types	90	9	2
Lite, 2 Tbsp, 1 oz	60	4	4
Nalley's all flavors, average	120	12	3
Naturally Fresh, all flavors, 1 oz	80	0	19
Old Dutch Cheddar, Nacho	35	3	3
Old El Paso: Black Bean	25	0	5
Cheese'n Salsa: Mild; Medium	40	3	3
Low-Fat, medium	30	1.5	3
Chunky Salsa varieties	15	0	3
Jalapeno Dip	30	1	4
Olys Bagel Spread: Berry	100	8	3
Honey Cinnamon; Raisin	100	8	6
Garden Veg; Garlic & Herb	90	9	1
Prices Orig. Pimiento Cheese Spr.	80	7	2
Rite Cream Cheese & Lox Spread	90	8	1
Ruffles French Onion; Ranch	70	6	4
Sealtest French Onion	50	4	2
Snyder's Mustard Pretzel	90	4	13
Stop & Shop: Veggie Dip, 2 Tbsp	110	10	3
Sour Crm French Onion, 2 T.	60	5	2
Supremo Chihuahua: Quéso Bianco	100	8	0
Quéso Fresco; Rancherito	80	6	0
TGI Fridays: Spinach,Chse,Artichoke	45	3.5	2
Black Bean & Cheese Dip	50	2.5	5
T. Marzetti: Blue Cheese	200	21	1
Light Ranch Veggie	70	6	3
Other flavors, average	130	13	2
Tostitos Dip: Con Quéso	40	2	5
Medium/Mild/Hot	15	0	3
Wise: Jalapeno Bean	25	0	5
Taco	12	0	3

Salsa: *See Page 85*

Egg & Egg Dishes

Chicken Eggs

Fresh Eggs	C	F	Cb
Raw (weight with shell):			
Small, 40g	65	4	0
Medium, 44g	70	4	0
Large, 50g	75	4.5	0
Extra Large, 56g	80	5	0
Jumbo, 63g	90	5.5	0
Egg Yolk, 1 extra large	63	5	0
Egg White, 1 extra large	16	0	0
Dried Egg Powder			
Whole Egg: ¼ cup, 1 oz	170	12	0
1 Tbsp	30	2	0
Egg White, ¼ cup, 1 oz	105	0	0
Egg Yolk, ¼ cup, 1 oz	195	18	0

Egg Substitutes

¼ Cup (Equivalent to 1 Egg) ~ Zero Cholesterol.

	C	F	Cb
Better 'n Eggs (*Papetti*),			
¼ cup, 2 oz	30	0	0
Egg Beaters *(Fleischmann's)* Frozen/Liquid			
Regular/Flavors, ¼ cup (61g)	30	0	1
Egg Watchers *(Tofutti)*, 2 oz	30	0	1
Eggstra, ½ envelope	50	2	0
Ener-G, Egg Replacer, 1½ tsp, 4 g	15	0	4
Healthy Choice, ¼ cup, 2 oz	25	0	0
Egg Substitute *(Jewel)*, ¼ cup	30	0	1
Scramblers *(Morn Star)*, ¼ cup	35	0	0
Second Nature: Regular, ¼ cup	60	2	3
Fat-Free, ¼ cup, 60ml	30	0	1
Simply Eggs, ¼ cup	35	1	1

Other Eggs

	C	F	Cb
Duck, 1 large, 2½ oz	130	9.5	0
Goose, 1 large, 5 oz	280	19	0
Quail, 3 eggs, 1 oz	42	3	0
Turkey, 1 large, 3 oz	135	9.5	0
Turtle, 1 egg, 1¾ oz	75	5	0

Omega-3 Fat Enriched

	C	F	Cb
Eggs Land's Best, 1 large	70	4.5	0
Eggs Plus *(Pilgrim's Pride)*, 1 large	70	4.5	0

Note: Cholesterol content same as regular eggs, but Omega-3 fats inhibit blood cholesterol increase.

Also see Cholesterol: *Page 271*

Cooked Eggs

	C	F	Cb
Boiled Egg: Same as raw egg			
Fried Egg:			
With fat: 1 large egg	100	8	0.5
2 small eggs	175	13	1
No fat/nonstick pan, 1 large	80	5.5	0
Deviled Egg, 2 halves	145	13	0.5
Eggs Benedict (2) on toast			
or English muffin	860	56	25
Eggs Florentine (2) on toast			
or English muffin	890	59	25
Pickled Egg, 1 large	80	5.5	0
Poached Egg, 1 large	80	5.5	0
Scotch Egg, 1 egg	300	21	16
Scrambled Eggs: 1 large egg:			
w. 1 Tbsp milk + 1 tsp fat	120	9	1
w. 1 Tbsp skim milk/no fat	85	5.5	1
2 large eggs:			
w. 2 Tbsp milk + 2 tsp fat	260	20	2
w. 2 Tbsp skim milk/no fat	180	11	2

Omelets

	C	F	Cb
1 Egg: Plain (w. 1 tsp fat)	125	10	0.5
with ½ oz cheese	175	15	0.5
w. ½ oz cheese + ½ oz ham	200	16	0.5
2 Eggs: Plain (w. 2 tsp fat)	250	20	1
with 1 oz cheese	360	29	2
w. 1 oz cheese+1 oz ham	410	32	2
3 Eggs: Plain (w. 1 Tbsp fat)	360	29	1.5
w. 2 oz cheese	580	47	2.5
w. 2 oz cheese+2 oz ham	680	53	2.5
Extras: Tomato/Onion/Veges	20	0	4.5
Egg Substitute *(Eggbeaters)*:			
2 eggs (½ cup) + 1 tsp fat	100	4	2
3 eggs (¾ cup) + 2 tsp fat	160	8	3
Extras: 1 oz cheese	110	9	1
1 oz ham	50	3	1
Tom./Onion/Veges	20	0	4.5

Egg Nog

~ Per ½ Cup (4 fl.oz)

	C	F	Cb
Regular: Borden	160	9	16
Crowley	190	9	23
Hood (Golden)	180	8	22
Light/Low-fat: Borden	120	2	23
Horizon; Hood	140	3	23
Fat-Free: *Hood*	100	0	21

Breakfast Sides

	C	F	Cb
Toast: Plain, 1 thick slice	85	1	13
with 2 tsp butter/marg.	155	9	13
with 3 tsp/1 Tbsp fat	190	13	13
English Muffin: Plain, 2 oz	130	1	26
with 3 tsp fat	230	12	26
Bacon, 2 strips	70	5	0
Ham, Lean, 2 oz	100	3	0
Hash Browns: ½ cup	125	6.5	14
1 cup serving	250	13	28
Sausages, 2 links (1 oz ea.)	180	16	1.5

Frozen Egg Breakfasts

	C	F	Cb
Jimmy Dean: **Breakfast Sandwiches,**			
Sausage Biscuit (2) 113g	400	28	27
Sausage, Egg & Cheese Muffin	380	25	26
Sausage, Egg & Cheese Biscuit	380	24	27
Bacon, Egg & Cheese Biscuit	290	15	26
Pillsbury: **Toaster Scrambles,**			
Cheese, Egg & Bacon/Ham	180	12	14
Cheese, Egg & Sausage	180	12	14
Swanson Great Starts: *Per Package*			
Egg, Bacon & Cheese Muffin	270	12	27
Egg, Chse & Bacon Biscuit	340	22	24
Sausage, Egg & Chse Biscuit	480	31	31
Sausage, Egg & Chse Croissant	470	33	27
Scrambled Eggs & Saus. Bkfst	370	27	17
French Toast & Sausage Bkfst	420	25	38
Pancakes & Sausage Breakfast	490	25	52
Uncle Ben's: *See Page 67*			
Weight Watchers: Omelet	220	5	30

Frozen Egg Rolls

	C	F	Cb
Chun King/La Choy: *Average All Brands*			
Chicken Egg Rolls: Mini, 6 rolls	210	9	25
Restaurant Style, 1 roll, 3 oz	210	9	25
Pork & Shrimp Egg Rolls:			
Mini, 6 rolls, 3 oz	210	9	27
Shrimp Egg Rolls: Mini, 6 rolls	190	6	28
Restaurant Style, 1 roll, 3 oz	180	7	25
Lotus: Pork, 3 oz	180	7	18
Vegetable, 3 oz	70	1.5	13
Kahiki: Pork, 3 oz	190	6	25
Chicken, 3 oz	120	2	16
Vegetable, 3 oz	120	2	23

Fast Food/Restaurants

	C	F	Cb
Au Bon Pain, Egg on a Bagel	390	4	63
Bojangles:			
Bacon/Egg/Cheese S'wich	550	42	27
Burger King:			
Egg'wich Bacon/Egg/Cheese	420	23	36
Croissan'wich Saus./Egg/Cheese	520	39	24
Carl's Jr, Scrambled Eggs	180	14	1
Denny's: Two Egg Breakfast	825	67	24
Omelette: Ham 'n Cheddar	605	47	5
Veggie-Cheese	510	39	11
Sirloin Steak & Eggs	655	45	1
Hardees: Bacon Egg, Chse Bisc.	520	30	45
Sausage & Egg Biscuit	620	40	45
Omelet	550	32	45
McDonald's: Egg McMuffin®	300	12	29
Bacon, Egg & Cheese Biscuit	480	31	31
Scrambled Eggs (2)	160	11	1
Perkins, Country Club Omelet	930	79	6
Whataburger:			
Breakfast Platter w. Bacon	685	42	52

New Diet Aid...
The Refrigerator Air-Bag!

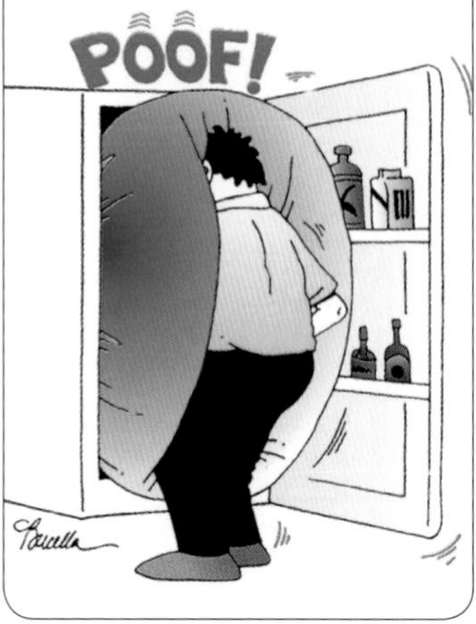

Meat & Beef

Note: Cooking reduces weight of meat by 20-45% due to water and fat losses. Average weight loss is 30%. Actual loss depends on cooking method and cooking time. Examples:

4 oz raw wt. = approx. 3 oz cooked wt.
4 oz cooked wt. = approx. 5½ oz raw wt.

What 3 oz Cooked Meat Looks Like

- Half the size of this book (4¼" x 3" x ³/₈" thick)
- Rectangular piece (4" x 2½" x ½" thick)
- Deck of cards (3½" x 2½" x ⁵/₈" thick)

Quick Guide

Steak
Sirloin (Choice Grade)
External fat trimmed to ¼"
Broiled, Edible Portion (no bone)

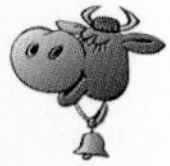

Small Serving, 3 oz (cooked)	C	F	Cb
(3 oz cooked, from 4-4½ oz raw)			
Lean + fat (¼"), 3 oz	**230**	14	0
Lean + marbling, 3 oz	**195**	10	0
(External fat trimmed **before** cooking)			
Lean only, 3 oz	**170**	7	0
(No external fat or marbling)			
Medium/Regular Serving, 5 oz (cooked wt)			
(from approx. 7 oz raw)			
Lean + fat (¼"), 5 oz	**470**	29	0
Lean + marbling, 5 oz	**400**	20	0
Lean only, 5 oz	**350**	14	0
Large Serving, 8 oz (cooked wt)			
(from 11-12 oz raw)			
Lean + fat, 8 oz	**610**	38	0
Lean + marbling, 8 oz	**520**	26	0
Lean only, 8 oz	**454**	18	0
Extra Large Serving, 12 oz (cooked wt)			
(from approx. 16-17 oz raw)			
Lean + fat (¼"), 12 oz	**915**	57	0
Lean + marbling, 12 oz	**780**	39	0
Lean only, 12 oz	**680**	27	0
Pan Fried			
Sirloin (choice), medium serving:			
Lean + fat (¼"), 5 oz	**450**	32	0
Lean only, 5 oz	**330**	15	0

Other Steaks

	C	F	Cb
Filet Mignon (Tenderloin):			
1 medium steak, 6 oz raw wt.			
Broiled, with ¼" fat trim			
Lean + fat (¼"), 4 oz	**340**	24	0
Lean only, 3½ oz	**210**	10	0
Broiled, (¼" fat removed before cooking)			
Lean + marbling, 3¼ oz	**220**	12	0
Lean only, 3 oz	**180**	8	0
New York/Club Steak:			
Top Loin/Short Loin			
1 steak, regular (9¼ oz raw, ¼" fat)			
Broiled: Lean + fat (¼"), 6¼ oz	**510**	35	0
Lean + marbling, 5½ oz	**330**	16	0
Lean only, 5¼ oz	**310**	14	0
Porterhouse Steak:			
1 medium, 6 oz raw wt. (no bone), broiled			
Lean + fat (¼"), 4¼ oz	**370**	27	0
Lean only, 3½ oz	**220**	11	0
With Bone: *See T-Bone Steak*			
T-Bone Steak (Broiled/Grilled)			
Medium, 8 oz raw wt.			
Lean + fat (¼")	**380**	27	0
Lean only	**220**	10	0
Large, 12 oz raw wt.	**570**	41	0
Supersize, 20 oz raw wt. (¼" fat)	**950**	68	0

Also See Fast-Foods & Restaurants Section ~
LoneStar Steakhouse, Outback Steakhouse, WesterN SizzliN

Beef - Average All Cuts

Average All Retail Cuts
Edible weight (no bone)

Raw	C	F	Cb
(1 lb raw yields approx. 11-12 oz cooked)			
Lean + fat (¼" trim), 1 oz	**70**	5.5	0
½ Pound, 8 oz	**560**	44	0
Lean only, 1 oz	**40**	2	0
½ Pound, 8 oz	**320**	16	0
Fat only, 1 oz	**190**	20	0
Cooked (No Added Fat)			
Lean + fat (¼"), 1 oz	**86**	6	0
Small serving, 3 oz	**260**	18	0
Lean + marbling, (no ext. fat), 1 oz	**78**	5	0
Small serving, 3 oz	**235**	15	0
Lean only, 1 oz	**60**	3	0
Small serving, 3 oz	**180**	9	0
Fat only, 1 oz	**193**	20	0

Beef - Individual Cuts

Average All Grades Edible Weight (no bone)	C	F	Cb
Brisket, whole, braised:			
Lean + fat ¼"), 3 oz	330	27	0
Lean + marbling, 3 oz	250	17	0
Lean only, 3 oz	205	11	0
Chuck, blade, braised:			
Lean + fat (¼"), 3 oz	290	22	0
Lean + marbling, 3 oz	285	20	0
Lean only, 3 oz	210	11	0
Flank: Raw, 4 oz	200	12	0
Braised, 3 oz	225	14	0
Broiled, 3 oz	190	11	0
Ribs, whole (ribs 6-12): Roasted (1 lb raw yields 10¼ oz roasted)			
Lean + fat (¼") (3.6 oz w. bone, 3 oz no bone)	300	25	0
Lean only, 3 oz (no bone)	200	11	0
Round, bottom, braised:			
Lean + fat (¼"), 3 oz	235	14	0
Lean only, 3 oz	180	7	0
Round, eye/tip, roasted:			
Lean + fat (¼"), 3 oz	200	11	0
Lean, 3 oz	150	5	0
Round, top: *Per 3 oz (cooked wt)*			
Braised, Lean + fat	210	10	0
Lean only	175	5	0
Broiled, Lean + fat	185	8	0
Lean only	155	4	0
Pan-fried, Lean + fat	235	13	0
Lean only	190	7	0

Ground Beef

	C	F	Cb
Ground Beef, Raw: *Per 4 oz*			
Regular: 70% lean (30% fat)	380	34	0
73% lean (27% fat), 4 oz	350	30	0
80% lean (20% fat), 4 oz	300	24	0
Reduced Fat, 85% lean (15% fat)	250	17	0
Lean, 90% lean (10% fat), 4 oz	190	8	0
Extra Lean, 96% lean (4% fat)	150	4.5	0
Rinsed (boiled/skimmed): 4 oz	180	12	0
Healthy Choice (97% lean), 4 oz	130	4	0
Baked/Broiled: Reg., 3 oz	250	18	0
Lean, 3 oz	230	16	0
Extra lean, 3 oz	200	12	0
Pan-fried: Regular, 3 oz	260	19	0
Lean, 3 oz	230	16	0
Extra lean, 3 oz	200	12	0
Ground Beef Patties: Average (20% Fat)			
Frozen, raw, 4 oz	290	22	0
Broiled, 3 oz	240	17	0

Quick Guide

Roast Beef	C	F	Cb
Round (Eye/Tip, average) Average All Cuts			
Small Serving, 3 oz (2 thin slices/1 thick slice)			
Lean + fat (¼"), 3 oz	200	11	0
Lean only, 3 oz	150	5	0
Medium Serving, 5 oz (3-4 thin slices)			
Lean + fat, 5 oz	330	18	0
Lean only, 5 oz	250	8	0
Large Serving, 8 oz (3 thick slices)			
Lean + fat, 8 oz	530	29	0
Lean only, 8 oz	400	13	0

Roast Dinner Extras

	C	F	Cb
Gravy: Thin, 2 Tbsp	20	1	0.5
Thick, 2 Tbsp	50	2	0.5
1 Ladle/4 Tbsp	100	4	1
Veges: Beans, green, ½ cup	20	0	5
Cauliflower w. cheese sauce, 4 oz	135	9	15
Corn, kernels, ¼ cup	35	0	9
Carrots, ¼ cup	20	0	3
Peas, ¼ cup	35	0	6
Pumpkin baked: w. fat, 4 oz	90	7	5
No added fat, 2 pces, 4 oz	25	0	5
Potato: Roasted w. fat, 1 small	155	8	30
Baked in Jacket, 1 large	220	0	50
with 1 Tbsp whipped butter	295	8	50
with Sour Cream, 2 Tbsp	270	6	51
Sweet Potato/Yam, 1 medium	80	0	20
Beef Kabobs: Beef & Veggies, 2 oz	160	10	4
If very lean meat	100	4	4

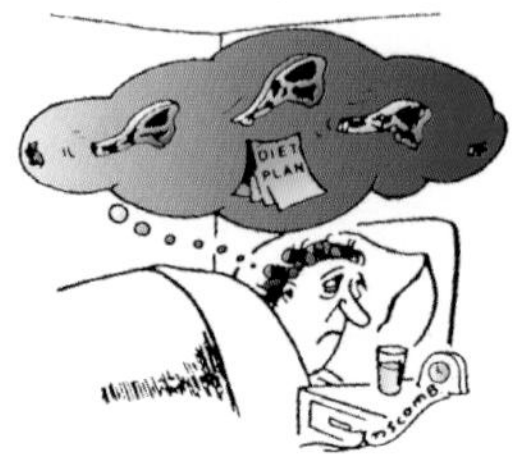

"347 ~ 348 ~ 349..."

Lamb

	C	F	Cb
Choice Grade			
Leg (Whole), roasted:			
Lean + fat, 3 oz	**220**	14	0
Lean only, 3 oz	**160**	7	0
Leg (Sirloin Half), roasted:			
Lean + fat, 3 oz	**250**	18	0
Lean only, 3 oz	**175**	8	0
Leg (Shank Half), roasted:			
Lean + fat, 3 oz	**190**	11	0
Lean only, 3 oz	**155**	6	0
Loin Chop, broiled:			
1 chop (raw wt., 4¼ oz):			
Lean + fat (2¼ oz edible)	**200**	15	0
Lean only (1.6 oz edible)	**100**	5	0
Rib Chop, broiled/roasted:			
1 chop (raw wt., 3½ oz)			
Lean + fat (2½ oz edible)	**255**	21	0
Lean only (1¾ oz edible)	**120**	7	0
Shoulder (Arm/Blade):			
Braised: Lean + fat, 3 oz	**290**	21	0
Lean only, 3 oz	**240**	14	0
Broiled: Lean + fat, 3 oz	**240**	16	0
Lean only, 3 oz	**180**	9	0
Roasted: Similar to Broiled			
Cubed Lamb (Leg/Shoulder):			
For stew or kabob			
Raw, lean only, 8 oz	**310**	12	0
Braised, lean only, 3 oz	**190**	8	0
Broiled, lean only, 3 oz	**160**	6	0
New Zealand Lamb (Imported):			
Similar calories and fat to domestic.			

Veal

Edible Weights	C	F	Cb
Leg (Top Round):			
Braised: Lean + fat, 3 oz	**180**	6	0
Lean only, 3 oz	**170**	5	0
Pan-fried, breaded:			
Lean + fat, 3 oz	**195**	8	9
Lean only, 3 oz	**175**	6	9
Pan-fried, not breaded:			
Lean + fat, 3 oz	**180**	7	0
Lean only, 3 oz	**155**	4	0
Roasted: Lean + fat, 3 oz	**135**	4	0
Lean only, 3 oz	**130**	3	0

Veal (Cont)

	C	F	Cb
Loin Chop: 1 chop, 7 oz raw wt.			
Braised: Lean + fat	**230**	14	0
Lean only	**155**	6	0
Roasted: Lean + fat	**175**	10	0
Lean only	**125**	5	0
Rib, roasted: Lean + fat, 3 oz	**195**	12	0
Lean only, 3 oz	**150**	7	0
Shoulder, Arm/Blade, roasted:			
Lean + fat, 3 oz	**155**	7	0
Lean only, 3 oz	**145**	6	0
Sirloin, roasted:			
Lean + fat, 3 oz	**170**	9	0
Lean only, 3 oz	**145**	6	0
Cubed for Stew, braised:			
Leg/Shoulder, lean only, 3 oz	**160**	4	0
(1 lb raw yields approx. 9¼ oz cooked)			

Pork

Figures based on NLMB data (1990)

	C	F	Cb
Fresh Pork (Cooked Wt., no bone)			
(4 oz raw wt. = approx. 3 oz cooked wt.)			
Blade Steak, broiled:			
Lean + fat, 3 oz	**220**	15	0
Lean only, 3 oz	**190**	11	0
Country Style Ribs, broiled:			
Lean + fat, 3 oz	**270**	22	0
Lean only, 3 oz	**205**	13	0
Spareribs, braised: lean & fat, 6 oz			
(from 1 lb raw wt)	**700**	53	0
Leg (Ham), roasted:			
Lean + fat, 3 oz	**250**	18	0
Lean only, 3 oz	**180**	9	0
(Ham, cured ~ See Cold Meats)			
Loin Chops, broiled: Average			
(From 1 chop: 5 oz raw wt. w. bone or 4 oz raw wt., no bone)			
Lean + fat, 3 oz	**200**	11	0
Lean only, 3 oz	**165**	7	0
Rib Chops, broiled:			
Lean + fat, 3 oz	**215**	13	0
Lean only, 3 oz	**180**	7	0
Rib Roast, roasted:			
Lean + fat, 3 oz	**210**	13	0
Lean only, 3 oz	**175**	9	0
Loin Roast, roasted:			
Lean + fat, 3 oz	**190**	10	0
Lean only, 3 oz	**160**	7	0

Pork (Cont)

	C	F	Cb
Sirloin Chop, broiled:			
Lean + fat, 3 oz	175	8	0
Lean only, 3 oz	155	6	0
Sirloin Roast, roasted:			
Lean + fat, 3 oz	215	14	0
Lean only, 3 oz	180	9	0
Tenderloin, roasted:			
Lean + fat, 3 oz	147	5	0
Lean only, 3 oz	140	4	0
Ground Pork			
Raw: Average, ¼ lb, 4 oz	300	24	0
Broiled, 3 oz	245	18	0
Pan-fried, drained, 3 oz	250	19	0

Bacon

Raw: 1 med. slice (20 lb), ¾ oz	125	13	0
1 thick slice (12 lb), 1⅓ oz	210	22	0
(1 lb raw yields approx. 5 oz cooked)			
Broiled/Pan-Fried: 1 med. sl., 6 g	36	3	0
3 medium slices, 18g	110	9	0
2 thin slices, ½ oz	80	7	0
1 thick slice, 12g	70	6	0
Canadian-style: Cooked, 1 slice	43	4	0
As purchased, 1 slice, 1 oz	45	4	1
Bacon Bits, 1 Tbsp, ¼ oz	20	1	0
Breakfast Strips: Broil., 1 sl., 12 g	50	4	0

Ham

	C	F	Cb
Boneless Ham, cooked:			
Regular, (approx. 11% fat):			
Unheated (as purch.), 1 oz	52	3	0
Roasted, 3 oz	150	8	0
Extra Lean (5% fat):			
Unheated, 1 oz	37	2	0
Roasted, 3 oz	125	5	0
Whole Ham, cooked:			
Lean + fat (as purchased)			
Unheated, 1 oz	70	5	0
Roasted, 3 oz	345	26	0
Lean only, unheated, 1 oz	40	2	0
Roasted, 3 oz	135	5	0
Canned Ham: Similar to boneless ham			
Chopped, canned, 3 oz	260	21	0
Ham Patties, ckd, 1 pty, 2¼ oz	205	18	1
Ham Steak, extra lean, 2 oz	70	2	0

Luncheon Slices: *See Deli Meats, Page 53*

Game & Other Meats

	C	F	Cb
Bison Steak,			
lean, 6 oz (raw)	210	4	0
Boar (wild), roasted, 3 oz	140	4	0
Buffalo Steak: *New West Foods*, 4 oz	70	3	0
Trader Joes, 1 patty	430	30	1
Caribou, roasted, 3 oz	140	4	0
Deer/Venison, roasted 3 oz	135	3	0
Goat (Capretto): Raw, 3 oz	110	2.5	0
Roasted, 3 oz	150	3	0
Ostrich: *Blackwing Ostrich Meats,*			
Sport Jerky, ½ oz pce	25	0	0
Sausage Patties (2) 2 oz	60	0.5	0
New West Foods:			
Ground Ostrich, 4 oz	110	2	0
Ostrich Steak, 4 oz steak	130	2.5	0
Rabbit: Roasted, 3 oz	130	6	0
Stewed, 1 cup, diced, 5 oz	300	14	0

Variety & Organ Meats

Brains: Braised, 3 oz	130	9	0
Pan-fried, 3 oz	200	14	0
Chitterlings, pork, simmered, 3 oz	260	25	0
Ears, pork, simmered, 1 ear	180	12	0
Feet, pork: Simmered, 3 oz	165	11	0
Cured, pickled, 3 oz	170	14	0
Hormel, 2 oz	80	6	0
Head Cheese (Pork Snouts/Ears/Vinegar/Spices):			
1 oz slice	50	4	0
Heart: Average, braised, 3 oz	140	5	0
Jowl, pork, raw, 4 oz	750	80	0
Kidneys, simmered, 3 oz	130	4	0
Liver: Raw, 4 oz	160	5	3
Braised, 3 oz	140	4	3
Pan-fried, 3 oz	200	9	3
Pancreas, braised, 3 oz	200	13	0
Pork Cracklins, 0.5 oz	80	6	0
Pork Hocks, 1 piece, 6 oz	340	23	0
Scrapple, pork, 1 oz	60	4	4
Spleen, braised, 3 oz	130	4	0
Stomach, pork, raw, 4 oz	180	11	0
Sweetbreads: Beef, ckd., 3 oz	270	20	0
Lamb, cooked, 3 oz	150	5	0
Tail, pork, simmered, 3 oz	340	31	0
Tongue, braised, 3 oz: Veal	170	9	0
Beef/Lamb/Pork, average	240	17	0
Tripe, beef, raw, 4 oz	110	5	0
Lean + fat	310	25	0

Sausages, Franks

Quick Guide

Franks & Weiners

Beef: *Average All Brands*	C	F	Cb
Regular/Smoked: *Per Frank*			
4 oz link	**280**	22	5
2.6 oz link	**240**	19	2
2 oz link (8/16 oz pkg)	**180**	17	2
1.6 oz link (10/16 oz pkg)	**140**	13	1
1.5 oz link (8/12 oz pkg)	**135**	12	1
1.2 oz link (10/12 oz pkg)	**110**	10	1
1 oz link (16/16 oz pkg)	**90**	8	0.5
Small/Cocktail (50/lb), each	**30**	3	0.5
Beef Light/Reduced Fat Franks:			
Ball Park, 1 frank, 2 oz	**100**	7	3
Best's Kosher	**50**	1	5
Boar's Head, 1.5 oz link	**80**	6	0
Oscar Mayer, 2 oz link	**110**	8	2
Hebrew National: 97% Fat Free	**50**	1.5	3
Reduced Fat, 1	**115**	10	0
Healthy Choice, low-fat, 1.8 oz	**60**	2.5	7
Beef Fat-Free Franks: *Oscar Mayer*	**40**	0	3
Ball Park (1),1.76 oz	**55**	0	7
Pork Franks:			
Boar's Head, 2 oz link	**155**	14	0
Country Style, 2 oz panfried	**240**	22	1
Chorizo, 5 sausages, 2.5 oz	**280**	26	3
El Popular, 2 oz cooked	**210**	17	3
Jimmy Dean, cooked, 2 oz	**240**	21	0
Oscar Mayer (2), 1.7 oz, ckd	**170**	15	1
Light, 2 oz link	**110**	8	2
Turkey Franks:			
Butterball, 1 frank, 1.75 oz	**45**	5	7
Empire Kosher, 2 oz	**90**	6	1
Foster Farms, 2 oz	**130**	11	0
Jennie-O, 2 links, 2 oz	**130**	11	0
Louis Rich: Orig., Lower Fat (1)	**100**	8	2
Bun Length (1)	**120**	10	3
Mr Turkey, smoked, 2 oz	**90**	5	3
Shelton's, 1 frank, 1.2 oz	**80**	6	1
Chicken Franks:			
Empire Kosher, 2 oz	**100**	7	1
Foster Farms, 2 oz	**140**	12	0
Scott Petersen, 1.2 oz	**80**	6	1
Shelton's, 1.2 oz	**95**	8	1
Zacky Farms, 2 oz	**150**	13	0

Vegetarian Sausages

See Frozen/Canned & Packaged Meals

Quick Guide

Fresh Sausages

Pork/Beef: *Average All Types*	C	F	Cb
Small: Raw, 4" link, 1 oz	**120**	12	1.5
Broiled/Pan-fried	**50**	4	1.5
Medium: Raw, 2 oz	**235**	23	2.5
Broiled/Pan-fried	**100**	8	2.5
Large: Raw, 3 oz	**360**	36	3.5
Broiled/Pan-fried	**150**	12	3.5
Italian: Raw, 3.2 oz	**315**	28	1.5
Cooked, 2.4 oz	**215**	17	1.5
Chorizo: Beef Chorizo, 2.5 oz pce	**320**	31	3
Pork Chorizo, 2.5 oz piece	**250**	22	4

Note: Fat is lost in broiling/pan frying. (Cooked wt. = approx. 60-70% raw wt.)

Smoked Sausage

Average All Brands: 2 oz link	**180**	16	4
3 oz link	**270**	24	6
Ball Park, Bun Size, 2 oz	**190**	17	4
Butterball (w. Turkey), 2 oz	**60**	0	6
Eckrich, 2 oz	**180**	16	4
Healthy Choice, Beef/Polska, 2 oz	**70**	2.5	6

Breakfast Sausages/Patties

Butterball: Turkey Brkfast Pats (2)	**100**	7	2
Turkey Breakfast Links (3)	**120**	8	2
Healthy Choice, Patties/Links (3), 2 oz	**70**	3	3
Jenny-O, Italian Turkey Saus. (2)	**160**	10	0
Jimmy Dean: Pork Saus. Patties (2)	**270**	25	0
Pork Sausage Links: Original (3)	**290**	28	0
Country Maple (3)	**230**	20	3
Breakfast Sandwiches: *See Page 47*			
Jones/Golden Brown:			
Pork Sausage Patties: Original (1)	**150**	14	0
All Natural (1)	**130**	12	0
Sandwich Patties (1)	**170**	16	1
Pork Sausage Links: 2 links	**190**	18	1
Light, 2 links	**100**	8	1
Swanson 'Great Starts': *See Page 47*			
Swift Premium Brown 'n Serve			
Pork/Turkey, 3 links, 2.1 oz	**210**	19	2
Lite Original, 3 links	**120**	8	3
Beef Sausage, 3 links, 2 oz	**230**	22	1

Vegetarian Patties:

Boca: *See Page 61*
Garden Burger: *See Page 62*

Bagel, Corn & Hot Dogs

Hot Dogs, Ready-To-Go	C	F	Cb
(Includes Ketchup/Relish; No Mayo)			
Small (1 oz frank/ 1 oz roll)	**200**	8	24
Regular (1½ oz frank/ 2 oz roll)	**310**	13	39
Large (2 oz frank/ 2 oz roll)	**360**	18	40
Super/Giant (3 oz frank/3 oz roll)	**540**	26	59
Weinerschnitzel: See Fast-Foods			
Corn Dogs			
Beef/Pork Frank: Average, 2.6 oz	**170**	10	16
Turkey: *Gobblers! (Shelton's)*	**220**	11	27
Foster Farms Chicken Franks:			
1 dog, 2.6 oz (75g)	**180**	10	15
Chili Cheese, 1 dog, 2.6 oz (75g)	**200**	9	24
Mini Corn Dogs, (4) 2.68 oz	**210**	12	18
Oscar Mayer Turkey & Pork, 3.2 oz	**260**	15	25
State Fair w. Ball Park Franks,			
Corn Dogs, 1 dog, 2.7 oz (76g)	**180**	12	15
Mini Corn Dogs (4)	**230**	13	22
Bagel Dogs			
Best's Kosher: 1 dog, 1 oz	**320**	11	43
Mini, 1 piece, 0.8 oz	**60**	2	8
Vienna Beef: 1 piece, 1 oz	**85**	3.5	7

Hot Dog Toppings/Extras:

American Chse, 1 slice, 1 oz	110	9	1
Catsup, 1 Tbsp	16	0	4
Chili (w. Beans), ¼ cup	70	3.5	9
Mustard, 1 Tbsp	20	0	1
Pickle Relish, 1 Tbsp	20	0	5
Sauerkraut, ½ cup	20	0	5

WILL-POWER TONIC
~ RECIPE ~

- 1 Cup of Desire
- 1 Quart of Determination
- 1 Tbsp of Common Sense
- 1 Tbsp of Stick-to-itiveness
- 1 Tbsp of Foresight
- 1 Cup of Energy

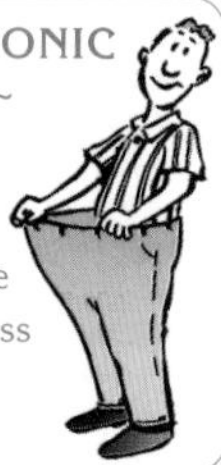

Deli & Luncheon Meats

Beef Jerky:	C	F	Cb
Bridgeford Beef Jerky, 1 oz	**50**	1	3
Beef Stick (5.5 oz stick), 1 oz	**140**	12	0
Beef Steak, 1 oz	**50**	1	0
Beef & Cheese (Giant Size), ½ pkg, 1.5 oz	**170**	14	1
Pepperoni Sticks, 2, 1 oz	**140**	12	0
Pepperoni (1" diam.), 1 oz	**130**	12	0
Teriyaki, 1.25 oz pkg	**80**	1	8
Original; Hot 'n Spicy	**70**	1	5
Berliner (pork/beef), 1 oz	**65**	4	0.5
Beerwurst (Beef):			
Small (2.75"diam), 1/16" slice	**20**	2	0
Large (4"diam), 1/8" slice	**75**	7	0.5
Beerwurst (Pork):			
Small (2.75"diam), 1/16" slice	**15**	1	0
Large (4"diam), 1/8" Slice	**55**	4	0.5
Bologna, Beef & Pork:			
Regular: 1 thin slice, 1 oz	**90**	8	1
1 thick slice, 1.6 oz	**145**	13	1
Light *(Oscar Mayer),* 1 sl., 1 oz	**60**	4	2
Red. Fat *(Hebrew Nat.),* 2 sl.,1 oz	**40**	2.5	0.5
Fat Free *(Osc. M.),* 2 sl., 1.6 oz	**40**	0	1
Healthy Choice, 1 oz	**35**	1	3
Weight Watchers, 2 sl., ¾ oz	**35**	2	0
Turkey, average, 1 oz	**60**	5	0.5
Chicken *(Tyson),* 1 slice	**45**	4	0.5
Ring *(Boar's Head),* 2 oz	**145**	13	0
Blood Sausage, 1 oz	**100**	9	0.5
Bratwurst:			
Average, 1 oz	**90**	8	0.5
Boar's Head, cook., 1 wurst, 4 oz	**300**	25	0
Bob Evan's, Beer, 2.6 oz link	**270**	21	1
Braunschweiger (Pork/Liver/Sausage), *Oscar Mayer,* 1 oz slice	**100**	9	1
Chicken, *Average All Brands*			
1 thick or 2 thin slices, 1 oz	**30**	1	1
Chicken Roll, 1 slice, 1 oz	**90**	4	1.5
Corned Beef:			
Average, full fat, 1 oz	**70**	5	1.5
Healthy Choice, Hillshire Farm, 1oz	**30**	1	0.5
Hebrew National, 4 slices, 2 oz	**90**	4.5	0
Loaf, jellied, 1 oz	**45**	2	0
Hash, canned, average, 1 oz	**50**	3	2
Dutch Brand Loaf, average, 1 oz	**70**	5	1.5

Continued Next Page

Deli & Luncheon Meats

Ham, Luncheon:	C	F	Cb
Baked/Boiled, sliced, 1 oz	30	1	0.5
Chopped: *Eckrich* (97% FF), 1 oz	25	1	1
Armour: Canned, 1 oz	35	1.5	0.5
97% Fat Free, 1 oz	25	1	1.5
Healthy Choice, 2 sl., 2 oz	60	1.5	2
Hormel (Black Label), 1 oz	70	6	0
Oscar Mayer, 1 oz slice	60	3	1
Honey/Brown Sugar: Avg., 1 oz	30	1	0.5
Healthy Choice Deli Traditions:			
2 slices, 2 oz	60	1.5	2
Prosciutto, average, 1 oz	70	5	1
Ham & Cheese Loaf, avg., 1 oz	70	5	0.5
Head Cheese *(Osc. Mayer),* 1 oz sl.	50	4	0
Honey Loaf *(Osc. Mayer),* 1 oz sl.	35	1	2
Italian Sausage, 2.6 oz	270	21	1
Kielbasa (Polish Sausage), 1 oz	85	7	0.5
Scott Petersen, 3.4 oz link	320	27	4
Beef, 2.8 oz link	290	25	4
Boar's Head, 1 oz	60	5	0
Kippered Beefsteak:			
Hickory Farms, 3 slices, 0.75 oz	50	1	1
Knackwurst, 1 oz	90	8	0.5
Linguica (Gaspar's), 2 oz	120	9	1
Liverwurst, 1 oz	95	8	0.5
Liver Pate, fresh, average, 1 oz	110	10	3.5
Luncheon Loaf (Foods Co), 1 oz	80	7	2
Mortadella, 1 oz	90	7	0.5
Olive Loaf, average, 1 oz	70	5	3
Oscar Mayer, 1 oz slice	70	6	2
Pastrami (Beef): Average, 1 oz	40	2	0.5
Healthy Deli, 1 oz	34	1	0.5
Hillshire (DeliSelect), 6 sl., 2 oz	60	1	1
Boar's Head, 2 oz	90	4	2
Peppered Beef, 1 oz slice	40	2	1
Pepperoni, 5 slices, 1 oz	135	12	0
Pickle Loaf, average, 1 oz	80	6	1
Pickle & Pimiento Loaf			
Oscar Mayer, 1 oz	80	6	3
Polish Sausage: *See Kielbasa*			
Proscuitti: Average, 1 oz	70	5	1
Hormel, 1 oz	90	7	1
Roast Beef: Lean, 1 oz	40	1	0.5
Healthy Choice, all types, 2 oz	60	1.5	1
Salami: Beef, average, 1 oz	80	7	1
Beer Salami, average, 1 oz	70	6	0.5
Cotto: *Oscar Mayer,* 1 slice, 1 oz	70	5	1
Dry: Hard, avg., 3 slices, 1 oz	110	10	0.5
Oscar Mayer, 2 slices, 1.6 oz	120	10	1

Salami (Cont):	C	F	Cb
Genoa: Average, 1 oz	110	10	0
Stick *(Best's Kosher),* 2, 1.75 oz	180	15	2
Italian *(Bridgeford),* 1 oz	120	11	0
Turkey, average, 1 oz	55	4	1
Spam *(Hormel):*			
Regular: ¼" slice, 1 oz	90	8	0
½" slice, 2 oz	180	16	1
Lite: ¼" slice, 1 oz	55	4	0
½" slice, 2 oz	110	8	1
Turkey: ¼" slice, 1 oz	40	2	0.5
½" slice, 2 oz	80	4	1
Summer Sausage:			
Bridgeford, 1 oz	100	9	0
Oscar Mayer, 1 slice, 0.8 oz	70	7	0
Treet (Armour), canned, 1 oz	100	9	1.5
Turkey: Average, 1 oz slice	30	1	0.5
¾ oz slice	22	0.5	0.5
Turkey Breast:			
Butterball Fat Free, 4 sl., 2 oz	50	0	2
Deli Thin Smoked, 1 sl., 1 oz	30	5	1
Hillshire Deli Select, 6 sl., 2 oz	60	0.5	2
Louis Rich Carvery Board,			
2 slices, 1.8 oz (52g)	50	0	2
Free, 2 slices, 2 oz	50	0	2
Healthy Choice: Deli Thin: *Per 4 Slices, 52g (1.8 oz)*			
Oven-Roasted	60	1.5	2
Smoked/Rotisserie Seasoned	60	1.5	2
Honey Roasted & Smoked	60	1.5	3
Hearty Deli Sliced:			
Oven Rstd Turkey Brst. 1 sl., 1 oz	30	1	1
Turkey Ham, 1 slice, 1 oz	35	1.5	0.5
Turkey Pastrami, 1 oz	35	1.5	0.5
Turkey Roll, 1 oz	40	2	0.5
Turkey Loaf, 1 oz	30	1	0.5

Vegetarian Deli *(Worthington, Yves):* *See Page 76*

Meat Spreads

Average All Brands: *Per ¼ Cup (2 oz)*	C	F	Cb
Chicken	120	8	2
Ham, deviled	160	14	0
Liverwurst	170	14	3
Roast Beef	140	11	0
Sandwich Spread	140	10	8
Turkey	110	7	2

Paté

Paté	C	F	Cb
Canned: *Average All Brands*			
Chicken Liver, 2 Tbsp, 1 oz	**60**	4	2
Paté de Foie Gras, goose liver, 1 oz	**130**	12	2
Fresh (Refrigerated):			
Average all types, 1 oz	**110**	10	1
Boar's Head Liverwurst Pate, 2 oz	**145**	12	0
Marcel Henri: Pate de Champagne	**210**	18	2
Chicken Liver w. Port Wine, 2 oz	**210**	18	2
Duck Truffle w. Port Wine, 2 oz	**240**	24	2
Old Wisconsin Pate, all types, 1 oz	**105**	9	1.5
Vegetable Pate; Spin/Mushr.m 2 oz	**105**	7	10
Toby's Tofu Pate: Original, 2 Tbsp	**90**	8	2
Lite, all flavors, 2 Tbsp, 1 oz	**40**	2	2
Trois Petit Cochons: Medit., 2 oz	**130**	11	3
Smoked Salmon, 2 oz	**115**	9	2
Wegmans: Alexian Wild, 2 oz	**270**	27	1
Cognac; Black Peppercorn, 2 oz	**160**	17	4

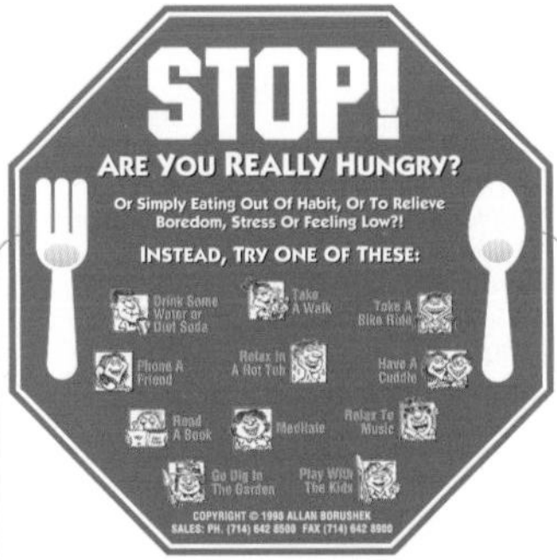
STOP!
ARE YOU REALLY HUNGRY?
Or Simply Eating Out Of Habit, Or To Relieve Boredom, Stress Or Feeling Low?!
INSTEAD, TRY ONE OF THESE:
Drink Some Water or Diet Soda
Take A Walk
Take A Bike Ride
Phone A Friend
Relax In A Hot Tub
Have A Cuddle
Read A Book
Meditate
Relax To Music
Go Dig In The Garden
Play With The Kids

Do you snack compulsively when you are bored, stressed or irritable?

If so, place this magnetic STOP! poster on your fridge.

To Order, See Page 303

Lunch Packs

Lunch Packs	C	F	Cb
Funny Bagels: *Per Package w. Drink, Yogurt*			
Honey Ham; Cheese Pizza, avg.	**435**	9	72
PB & J	**490**	14	82
Cream Cheese and Jelly	**470**	14	77
Lunchables *(Oscar Mayer): Per Package*			
Cracker Stackers Ham & Cheddar	**420**	23	37
Deluxe Turkey Breast & Ham	**365**	20	25
Nachos Cheese & Salsa, 4.4 oz	**375**	21	39
Pizza varieties, avg. 4.5 oz	**300**	13	28
Ham Turkey & Cheddar S'wiches	**465**	22	47
Taco Bell Beef Tacos, 5.35 oz	**310**	11	34
Fun Fuel: Ham Bagels, 5.6 oz	**410**	10	64
Chicken/Ham Wraps, 5.5 oz	**435**	13	64
Pile-Ups: Pizza Thin Crusts	**475**	13	75
Peanut Butter Soft White Bread	**600**	19	85
Turkey Bagels, 5.6 oz	**410**	10	64
Fun Pack: All Star Burgers/Juice	**215**	7	30
All Star Hot Dogs/Juice	**465**	19	64
Cracker Stackers: Ham & Chse	**440**	19	52
Lean Ham & Cheddar, 5.8 oz	**390**	11	56
Pancakes & Bac'n Bites, 4.9 oz	**530**	10	102
Pizza Dunks Soft Breadsticks	**500**	13	84
Beef Taco, 5.7 oz	**495**	15	69
Waffles & Sausage, 4.8 oz	**470**	16	66
Fun Snacks: Chips Ahoy!, 3.1 oz	**205**	9	30
Fudge Brownie, 4.3 oz	**255**	9	42
Oreo Cookies 'N Frosting, 3.7 oz	**235**	9	37
S'Mores, 3.4 oz	**200**	6	35
Star Cookies 'N Frosting, 3.6 oz	**230**	10	34
Mega Pack: Combo Ham & Ched.	**765**	32	101
Combo Turkey & Cheddar, 5.4 oz	**755**	31	101
Pizza: Pepperoni, 6.85 oz	**760**	28	105
Extra Cheesy, 6.8 oz	**725**	25	104
Pizza Stix, 7.15 oz	**695**	16	118
Ultimate Nachos Cheese & Salsa	**775**	32	113
Lunch Bucket *(Armour)*			
Beans 'n Weiners, 7.5 oz	**290**	10	37
Chili w. Beans, 7.5 oz	**235**	9	25
Hearty Beef Stew, 7.5 oz	**155**	8	15
Rings 'n Franks, 7.5 oz	**225**	9	30
Lunchmakers *(Armour):*			
Loco Nachos	**370**	13	59
Cheese Pizza	**310**	13	36
CrackerCrunchers: Bologna	**280**	19	19
Other varieties, average	**240**	15	18
Munch-A-Bunch *(Jewel): Per 4 oz Package*			
Bologna/Chse/Crackers/Cookies	**430**	29	27
Other varieties, average	**350**	19	29
Smuckers: Snackers, 3.3 oz pkg	**410**	20	47
Uncrustables, 1 sandwich	**210**	8	26

Chicken

Quick Guide

Chicken	C	F	Cb
From 3lb ready-to-cook chicken			
Breast/Wing Quarter			
Roasted: With skin	**300**	15	0
Without skin	**190**	5	0
Fried, batter dipped	**480**	26	18
Leg Quarter: Thigh & Drumstick			
Roasted: With skin	**265**	15	0
Without skin	**180**	8	0
Fried, batter dipped	**430**	26	16
KFC: *See Fast-Foods Section*			

Average - All Meats

Average of Light & Dark Meats	C	F	Cb
Per 4 oz Serving (no bone)			
Roasted: With skin	**270**	15	0
Without skin	**215**	8	0
Stewed: With skin	**250**	14	0
Without skin	**200**	8	0
Fried: Batter-dipped	**330**	20	11
Flour coated	**305**	17	3.5

Chicken Parts

Broilers or Fryers: Edible Weights (no bone)	C	F	Cb
Breast: *Per ½ Breast*			
Raw: With skin, 5 oz	**245**	13	0
Without skin, 4¼ oz	**130**	2	0
Roasted: With skin, 3½ oz	**195**	8	0
Without skin, 3 oz	**140**	3	0
Stewed: With skin, 4 oz	**210**	8	0
Without skin, 3¼ oz	**140**	3	0
Fried: Batter-dipped, 5 oz	**370**	19	12
Flour coated, w. skin, 3½ oz	**220**	9	7
Drumstick: *Per Drumstick*			
Roasted: With skin, 2 oz	**125**	6	0
Without skin, 1½ oz	**75**	2	0
Fried: Batter-dipped, 2½ oz	**195**	11	7
Flour coated, 1¾ oz	**120**	7	1
Stewed: With skin, 2 oz	**115**	6	0
Without skin, 1½ oz	**80**	3	0
Thigh Portion: Edible Wt. (no bone)			
Raw: With skin, 3.3 oz (4¼ oz with bone)	**200**	14	0
Without skin, 2.4 oz	**80**	3	0
Roasted: With skin, 2¼ oz	**155**	10	0
Without skin, 2 oz	**110**	6	0

Thigh Portion (Cont)	C	F	Cb
Stewed: With skin, 2½ oz	**160**	10	0
Without skin, 2 oz	**105**	5	0
Fried: Batter-dipped, 3 oz	**240**	14	8
Flour coated, 2¼ oz	**165**	9	2
Wing: *Per Wing*			
Raw Weight 3.2 oz (with bone)			
Raw: With skin	**110**	8	0
Without skin	**35**	1	0
Roasted: With skin	**105**	7	0
Without skin	**45**	2	0
Fried: Batter-dipped	**160**	11	5
Flour coated	**105**	7	1
Stewed: With skin, 4 oz	**100**	7	0
Buffalo Wings: *See Fast-Foods Section (Denny's, Domino's, O'Charleys, Pizza Hut)*			
Neck: Simmered, with skin	**95**	7	0
Without skin	**30**	2	0
Skin Only: *Skin from ½ Chicken*			
Raw skin, 2¾ oz	**275**	26	0
Roasted skin, 2 oz	**255**	22	0
Stewed skin, 2½ oz	**260**	24	0
Fried, Flour coated, 2 oz	**280**	24	5
Fried, Batter-dipped, 6¾ oz	**750**	55	45
Roasters			
Average of Light & Dark Meat:			
Roasted: With skin, 4 oz	**250**	15	0
Without skin, 4 oz	**190**	8	0
Light Meat: Without skin, roasted	**175**	5	0
Dark Meat: Without skin, roasted	**206**	10	0
Stewing Chicken			
Stewed: *Per 4 oz Serving*			
Average of Light & Dark Meat:			
With skin	**325**	21	0
Without skin	**270**	14	0
Light Meat: Without skin	**240**	9	0
Dark Meat: Without skin	**295**	17	0
Capon Chicken			
Roasted: With skin, 4 oz	**260**	13	0
½ Chicken, with skin	**1460**	74	0
Chicken Offal & Stuffing			
Giblets, simmered, 1 cup	**230**	7	1.5
Fried, flour-coated, 1 cup	**400**	20	6
Gizzard, simmered, 1 cup	**220**	5	1.5
Heart, simmered, 1 cup	**270**	12	0.5
Liver: Raw, 4 oz	**140**	5	3.5
Simmered, 1 cup	**220**	8	1
Liver Pate Fresh, 1 Tbsp, ½ oz	**60**	8	2
Stuffing: Average, ½ cup	**200**	2	22

Chicken Products

	C	F	Cb
Shop Stop			
Blazing Chicken Wings, 3 oz	200	12	1
Breaded Tenderloins, (3) 4 oz	240	12	15
Boneless Skinless Breasts, (1) 8 oz	210	5	3
Stove Top			
Chicken Stuffing Mix: 1 oz	110	1	20
½ cup prepared	170	9	20
Tyson: Breaded Nuggets (6)	250	18	12
Chicken Chunks: Reg., (6)	280	20	19
Breast, (6)	220	19	11
Southern Fried, (6)	260	19	11
Breast Patties: Regular, each	190	12	11
Chick 'n Quick/Chedd., 74g ea.	220	14	12
Crispy Baked, each	80	0	9
Thick 'n Crispy, each	200	19	10
Southern Fried, each	180	12	8
Wings: Flavored, average (3)	170	10	1
BBQ Style (3)	200	13	2
Stir Fry Kit: Chicken, 2¾ c. froz.	430	4.5	73
M/wave S/wiches: Breast, 119g	320	15	33

Duck, Goose, Quail

Duck: Roasted, with skin, 3 oz	285	24	0
Without skin, 3 oz	170	10	0
½ whole duck, with skin	1300	108	0
Goose: Roast, with skin, 3 oz	260	19	0
Without skin, 3 oz	200	11	0
Pheasant: ½ bird, raw	720	37	0
Quail: 1 whole, raw	210	13	0

Turkey

Fryer-Roasters: *Per 3 oz Serving*			
Roasted: Light Meat, with skin	140	4	0
without skin	120	1	0
Dark Meat: with skin	155	6	0
without skin	140	4	0
¼ of Whole Turkey: (Approx. 3¼ lbs raw wt. w/out neck and giblets; 2 lb 6 oz cooked wt.)			
Roasted: With skin	1400	46	0
Without skin	1030	18	0
Ground Turkey, Raw: (4 oz raw wt. = 3 oz ckd wt.)			
Regular (85% lean), 4 oz	180	10	0
Lean (90% lean), 4 oz	160	8	0
Foster Farms, (94% lean), 4 oz	150	7	0
Jennie-O, (93% lean), 4 oz	160	8	0
Breast, no skin, 4 oz	115	1	0
Patties: Small, 3 oz	110	6.5	0
Large, 5.3 oz	175	10	0

Turkey Parts

	C	F	Cb
Roasted, Edible Weights (no bone)			
Breast (¼): (from 17¼ oz raw wt. w/bone)			
With skin, 12 oz (no bone)	525	11	0
Without skin, 10¾ oz	415	2	0
Back (½): With skin, 4½ oz	265	13	0
Without skin, 3½ oz	165	5	0
Leg (Thigh & Drumstick): (from 1 lb raw wt. w/bone)			
With skin, 8½ oz (no bone)	420	13	0
Without skin, 7¾ oz	355	8	0
Wing: (from 7¼ oz raw wt. w/bone)			
With skin, 3 oz (no bone)	185	9	0
Without skin, 2 oz	100	2	0
Neck: Simmered, 1 neck, (9 oz w. bone)	275	11	0
Giblets, simm., 1 cup, 5 oz	240	7	3

Young Hens (Roasted)

Light Meat: With skin, 3 oz	175	8	0
Without skin, 3 oz	135	3	0
Dark Meat: With skin, 3 oz	200	11	0
Without skin, 3 oz	165	7	0
Young Toms – Similar to Young Hens			

Turkey Products

Banquet: *See Frozen Meals, Page 61*			
Circle L: Boneless Bacon, 3 oz	120	9	1
Jenny-O: Turkey Bacon, 2 slice	40	1.5	0
Louis Rich: Fat Free Breast of Turkey			
Rotiss'd/Smoked/Rstd, 2 oz	60	0	1
Turkey Ham & Chunks, cooked:			
Breast & White Turkey, 2 oz	60	1	2
Turkey Ham/Pastrami, 2 oz	70	3	1
Turkey Salami, 2 oz	100	8	0
Luncheon Slices: *See Deli Meats, Page 54*			
Franks: Medium, 1½ oz	80	6	2
Large, 2 oz	110	8	3
Smoked Sausage/Kielbasa, 1 oz	45	2	1
Turkey Bacon, 1 oz	35	2.5	0
Turkey Nuggets/Sticks, ckd, ea.	75	5	4.5
Turkey Patties, cooked, each	220	13	13
Swanson: *Frozen Meals, Page 67*			
Turkey Store			
Gobble Stix, Honey, each	25	0	1
Lean Burger Patties, 1 patty	180	8	5
Lean Italian Sausage, 1 link	190	8	2

Fish ~ Fresh & Canned

Quick Guide

Fresh Fish

	C	F	Cb
Low Oil (Less than 2.5% fat)			
White/pale colored flesh. Examples: Cod, Flounder, Haddock, Halibut, Mahi Mahi Perch, Pike, Pollock, Snapper, Sole, Whiting.			
Per 4 oz Edible Portion			
Raw, 4 oz (no bones)	90	1	0
Steamed, Broiled, Baked	130	1	0
Fried: Lightly Floured	210	8	3.5
Breaded	260	12	8
In Batter	320	16	27
Medium Oil (2.5-5% fat)			
Pale colored flesh. Examples: Bluefin Tuna, Catfish, Kingfish, Orange Roughy, Salmon (Pink), Swordfish, Rainbow Trout, Yellowtail.	C	F	Cb
Raw, 4 oz (no bones)	140	5	0
Baked, Broiled, 4 oz	175	6	0
Fried, 4 oz	230	11	8
High Oil (Over 5% fat)	C	F	Cb
Darker colored flesh. Examples: Albacore Tuna, Bluefish, Herring, Mackerel, Salmon (Atl./Chinook/Sockeye), Sardines, Trout, Whitefish.			
Raw, 4 oz (no bones)	230	16	0
Baked, Broiled, 4 oz	275	17	0
Fried, 4 oz	340	23	12

Cooking Yields (Fin Fish):
4 oz Raw wt. = 3 ½ oz Cooked wt.
4 oz Cooked wt. = 5 oz Raw wt.

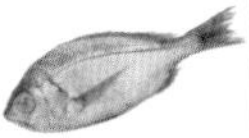

Calorie & Fat Variations

The amount of fat/oil in fish varies with the species, season and locality. Within the same fish, fat/oil content is generally higher towards the head.

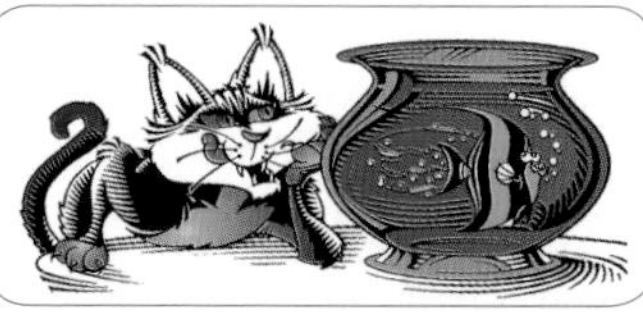

Fish & Shellfish

Edible Weights: (no bones/shell)	C	F	Cb
Abalone: Raw, 4 oz	120	1	7
Ahi Tuna, grilled, 6 oz fillet (no fat)	220	2	0
Anchovy: Paste, 1 Tbsp, ¼ oz	15	1	0.5
Cnd. in oil, drnd., 5 only, ¾ oz	40	2	0
Pickled, 1 oz	50	3	0
Barracuda (Pacific), raw, 4 oz	130	3	0
Bass: Black, raw, 4 oz	105	1	0
Striped: Raw, 1 fillet, 5½ oz	150	4	0
Baked, 3 oz	105	3	0
Blue Fish: Raw, 1 fillet, 5¼ oz	185	6	0
Baked, 3 oz	130	5	0
Butterfish, raw, 4 oz	165	9	0
Cajun & Creole Dishes: *See Page 175*			
Calamari, breaded/fried, 1 serve	360	21	10
Carp, raw, 4 oz	145	6	0
Catfish: Raw Frozen, 4 oz	150	9	0
Fried, breaded, 1 fillet, 3 oz	200	12	7
Baked, 3 oz	120	5	0
Caviar: black/red, 1 Tbsp, 16g	40	3	0.5
Clams: Raw, 3 oz (4 lge/9 small)	65	1	2
Fried, breaded, ¾ cup, 4 oz	450	26	39
Canned *(Snow's)* in clam jce 2 oz	25	0	2
Minced, ¼ cup, 2 oz	25	0	0.5
Clam Juice: (*Snow's*) 1 Tbsp	0	0	0
Cod, Atlantic/Pacific: Raw, 4 oz	95	1	0
Baked/Broiled, 1 fillet, 6¼ oz	135	2	0
Canned, 3 oz	90	1	0
Minced, ¼ cup, 2 oz	25	0	0
Smoked, 3 oz	95	1	0
Crab: Alaska King, raw, 4 oz	95	1	0
1 leg, cooked, 4¾ oz	130	2	0
Blue: Raw, 1 crab			
(⅓ lb whole crab, ¾ oz flesh)	18	0.5	0
Steamed, 3 oz	85	1	0
Canned, ½ cup, 2½ oz	65	0.5	0
Dungeness, 1 crab, 5¾ oz edible			
(from 1½ lb whole crab)	140	2	2
Imitation Crab Legs/Stix, 3oz	80	1	8.5
Crab Cakes (Low-fat), (1), 2 oz	100	4	12
Regular (1), 3 oz	190	12	16
Crayfish, raw, 4 oz (edible)	100	1	0
Croaker, raw, 4 oz	120	3	0
Cuttlefish, raw, 3 oz	70	1	1
Dolphinfish, raw, 4 oz	95	1	0
Eel: Raw, 4 oz	210	13	0
Smoked, 2 oz	190	16	0
Fish & Chips: *Arthur Treachers*	1565	101	132
Denny's	955	54	83
Fish S'wich, w. Tartar Sce, 5½ oz	430	23	41
Fish Sticks, frozen, breaded, ½ oz	35	2	3

Fish & Shellfish (Cont)

Edible Weights: (no bones/shell)	C	F	Cb
Fish Oil, 1 Tbsp, ½ oz	125	14	0
Flounder/Sole: Raw, 4 oz	120	0.5	0
Baked, 3 oz	90	2	0
Frozen Fish & Entrees: *See Page 60*			
Gefilte Fish: *See Kosher/Deli Foods, Page 179*			
Grouper, raw, 4 oz	105	1	0
Haddock: Raw, 4 oz	100	0.5	0
Broiled, 1 fillet, 5¼ oz	170	1	0
Smoked, 2 oz	22	0.5	0
Baked, 3 oz	90	1	0
Halibut: Raw, 4 oz	125	3	0
Baked, 3 oz	105	2	0
Herring: Atlantic, raw, 4 oz	180	10	0
Pickled, 2 pieces, 1 oz	60	4	2
In Sour Cream, 1 oz	75	5	1
Party Snacks, ¼ cup, dr., 2 oz	120	5	0
Rollmops, 1½ oz	110	8	6
Canned: Plain w. liq., 4 oz	235	15	0
in Tomato Sauce, 4 oz	200	12	1
Smoked, kippered, 4 oz	245	14	0
Jellyfish: Raw, 4 oz	30	0	0
Dried, Salted, 1 cup, 2 oz	20	1	0
Kingfish, raw, 4 oz	120	3.5	0
Ling, raw, 4 oz	100	0.5	0
Lobster, Northern: Raw, 4 oz	105	1	0.5
1 Lobster, 6¼ oz (from 1½ lb whole lobster)	135	1.5	0.5
Cooked, 1 cup, 5 oz	140	1	2
Lobster Newberg, ¾ cup	360	20	9
Lobster Thermidor, 1 serving	370	22	15
Lobster Salads, ½ cup	220	13	5
Lomi Salmon, ¼ cup, 4 oz	20	1	3
Lox, Regular/Nova, 2 oz	65	2.5	0
Mackerel: Atlantic, raw, 4 oz	235	16	0
Broiled, 3 oz	190	12	0
Jack, canned, ½ c., 3⅓ oz	150	6	0
King, raw, 4 oz	120	2	0
Pacific/Jack: Raw, 4 oz	180	9	0
Broiled, 3 oz	190	12	0
Spanish, raw, 4 oz	160	7	0
Mahi-Mahi, raw, 4 oz fillet	100	1	1
Milkfish, raw, 4 oz	165	7.5	0
Monkfish: Raw, 4 oz	75	1	0
Baked, 3 oz	80	2	0
Mullet, striped, raw	135	4	0
Mussels: Raw, 4 oz (edible wt.)	100	2	4
1 cup, 5¼ oz (edible wt.)	130	3	5
Cooked, moist heat, 3 oz	150	4	6

	C	F	Cb
Ocean Perch: Raw, 4 oz	90	1.5	0
Baked, 3 oz	100	20	0
Octopus, common, raw, 4 oz	95	1	2
Orange Roughy, raw, 4 oz	145	9	0
Oysters: Common, raw, 3 oz	70	1	3.5
Eastern raw: 6 medium, 3 oz	60	2	3
1 cup, 8¾ oz	170	6	8.5
Fried/breaded, 6 med., 3 oz	170	11	10
Pacific, raw, 1 med., 1¾ oz	40	1	2
Oysters Rockerfeller, 3 oysters	220	13	12
Perch, average, raw, 4 oz	105	2	0
Pike: Northern, raw, 4 oz	100	1	0
Walleye, raw, 4 oz	105	2.5	0
Pollock, raw, 4 oz	100	1	0
Pout, (Ocean), raw, 4 oz	90	1	0
Pompano, Florida, raw, 4 oz	190	10	0
Porgy/Scup, raw, 4 oz	130	4	0
Quahogs ~ See Clams			
Red-Snapper, raw, 4 oz	115	1.5	0
Rockfish, Pacific, raw, 4 oz	110	2	0
Roe, raw, 2 Tbsp, 1 oz	40	2	0.5
Sablefish: Raw, 4 oz	220	17	0
Smoked, 3 oz	220	17	0
Salmon:			
Raw: Chinook, 4 oz	205	7	0
Atlantic; Coho/Silver, 4 oz	160	7	0
Chum; Pink, 4 oz	135	4	0
Red/Sockeye, 4 oz	190	10	0
Baked: Atlantic/Coho, 3 oz	150	7	0
Smoked Salmon: Chinook, 3 oz	100	4	0
Pacific Supreme, 2 oz	100	4	0
Wild Oats, Pastrami Style, 2 oz	130	9	0
Canned Salmon: *Average All Brands*			
Pink: 1 oz	40	2	0
¼ cup, 63g (2.2 oz)	90	5	0
3¾ oz can, whole	155	8.5	0
7½ oz can, whole	300	17	0
Skinless/boneless, ¼ c., 2 oz	70	2	0
Red Sockeye: 1 oz	50	3	0
¼ cup, 63g (2.2 oz)	110	7	0
3¾ oz can, whole	190	12	0
Atlantic, ½ cup, 3½ oz	230	14	0
Chinook/King, ½ cup	210	14	0
Chum, ½ cup, 3½ oz	140	5	0
Coho/Silver, ½ cup	155	5	0
Atlantic Steaks: Small, 8 oz	320	14	0
Medium, 12 oz	480	21	0
Large, 16 oz	640	28	0
Salmon Cake, take-out, 3 oz	240	15	6

Fish ~ Fresh & Canned (Cont)

Fish (Cont)

	C	F	Cb
Sardines (Canned): *Average All Brands*			
In Oil, undrained, 1 oz	**85**	7	0
Drained of oil, 1 oz	**60**	3	0
3¾ oz can, drained, (3¼ oz)	**190**	11	0
1 lrg/2 med. 3/5" small, 0.8 oz	**50**	3	0
In Tom./ Mustard Sce, 1 oz	**45**	3	0
3¾ oz can (8 sardines)	**170**	11	0
Sashimi: *See Japanese Foods, Page 178*			
Scallop: Raw, 6 lge/10 small, 3 oz	**75**	0.5	2
Breaded/fried, 6 pces, 5 oz	**380**	19	38
Seabass, raw, 4 oz	**110**	2	0
Seafood Salad, 1 scoop (#16)	**140**	10	8
Shark: Raw, 4 oz	**150**	6	0
Batter-dipped, fried, 4 oz	**260**	16	7
Baked, 3 oz	**135**	5	0
Shark Fin, dried, 1 oz	**30**	0	0
Shrimp: Raw, in shell, ½ lb	**140**	2	1.5
Raw, shelled, 3 oz (12 lge)	**90**	1.5	0.5
Breaded/fried, 3 oz (11 lge)	**210**	11	10
Canned, 2 oz	**45**	0	0.5
Tiger, cooked, 1 shrimp, ½ oz	**15**	0.5	0
Battered, fried, 1 shrimp	**60**	4	3
Smelt, Rainbow, raw, 4 oz	**115**	3	0
Snapper, raw, 3 oz	**85**	1	0
Cooked, 1 fillet, 6 oz	**215**	3	0
Sole, Lemon, raw, 4 oz	**90**	1	0
Squid: Raw, 4 oz	**105**	1	3.5
Fried, 3 oz	**140**	6	7
Surimi (Imitation Crab), 4 oz	**110**	1	7.5
Sweet & Sour Fish, ½ dish, 10 oz	**580**	29	53
Swordfish raw:			
Small Steak, 4 oz	**135**	4.5	0
Medium Steak, 6 oz	**200**	7	0
Tilapia, Rain Forest Fillets, 4 oz	**95**	1	0
Trout, Rainbow: Raw, 4 oz	**135**	4	0
Broiled, 3 oz	**125**	4	0
Smoked, 2 oz	**110**	6	0
Tuna: *Average All Brands*			
Raw: Albacore, 4 oz	**190**	8	0
Bluefin, 4 oz	**160**	5.5	0
Skipjack, Yellowfin, 4 oz	**120**	1	0
Broiled, 3 oz	**110**	1	0
Canned:			
In Water, drained:			
Chunk/Solid, 2 oz can	**60**	0.5	0
3 oz can	**90**	1	0
6 oz can	**150**	1.5	0
In Oil, drained:			
Chunk Light, 2 oz	**110**	5.5	0
6 oz can, drained	**275**	14	0

Tuna (Cont)	C	F	Cb
Solid White, 2 oz	**90**	2.5	0
6 oz can, drained	**225**	6.5	0
Tuna Salad: Deli Style, ½ c., 4oz	**300**	24	15
Lower fat, 4 oz	**210**	10	11
Whitefish: Raw, 4 oz	**150**	6.5	0
Baked, 3 oz	**140**	6	1
Smoked, 3 oz	**90**	1	0
Whiting: Raw, 4 oz	**100**	1.5	0
Baked, 3 oz	**85**	1	0
Yellowtail: Raw, 3 oz	**125**	4.5	0
Grilled, 3 oz (from 4 oz raw)	**160**	6	0

Other Canned/Packaged Fish

	C	F	Cb
Bumble Bee: *Incl. Mayo & Crackers*			
Tuna Salad Kit	**420**	22	24
Fat-Free Kit	**150**	2	24
Chicken of the Sea			
Tuna Salad Kits: *Per 5 oz*			
Light Tuna: in Mayo/Onion	**365**	23	18
w. Sweet Pickle Relish	**315**	17	19
Libby's: Crab Delights, 2 oz	**30**	0	5
Shrimp/Lobster Delight, 2 oz	**35**	0	4
Starkist			
Pouch: *Per 3 oz*			
Tuna Chunk Light, in water	**90**	1	0
Albacore Tuna, in water	**105**	1.5	0
Lunch-To-Go: Chunk Light Tuna			
w. Mayo/Crackers, 4.5 oz	**210**	9	27
Tuna Creations: Chunk Light Tuna			
w. Mayo/Crackers, 4.5 oz	**210**	9	27
Hickory Smoked (Tuna only), 2 oz	**60**	0	0

Frozen Fish Products

Gorton's: *See Page 62*
Kroger: *See Page 64*
Mrs Paul's: *See Page 65*
SeaPak: *See Page 66*
Van De Kamp's: *See Page 68*
Fast-Foods & Restaurant Chains: *See Page 183*
Captain D's Seafood: *See Fast-Food Section*
Long John Silvers: *See Fast-Food Section*
Shoney's: *See Fast-Food Section*

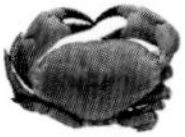

Amy's (Vegetarian)

	C	F	Cb
Per Serving			
Bowls: Brown Rice & Vegs, 10 oz	**240**	8	42
Santa Fe Enchilada, 10 oz	**340**	9	47
Other varieties, average	**300**	12	35
Asian Meals: Thai Stir Fry, 9.5 oz	**270**	11	36
Asian Noodle Stir Fry, 10 oz	**240**	4.5	52
Entrees: Chse Enchilada, 4.75 oz	**210**	12	13
Cheese Lasagna, 10.25 oz	**330**	12	36
Macaroni & Cheese, 9 oz	**410**	16	47
Macaroni & Soy Cheeze, 9 oz	**370**	14	42
Ravioli w. Sauce, 8 oz	**340**	12	43
Whole Meals: Chse Enchilada, 9 oz	**330**	14	38
Black Bean Enchilada, 10 oz	**320**	6	55
Veggie Loaf, 10 oz	**280**	7	47
Pot Pies: Country Vege, 7½ oz	**370**	16	47
Mex. Tamale; Shepherd's Pie, avg.	**160**	4	27
Vegetable (Non Dairy), 7½ oz	**320**	9	50
Burgers: Californian, 2½ oz	**130**	3	19
Other varieties, avg., 2½ oz	**120**	2.5	14
Burritos: Bean & Rice, 6 oz	**280**	8	43
Breakfast Burrito, 6 oz	**210**	6	38
Non Dairy, 6 oz	**270**	6	48
Snacks: Mini Pockets, 5-6 pc, 3 oz	**180**	6	22
Tofu Scramble, Vege Pie, 5 oz	**300**	9	45

Atkins

	C	F	Cb
Entree: Meatloaf, ¼ loaf	**290**	20	2
Beef Stroganoff, ½ tray, 5 oz	**200**	8	9
Chicken Marsala, ½ tray, 5 oz	**160**	4.5	10
Four Cheese Macaroni, 5 oz	**240**	13	10
Italian Entree: *Per Serving (½ Tray, 5 oz)*			
Baked Ziti, ½ tray	**195**	8	10
Chicken Cacciatore, ½ tray	**95**	1	10
Meatballs & Pasta, ½ tray	**160**	6	10
Menu Classics: Beef Teriyaki	**205**	7	9
Chicken Teriyaki	**155**	5	9
Chicken Tetrazzini	**355**	16	9
Pasta Sides, avg., 1 cup	**260**	7	17
Quiche: *Per 3½ oz*			
Bacon & Onion Crustless	**325**	27	2
Other varieties, avg.	**310**	24	2
Souffle: Crab & Cheddar, 3½ oz	**285**	25	2
Broccoli, Cheddar & Bacon, 3½ oz	**195**	15	3
Spinach, Tomato & Feta, 3½ oz	**175**	13	4

Banquet

	C	F	Cb
Pot Pies: Beef, 7 oz	**330**	25	38
Chicken, 7 oz	**195**	23	35
Chicken: Breast Patties (1)	**260**	19	13
Chicken Breast Tenders (5)	**280**	19	14
Chicken Breast Nuggets (5)	**290**	21	15
Fried Chicken Breasts, 1 piece	**230**	17	10
Crispy Chicken, Skinless, 3 oz	**260**	16	9
Buffalo Style Jumbo Wings, 3 oz	**170**	10	0.5
Popcorn Chicken, 11 pieces	**110**	9	18
Crock Pot Classics: *Per Cup*			
Stroganoff Beef & Noodles	**350**	12	38
Chicken & Red Potatoes	**240**	11	21
Chicken & Dumplings	**310**	14	27
Meals: Boneless Pork Rib	**400**	19	39
Beef Patty w. Country Style Veg	**265**	15	22
Corn Dog Meal, 7.5 oz	**485**	19	68
Country Fried Pork	**430**	24	40
Fettuccine Alfredo	**450**	20	53
Fried Rice w. Chicken & Egg Roll	**315**	9	46
Lasagna w. Meat Sauce, 11 oz	**325**	9	46
Mexican Style Enchilada Combo	**370**	11	55
Our Original Fried Chicken	**470**	27	35
Pot Roast	**215**	8	21
Salisbury Steak Meal, 9.5 oz	**400**	25	28
Spaghetti & Meatballs, 10.5 oz	**440**	20	43
Swedish Meatballs, 10.25 oz	**390**	19	33
Turkey Mostly White Meat	**290**	10	34

Birds Eye – Voila!

	C	F	Cb
Per Cup, Cooked (2 Cups Frozen)			
Chicken Voila!: Garlic Chicken	**240**	8	29
Other varieties, average	**240**	9	24
Steak Voila! Beef Sirloin/Potato	**240**	9	26
Turkey Voila! Turkey w. Potato	**200**	6	24

Birds Eye Hearty Spoonfuls Soup Bowls: *See Page 78*

Boca (Vegetarian)

	C	F	Cb
Burger: Cheeseburger, 1 patty	**115**	5	5
All American Flame Grilled (1)	**110**	4	5
Vegan, Original, 1 patty	**85**	1	6
Organic Burgers: Vegan, Orig. (1)	**105**	2	9
Roasted Garlic/Onion, 1 patty	**125**	3	9
Chik'n: Nuggets (4), 3 oz	**180**	6	17
Hot & Spicy Buffalo Wings (4)	**175**	7	14
Patties (1), 2.5 oz	**140**	6	11
Sausages: Bratwurst (1), 2.5 oz	**145**	7	6
Italian; Smoked, 2.5 oz	**130**	6	6
Organic Pizza, ⅓ Pizza	**260**	8	36

Budget Gourmet (Michelina's)

Bistro: *Per Bowl*	C	F	Cb
Grilled Chicken Caesar	**300**	4.5	46
Spicy Beef & Broccoli	**300**	2	49
Shrimp & Vegetables	**320**	8	43
Shrimp Fried Rice; Teriyaki Chicken	**300**	3	56
Lean Gourmet: Cheese Lasagna	**230**	5	36
Garden Bistro Italian Style Bowl	**180**	5	39
Macaroni & Cheese, 10 oz	**305**	5	51
Salisbury Steak w. Pot. & Gravy	**205**	7	23
Santa Fe Style Rice & Beans	**340**	9	56
Shrimp w. Pasta & Veges, 8 oz	**255**	6	37
Spaghetti & Meat Sauce, 9 oz	**275**	5	45
Swedish Meatballs, 9 oz	**290**	7	40

Claim Jumper

Meals: Baby Back Pork Ribs (3)	**215**	14	8
Buffalo Wings (2)	**155**	9	5
Chicken Pot Pie, ½ pie, 8 oz	**565**	39	37
Country Fried Beef Steak (1)	**945**	58	80
Country Fried Chicken, 19 oz	**710**	24	86
Lasagna w. Meat Sauce, 8 oz	**275**	13	22
Meatloaf Dinner	**665**	41	45
Rst Turkey Brst w. Gravy & Dressing	**540**	23	51
Salisbury Steak	**535**	15	39
Spicy Chicken Tenderloins, 3 oz	**180**	7	17
Turkey Pot Pie, ½ pie, 8 oz	**575**	41	35
Sauce: Hot Sauce, ½ Tbsp	**0**	0	0
Original Barbecue, 4 Tbsp	**70**	0.5	17

Croissant Pockets

Egg, Sausage & Cheese	**350**	18	38
Ham & Cheddar	**340**	16	36
Pepperoni Pizza	**370**	19	40
Philly Steak & Cheese	**360**	20	34

El Monterey

Burritos: Bean & Cheese, 5 oz	**295**	9	44
Beef & Bean/Chili, 5 oz	**360**	17	42
Cruncheros: Beef, 5 oz	**185**	9	18
Cream Cheese Jalapenos (3)	**370**	24	32
Nacho Cheese Beef (3)	**325**	16	35
Enchiladas (w. Sauce): Beef, 5 oz	**185**	9	18
Cheese, 5 oz	**220**	13	16
Chicken, 5 oz	**220**	11	19
Quick Classics Chimichanga:			
Beef & Cheese, 3-Count, 5 oz	**360**	18	37
Chicken & Chse, 3-Count, 5 oz	**310**	11	39
Taquitos: Chicken & Cheese (3)	**360**	18	38
Shredded Beef & Cheese (3)	**375**	20	37

Essensia (Albertson's)

Entrees: *Per Serving*	C	F	Cb
Beef Pot Roast, ⅓ pkg	**200**	7	29
Herbed Chicken, ⅓ pkg	**180**	4.5	17
Chicken Potstickers, ⅓ pkg	**230**	3	42
Six Cheese Cannelloni (1)	**190**	6	22
Vegetable Lasagna, 1 cup	**220**	7	29
Jambalaya, 1 cup	**220**	4.5	26
Six Cheese Sacchettini, 1 cup	**220**	11	22
Sides: Cheese Hors D'oeuvres (7)	**460**	32	33
Puffs/Triangles, 1 pce, avg.	**70**	4.5	5
Vegetable Spring Rolls w. Sce (1)	**170**	7	23

GardenBurger (Vegetarian)

Burgers:			
BBQ Chicken (1) & Sauce, 5 oz	**250**	8	30
Diner Deluxe (1, 2½ oz	**115**	5	6
Garden Vegan (1), 2½ oz	**90**	0	12
Savory Portabella Burger (1), 2½ oz	**120**	2.5	18
Meals: Country Fried Chicken, 5 oz	**180**	9	16
Herb Crusted Cutlet (1), 2½ oz	**170**	9	12
Meatless: Meatloaf, slice w. gravy	**130**	3.5	12
Riblets w. BBQ Sauce (1)	**155**	5	11
Sweet & Sour Pork, ½ pouch	**170**	2	30

Gorton's

Crunchy Fish Fillets: *Per Fillet*			
Battered: Lemon Pepper, 1 fillet	**135**	9	9
Crispy, 1 fillet	**135**	10	8
Breaded: Lemon Pepper, 1 fillet	**135**	9	9
Garlic & Herb; Hot & Spicy	**125**	7	10
Crunchy Golden, 1 fillet	**135**	7.5	12
Grilled: It. Herb; Lemon Pepper	**130**	6	2
Cajun Blackened; Lemon Butter	**120**	6	1
Grilled Fillets, avg. all (1)	**100**	3	1
Shrimp Bowl: Alfredo, 1 bowl	**290**	5	49
Fried Rice, 1 bowl	**320**	2	65
Garlic Butter, 1 bowl	**280**	5	46
Primavera, 1 bowl	**270**	6	41
Teriyaki, 1 bowl	**320**	6	57
Fish Portions, 1 portion, 2½ oz	**170**	11	12
Fish Sticks, Breaded, 6, 3 oz	**210**	12	17
Popcorn Shrimp, 20 shrimp, 3 oz	**240**	12	26
Tenders: Extra Crunchy, 3½ pcs	**260**	12	29
Original, 3½ pieces, 4 oz	**260**	15	22

Green Giant

	C	F	Cb
Create A Meal: *Prepared with Meat & Oil (Prepared Wt. ~ Approx 10 oz)*			
Oven Rstd: Garlic Chkn, 1¾ cup	350	9	35
Lemon Pepper Chicken, 1⅔ c.	310	8	30
Parmesan Herb Chicken, 1¾ c.	340	11	29
Pasta Creations: *Per Cup (Prepared)*			
Creamy Cheddar	250	8	36
Garlic	260	10	36
Stir Fry: Beef & Broccoli, 1⅓ cup	290	13	15
Lo Mein, 1¼ cup	320	7	33
Szechuan, 1¼ cup	310	14	20
Teriyaki, 1¼ cup	230	6	18
Complete Skillet: *Per 1¼ Cup (Prep.)*			
Beef Stew	180	3.5	27
Chicken Alfredo/& Cheesy Pasta	270	7	39
Chicken Lo Mein; Garlic Chkn Pasta	250	7	30
Sweet & Sour Chicken	320	1.5	62
Pasta Accents: *Per Cup (Cooked)*			
Creamy Cheddar	250	11	33
Garlic	240	10	31

Healthy Choice

	C	F	Cb
Mixed Grills: *Per Serving*			
Chicken: w. BBQ/Honey Dipping Sce	390	9	46
w. Roasted Garlic Tomato Sce	420	9	47
Steak: w. Teriyaki Dipping Sce	450	10	62
w. Zesty Dipping Sce	340	10	37
Entrees/Familiar Favorites: *Per Meal*			
Cheesy Rice & Chicken	250	5	27
Chicken Enchilada	300	7	46
Lasagna Bake	270	7	38
Macaroni & Cheese	290	7	44
Roast Turkey Breast	220	6	23
Salisbury Steak & Mashed Potatoes	200	6	20
Sesame Chicken	260	6	34

"He misses the way you used to bend over and pat him."

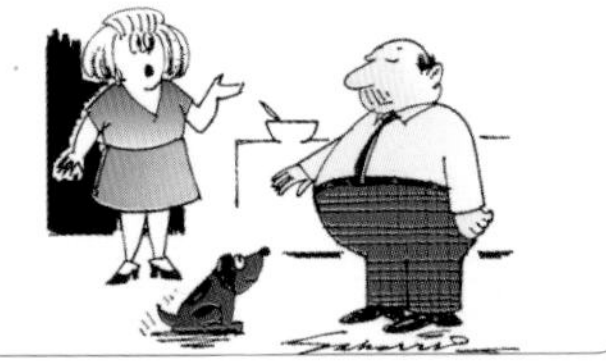

Healthy Choice (Cont)

	C	F	Cb
Dinners: Beef Pot Roast	315	9	39
Beef Tips Portabello	275	8	28
Chicken Enchilada Supreme	350	7	59
Chicken Parmigiana	315	9	40
Chicken Teriyaki w. Rice	265	6	37
Herb Baked Fish	355	8	55
Lemon Pepper Fish	285	5	49
Meatloaf	295	9	36
Roasted Chicken Breast	270	8	32
Salisbury Steak	355	9	45
Sweet & Sour Chicken	340	7	54
Flavor Adventures: Beef Merlot	240	8	25
Chicken Tuscany	240	9	39
Grilled Chicken Caesar	360	8	33
Oriental Style Beef	310	9	33

Hot Pockets

	C	F	Cb
Per Pocket			
Breakfast Pastries: Ham, Egg & Chse	155	7	17
Bacon/Sausage, Egg & Cheese	165	7	20
Fruit Pastries: Apple/Strawberry	250	9	39
Cream Cheese & Strawberry w. Icing	240	10	34
Pizza Mini's, avg., 5 pces, 3 oz	240	11	30
Sandwiches: *Per Serving (4.5 oz)*			
Barbecue Sce with Beef; Italian	355	17	39
Beef Taco; Three Cheese	320	13	37
Chicken Melt with Bacon	350	17	36
Four Cheese Pizza (no meat)	390	20	41
Ham 'N Cheese	305	13	33
Jalapeno Steak & Cheese	320	14	39
Pepperoni Pizza; Philly Steak	365	18	40
Steak Fajita	280	11	34
Turkey & Ham with Cheese	300	13	34

Impromptu Gourmet (Schwan's)

	C	F	Cb
Entrees: Choice Beef Filet Mignon	610	50	0
Choice Beef Rib Eye Steak	355	31	0
French Cut Rack of Pork	135	5	1
Fully Cooked Cajun Turkey	140	7	2
Gourmet Chicken Wellington	420	18	13
New York Strip	650	48	0
Orange Ginger Mahi Mahi	240	6	9
Prime Rib Roast	140	12	0
Prosciutto Chicken Breast	195	7	7
Spiral Sliced Ham	90	7	7
Stuffed Chkn Breast Saltimbocca	325	14	3
T-Bone Steak	240	17	0

Frozen Entrees & Meals (Cont)

José Olé

	C	F	Cb
Taquitos: Chicken in Corn, 3 pces	**190**	9	21
Shredded Beef, 3 pces	**180**	9	20
Mexi-Minis: Beef & Chse Tacos (4)	**200**	11	18
Cheese Burritos, 3 pces	**160**	4.5	25
Chimichangas, 3 pces	**230**	11	25
Taquitos, 4 pces	**190**	9	20
Quesadillas, 3 pces	**220**	8	28
Chicken & Cheese Tacos, 4 pces	**150**	5	19
Burrito: Beef & Cheese (1)	**330**	11	44
Chicken Monterey (1)	**300**	7	46
Chimichanga: Beef, 1 pce	**380**	17	42
Chicken , 1 pce	**340**	12	45

Kid Cuisine

	C	F	Cb
Cheese Pizza	**410**	10	70
Chicken Nuggets	**500**	24	54
Fun Nuggets	**390**	18	46
Macaroni & Cheese	**380**	13	54
Pepperoni Pizza	**610**	22	88
Taco Roll-Up, 7.35 oz	**360**	13	50

Kroger

	C	F	Cb
Meals: Herb Roasted Chicken Rice	**240**	6	30
Sliced Rstd Turkey Brst w. Gravy	**295**	4	48
Swedish Meatballs & Egg Noodles	**325**	8	41
Rice Bowls: Honey Dijon Chicken	**390**	6	70
Spicy Beef & Broccoli	**410**	5	73
Sweet & Sour Chicken	**370**	3	71
Teriyaki Stir Fry Vegetables	**360**	5.5	69

Lean Cuisine

	C	F	Cb
Cafe Classics Bowls: *Per Bowl*			
Chicken Teriyaki	**340**	2.5	63
Grilled Chicken Caesar	**240**	5	30
Three Cheese Stuffed Rigatoni	**280**	6	46
Cafe Classics: Baked Chicken	**235**	4.5	32
Beef Portabello	**220**	7	25
Cheese Lasagna w. Chicken	**285**	8	36
Chicken in Peanut Sauce	**275**	7	32
Honey Roasted Pork	**230**	4	34
Meatloaf & Whipped Potato	**270**	8	30
Roasted Turkey Breast	**275**	2.5	51
Salisbury Steak	**275**	9	24
Sweet & Sour Chicken	**290**	2.5	51
Dinnertime Selections: *Per Meal*			
Beef Steak Tips Dijon	**310**	7	44
Grilled Chicken & Penne Pasta	**340**	6	46
Roasted Chicken	**315**	4.5	48
Salisbury Steak	**320**	9	35

Lean Cuisine (Cont)

	C	F	Cb
Everyday Favorites: Rstd Chicken	**260**	7	33
Angel Hair Pasta	**260**	4	48
Chicken Enchilada	**285**	5	48
Lasagna w. Meat Sauce	**310**	7	43
Macaroni & Cheese	**295**	7	42
Santa Fe Rice & Beans	**300**	5	53
Stuffed Cabbage	**185**	5	26
Swedish Meatballs	**290**	7	36
Teriyaki Stir-Fry	**305**	4.5	49
Skillet Sensations: Chkn Alfredo	**180**	4	23
Chicken Primavera	**180**	2.5	28
Garlic Chicken	**240**	4.5	36
Herb Chicken & Roasted Potatoes	**170**	3	24

Lean Pockets

	C	F	Cb
BBQ Sauce w. Beef	**290**	7	48
Cheeseburger; Chicken Parmigiana	**290**	7	45
Chicken Fajita	**260**	7	38
Ham & Cheddar, 1 pce	**280**	7	40
Meatballs & Mozzarella	**280**	7	44
Pepperoni/Saus. & Pepperoni Pizza	**290**	7	42
Philly Steak & Cheese, 1 pce	**280**	7	42
Steak Fajita	**240**	7	22
Turkey/Broccoli/Cheese	**270**	7	39

Life Choice

	C	F	Cb
Meals: *Per Package*			
Beef Pot Roast	**280**	9	12
Cheesy Chicken Florentine	**310**	13	12
Chicken Parmesan	**300**	10	13
Hearty Meatloaf	**360**	16	16
Herb Roasted Chicken	**390**	19	15
Homestyle Baked Chicken	**220**	8	11
Oven Roasted Turkey	**250**	6	17
Roasted Turkey Breast	**260**	4.5	15
Salisbury Steak	**360**	12	18
Slow Roasted Beef Tips	**260**	8	12
Three Meat Alfredo	**380**	16	12

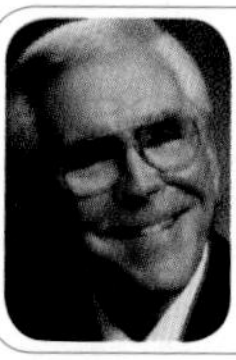

"If it's going to be, it's up to me!"

Rev. Dr. Robert Schuller

Marie Callender's

	C	F	Cb
Meals & Dinners: *Per Serving*			
Beef Stroganoff	**410**	14	39
Beef Tips in Mushroom Sce, 13.6 oz	**405**	19	34
Chicken Cordon Bleu, 1 dinner	**490**	23	38
Chicken Fried Beef Steak	**630**	41	45
Chicken Parmigiana, 1 dinner	**575**	33	40
Country Fried Chick. & Gvy, 1 din.	**660**	34	63
Fish w. Mac & Cheese	**400**	16	36
Grilled Chkn & Mashed Pot., 15 oz	**470**	25	30
Ham Steak w. Macar. & Chse, 1 din.	**410**	13	43
Herb Rstd Chicken & Mashed Pot.	**570**	35	24
Meatloaf & Gravy w. Mashed Pot.	**510**	30	34
Pork Chop, 1 dinner	**620**	36	53
Roast Beef w. Mashed Potato	**370**	19	27
Salisbury Steak & Gravy, 14 oz	**440**	22	34
Sweet & Sour Chicken, 1 dinner	**570**	15	86
Pot Pies: Beef	**510**	32	40
Chicken Au Gratin, 1 cup	**560**	37	41
Turkey, 1 cup	**545**	35	45
One Dish Classics: Cheese Ravioli	**590**	20	80
Cheesy Chicken Breast & Rice	**465**	20	39
Chicken and Rice w. Broccoli	**440**	14	47
Chili Cornbread, 16 oz	**495**	21	49
Country Beef Stew w. Cornbread	**425**	9	69
Fettucini Alfredo, 14 oz	**880**	55	73
Grilled Chicken Breast w. Pasta	**565**	21	64
Macaroni & Cheese, 8 oz	**335**	13	39
Meat Lasagna, 8 oz	**270**	12	25
Swedish Meatballs, 14 oz	**555**	25	56
Tuna & Noodles, 14 oz	**605**	35	46
Turkey Breast Medallions w. Pasta	**630**	32	58

Michael Angelos

	C	F	Cb
Entrees: *Per 1 Cup*			
Chicken Parmesan	**260**	10	25
Eggplant Parmesan	**285**	19	23
Fettuccine Alfredo	**290**	8	40
Manicotti w. Sauce	**225**	12	11
Saus. & Pepper & Onion Lasagna	**225**	7	31
Spaghetti & Meatballs	**235**	9	26
Bowls: Angel Hair & Shrimp	**200**	6	28
Angel Hair Pasta Pomodoro	**200**	5	34
Chicken Milano Pasta	**290**	11	30
Chicken Rosemary Pasta; Sausage	**250**	8	30
Lasagna: Chicken, 8 oz	**295**	7	37
Four Cheese Sausage, 8 oz	**445**	25	24
Meat Lasagna, 8 oz	**290**	10	26
Vegetable, 8 oz	**235**	7	23
Snacks: Four Chse Calzone (1)	**375**	13	50
Meatball Calzone (1), 5 oz	**380**	15	45
Mini Calzone (1), avg. 0.7 oz	**55**	2.5	6

Morningstar Farms

	C	F	Cb
Better'n Burger (1), 3 oz	**80**	0	6
Better'n Eggs, ¼ cup, 2 oz	**20**	0	0
Breakfast Links, 2 links, 1½ oz	**80**	3	3
Breakfast Strips, 2 strips	**60**	4.5	2
Buffalo Wings, 5 nuggets, 3 oz	**200**	9	18
Burger-Style Recipe Crumbles, ⅔ c.	**80**	2.5	4
Chik Patties, 1 pattie	**150**	6	16
Grillers: Original, 1 pattie, 2¼ oz	**140**	6	5
Prime (1) 2½ oz	**170**	9	5
Grnd Meatless Crumbles, ½ c., 2 oz	**60**	0	4
Mushroom & Pepper Burger, (1)	**120**	4	9
Pot Pie: Hearty Chik'n	**350**	14	45
Homestyle Chili Pie	**330**	9	49
Saus. Recipe Crumbles, ⅔ c., 2 oz	**90**	3	5
Scramblers, ¼ cup, 2 oz	**35**	0	2
Spicy Black Bean Burger, 1 pattie	**150**	4.5	16
Supreme Pizza, ½ pizza	**300**	9	38
Tom. & Basil Pizza Burger, ⅔ oz	**130**	6	7
Veggie Dog, 1 link, 2 oz	**80**	0.5	6
Breakfast Sandwiches:			
Muffin/Scramblers/Pattie/Chse	**280**	3	35
Muffin/Scramblers/Pattie	**240**	2.5	32

Mrs Paul's

	C	F	Cb
Bowls: Shrimp Stir-Fry	**330**	1	67
Shrimp Alfredo	**300**	9	39
Sweet & Sour Shrimp	**310**	1	65
Shrimp & Tortellini	**340**	4	58

Ore-Ida

	C	F	Cb
Bagel Bites: *Per 4 Pieces (3 oz)*			
Cheese/Pepperoni, average	**200**	6	27
Spicy Nacho	**240**	10	26

Quorn (Vegetarian)

	C	F	Cb
Turkey Style Roast, 3 oz	**115**	2.5	8
Garlic & Herb Ckn-Style Cutlets (1)	**190**	8	20
Nuggets, 3-4 pieces, 3 oz	**175**	8	18
Patties (1), 2.6 oz	**145**	7	12
Tenders, 1 cup, 3 oz	**100**	2	8
Meat-free Dogs (1), 1.5 oz	**70**	4	3
Meat-free Links (2), 1.6 oz	**70**	3	2
Meat-free Meatballs (4), 2.4 oz	**110**	3	7
Naked Cutlets (1), 2.4 oz	**80**	2.5	5
Riblets (1), 1.5 oz	**60**	2	3

Rosina Presents Celentano

Entree: *Per Serving*	C	F	Cb
Eggplant Parmigiana, 10 oz	485	35	30
Eggplant Rolletts, 10 oz	340	17	38
Manicotti, 10 oz	320	14	35
Ravioli Stuffed Cheese, Mini, 4 oz	215	4	36
Stuffed Shell: 10 oz	305	15	31
Light Broccoli, 10 oz	230	4	39

Safeway Select

Gourmet Club Meals: *Per Serving*			
Beef Meatloaf	180	9	9
Beer Battered Cod Fillets	160	7	13
Chicken Enchiladas	180	12	13
Chicken Nuggets, 6 pces	210	12	10
Chicken Strips	230	13	11
Chicken Stew w. Veges, 1 cup	400	15	38
Grilled Chicken Quesadillas, 2 pces	330	16	28
Low Fat Turkey Lasagna	300	3	48
Macaroni & Cheese	350	18	30
Meat Lasagna	290	11	30
Mexican Style Lasagna	390	22	26
Pot Roast & Vegetables	210	6	15
Salisbury Steak w. Gravy, 1 steak	380	26	9
Scalloped Potatoes, ⅔ cup	250	16	20
Shrimp Fried Rice, 1 cup	300	13	33
Southwestern Quesadilla	280	15	21
Stuffed Baked Potatoes, 1 potato	280	11	35
St Louis Style Pork Spareribs	370	23	17
Tamale Bake	400	23	32
Turkey Pot Pie, 1 cup	520	30	45
Vegetable Lasagna, 1 lasagna	310	17	27
Stir Fry: Chicken Fajita	130	2	14
Shrimp & Vegetable	150	2	24
Shrimp Primavera	270	6	39
Teriyaki Beef	190	3	28
Eating Right: *Per ½ Package*			
Burgundy Beef Stew	250	9	38
Chicken Penne Pasta	280	8	34
Chicken Tamales Verde	220	9	25
Creamy Broccoli Beef	290	7	40
Ginger Chicken	350	6	49
Meatloaf Dinner	230	6	31
Orange Glazed Chicken	350	5	56

SeaPak

Coconut Shrimp, 4 pces	270	17	19
Jumbo Butterfly Shrimp, 4 pces	200	9	20
Popcorn Shrimp, 15 pces, 3 oz	240	11	25
Shrimp Scampi, 8 pces	350	32	4

Seeds of Change

Per Bowl (11 oz)	C	F	Cb
Bowtie Primavera	380	12	51
Creamy Spinach Lasagna	370	16	36
Macaroni & Cheese	420	16	52
Mushroom Wild Pilaf	350	16	40
Penne Marinara	290	7	44
Seven Grain Pilaf	390	14	52
Spicy Peanut Noodles	370	12	53
Teriyaki Stir-Fried Rice	340	8	56

Stouffer's

Entrees: Beef Stroganoff, 9.75 oz	350	15	37
Creamed Chipped Beef	175	13	10
Grilled Teriyaki Chicken	300	3.5	45
Chicken a la King	370	12	45
Cheesy Spaghetti Bake	430	21	39
Lasagna w. Meat Sce, 10½ oz	370	14	35
Macaroni & Beef w. Tomatoes	350	12	41
Macaroni & Cheese, 1 cup, 8 oz	335	16	33
Maxaroni, Macaroni & Cheese	395	17	44
Spaghetti w. Meat Sauce	350	15	56
Stuffed Pepper, 10 oz	240	12	24
Swedish Meatballs w. Pasta	520	25	49
Tuna Noodle Casserole	360	16	36
Turkey Tetrazzini	400	19	36
Family Style Recipes: *Per Serving*			
Grandma's Chkn & Vege Bake	360	15	36
Lasagna w. Meat Sce, 1/12 pkg	265	10	28
Macaroni & Cheese, 1 cup	370	18	37
Italian Style: 3 Cheese Manicotti	335	13	39
Cheese Stuffed Rigatoni, 8.2 oz	475	22	51
Italian Sausage Stuffed Rigatoni	375	16	41
Roasted Chicken Ravioli, 8.2 oz	360	13	42
Homestyle Dinners: *Per Serving*			
Chicken Fettucini, 10.5 oz	350	14	34
Country Fried Beef Steak, 16 oz	675	37	60
Grilled Lime Chicken, 14 oz	485	13	67
Meatloaf, 17 oz	360	32	38
Monterey Chicken, 14.25 oz	575	21	68
Roast Turkey Breast, 16 oz	460	16	55
Salisbury Steak, 16 oz	550	27	49
Homestyle: *Per Serving*			
Breaded Boneless Pork Cutlet	370	20	34
Fish Fillet w. Mac Cheese, 9 oz	410	16	44
Roasted Pork, 9.5 oz	400	18	46
Skillet Sensations: *Per Bowl*			
Homestyle Beef	360	15	37
Teriyaki Chicken, 12.5 oz	340	2.5	40

Swanson

	C	F	Cb
Standard Meal: Salisbury Steak	470	19	33
Boneless White Meat Fr. Chkn	450	18	50
Breaded Fish fillet, 10 oz	405	15	51
Chicken Strips w. Fries	650	30	80
Chicken Teriyaki (Standard)	340	7	49
Classic Fried Chicken, 11½ oz	640	36	41
Grilled Glazed Turkey Medallions	380	11	45
Turkey Breast w. Stuffing & Gravy	420	15	39
White Meat Chicken w. Penne	310	11	31
Hungry Man Dinners: Mexican	690	27	87
Boneless Pork Rib	840	39	99
Boneless White Meat Fried Chkn	640	24	72
Buffalo Chicken Strips	870	28	106
Classic Fried Chicken, 16½ oz	790	40	75
Hearty Breakfast	1170	61	125
Meatloaf Angus Beef	560	25	52
Mexican Style Fiesta	710	29	87
Salisbury Steak	470	19	33
Turkey Breast	630	20	82
Hungry Man XXL: Backyard BBQ	1160	48	110
Roasted Carved Turkey Dinner	1450	58	174
Southern Fried Boneless Chicken	1160	48	110
Sports Grill: *Per Serving*			
Beer Battered Chkn & Fries	665	26	63
Chicken Quesadilla & Potato Skins	765	35	72
Pulled Pork w. BBQ Sauce in Flatbrd & Chse Fries, 16 oz	810	44	96
Steak House: *Per Serving (20 oz)*			
Grilled: BBQ Chicken	875	28	116
Beef Steak Strips	580	16	75
Smothered Chicken	595	24	56
Pot Pies: Flaky Crust Chicken/Turkey	380	21	38
Meals: *Per Serving*			
Bean & Rice Burrito, 6 oz	350	12	51
Bean, Rice & Cheese Burrito, 6 oz	360	14	49
Brown & Serve Links (2)	115	8	1
Burger, Meat Free: Garlic, 2.5 oz	85	1	7
Gourmet, 2.5 oz	105	2	9
Vegan, 2.5 oz	85	0	8
Cheese Enchilada (2)	405	21	37
Chicken Enchilada (2)	355	15	38
Chicken Taquitos (5)	270	5	40
Macaroni & Cheese: Alfredo, 2 oz	210	3	39
Traditional Cheddar, 2 oz	200	2	39
White Cheddar, 2 oz	210	3.5	38

TGI Friday's

	C	F	Cb
Buffalo Wings (3)	175	13	2
Honey BBQ Wings (3)	165	10	7
Mozzarella Sticks & Sce, 1 Serve	120	6	15
Quesadilla Rolls: Chicken (2)	245	11	26
Steak (2)	215	11	21
Sides: Spinach Dip, , 2 Tbsp (1 oz)	50	3.5	2

Tyson

	C	F	Cb
Barbeque Style Chicken Wings (3)	200	13	7
Breaded Chkn Breast Tenders, 5 pces	220	11	15
Breaded Chicken Nuggets, 5 pces	240	14	16
Breaded Pork Chops, 1 chop	180	7	10
Buffalo Style Chicken Strips, 2 pces	230	10	21
Centre Filets	190	5	0
Chicken Breast Patties, 1 patty	180	11	12
Flat Iron Grillers, 1 steak	160	2	0
Hot'n Spicy Chicken Wings, 3 pces	220	15	1
Popcorn Chicken Bites, 6 pces	210	9	17
Stuffed Pork Chops, 1 chop	240	10	11
Southern Style Chkn Nuggets, 6 pces	270	21	11

Uncle Ben's

	C	F	Cb
Breakfast Bowls: *Per Bowl*			
French Toast & Sausage	420	22	45
Seven Grain Cereal & Fruit	350	2	76
Chili Bowl w. Beans & Rice	360	7	48
Mexican Style Bowls: Beef Fajita	310	4.5	45
Chicken varieties, avg.	360	6	55
Mini Bowls: Sizzlin Saus. Pizzeria	320	12	36
Noodle Bowls: Honey Ging. Chkn	420	5	69
Spicy Peanut Chicken	415	8.5	58
Thai Style Chicken	400	8	60
Pasta Bowls: 4-Cheese Lasagna	340	7	41
Chicken Fettuccini	360	7	47
Lasagna varieties, avg., 12 oz	330	7	42
Parmesan Shrimp Penne, 12 oz	390	7	58
Savory Beef Portabello	300	6	43
Three Cheese Ravioli, 12 oz	365	7	55
Rice Bowls: Roasted Chicken Vege	360	4.5	52
Broccoli, Cheese & Ham	420	12	56
Chicken Fried Rice	420	7	65
Chicken & Vegetable	350	4.5	56
Spicy Beef & Broccoli	375	4.5	62
Sweet & Sour Chicken	355	3	61
Teriyaki Chicken	375	3.5	66
Turkey, Stir Fry Vegetable	355	3	74

Van De Kamp's

	C	F	Cb
Butterfly Shrimp, 7 pces, 4 oz	**300**	15	30
Crispy Battered Halibut, 3 fillets	**240**	12	22
Crispy Fish Tenders, 4 pces, 4 oz	**260**	14	23
Crispy Fish Portions, 1 pce	**150**	8	14
Popcorn Shrimp, 20 pces, 4 oz	**270**	12	30
Fish Sticks, Breaded, 6 stix, 4 oz	**290**	17	23
Battered Fillets, 2.6 oz fillet	**180**	11	12
Crispy Fish Fillets, 1 pce, 2.6 oz	**160**	8	15
Crisp & Healthy, Breaded (1), 1.8 oz	**85**	1.5	12

Weight Watchers

	C	F	Cb
Smart Ones: *Per Meal*			
3 Cheese Ziti Marinara	**290**	7	47
Fettucini Alfredo w. Broc., 9.25 oz	**270**	6	39
Fiesta Chicken, 8.5 oz	**210**	2	35
Grilled Salisbury Steak	**260**	6	25
Lasagna Bolognese	**270**	7	38
Lasagna Florentine, 10.5 oz	**290**	8	36
Lemon Herb Chicken Piccata	**250**	5	36
Mac. & Chse; Lasagna Bolognese	**240**	2.5	45
Radiatore Romano	**280**	8	40
Ravioli Florentine, 8.5 oz	**220**	2	43
Santa Fe Style Rice & Beans, 10 oz	**300**	8	49
Southwestern Style Chkn Bowl	**230**	2.5	35
Spaghetti Bolognese	**280**	5	43
Spaghetti Marinara, 9 oz	**280**	7	46
Spicy Szechuan Veg. & Chicken	**230**	5	34
Swedish Meatballs, 9 oz	**280**	7	34
Three Cheese Macaroni	**290**	7	45
Tuna Noodle Gratin	**240**	2.5	43
Smartwiches: Ham & Cheddar	**260**	7	36
Average other varieties	**265**	7	38
Smart Ones Bistro Selections:			
Basil Chicken	**270**	6	34
Chicken Parmesan	**300**	5	32
Chicken Tenderloins w. BBQ Sce	**300**	8	30
Fire-Grilled Chkn & Vegetables	**280**	5	40
Golden Baked Garlic Chicken	**280**	6	40
Meat Loaf w. Gravy & Potatoes	**260**	8	22
Peppercorn Beef Fillet	**230**	8	24
Roast Beef w. Gravy	**220**	7	19
Roast Chicken w. Sour Crm & Chives	**190**	3.5	23
Slow Roasted Turkey Breast	**220**	7	20
Thai Style Chkn & Rice Noodles	**290**	4	39

Weight Watchers (Cont)

	C	F	Cb
Truth About Carbs: *Per Package (9 oz)*			
Chicken Marsala w. Broccoli	**170**	5	12
Creamy Chicken Tuscan	**205**	9	9
Creamy Parmesan Chicken	**230**	8	12
Grilled Chicken in Garlic Sce	**210**	9	9
Sirloin Beef & Asian Style Vege	**225**	9	11
Turkey Medallions w. Gravy	**195**	8	10

White Castle

	C	F	Cb
Cheese Burger, Microwaveable, 1 pkg, 3.7 oz	**310**	17	23
Hamburgers, 1 pkg	**270**	14	23

Worthington (Vegetarian)

	C	F	Cb
Bolono, 3 slices, 2 oz	**85**	3	3
Chic-ketts, 2 3/8 slice, 1.9 oz	**125**	7	2
Chicken Diced, ¼ cup, 1.9 oz	**55**	0	3
Chicken Roll, 3/8 slice, 1.9 oz	**85**	4.5	2
Chicken Slices, 3 slices, 2 oz	**85**	4.5	2
ChikSticks, 1 pce, 1.6 oz	**110**	6	4
Corned Beef Roll, 3/8 slice, 1.9 oz	**140**	9	5
Corned Beef Slices, 3 slices, 2 oz	**140**	9	5
Crispy Chik Patties (1), 2.5 oz pattie	**155**	6	16
Fillets, 2 pieces, 2.9 oz	**175**	9	8
FriPats, 1 pattie, 2.25 oz	**135**	6	5
Golden Croquettes, 4 pieces, 2.9 oz	**215**	11	14
Leanies, 1 link, 1.4 oz	**105**	7	2
Prosage: Links, 2 links, 1.6 oz	**75**	3	3
Patties, 1.3 oz Pattie	**80**	3	3
Vegetable Roll, 5/8 slice	**140**	10	2
Salami, 3 slices, 2 oz	**125**	7	3
Smkd Turkey Roll, 3/8 slice, 1.9 oz	**135**	9	4
Smkd Turkey Slices, 3 slices	**140**	9	5
Stakelets, 2.5 oz piece	**145**	7	7
Wham Vege Roll, 3/8 slice	**105**	6	3
Wham Vege Slices, 2 slices	**115**	7	3

Zatarain's

	C	F	Cb
Blackened Chicken Alfredo, 10.5 oz	**535**	30	44
Jambalaya seasoned w. Chicken	**360**	8	53
w. Sausage	**390**	12	58
Red Beans & Rice w. Sausage	**565**	19	76

Frozen Pizzas

	C	F	Cb
Amy's: *Per ⅓ Pizza*			
Cheese; Spinach; Pesto	300	12	38
Roasted Vegetable, 4 oz	270	8	43
Soy Cheese; Veggie Combo, avg.	280	10	37
Mushroom & Olive	250	9	33
California Pizza Kitchen			
Barbeque Chicken, ⅓ pizza	100	3	13
Five Chse & Fresh Tom., ⅓ pizza	105	5	9.5
Garlic Chicken Pizza, ⅓ pizza	95	4	10
Jamaican Jerk Chicken, ⅓ pizza	270	9	33
Portobello Mixed Mushr., ½ pizza	180	6	23
Sausage, Pepperoni & Mushr., ⅓	100	4.5	10
Thai Chicken Pizza, ½ pizza	95	3.5	11
Celeste			
Pizza For One: Cheese, 1 pizza	390	19	42
Deluxe	440	23	42
Original Four Cheese	430	21	40
Pepperoni	420	23	39
Sausage & Pepperoni; Suprema	500	28	44
Zesty Chicken Supreme	360	16	40
Di Giorno			
Rising Crust (Large): *Per ⅙ Pizza*			
Four Cheese	320	11	40
Pepperoni/& Sausage; 3 Meat	360	16	40
Spicy Chicken Supreme	320	10	40
Spinach, Mushroom & Garlic; Vege	300	9	41
Supreme	370	15	41
Rising Crust (Small): *Per ⅓ Pizza*			
Four Cheese	270	9	34
Pepperoni	310	14	35
Sausage & Pepperoni; 3 Meat	320	14	35
Spicy Chicken Supreme	280	9	35
Spinach, Mushr. & Garlic; Vege	260	8	36
Supreme	330	14	35
Deep Dish: Three Meat, ⅛ pizza	300	16	25
Supreme, ⅛ pizza	310	17	25
Pepperoni, ⅙ pizza	390	22	32
Cheese Stuffed Crust:			
Supreme, ⅛ pizza	300	14	30
Pepperoni, ⅙ pizza	390	20	35
Half & Half: *Per ⅙ Large Pizza*			
Supreme/Pepperoni: Supreme	360	15	40
Pepperoni	370	16	41
Supreme/Cheese: Supreme	390	18	41
Cheese	320	11	41
Pepperoni/Cheese: Pepperoni	390	18	41
Cheese	310	11	40
Thin Crispy Crust: *Per ⅕ Large Pizza*			
Four Meat	320	13	37
Pepperoni	310	12	34
Supreme; Four Cheese, avg.	300	12	35

	C	F	Cb
Freschetta			
Bake & Rise (Large): 4 Cheese, ⅕	390	16	46
4 Meat, ⅙ pizza	350	15	40
Pepperoni, ⅙ pizza	360	17	38
Special Delux, ⅙ pizza	370	16	40
Supreme, ⅙ pizza	370	17	39
Vegetable Primavera, ⅙ pizza	310	11	40
Brick Oven 8": BBQ Chicken, ⅓ pizza	290	12	30
Ham & Mushroom, ½ pizza	325	11	39
Potato, Bacon & Cheese, ½ pizza	395	17	43
Thai Chicken, ⅓ pizza	300	14	27
Italian Style Pepperoni, ¼ pizza	420	22	37
Sauce Stuffed Crust: 4 Chse, ⅕ pizza	355	12	43
Sausage & Pepperoni, ⅕ pizza	370	15	44
Supreme, ⅕ pizza	360	15	42
Grilled Vege, ⅕ pizza	310	9	44
Small Pizzas: Pepperoni, ½ pizza	440	20	47
Rstd Garlic Chicken, ½ pizza	370	12	49
Mozzarella & Basil, ½ pizza	370	15	46
Southwest Chkn Supreme, ½ pizza	350	12	47
Healthy Choice: French Bread Pizza			
Solos: Cheese; Pepperoni, 6 oz	355	5	57
Sausage	345	5	55
Supreme, 6.35 oz	355	5	58
Vegetable, 6 oz	315	5	58
Jeno's: Crispy & Tasty			
Combination, 1 pizza	500	28	50
Cheese, 1 pizza	460	21	51
Pepperoni; Supreme, 1 pizza	510	27	50
Three Meat, 1 pizza	490	25	49
Heaven's Bistro: *Per ⅓ Pizza*			
Chicken w. BBQ Sauce	270	2	48
Chicken Sausage Pizza	250	3	42
Grilled Vegetable	230	1	42
Pepperoni Pizza	250	2	42
Three Cheese Pizza	240	2	42
Jewel (Albertson's):			
Cheese, ⅓ pizza	310	11	40
Pepperoni, ¼ pizza	290	13	32
Supreme, ¼ pizza	320	15	32
Lean Cuisine			
French Bread Pizza: Cheese, 6 oz	325	7	47
Deluxe, 6 oz	320	9	44
Pepperoni, 6 oz	305	7	44

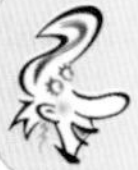

"...and could you please cut the pizza into only 6 pieces - I couldn't possibly eat 8!"

	C	F	Cb
Ralph's			
Large (Self-Rising Crust):			
Four Cheese, ⅙ pizza	330	10	48
Pepperoni, ⅙	390	15	49
Supreme, ⅙	390	15	49
Small: Cheese, 1 pizza	440	11	62
Combination, 1 pizza	520	20	61
Pepperoni, 1 pizza	510	19	62
Red Baron			
Classic (Large): 4 Cheese, ¼ pizza	420	23	36
Pepperoni, ¼ pizza	440	26	36
Sausage & Pepperoni, ⅕ pizza	360	21	29
Supreme, Special Deluxe, ⅕ pizza	350	20	30
Deep Dish Pan Style:			
4 Cheese, ⅓ pizza	370	17	39
Pepperoni; Meat Trio, avg., ⅓ pizza	400	21	39
Supreme, ⅓ pizza	410	21	40
Deep Dish Singles: 4 Cheese, 1	440	23	41
Pepperoni, 1 pizza	460	25	41
Cheese; Meat Trio, avg., 1 pizza	420	21	42
Special Deluxe, 1 pizza	430	24	40
Supreme, 1 pizza	470	27	40
French Bread Pizzas: Supreme (1)	370	15	43
5 Cheese & Garlic (1)	420	23	39
Pepperoni	360	15	42
Pizzeria Style, average, ⅓ pizza	380	16	44
Reggio's			
Family Size: Cheese, ⅙ pizza	320	12	38
Sausage , ⅙ pizza	330	12	38
Dinner Size: Cheese, ¼ pizza	330	12	41
Pepperoni & Sausage, ¼ pizza	400	18	41
Sausage, ¼ pizza	380	16	41
Stop & Shop			
Single Serving: Cheese, 1	390	19	42
9 Slices: Cheese, 2 slices	350	10	49
Stouffer's French Bread Pizzas			
Cheese, 1 piece (½ pkg)	370	16	43
Deluxe, 1 piece	420	19	50
Extra Cheese, 1 piece	400	16	49
Pepperoni, 1 piece	410	20	47

	C	F	Cb
Tombstone			
Original Pizza, 12 inch: *Per Serving*			
BBQ Chicken, ¼ pizza	320	12	38
Extra Cheese, ¼ pizza	350	15	35
4-Meat, ⅕ pizza	310	15	30
Pepperoni, ¼ pizza	380	19	37
Sausage & Pepperoni, ⅕ pizza	320	16	29
Supreme, ¼ pizza	300	12	38
Half & Half Pepperoni & Cheese:			
Pepperoni, ¼ pizza	420	22	37
Cheese, ¼ pizza	340	15	37
Deep Dish: *Per ½ Package*			
Cheese; Pepperoni; Supreme, avg.	500	25	51
Tony's			
Original: Cheese, ⅓ pizza	390	22	33
Pepperoni, ⅓ pizza	410	22	37
Sausage & Pepperoni, ⅓ pizza	420	23	38
Supreme, ⅓ pizza	420	22	39
Thin Crust: Cheese, ⅓ pizza	290	12	31
Sausage &/Pepperoni, ⅓ pizza	350	18	33
Supreme, ⅓ pizza	340	17	33
Totino's			
Crisp Crust Party Pizza: *Per ½ Pizza*			
Cheese	320	14	34
Pepperoni; Supreme	380	21	35
Verdi (Safeway Select)			
Self-Rising Crust (Large): *Per Serving*			
Chicken Parmesano, ⅙ pizza	310	11	39
Ham & Fire-Roasted Pineapple, ⅙	310	10	40
Meat Magnifico, ⅙ pizza	370	15	41
Self-Rising Crust (Small): *Per Serving*			
Primo Pepperoni, ⅓ pizza	300	13	32
Weight Watchers (Smart Ones): *Per Pizza*			
Deluxe, 6.6 oz	380	9	40
Four Cheese, 6.5 oz	400	7	65
Pepperoni, 7 oz	400	9	58
Veggie Ultimate, 7.7 oz	405	5	39

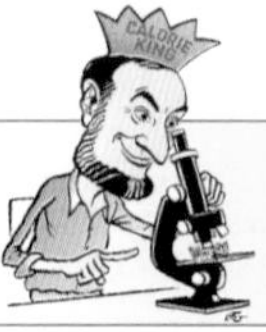

For full nutritional data and product updates check the food database of the author's website www.CalorieKing.com

Canned & Packaged Meals

	C	F	Cb
Annies Homegrown: *Per Cup*			
Arthur Mac & Cheese	370	14	50
Cheeseburger Macaroni	350	13	27
Beef Stroganoff	320	13	24
Shells & Cheddar	290	5	49
B & M: *Per ½ Cup (4½ oz)*			
Baked Beans: Original	170	2	30
Barbeque	210	1	42
Brown Raisin Bread, ½" slice, 2 oz	130	0.5	29
Banquet			
Homestyle Bakes: *Per Serving (Prepared)*			
BBQ Baked Beans & Chkn, 7.2 oz	350	7	58
Beef & Sour Cream Sauce, 7 oz	380	11	54
Chicken & Dumplings, 7.8 oz	250	9	32
Creamy Chkn & Biscuits, 7.4 oz	340	16	40
Tuna Mac & Cheese, 7.7 oz	420	20	44
Meal Toppers, Chicken flavor, ½ cup	50	1	8
Betty Crocker			
Potato Bakes: *Per Serving (Prepared As Directed)*			
Cheesy Scalloped; Au Gratin	150	6	21
Other varieties, average	125	4	22
Complete Meals: *Per Serving (⅕ Box)*			
Chicken & Buttermilk Biscuits	320	13	41
Chicken Fettuccini Alfredo	310	11	38
Ham & Au Gratin Potatoes	300	13	37
Homestyle Chkn & Dumplings	250	9	33
Lasagna Bake	240	8	35
Oven Favorites: *Per Serving (Prepared As Directed)*			
Chicken Helper: Pot. Au Gratin	270	7	25
Cheddar & Mozz; Crmy Chicken	320	12	30
Homestyle Chicken	290	10	21
Hamburger Helper: *Per Serving (Prep. As Directed)*			
Cheesy Baked Potato	320	15	28
Four Cheese Lasagna	330	15	27
Cheeseburger Macaroni	350	16	31
Cheesy Enchilada	370	15	27
Other varieties, average	300	13	27
Tuna Helper: *Per Serving (Prep. As Directed)*			
Creamy Parmesan	260	9	32
Other varieties, average	300	13	33
Pork Helper: *Per Serving (Prep. As Directed)*			
Pork Chops & Stuffing	320	2	23
Pork Fried Rice	340	0.5	24
Chicken Helper: *Per Serving (Prep. As Directed)*			
Cheesy Chicken Enchilada, 1 cup	350	9	40
Chicken Fried Rice, 1 cup	260	8	22
Homestyle Chicken & Dumpling	290	10	27
Chicken & Potatoes Au Gratin	270	7	25
Fettuccini Alfredo	300	8	27

Betty Crocker (Cont)	C	F	Cb
Slow Cooker Helper: *Per Cup (Prepared)*			
Beef Stew, 1 cup	200	5	24
Pot Roast	290	12	27
Chicken & Dumpling	240	6	26
Suddenly Salad: *Prepared*			
Caesar, ½ cup dry	170	1	34
Classic, ⅔ cup	240	7	37
Ranch & Bacon, ¾ cup	330	20	31
Rstd Garlic & Parmesan, ¾ cup	260	11	33
Bowl Appetit: *Per Bowl*			
Pasta Alfredo	360	12	53
Three Cheese Rotini	360	10	56
Cheddar Broccoli Rice	390	7	51
Bush's Best: *Per ½ Cup*			
Chili Beans	120	1	20
Dark Red Kidney Beans, ½ cup	130	1	21
Frijoles Negras, ½ cup	100	0.5	20
Frijoles Pintos, ½ cup	110	0	19
Garbanzo Beans/Chick Peas, ½ c.	130	2	22
Refried Beans: Traditional	150	3	24
Fat Free	130	0	24
Baked Beans: Vegetarian	130	0	24
Other flavors, average	160	1	30
Campbell's: *Per ½ Cup (4½ oz)*			
Chunky Chili: Roadhouse; Firehouse	110	4	13
Tantalizin Turkey	95	1	14
Pork & Beans in Tomato Sauce	140	1	27
Spaghetti O's w. Meat Sauce	85	1	16
Spaghetti O's Meatballs	120	4	16
Sliced Franks	115	5	14
Supper Bakes: *Per ⅙ Box (Prepared As Directed)*			
Cheesy Chicken	320	10	28
Savory Pork Chops	380	18	31
Southwestern Style Chicken	290	7	32
Other varieties, average	340	7	43
Carb Monitor			
Mashed Potatoes: Rstd Garlic, ½ c.	150	7	22
Other varieties, avg., ½ cup	160	7	20
CarbSense: *Per Cup (Prepared As Directed)*			
Aramana Pasta: Mild Mexican	260	16	12
Cheddar Cheeseburger	260	17	11
Creamy Chicken Alfredo	260	16	12
Cedarlane (Vegetarian)			
Burrito, Beans, Rice, Chse, (1) 6 oz	260	1	48
Eggplant Parmesan, ½ pkg, 5 oz	165	8	16
Carb Buster: 4 Cheese Quiche, 6 oz	500	38	5
Chili Relleno Pie, 9.5 oz	525	40	9
Spinach Enchilada, 9 oz	490	37	11
Enchilada: Garden Vege, (1) 4.8 oz	140	3	20
Three-Layer Pie, ½ pkg, 5.5 oz	225	7	27
Lasagne: Cheese, ½ ctn, 5 oz	190	6	22
Garden Vege, ½ ctn, 5 oz	180	3	26

Canned & Packaged Meals (Cont)

Chef Boyardee	C	F	Cb
Beefaroni, all types, 1 cup	260	10	33
Deep Dish Meals: *Per ⅙ Package*			
Cheese Lover's Lasagna	290	14	38
5 Chse Ravioli; Cheesy Burger Mac	270	12	39
Pepperoni & Sausage Rotini	250	9	41
Mini Bites (14.75 oz Can): *Per Cup*			
Mini Beef Ravioli w. Meatballs	300	13	36
Mini Pasta Shells w. Meatballs	270	12	32
Mini Spaghetti w. Meatballs	280	13	31
Jumbo (15 oz Can): *Per Cup*			
99% Fat Free: Beef Ravioli	190	1.5	37
Cheese Ravioli	240	2.5	45
Lasagna	270	10	36
Mini Ravioli	240	7	35
Spaghetti w. Jumbo Meatballs	280	13	30
Overstuffed Ital. Sausage Ravioli	280	4	50
Twistaroni: Cheesy Nacho, 1 cup	250	6	40
Chili Cheese Dog, 1 cup	220	7	30
Tomato & Beef, 1 cup	280	13	31
Dennison's Chili *(15 oz Can): Per Cup*			
Chili Con Carne With Beans:			
Original; Hot, 1 cup	350	15	33
Chunky	310	11	32
99% Fat Free: Beef Chili w. Beans	220	2	27
Turkey Chili w. Beans	210	3	29
Dinty Moore *(Hormel Foods)*			
1½ lb Can: Beef Stew, 1 cup	180	8	17
7½ oz Can: Beef Stew, 1 cup	180	8	17
American Classics: *Per Microwave Bowl (10 oz)*			
Beef Stew	250	11	22
Chicken w. Mashed Potatoes	230	5	27
Noodles & Chicken	250	8	28
Microwave Cup: Beef Stew, 1 cup	160	7	16
Corned Beef Hash, 1 cup	350	22	19
Chicken & Dumplings	190	6	24
Other varieties, average	240	13	19
Dr. McDougall's: *Per Cup*			
Pinto Beans & Rice, Sthwestern	180	1	36
Ramen Noodles	150	0.5	29
Rice & Pasta Pilaf	190	1	41
Eden Soy (Vegetarian): *Per ½ Cup (4½ oz)*			
Baked Beans w. Sorghum, Mustard	140	0	27
Black Eyed Peas	95	1	16
Black Soybeans	130	6	8
Refried Black/Pinto/Kid. Beans, avg.	130	1.5	18
Other varieties, average	125	0	21

Fantastic: *Per Packet*	C	F	Cb
3-Bean Chili, 1 cup	190	4	28
Spanish Paella, 1 cup	290	5	55
Tuscan Mushroom Risotto, 1 cup	250	1.5	50
Cup Meals: Cajun w. Red Beans	185	1.5	35
Bombay Curry w. Lentils	200	1.5	39
Broccoli & Cheddar	115	2	20
Spicy Jamaican w. Beans	195	1	39
Tex Mex w. Pinto	185	3	34
Rice Noodles: Pad Thai, 7.8 oz	405	11	59
Ginger Shiitake, 7.8 oz	355	10	58
Carb 'Tastic: Penne Alfredo	335	15	25
Vegetarian Chili Mac	320	18	19
Vegetarian Teriyaki	290	10	29
Other varieties, avg.	295	14	22
Farmhouse			
Creamy Garlic; Herb Butter, ¾ cup	450	22	53
Four Cheese Pasta, ¾ cup	420	20	48
Long Grain & Wild Rice, 1 cup	200	1.5	43
White Cheddar Pasta, ¾ cup	370	13	52
Other varieties, avg., ¾ cup	290	11	41
Health Valley (Vegetarian)			
Fat-Free Beans & Chili:			
Chili in a Cup, all types, ⅓ cup	120	1	21
Vegetarian/Chili, 1 cup	160	1	28
Turkey w. Chili Beans, 1 cup	220	3	34
Other varieties, ½ cup	80	0	15
Meal Cups, average all varieties	140	1	27
Heinz Vegetarian Beans, ½ cup	140	0.5	27

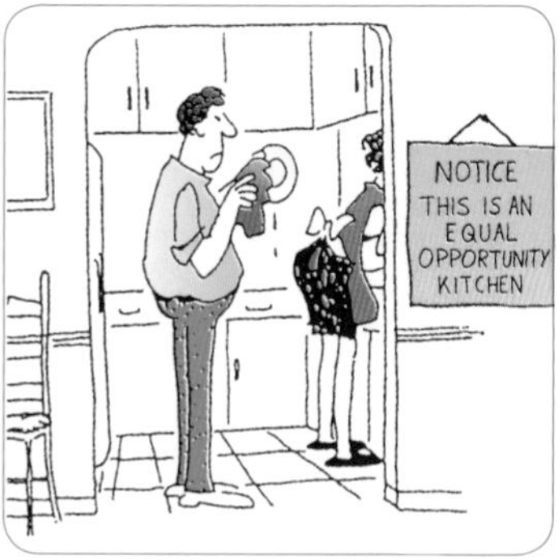
NOTICE
THIS IS AN
EQUAL
OPPORTUNITY
KITCHEN

Hormel: *Per Cup*	C	F	Cb
Kid's Kitchen: Beans & Wieners	**350**	20	28
Cheesy Mac'N Cheese	**260**	11	30
Mini Beef Ravioli	**240**	7	34
Noodle Rings & Chicken	**140**	4	18
Chili (15 oz Can): *Per Cup*			
With Beans: Homestyle Chili	**330**	20	28
Reg./Hot/Chunky/Less sodium	**270**	7	34
Turkey (99% Fat Free)	**200**	3	26
Vegetarian (99% Fat Free)	**200**	1	38
Without Beans: Hot/Chili, 1 cup	**210**	9	17
Turkey No Beans	**190**	3	17
Tamales (15 oz Can), 2 Tamales	**140**	7	15
Hungry Jack Potatoes			
Instant Potato Flakes, ⅓ cup	**80**	0	18
Hunt's			
Chilli Beans, ½ cup	**90**	1	17
Manwich Sloppy Joe, ¼ cup	**30**	0	6
Ken & Robert's (Vegetarian)			
Veggie Burger	**130**	1	26
Veggie Pockets, average, 4.5 oz	**250**	8	39
Keto: Ketatoes Mix, all types, ¼ cup dry (makes ½ cup)	**95**	2	11
Knorr			
Hash Browns w. Cheese Blend	**120**	3	22
Scalloped Potatoes, ½ cup, dry	**110**	2	18
Skillet Potatoes, ⅓ cup, dry	**100**	0.5	20
Sliced Potatoes in Crm Sce, ⅓ c., dry	**100**	0.5	20
w. Roasted Garlic, ⅔ cup, dry	**120**	1	23
Rice: *Per Cup (Prepared As Directed)*			
Broccoli Au Gratin Risotto	**265**	2.5	54
Onion Herb Risotto	**300**	1.5	66
Risotto Milanese	**260**	1	59
Risotto Mushroom	**280**	1	62
Vegetable Risotto Primavera	**275**	1	61
Pilaf Rice: Chicken, ⅓ cup, 2.1 oz	**210**	1	45
Lemon Herb w. Jasmine, ⅓ cup	**260**	2	55
Original, ⅓ cup, 2.1 oz	**210**	0.5	46
Pasta: *Per ½ Cup*			
Bow Tie w. Chicken Vege Sauce	**110**	1.5	20
Fettuccine w. Alfredo Sauce	**280**	7	43
Rotini w. Four Cheese Sauce	**130**	3.5	21
Rotini w. Mushroom Sauce, ½ cup	**260**	1.5	50
Kraft			
Minute White Rice, ¾ cup	**160**	0	36
It's Pasta Anytime Meals: *Per Package*			
Fettuccine w. Classic Alfredo Sauce	**580**	22	74
Spaghetti w. Tomato Sauce	**500**	9	88

Kraft (Cont)	C	F	Cb
Dinners: *Per Serving (Prepared As Directed)*			
Macaroni & Cheese: Orig., ⅓ box	**410**	18	49
Scooby-Doo Spirals	**390**	20	49
Mac & Chse: Crazy Noodles, ½ box	**390**	20	49
Thick'n Creamy, ½ box	**390**	20	51
Easy Mac, avg. all varieties., 1 pouch	**250**	8	38
Deluxe: Orig.; Sharp Chedd., ¼ box	**320**	10	45
Rotini White Cheese Sce, ½ box	**400**	15	48
Velveeta Shells & Cheese, ⅓ box	**360**	13	47
Cheesy Potatoes: *Per ½ Cup (Prep. As Directed)*			
Au Gratin Potatoes	**200**	7	27
Bacon Scalloped Potatoes	**200**	9	24
Mashed Potatoes	**200**	12	20
Lipton Packet Meals			
Fiesta Sides: *Per Cup (Prepared As Directed)*			
Taco Rice	**300**	6	52
Smoked Chipotle Rice	**310**	6	55
Nacho Pasta	**320**	10	47
Carb Options: *Per ¾ Cup (Prepared As Directed)*			
Sundried Tomato Pesto	**160**	8	12
Classic Basil Pesto	**220**	16	12
Pasta Sides: *Per Cup (Prepared As Directed)*			
Alfredo; Parmesan	**330**	14	40
Butter	**300**	13	40
Stroganoff	**290**	11	40
Asian Sides: *Per Cup (Prepared As Directed)*			
Beef Lo Mein; Thai Ses. Noodles	**230**	2.5	43
Teriyaki/Swt & Sour Noodles, avg.	**250**	3	46
Loma Linda (Vegetarian)			
Big Franks: 1 link, 1.8 oz	**110**	4.5	2
Low-fat, 1 link, 1.8 oz	**80**	3	3
Chicken Supreme Mix, ⅓ cup mix	**90**	1	6
Dinner Cuts, 2 sl., 1.4 oz (41g)	**90**	1.5	3
Fried Chik'n/Gravy, 2 pcs, 3 oz	**160**	9	14
Gravy Quik, 1 Tbsp mix (¼ pkt)	**20**	0	4
Linketts, (1), 1¼ oz	**70**	4.5	1
Little Links, 2 links, 1.6 oz	**70**	4.5	1
Nuteena, ⅜" slice, 2 oz	**160**	13	6
Ocean Platter, ⅓ c. dry mix, 1 oz	**90**	1	8
Patty Mix, ⅓ cup dry mix, 1 oz	**90**	1	7
Redi-Burger, ⅝" slice, 3 oz	**120**	2.5	7
Sandwich Spread, ¼ cup, 2 oz	**80**	4.5	7
Savory Din. Loaf, ⅓ cup, dry mix	**90**	1.5	7
Soyagen, ¼ c. (1 oz) dry (make 1 c.)	**130**	6	12
Swiss Steak, 1 piece, 3¼ oz	**140**	9	4
Tender Bits, 6 pieces, 3 oz	**110**	2.5	7
Tender Rounds, 6 pieces, 2¾ oz	**120**	5	5
Vege-Burger, ¼ cup, 2 oz	**70**	1.5	2
Vita-Burger Granules, 3 T., ¾ oz	**70**	1	6

Maruchan	C	F	Cb
Ramen Noodles: *Per Serving*			
Beef/Chicken/Shrimp Flavors, ½ block, 1½ oz	**190**	7	26
Noodles: Fat Fried Shrimp, 1½ oz	**170**	6	26
Other Flavors, 1½ oz	**160**	6	26
Fried Cup Beef, 1 packet, 2.2 oz	**300**	13	38
Low-fat varieties, average, 2 oz	**215**	1.5	45
Natural Touch (Vegetarian)			
Gravy Mix, average all types, 1 Tbsp (makes ¼ cup)	**20**	0	4
Kaffree Roma, 1 rounded tsp, 2g	**10**	0	2
Roasted Soy Butter, 2 Tbsp, 1.1 oz	**170**	11	10
Vegetarian Tuno, ⅓ cup, dr., 2 oz	**60**	2	2
Vegetarian Chili, 1 cup, 8 oz	**170**	1	21
Near East			
Couscous: *Per 2 oz (Dry)*			
Original Plain	**225**	1	46
Parmesan; Rst Garlic & Oil	**210**	1.5	41
Toasted Pine Nut	**210**	2.5	40
Other varieties, avg.	**200**	0.5	42
Creative Grains: *Per ⅓ Cup (Prepared)*			
Chicken & Herbs w. Brown Rice	**255**	2	51
Creamy Parmesan w. White Rice	**250**	3	48
Roasted Garlic w. Brown Rice	**205**	2	41
Roasted Pecan & Garlic w. Brown	**215**	5	37
Pasta, all types	**240**	6	41
Falafels, ¼ cup (Prepared)	**120**	1	18
Rice Pilaf: *Per 2 oz (Dry)*			
Spanish Mix	**240**	0.5	54
Tabouli Mix, Wheat Salad	**95**	0	21
Toasted Almond Mix	**210**	3	40
Wheat Mix; Brown Rice Mix	**195**	1	40
Other varieties, avg.	**200**	0.5	44
New Menu (Vitasoy) Vegetarian			
VegiBurgers, 3 oz	**110**	1	12
VegiDogs, 1 link, 1.5 oz	**45**	0	1
Tofumate (Season. Mixes), ¼ pkt	**25**	0	4
Nile Spice: *Per Cup*			
Couscous: Almondine	**200**	2.5	37
Lentil Curry	**200**	1.5	36
Minestrone	**140**	1	3
Parmesan	**200**	3	34
Nissan: Cup Noodles, all types, avg.	**300**	14	38

Old El Paso	C	F	Cb
Dinner Kits: *Per Serving (Prepared)*			
Soft Taco	**390**	19	33
Burrito (1)	**270**	12	27
Hard & Soft Taco (2)	**360**	17	32
Shells, Taco Sce, Seasoning (2)	**310**	18	19
Fajita (2)	**330**	10	35
Taco Dinner (2)	**300**	17	19
Side Dishes: Chili Beans, 1 cup	240	11	19
Boxed: Chsy Mexican Rice ⅓ pkt	**250**	2	55
Spanish Rice, ⅓ pkt	**280**	4.5	55
Refried Beans: Regular, ½ cup	**100**	0.5	17
w. Green Chilies, ½ cup	**100**	0.5	19
w. Cheese, ½ cup	**130**	3.5	18
w. Sausage, ½ cup	**200**	13	14
Fat Free varieties, ½ cup	**100**	0	18
Mexe/Pinto Beans, ½ cup	**110**	0.5	19
Pasta-Roni: *Per Cup (Prepared)*			
Angel Hair Pasta varieties, avg.	**320**	14	40
Fettuccine Alfredo	**460**	25	48
Chicken (flavor)	**310**	13	41
Chicken; Shells & White Cheddar	**310**	13	41
Chicken & Broccoli	**370**	16	49
Homestyle Deluxe: Creamy Garlic	**350**	17	40
Four Cheese; Parmesano	**390**	17	50
Homestyle Chicken	**310**	13	31
Ragu			
Express! Pasta Snacks: *Per ⅙ Box (4.2 oz)*			
Classic Meat Flavor; Tomato	**200**	3	37
Sweet Tomato & Garlic	**200**	2	39
Rice Pride			
Rice Bowls: Spicy Shrimp	**230**	0.5	48
Teriyaki Beef	**260**	1	56
Tex Mex Beef	**250**	2	52
Rice-A-Roni: *Per Cup (Prepared)*			
Beef; Herb & Butter; Rice Pilaf	**310**	9	52
Broccoli Au Gratin	**370**	17	46
⅓ Less Salt	**320**	11	50
Chicken	**310**	9	51
⅓ Less Salt	**280**	5	53
Low-fat	**210**	3	41
Chicken & Broccoli	**230**	5	41
Chicken & Garlic; Chkn Teriyaki	**260**	8	41
Fried Rice	**320**	11	50
Spanish Rice	**270**	8	46

(Reduced Fat Recipe: If only 1 Tbsp fat is used instead of 2 Tbsp, deduct 35 calories and 4g fat.)

Rosarita	C	F	Cb
Refried Beans: *Per ½ Cup*			
Traditional; Vegetarian; Spicy	**100**	2	18
Low-fat Black Bean	**90**	0.5	18
Fat-Free varieties	**90**	0	18

Slim-Fast	C	F	Cb
Hot Meal Options: *Per Package (Prepared)*			
Fettucine Alfredo	240	6	41
Shells & Creamy Cheese Sauce	245	6	40
Stagg Chili			
15 oz Can: *Per Cup (8.7 oz)*			
Chili w. Beans: Classic/Dynamite	310	17	24
Country/Laredo	310	16	25
Fiesta Grille	240	9	25
Ranch House Chicken	270	11	26
Rio Blanco Chicken	250	12	19
No Beans: Steakhouse/Double	330	21	16
99% Fat Free: Veg. Gdn/4 Bean	200	1	37
Turkey Ranchers/Silvarado Beef	240	3	31
S & W: *Per ½ Cup*			
Baked Beans, avg. all types	145	0.5	29
Caribbean Black Beans	90	0	18
Kidney Beans	100	0.5	23
Red Beans Louisiana Style	80	0	20
San Antonio; Santa Fe Beans	90	0.5	20
White Beans	80	0.5	19
Sun Bird: *Noodle/Rice Mix (Prepared)*			
Chow Mein; Hunan Beef, ¼ cup	110	1	24
Kung Pao Chicken, ¼ cup	130	2	2
Mongolian Beef, ¼ cup	120	0.5	28
Teriyaki Beef; Sweet & Sour, ¼ cup	155	0	39
Thai Beef, ¼ cup	140	1.5	28
Sesame Chicken, ¼ cup	150	0	34
Taco Bell: *Per ½ Cup*			
Home Originals: Refried Beans	120	1	20
Fat Free Beans w. Green Chilles	100	0	18
Tasty Bite			
Ready Meals: *Per Package (w. Rice)*			
Peas Paneer	425	15	54
Spinach Dahl	370	9	62
Beans Masala	425	8	75
Sprouts Curry	365	6	63
Vegetable Supreme	315	6	55
Vegetarian Entrees: *Per ½ Package*			
Agra Peas & Greens	140	10	9
Bengal Lentils	160	8	16
Bombay Potatoes	105	4	13
Jaipur Vegetables	170	11	7
Jodhpur Lentils	105	4	12
Kashmir Spinach	115	8	8
Madras Lentils	125	5	14
Punjab Eggplant	110	9	13
Simla Potatoes	120	7	12

Tasty Bite (Cont)	C	F	Cb
Chicken Entrees: *Per Package*			
Chicken Moglai	320	15	29
Chicken Roganjosh	300	16	28
Chicken Vindaloo	350	17	29
Thai Kitchen			
Bowls, avg. all types, 1.7 oz	170	2	35
Rice Noodles: *Per Serving*			
Pad Thai varieties, ½ package	260	0	63
Savory Garlic, ½ package	270	6	51
Thai Peanut, ½ package	243	3	50
Thin/Stir Fry, 2 oz	195	0	46
The Spice Hunter: *Per Package*			
Risotto: Wild Mushroom	230	1	47
Three Cheese; Spinach, avg.	245	2.5	46
Stuffed Potato: Creamy Butter	140	3	25
Bacon & White Cheddar	160	3	29
Sour Cream & Chives	160	2	31
Quick Hot Pasta: *Per Cup (Prepared)*			
Primavera Pasta	250	3	45
Roasted Peppers & Garlic	225	3	40
Tomato & Basil	200	1	42
Quick & Natural: Potato Leek, 1 pkg.	150	3	25
Creamy Thai Noodle, 1 bowl	180	4.5	29
Tofurky			
Deli Slices, average all	105	3	8
Holiday: Dumplings (2), 4 oz	215	1	45
Tofurky Roast, 4 oz	190	5	10
Tofurky Wild Rice Stuffing, ½ cup	140	5	21
Tofurky Wishstix, ½ piece	10	0	1
Jurky, 4 pieces	100	2	9
Sausages: Beer Brats (1), 3.5 oz	245	11	8
Kielbasa (1), 3.5 oz	245	12	8
Sweet Italian Sausages (1), 3.5 oz	280	13	12
Trader Joe's			
Bean Medley, ½ cup	150	1	26
Beef/Turkey Chili w. Beans, 1 cup	230	3	33
Black Bean Chili, 1 cup	230	1.5	37
Chicken Chili w. Beans, 1 cup	290	9	32
Refried Beans, avg., ½ cup	120	0	22
Organic Beans, avg., ½ cup	110	0	21
Black Beans: Regular, ½ cup	130	0.5	22
Cuban Style, ½ cup	130	2	21
Premium: Beef Stew, 1 cup	130	2	21
Chicken Stew, 1 cup	230	14	16
Quiche: Broccoli & Cheddar, 6 oz	490	33	33
Mexicaine, 6 oz	510	36	29
Spinach & Mushroom, 6 oz	470	30	32

Tuna Helper: *See Betty Crocker, Page 71*

Uncle Ben's	C	F	Cb
Flavorful Rice: *Per Cup (Prepared w. Margarine)*			
Average all varieties	**295**	12	42
Country Inn: *Per Cup (Prepared w/out Margarine)*			
Broccoli Rice Au Gratin	**205**	2	43
Three Cheese Rice	**205**	2.5	41
Other varieties, avg.	**200**	1	43
Ready Rice: *Per ½ Pouch (Prepared)*			
Spanish Style	**195**	4	36
Other varieties, avg.	**185**	2.5	38
Valley Fresh			
Chicken: *Per ½ Can*			
White & Dark Chunk	**80**	2	0
Premium Chunk White	**70**	1	0
Turkey, Premium Chunk White, ¼ can	**80**	1.5	0
Van Camps			
Pork & Beans, ½ cup	**110**	1	23
Original Baked Beans, ½ cup	**140**	1	30
Beanie Weanie Original, 7¾ oz	**220**	8	29
Baked Beans: w. Hot Dog, 1 cup	**340**	6	47
w. Ground Beef, 1 cup	**370**	7	57
w. Chicken, 1 cup	**360**	2	62
Spanish Rice, 1 cup	**180**	3	37
Westbrae (Vegetarian)			
Vegetarian Chili, ½ cup	**100**	0	19
White Wave (Vegetarian)			
Seitan: Chicken w. Broth, 5 oz	**130**	0	12
Traditional, 4 oz	**140**	0	4
Tofu: Baked, all flavors, 2 oz	**120**	6	3
Organic, Soft/Firm, ⅕ pkg, 3.2 oz	**90**	6	1
Fat-Reduced, ⅕ pkg, 3.2 oz	**90**	4	4
Extra Firm, ¼ pkg, 3 oz	**80**	5	1
Soy Milks & Yogurts: *See Pages 27, 30*			
Wolf			
Chili w. Beans: 227g Can	**300**	16	27
1 cup, 254g	**330**	18	30
Chili No Beans: 227g Can	**390**	27	18
1 cup, 248g	**420**	30	20
Chunky Beef w. Beans:			
1 cup, 254g	**300**	15	28
No Beans, 1 cup, 246g	**330**	22	18
Worthington (Vegetarian)			
Chik, 3 slices, 3.1 oz	**115**	5	3
Chili: Regular, 1 cup, 8 oz	**295**	15	21
Low Fat, 8 oz	**165**	1	21
Country Stew, 1 cup, 8.4 oz	**130**	7	5
Diced Chik, ¼ cup drained, 1.9 oz	**60**	3.5	1
Dinner Roast, ¾ slice, 2.9 oz	**180**	11	6

Worthington (Cont)	C	F	Cb
FriChik: Regular, 2 pieces, 3.1 oz	**120**	8	1
Low Fat, 2 pieces, 2.9 oz	**80**	3	2
Numete, ⅜ slice, 1.9 oz	**135**	10	5
Prime Stakes, (1), 3.2 oz	**140**	9	6
Protose, ⅜ slice, 1.9 oz	**135**	7	5
Saucettes (4), 3 oz	**90**	6	1
Savory Slices, 3 slices, 2.9 oz	**150**	8	7
Sloppy Joe, ½ cup, 4.9 oz	**140**	2	21
Stroganoff, ½ cup, 4.9 oz	**115**	3.5	10
Super Links, 1 link, 1.6 oz	**130**	7	5
Tuno, ⅓ cup, 1.9 oz	**80**	4	4
Turkee Slices, 3 slices, 3.3 oz	**190**	14	3
Vegetable Scallops, ½ cup, 3 oz	**90**	1.5	3
Vegetable Steaks, 2 slices, 2.5 oz	**80**	1.5	3
Vegetarian Cutlets (1), 2.2 oz	**80**	1.5	3
Veja Links: Regular (1), 1 oz	**50**	3	1
Low Fat, 1 link, 1 oz	**40**	1.5	1
Yves Veggie Cuisine (Vegetarian)			
Chick'n Nuggets (4) 3 oz	**190**	7	17
Santa Fe Veggie Beef Bowl	**360**	9	57
Mac'n Soy Cheese	**340**	9	52
Breakfast: Brkfast Links (2) 1.8 oz	**70**	2	3
Breakfast Patties (1) 2 oz	**80**	2	4
Canadian Veg. Bacon, 3 slices	**75**	0.5	1
Burgers: Veggie (1) 2.6 oz	**110**	4	7
Garden Vege Patties (1) 3 oz	**90**	0	11
Veggie Chick'n Burger (1) 2.6 oz	**105**	2.5	5
Dogs: Jumbo Veggie Dog (1) 2.6 oz	**105**	1.5	7
Hot & Spicy Chili/Good (1) 1.8 oz	**70**	1	3
Veggie/Tofu Dog, avg. (1)	**50**	0	1
Veggie Ground Round: Orig., Ital.	**60**	0.5	5
Mexican, ⅓ cup, 1.93 oz	**90**	2.5	4
Slices: Bologna, 2 oz (62g)	**80**	1	4
Pizza Pepperoni, 1.7 oz (48g)	**70**	0	4
Veggie Ham/Salami, avg., 2 oz	**85**	0	6
Veggie Turkey, 2 oz (62g)	**90**	2	4
The Good Lunch: Taco	**360**	11	55
Bologna; Turkey	**390**	12	55
Pizza	**420**	8	63
Veggie Entrees: Chili, 10.5 oz	**240**	1	87
Lasagne, 10.5 oz	**300**	3	51
Meatballs (5), 2.6 oz	**115**	2.5	7
Zatarain's: *Pasta Dinner Mix (Prepared)*			
Alfredeaux, 1 cup	**140**	3.5	22
Gumbo, 1 cup	**110**	1	23
Jumbalaya, 1 cup	**130**	1	27
Scampi, 1 cup	**100**	1	27

Soybean Products	C	F	Cb
Cheeses (Soy): *See Page 44*			
Miso: ½ cup, 5 oz	**280**	8	39
Cold Mountain: Red, 1 tsp, 7g	**10**	0	1
Mellow White, 1 tsp, 7g	**15**	0	3
Natto, ½ cup, 3 oz	**190**	10	13
Tempeh, 1 piece, 3 oz	**170**	6	14
Fried, 3 oz	**250**	14	14
Seitan *(White Wave)*, Trad., 3 oz	**140**	1	3
Soybean Protein (TVP), 1 oz	**100**	0.5	9
Soy Bean Paste, 1 tsp	**10**	0	2
Soy Beans: *See Page 149*			
Soy Drinks: *See Page 27*			
White Wave: *See Page 76*			

Tofu ~ Packaged	C	F	Cb
Tofu Stir Fried, average all, 4 oz	**120**	8	3
Azumaya Tofu:			
Soft (Silken), 3 oz	**45**	2	4
Soft, Light (Silken), 3 oz	**40**	1	3
Firm, 3 oz	**70**	4	2
Extra Firm, 3 oz	**70**	4	2
Light Extra Firm, 3 oz	**60**	2	3
Seasoned Tofu, 3 oz	**90**	5	3

Tofu ~ Packaged (Cont)	C	F	Cb
Hinoichu Tofu:			
Soft, 3 oz, 1" slice	**50**	2.5	2
Reg. (Japanese), 3 oz, 1" slice	**60**	3	1
Firm (Chinese), 3 oz, 1" slice	**70**	3.5	2
Extra Firm, 3 oz	**80**	4	1
Mori-Nu Tofu (Silken):			
Soft, 3 oz, 1" slice	**45**	2.5	2
Firm, 3 oz, 1" slice	**55**	2.5	2
Extra Firm, 3 oz, 1" slice	**45**	1.5	2
Nasoya Tofu: Soft, 3 oz	**60**	3	1
Silken, 3 oz	**45**	2.5	2
Firm, 3 oz	**70**	3	2
Extra Firm, 3 oz	**80**	4	2
Chinese 5 Spice Tofu, 3 oz	**90**	5	3
Pulmuone Tofu: Soft, 3 oz	**70**	3	1
Firm, 3 oz	**70**	3	1
White Wave: Baked Tofu, 1 square	**90**	5	2
Soft/Firm Tofu, 1/5 block	**110**	6	4
Reduced Fat, 1/5 block	**90**	4	1
Firm, 3 oz	**70**	3	1

Homemade & Restaurant

Restaurant & Take-Out

Per 8 fl.oz

	C	F	Cb
Bean Medley	200	3	34
Beef Consomme	30	0	2
Borscht (w. Cream)	130	8	14
Bouillabaisse	400	15	10
Chicken & Corn	290	14	20
Chicken & Wild Rice	80	4	9
Chicken Consomme	50	0	2
Chicken Curry	180	8	18
Chicken Jambalaya	160	7	8
Chicken Noodle	80	2	12
w. Chicken	160	4	12
Chicken Soup	80	2	6
Chili with Beans	250	12	25
Clam Chowder	240	15	17
Corn & Crab	120	3	18
Corn Chowder	150	8	16
Cream of Broccoli	200	12	20
Cream of Potato	220	12	25
Cream of Mushroom	290	21	20
Creamy Pumpkin	210	10	26
Fish Chowder	220	15	6
French Onion	420	15	25
Gazpacho	60	0	13
Lentil Soup	250	9	28
Lobster Bisque	320	15	10
Matzo Ball (w. 1 large ball)	180	7	24
Minestrone	140	2	14
Mulligatawny	300	15	8
Pea & Ham	240	10	25
Potato & Bacon	170	7	19
Shark Fin Soup	220	6	4
Spicy Shrimp Soup, 1 bowl	160	7	10
Split Pea Soup	150	6	18
Vegetable (Fat Free)	75	0	18
Vegetable Beef	80	2	10
Vichyssoise	200	9	15
Watercress	90	4	13

Other Soups: *See International & Fast-Foods Sections*

(Arby's, Au Bon Pain, Boston Market, Dunkin' Donuts, Denny's, Schlotzsky's, Sizzler, Souplantation, Sweet Tomatoes)

Homemade Soups: Calculate calories, fat and carbohydrates from ingredients.

Bouillon Cubes & Powders

	C	F	Cb
Bouillon Cubes: *Average all Types*			
Regular, 1 cube	8	0	1
Low Sodium (LiteLine)	12	0	1
Powders: Average, 1 tsp	8	0	1
Herb-Ox: Instant Broth & Seasoning,			
Beef, 1 envelope	10	0	2
Chicken; Vegetarian	10	0	2
Herbs, Spices: 1 tsp	5	0	1
Soup Oyster Crackers			
40 small/3 large, ½ oz	60	2	8

Amy's

Per Cup (½ Can)

	C	F	Cb
Alphabet Soup	80	0.5	16
Black Bean Vegetable	130	1.5	25
Butternut Squash	100	2.5	20
Chunky Tomato Bisque	120	3.5	21
Cream of Mushroom, ¾ cup	140	9	13
Lentil Vegetable	150	4.5	19
Minestrone	90	1.5	17
Pasta & 3 Bean	130	5	19
Vegetable Barley	70	1	13

Andersen's

Per Cup

	C	F	Cb
Split Pea	130	0	24
Split Pea w. Bacon	135	1	22
Tomato	130	3	24

Bean Cuisine

Per Cup (Made as Directed)

	C	F	Cb
Barcelona Red Beans & Radiatore	155	1	29
Country French Beans w. Gemelli	0	0	0
Florentine Beans w. Bow Ties	0	0	0
Mediterranean Blk Beans & Fusilli	155	1	30
Island Black Bean	90	0	17
Soup Mix: *Dry Mix Only*			
Mesa Maize, 1 oz	95	0	18
White Bean Provencal, 1 oz	175	1	32

Birds Eye

Hearty Spoonfuls Soup Bowls (Frozen): *Per Bowl*

	C	F	Cb
Cheesy Cream of Broccoli	230	10	25
Chicken Noodle	140	1.5	19
Chicken, Rice & Vegetables	160	2	26
Italian Minestrone	240	4	37

Campbell's

	C	F	Cb
Classic Red & White: *Per ½ Cup*			
Bean w. Bacon	170	4	25
Beef Noodle	75	2.5	9
Beef w. Vegetables & Barley	95	1.5	15
Black Bean	115	2	19
Cheddar Cheese	100	4.5	12
Chicken & Dumplings	190	9	17
Chicken Won Ton	45	1	6
Classic Chicken Noodle	100	2.5	16
Cream of Asparagus	110	7	10
Cream of Broccoli	90	3.5	12
Cream of Chicken & Brocc./Mushr.	120	8	9
Cream of Mushroom	105	7	9
Cream of Onion	100	5	12
Cream of Potato	95	3	15
Cream of Shrimp	90	6	8
Creamy Chicken Noodle	130	7	13
Fiesta Chili Beef	175	5	25
French Onion	45	1.5	6
Green Pea	175	3	28
Hearty Vegetable w. Pasta	95	0.5	19
Manhattan Clam Chowder	60	0.5	12
Minestrone	95	1	17
New England Clam Chowder	240	14	21
Old Fashioned Vegetable	80	1.5	14
Split Pea w. Ham & Bacon	170	2.5	27
Tomato	90	0	20
Tomato Bisque	130	3.5	23
Tomato w. Rstd Garlic & Herbs	95	0	23
Turkey Vegetable	75	2	11
Vegetable	130	3	22
Chunky: *Per Cup*			
Baked Potatoes w. Bacon Bits	160	5	21
Clam Chowder Manhatten	130	3.5	19
Grilled Chicken & Sausage Gumbo	140	2.5	21
Hearty Veges w. Pasta	130	2	23
Seasoned Rib Roast	110	1	17
Tomato Cheese Ravioli	150	3.5	27
Healthy Request: *Per ½ Cup*			
Chicken Rice	80	2	13
Vegetable Beef	90	1	15
Other varieties, average	90	1.5	18
98% Fat Free, prep., avg., ½ cup	70	2	10
Carb Request: *Per Cup*			
Chicken Broccoli; Cheese	130	7	8
Mediterranean Style Meatball	90	4.5	5
Roasted Chicken w. Veges	70	1	7
Savory Beef & Mushroom	70	2	7
Spicy Sausage w. Chicken	100	4	7

Campbell's (Cont)

	C	F	Cb
Select: *Per Cup (8 fl.oz)*			
Bean & Ham	165	1	30
Beef w. Portabello Mushr. & Rice	105	1.5	15
Beef w. Roasted Barley	145	1.5	24
Chicken & Pasta w. Roasted Garlic	105	1.5	16
Chicken Rice	100	1	17
Chicken Vegetable	105	0.5	18
Chicken w. Egg Noodles	105	1.5	14
Creamy Chicken Alfredo	220	12	16
Creamy Potato w. Roasted Garlic	175	9	20
Fiesta Vegetable	115	0.5	24
Grilled Chicken w. Sundried Tom.	110	1	17
Herbed Chicken w. Rstd Vegetable	90	0.5	14
Honey Roasted Chkn w. Potatoes	100	1	16
Italian Style Wedding	120	2.5	16
Minestrone	100	0	20
New England Clam Chowder	200	11	19
Roasted Chicken w. Wild Rice	95	0.5	17
Rstd Chkn w. Rotini & Penne	100	1	16
Rosemary Chkn w. Rstd Potatoes	105	0.5	18
Savory Lentil	145	0.5	27
Split Pea w. Ham	165	1	29
Tomato Garden; Vegetable	100	0.5	21
Vegetable Beef	115	2	16
Simply Home: *Per Serving (8.6 oz)*			
Chicken & Pasta	90	1	14
Chicken Noodle	85	1	13
Chicken w. White & Wild Rice	105	1	19
Country Vegetable	110	0	25
Minestrone	120	0.5	24
Vegetable Garden	100	0.5	20
Soup at Hand: *Per Container*			
Chicken varieties, average	75	1.5	12
Creamy Mushroom	120	8	8
Creamy Tomato	180	4	34
Mexican Style Fiesta	130	3	22
New England Clam Chowder	110	6	12
Pizza Soup	130	0.5	27
Vegetable Beef	60	1	10
Velvety Potato	150	6	21
Soup to Go: *Per Serving (10.7 oz)*			
Chicken Rice	140	1.5	25
Garden Vegetable	130	0	27
Hearty Chicken Noodle	80	0.5	12
Minestrone	140	1	27
Vegetable Beef w. Pasta	115	1	19
Soup & Recipe Mixes (Dry): *Per Tablespoon*			
Chicken Noodle/w. Broth	30	0.5	5
Onion	20	0	5

Soups (Cont)

CarbSense

	C	F	Cb
Per Cup (Prepared)			
Miso	**35**	1	5
Thai Coconut Cream	**100**	6	9
Szechuan Beef	**25**	0.5	4

Dr McDougall's

	C	F	Cb
Per Serving (Mix)			
Split Pea w. Barley, 1.5 oz	**150**	2	28
Tortilla Soup w. Baked Chips. 1 oz	**80**	0.5	16
Vegetarian Vegetable, 1 oz	**80**	0.5	16

Fantastic Cup Soups

	C	F	Cb
Per Container (Mix): Split Pea	**160**	1	28
Cha Cha Chili	**220**	2	37
Corn & Potato Chowder	**130**	1	26
Couscous w. Lentils	**170**	1	35
Split Pea	**220**	1	38
Creamy Soups, average	**150**	2.5	27
Hearty Soup Cups: *Per ½ Ctn*			
Country Lentil; Five Bean	**180**	1.5	32
Jumpin' Black Bean	**230**	1.5	41
Minestrone	**140**	1.5	27
Vegetable Barley	**120**	0.5	27
Big Soup: *Per Cup*			
Hot & Sour	**130**	2	22
Italian Tomato Noodle	**130**	1	26
Mandarin Broccoli	**110**	0	20
Spring Vege; Vege Beef Noodle	**100**	0	20
Spicy Thai	**110**	1	22
Sesame Miso	**90**	1	17
Vegetarian Chicken Noodle	**90**	0.5	19
Carbtastic: Hot & Sour, 1 pkg	**70**	2.5	7
Vegetarian Beef w. Barley, 1 pkg	**90**	1	14
Broccoli Cheddar, 1 pkg	**110**	3	12

Hain

	C	F	Cb
All Natural (canned): *Per Cup*			
Black Bean	**90**	0	18
Chicken Broth	**25**	2	3
Chicken Noodle	**150**	3	24
Mushroom Barley	**130**	1.5	26
Vegetable Broth	**25**	0	6
Wild Rice	**80**	1.5	15

Healthy Choice

	C	F	Cb
Per Cup			
Bean & Ham	**170**	2.5	29
Beef and Potato; Chicken w. Pasta	**110**	1	19
Chicken & Dumplings; Vege Beef	**130**	2	22
Chicken w. Rice Soup	**90**	3	12
Country Vegetable	**100**	0.5	22
Fiesta Chicken	**100**	2	17
Garden Vegetable	**120**	1	25
Hearty Chicken	**120**	2	20
Hearty Chilli Beef	**170**	2	31
Italian Bean & Pasta; Crmy Tomato	**100**	1.5	18
New England Clam Chowder	**110**	1.5	21
Roasted Italian Chicken/ w. Garlic	**120**	2	18
Split Pea and Ham	**170**	2.5	30
Turkey w. Rice; Zesty Gumbo	**90**	1.5	16

Health Valley

	C	F	Cb
Per Cup			
Bean Vegetable	**140**	0	32
Beef Broth	**10**	0	0
Carotene varieties, average	**70**	0	16
Chicken Broth, Low-fat	**35**	1.5	0
Chicken Noodle/Rice	**130**	2	20
Corn & Vege; Super Broccoli	**70**	0	17
Garden/Tomato Vegetable	**80**	0	17
Italian Minestrone; Lentil & Carrots	**100**	0	20
Mushroom Broth	**10**	0	2
Real Minestrone; Italian Plus; Vege	**80**	0	20
Rotini & Vegetables	**100**	0	20
Split Pea	**110**	0	17
Pasta Soups, avg. all varieties	**115**	0	24
Organic: Black Bean; Split Pea	**130**	0	25
Mushroom Barley; Potato Leek	**70**	0	16
Lentil; Tomato; Minestrone	**70**	0	17
Dry Soups: ⅓ cup, average	**120**	0	24
Soup Cups: *Per Cup*			
Chicken Broth	**25**	0	0
Corn Chowder w. Tomato	**105**	0	21
Creamy Potato w. Broccoli	**80**	0	17
Garden Split Pea; Zesty Blk Bean	**115**	0	22
Lentil w. Couscous	**130**	0	28
Pasta Marianara/Parmesan	**100**	0	20
Spicy Black Bean w. Couscous	**100**	0	21

Home Again

	C	F	Cb
Soup Mix: *Per ¼ Cup (dry)*			
Chunky Potato	160	6	25
Country Noodle	100	0	23
Southwest Chili	120	1	23
Creamy Potato w. Bacon	170	6	25
Creamy Broccoli & Rice	160	5	25

Imagine

	C	F	Cb
Per Cup			
No Chicken/Vegetable Broth	30	0.5	5
Free Range Chicken Broth	15	0.5	2
Organic Creamy: Broccoli	65	1.5	10
Butternut Squash	120	2	23
Portobello Mushroom	85	3	10
Potato Leek; Sweet Corn, avg.	100	3	15
Tomato	90	2.5	14

Knorr

	C	F	Cb
Naturals Hearty Soup Mix: *Dry Mix*			
Chunky Pot. w. Rstd Onion, 2 Tbsp	95	1	20
Homestyle Chicken Noodle, 3 Tbsp	80	1.5	13
Roasted Vegetable w. Rice, 2 Tbsp	85	1	17
Savory Soup: *Per 3 Tbsp (Dry Mix)*			
Chicken Flavor Noodle	70	1.5	11
Cream of Chkn & Rice	90	2.5	14
Cream of Vegetable,	95	4.5	12
Mediterranean Style Minestrone	100	2	18
Recipe Classics: *Dry Mix*			
Beef Stew (Goulash), 1⅓ Tbsp	40	1.5	6
Cream of Broccoli, 3 Tbsp	70	2.5	10
Cream of Spinach, 2 Tbsp	70	2.5	10
French Onion, 2 Tbsp	35	1	6
Hot & Sour, 2 Tbsp	45	1.5	8
Leek Soup, 2 Tbsp	70	2.5	10
Pot Roast (Sauerbraten), 1 Tbsp	35	1	6
Roasted Garlic Herb, 3 Tbsp, 0.7 oz	75	1.5	13
Spring Vegetable, 2 Tbsp, 0.3 oz	25	0	5
Tomato w. Basil, 3 Tbsp, 0.7 oz	85	2.5	13
Vegetable, 2 Tbsp, 0.6 oz	60	1.5	10
Tasty Break: *Per Container*			
Chicken Noodle	130	2	23
Chicken Vegetable	130	2	23
Navy Bean	145	1	27
Three Cheese Macaroni	250	4.5	44

Lipton

	C	F	Cb
Cup-a-Soup: *Per Envelope*			
Cream of Chicken	70	2	12
Chicken Noodle	50	1	8
Carb Options: Chicken	35	1	6
Chicken Noodle	25	0	4
Recipe Secrets Mixes: *Per Serving*			
Beefy Onion; Onion Mushroom	25	0.5	5
Chicken Noodle	80	2	11
Onion	20	0	4
Savory Herb w. Garlic; Vegetable	30	0	7
Soup Secrets: *Per Cup (Prepared)*			
Chicken Noodle	80	2	11
Noodle Soup	60	1.5	9

Manischewitz

	C	F	Cb
Condensed: *Per ½ Cup (Unprepared)*			
Chicken	15	0.5	2
Chicken w. Kieplach	35	1	5
Chicken w. Matzo Balls	80	4	9
Four Bean	70	1	13
Lentil	140	2	24
Minestrone	90	1.5	16
Condensed: *Per 8 fl.oz (Prepared)*			
Borscht w. Beets	90	0	21
Borscht Low Calorie	25	0	6
Ready To Serve: Matzo Ball Soup	110	5	13
Matzo Balls in Broth	215	9	27
Whitefish & Pike in Broth	55	1.5	3
Dry Mixes: *Per Cup*			
Matzo Ball & Soup Mix	40	0.5	9
Split Pea Cello	140	0	25
Vegetable Soup Cello	120	0	22

Maruchan - *Per Cup*

	C	F	Cb
Instant Lunch, avg. all flavors	290	12	37
Ramen flavors, ½ pkt, 1½ oz	190	8	26

Miso Cup

	C	F	Cb
Original; Golden Seaweed, 1 cup	30	1	3
Traditional, 1 pkg	35	1	4
Reduced Sodium, 1 pkg	25	1	3

Nile Spice

	C	F	Cb
Per Cup: Black Bean; Lentil	170	1.5	36
Cheddar Broccoli	130	3	20
Chicken Flavored Vegetable	110	1.5	21
Country Mushroom	140	2.5	26
Minestrone	140	1	30
Red Beans & Rice	170	1	35
Split Pea	200	1	35
Couscous: Parmesan	200	3	34
Other varieties, average	190	2	36

Pacific Foods

	C	F	Cb
Per Cup:			
Chicken Broth	**10**	0	**1**
Natural, Beef Broth	**20**	0	**1**
Organic: French Onion	**35**	0	**6**
Creamy Butternut Squash	**90**	2	**17**
Creamy Tomato	**100**	2	**16**
Roasted Red Pepper & Tomato	**100**	2	**16**
Vegetable Broth	**0**	0	**0**

Pritikin

	C	F	Cb
Per Cup: Black Bean w. Rice	**200**	1	**37**
Chicken Pasta	**80**	0	**15**
Fat Free Chicken Broth	**10**	0	**0.5**
Hearty Vegetable	**90**	0.5	**16**
Minestrone	**90**	0.5	**18**
Potato Broccoli	**110**	0	**22**
Split Pea	**180**	0.5	**32**
Three Bean Chili	**230**	1	**39**
Vegetarian Vegetable	**100**	0	**21**

Progresso *- Per Cup*

	C	F	Cb
Beef Barley; Chickarina, avg.	**130**	4	**13**
Beef & Vegetable	**125**	2.5	**16**
Chicken & Herb Dumplings	**110**	2.5	**15**
Chicken & Rotini/ Vegetable	**100**	2	**12**
Chicken Vegetable	**90**	1.5	**13**
Chicken with Wild Rice/Barley	**100**	1.5	**17**
Creamy Mushroom	**180**	14	**12**
Green Split Pea	**170**	3	**28**
Grilled Chicken Italiano	**110**	2.5	**14**
Grilled Steak w. Veg. Penne	**120**	3.5	**13**
Hearty Black Bean	**170**	1.5	**30**
Hearty Tomato	**100**	2	**23**
Hearty Penne in Chicken Broth	**80**	1	**14**
Home Style Chicken; Turkey Noodle	**90**	1.5	**11**
Lentil	**180**	2	**31**
Macaroni & Bean	**160**	4	**23**
Manhattan Clam Chowder	**110**	2	**17**
Minestrone	**110**	1.5	**19**
New England Clam Chowder	**190**	13	**23**
Potato w. Broccoli & Cheese	**160**	6	**21**
Roasted Chicken varieties, avg.	**80**	1.5	**10**
Southwestern Style Chicken	**120**	2	**19**
Southwestern Style Corn Chowder	**200**	7	**29**
Split Pea w. Ham	**150**	4	**20**
Steak & Baked Potato	**130**	2.5	**18**
Steak & Mushrooms/Vegetables	**110**	2	**16**
Tomato; Tomato Basil	**100**	2	**19**
Tomato Rotini	**140**	5	**30**
Turkey Rice w. Vegetable	**110**	1	**18**
Vegetable	**80**	2	**15**

Progresso (Cont)

	C	F	Cb
Rich & Hearty: Chicken Pot Pie	**160**	4.5	**20**
Beef Pot Roast w. Veges	**130**	1.5	**17**
Creamy Chicken w. Rice	**160**	5	**19**
Other varieties, avg.	**120**	1	**17**
99% Fat Free: Chicken Noodle	**90**	1.5	**13**
Beef Barley; Lentil; Minestrone	**130**	2	**20**
New England Clam Chowder	**110**	1.5	**18**
White Cheddar Potato	**100**	1.5	**20**
Carb Monitor: *Per Cup*			
Bey Vegetable	**70**	1.5	**6**
Chicken Cheese Enchilada	**200**	16	**7**
Chicken Vegetable	**70**	2	**7**

Rokeach

	C	F	Cb
15 oz Can (Ready to Serve): *Per Serving*			
Barley & Mushroom; Vegetable	**110**	1	**23**
Chicken Consomme	**50**	4	**0**
Cream of Mushroom	**120**	7	**13**
Minestrone	**170**	1	**32**
Potato	**100**	1	**20**
Seven Bean	**130**	1	**24**
Split Pea & Egg Barley	**190**	1.5	**35**

Schwan's

	C	F	Cb
Soups: *Per Bowl (10 oz)*			
Cheesy Broccoli	**360**	27	**18**
Chicken Noodle	**175**	6	**18**
Chili w. Beans	**385**	19	**33**

Slim-Fast

	C	F	Cb
Creamy: Broccoli, 1 container	**210**	5	**30**
Chicken Flavored	**220**	5	**33**
Potato Cheddar & Chive	**220**	5	**35**

Swanson

	C	F	Cb
Per Cup			
100% Fat Free Chicken Broth	**15**	0	**1**
Beef Broth	**10**	0.5	**0**
Chicken Broth	**15**	0.5	**1**
Vegetable Broth	**15**	0	**3**

Tabatchnick

	C	F	Cb
Frozen: *Per Bag (7½ oz)*			
Pea	**240**	1	**45**
Barley Mushroom	**70**	0	**13**
Cream of Spinach	**90**	4	**11**
Old Fashioned Potato	**70**	0	**16**
Vegetable	**110**	1	**20**
Yankee Bean	**160**	2	**27**

Thai Kitchen

	C	F	Cb
7 oz Can: *Per Serving*			
Coconut Ginger	**190**	15	11
Hot & Sour	**40**	0.5	7
Instant Rice Noodle: *Per Serving (1.6 oz)*			
Bangkok Curry	**90**	3	16
Garlic & Vegetable	**80**	1.5	17
Lemongrass & Chili	**80**	1.5	17
Spring Onion, 1.6 oz	**90**	1.5	16
Thai Ginger	**80**	12	16
Other varieties	**120**	1.5	25
Rice Noodle Soup Bowls: *Per Serving*			
Curry, ½ pkg., 2.5 oz	**290**	6	55
Hot & Sour, ½ pkg., 2 oz	**115**	0.5	26
Lemongrass & Chili, ½ pkg., 2.5 oz	**115**	0.5	24

Trader Joe's

	C	F	Cb
Per Cup			
Barley w. Vegetables; Rich Onion	**95**	1	19
Chicken Broth	**15**	0.5	0
Chicken Noodle	**90**	1	14
Chunky Minestrone	**100**	2	16
Country Style Tomato	**75**	0.5	14
Creamy Corn Chowder	**165**	7	23
Lentil w. Vegetables	**175**	1.5	30
Mixed Vegetable	**105**	6	10
Mostly Unsplit Pea	**175**	0.5	32
Salmon Chowder	**165**	8	15
Spicy Bean	**200**	5	30
Spicy Black Bean	**230**	3	41
Split Pea, Low Fat	**145**	1	26
Condensed: Clam Chowder	**150**	4	22
Crab Bisque	**150**	6	18
Creamy Asparagus	**195**	13	16
Cups: Split Pea	**210**	0.5	37
Tortilla Salsa	**175**	1.5	33
Vegetarian Vegetable w. Pasta	**160**	1.5	31

Walnut Acres

	C	F	Cb
Per Cup (250g)			
Autumn Harvest	**100**	2	19
Country Corn Chowder	**150**	3	28
Cuban Black Bean; Four Bean Chili	**150**	1	30
Ginger Carrot	**100**	1	22
Classic Minestrone	**100**	0	22
Mediterranean Lentil	**130**	0	26
Savory Tomato	**120**	2	23

Weight Watchers

	C	F	Cb
Chicken Noodle, 10½ oz	**150**	2	25
Chicken & Rice, 10½ oz	**110**	1.5	17
Minestrone; Vegetable, 10½ oz	**130**	1	27
Instant Beef/Chicken Broth, 1 pkg	**10**	0	2

Westbrae

	C	F	Cb
Canned: *Per Cup (240g) Unless Indicated*			
Alabama; Mediterranean Lentil	**140**	0	24
Instant Miso Soup, 1 pkt	**35**	1.5	3
New York UnChicken Noodle	**60**	1	10
Old World Split Pea	**150**	0	28
Santa Fe Vegetable	**160**	0	31
Other varieties, average	**125**	0	25
Condensed: *Per ¾ Cup, Prepared*			
California UnChicken Broth, 180g	**15**	0.5	2
Monte Carlo Crmy Mushr., 180g	**70**	3	10
Tuscany Tomato, 180g	**70**	0	16

Wylers

	C	F	Cb
Dry Mix: Mrs Grass Onion, 10g	**30**	0	6
Homestyle Vegetable, 12g	**35**	0	7
Soup Starter: *Per Cup*			
Chicken Noodle	**70**	1	13
Beef Vegetable	**90**	0.5	18

Feedback Welcome

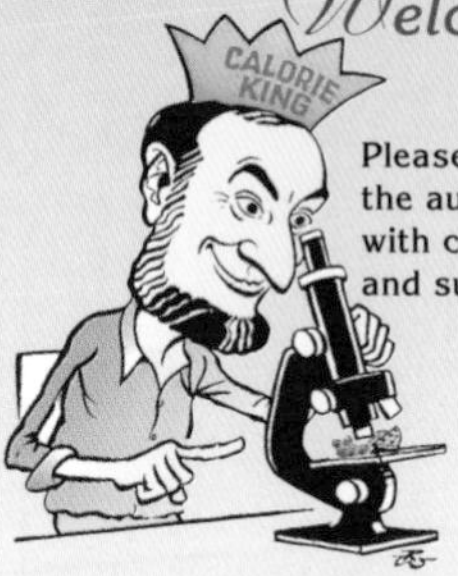

Please contact the author with comments and suggestions.

Write to: Allan Borushek
1001 West 17th St, Costa Mesa CA 92627
Email: allan@calorieking.com

Herbs & Spices

	C	F	Cb
Per Teaspoon: Average all types	5	0	1
Allspice, ground	5	0	1
Chili Powder	8	0	1
Cinnamon, ground	6	0	2
Curry Powder	6	0	1
Garlic Powder	9	0	2
Nutmeg, ground	12	0	1
Onion Powder	7	0	2
Parsley, dried	4	0	1
Pepper, black/red/white, avg.	6	0	1
Saffron	2	0	0
Tumeric, ground	8	0	1
Seeds: Fenugreek	12	1	2
Mustard, Poppyseed	15	1	1
Other types, average	7	0	1
Parsley Patch: Sesame, 1 tsp	16	1	1
Salt-free blends, average	10	0	2
All-purpose, 1 tsp	6	0	1

Seasonings & Flavorings

	C	F	Cb
Accent Flavor Enhancer, 1 tsp	10	0	0
Angostura Bitters, 1 tsp	12	0	3
Bacon Bits, average, 1 Tbsp	30	1	0
Bacon Chips *(Durkee)*, 1 Tbsp	45	1	2
Best O'Butter, 1 tsp	10	0.5	2
Bragg Liquid Aminos, 1 tsp	5	0	0
Butter Buds, 1 tsp	8	0.5	2
Garlic Bread Sprinkle, 1 tsp	8	0.5	1
Garlic Salt, 1 tsp	2	0	0
Italian Seasoning, 1 tsp	4	0	1
Lemon Pepper Seasoning, 1 tsp	7	0	1
Meat Tenderizer, avg., 1 tsp	7	0	1
Molly McButter, 1 tsp	5	1	1
Mrs Dash Blends, 1 tsp	0	0	2
Perc Salt-free Seasoning, 1 tsp	8	0	2
Potato Toppings *(Knudsen)*, 1 Tbsp	30	2.5	1
Salad Sprinkles *(Lawry's)*, 1 tsp	16	0.5	2
Salad Supreme *(McCormick)*, 1 tsp	10	0.5	2
Salt: Regular, Sea Salt, Lite Salt	0	0	0
Seasoning Mixes, avg., ¼ pkg	70	1	9
Taco Seasoning, avg., ¼ pkg	30	0.5	4
Old El Paso: Chili Season. Mix, 1 T.	15	0.5	3
Cheesy Taco Season. Mix, 1 Tbsp	15	0.5	3
Taco/Burrito Seasoning Mix, 2 tsp	15	0	4
Enchilada Seasoning Mix, 2 tsp	10	0	2
Fajita Seasoning Mix, 1 tsp	10	0	3
Vegit Seasoning Mix, 1 tsp	5	0	1

Condiments, Sauces

	C	F	Cb
Average of Brands & Homemade			
Apple Sauce: *Also see Page 146*			
Sweetened, ¼ cup, 2¼ oz	45	0	11
Unsweetened, ¼ cup, 2 oz	27	0	6.5
Bac O's *(Betty Crocker)*, 1 tsp, ½ oz	60	3	4
Barbecue, average	25	0	6
Bearnaise Sce, ¼ cup, 2½ oz	190	19	5
Buffalo Wing Sce: Honey Mustard, 1 T.	40	3	3
Average other varieties, I Tbsp	25	2	2
Catsup (Ketchup): Reg., 1 Tbsp	15	0	4
Cheese, h/made, ¼ cup, 2½ oz	150	10	12
Chili Sauce: *Heinz,* 1 Tbsp	15	0	4
Del Monte, 1 Tbsp	20	0	5
Wolf Hot Dog, 1 Tbsp	15	1	2
Cocktail Sauce, ¼ cup	110	0	15
Cranberry, all types, ¼ c., 2½ oz	110	0	27
Escoffier Sauces, 1 Tbsp	20	0	4
Honey Mustard *(French's)* 1 tsp	5	0	1
Horseradish: 1 tsp	2	0	0
Sauceworks Sauce, 1 tsp	20	2	0
Ketchup: Regular, 1 Tbsp	16	0	4
Heinz Lite, 1 Tbsp	8	0	2
Heinz Kick'rs, 1 Tbsp	20	0	4
Mushroom Sauce, ½ cup, 2 oz	50	2	5
Mustard, average, 1 tsp	5	0	0.5
Pesto, ¼ cup, 2 oz	35	3	2
Pizza Sauce, cnd., ¼ cup, 2 oz	25	0	5
Seafood Cocktail Sce, ¼ cup	60	0	14
Soy Sauce, all types, avg., 1 Tbsp	10	0	0
Sour Cream Sce, ½ cup	250	15	22
Spaghetti Sce, ½ cup, 4½ oz	135	6	19
Steak Sauce: *Heinz,* 1 Tbsp	15	0	3
Lea & Perrins, 1 Tbsp	25	0	6
Lawry's Low Carb, 1 Tbsp	5	0	1
Str'berry Puree Sce: Unsweet., 2 T.	9	0	2
Sweet & Sour Sauce:			
Contadina, 2 Tbsp	40	1	8
Kikkoman Lite Soy, 1 Tbsp	10	0	1
La Choy, 2 Tbsp, 34g	60	0	14
Tabasco Sauce, 1 Tbsp	2	0	0
Taco Sauce, average, 2 Tbsp	10	0	1
Tartar Sauce: *Heinz,* 2 Tbsp, 30g	140	14	4
America's Choice, 2 Tbsp, 27g	160	17	1
Hellman's: Regular, 2 Tbsp, 30g	80	7	3
Low-fat, 2 Tbsp, 30g	40	1.5	7
Teriyaki Sauce, *Kikkoman,* 1 Tbsp	15	0	2
Vinegar, White or wine, 1 fl.oz	4	0	1
White Sauce, ½ cup, 5 oz	130	7	12
Worcestershire Sauce, 1 tsp	5	0	1

Pickles & Relish

	C	F	Cb
Average All Brands			
Bread & Butter Pickles, 4 sl., 1 oz	20	0	5
Chutney, 2 Tbsp, 1¼ oz	40	0	12
Dill Pickle:			
Slices, 4 slices, 1 oz	3	0	0.5
1 large, (3¾"x 1¼" diam.), 2¼ oz	12	0	3
Extra lrg (4"x 1¾" diam.), 5 oz	30	0	6
Halves: Small, 1 oz	3	0	0.5
Large, 2½ oz	8	0	2
Sweet, small, ½ oz	22	0	6
Gherkins, sweet, 1 med., 1 oz	15	0	7
Green Chilies, chopped, 2 Tbsp	5	0	1
Horseradish, 1 Tbsp	10	0	2
Jalapenos, pickled, 2 whole	5	0	1
Jalapeno Relish, 1 Tbsp, ½ oz	5	0	1
Mustard, avg. all brands, 1 tsp	5	0	0.5
Peppers: Hot/Mild, 1 oz	8	0	2
Pickled: Beets, ½ cup, 4 oz	75	0	19
Onions, 1 medium, ¾ oz	10	0	2
Cocktail Onion, 1 onion	2	0	0
Red Cabbage, ½ cup, 3 oz	60	0	13
Pickles: Sweet, 2 Tbsp, 1 oz	35	0	0
Large (3" x ¾ diam.), 1¼ oz	40	0	10
Pickle in a Pouch, 1 large	12	0	3
Relishes: Sandwich Spread, 1 tsp	20	1	5
Cranberry-Orange, 1 Tbsp	30	0	7
Hot Dog *(Heinz)*, 1 Tbsp	17	0	28
Sweet Pickle, 1 Tbsp	20	0	5
Sauerkraut, ½ cup, 3½ oz	25	0	5
Sweet Cauliflower	35	0	8

Salsa

	C	F	Cb
Average all Types: *Per 2 Tablespoons*			
Regular, no oil, 2 Tbsp	15	0	3.5
Homemade w. Oil, 2 Tbsp	40	3	8
Chef's Kitchen, 2 Tbsp	10	0	2
Del Monte, all flavors, 2 Tbsp	10	0	2
Kaukauma, 2 Tbsp	15	0	3
La Victoria, 2 Tbsp	10	0	2
Wild Oats, 2 Tbsp, 1 oz	10	0	2

Gravy

	C	F	Cb
Homemade Gravy:			
Thin, little fat, 2 Tbsp, 1 oz	20	1	3
Thick, 2 Tbsp, 1¼ oz	50	2	9
¼ cup, 2½ oz	100	4	18
Franco-American (Canned)			
Au Jus Gravy, ¼ cup, 2 oz	10	0	2
Beef; Turkey Gravy, 2 oz	25	0.5	3
Chicken Gravy, ¼ cup, 2 oz	40	4	4
Franco-American (In Jars)			
99% Fat Free, ¼ cup, 2 oz	25	0.5	4
Pillsbury (Gravy Mixes)			
Brown; Homestyle, ¼ cup, 2 oz	15	0	3
Chicken, as prep., ¼ cup, 2 oz	20	0	4

Gravy-In-Jars-Homestyle

	C	F	Cb
Boston Market, ¼ cup, 2 oz	25	1	3
Heinz, reg., all types, ¼ c., 2 oz	25	1	3
Fat Free Rst. Turkey, ¼ c., 2 oz	10	0	2
Vons, all types, ¼ c., 2 oz	20	0.5	4

Tomato Products

	C	F	Cb
Whole/Chopped/Crushed/Diced			
1 cup, 8½ oz	50	0	10
In Aspic, ½ cup	50	0	12
w. Green Chili, 1 cup, 8½ oz	45	0.5	11
Stewed, ½ cup	40	2.5	9
Wedges in Tom Juice, 1 cup	70	0.5	15
Salsa, average, 1 Tbsp	15	0	3.5
Tomato Ketchup:			
Regular, 1 Tbsp	16	0	4
Green *(Heinz)*, 1 Tbsp	20	0	5
Tomato Paste, 2 Tbsp	25	0	5
Regular, 6 oz, ¾ cup	150	0	34
Tomato Puree, ½ cup	50	0	10
Tomato Sauce:			
Regular, ½ cup	40	0	9
Spanish Style, ½ cup	40	0	9
w. Mushrooms, ½ cup	40	0	9
w. Onions, ½ cup	50	0	11
Tomato Seasoning, 3 tsp	20	0	4
Sundried Tomatoes:			
Natural, 5-6 pces, 0.4 oz	22	0	5
In Oil, drained, 6 pces, ½ oz	60	4	5

Brands	C	F	Cb
A-1			
Steak Sauce: *Per Tablespoon*			
Original	10	0	3
Bold & Spicy	20	0	5
Smoky Mesquite	30	0	8
Barilla: *Per ½ Cup*			
Marinara; Sweet Peppers & Garlic	90	3	11
Roasted Garlic & Onion	90	3.5	11
Tomato & Basil	80	2.5	12
Bertolli/Five Brothers: *Per ½ Cup*			
Alfredo w. Mushrooms	160	12	6
Creamy Alfredo	220	20	6
Grilled Summer Vegetable	80	5	12
Imported Romano & Garlic	90	4	10
Marinara w. Burgundy Wine	80	3	12
Mushroom & Garlic	90	3	13
Olive Oil & Garlic	90	4	9
Olive w. Sundried Tomato	100	4	13
Oven Roasted Garlic & Onion	70	1.5	10
Roasted Red Pepper	80	3	13
Tomato Basil	80	2	10
Best Foods			
Dippin' Sauce: *Per Tablespoon*			
Honey Mustard Madness	30	1	5
Rockin' Ranch	45	3	4
Totally BBQ	55	6	0.5
Bookbinders: *Per ½ Cup*			
White Clam Sauce	300	30	4
Buitoni			
Pasta Sauce: *Per ½ Cup*			
Alfredo	140	12	5
Light Alfredo	80	5	5
Marinara	80	3	11
Roasted Garlic Marinara	60	1.5	9
Tomato Herb Parmesan	120	8	9
Bullseye			
BBQ Sauce: *Per 2 Tbsp*			
Grilled Onion w. Garlic, 1.3 oz	60	0	14
Sweet Hickory Smoke, 1.3 oz	65	0	15
Avg., other flavors	50	0	13
Carb Options: *Per Serving*			
Alfredo, ¼ cup	100	10	2
Barbeque varieties, 2 Tbsp	10	0	3
Double Cheddar, ¼ cup	90	8	2
Garden Style, ½ cup	75	4.5	7
Hickory Barbeque, 2 Tbsp	10	0	3
Marinades: Italian Garlic, 1 Tbsp	0	0	0
Steak, 1 Tbsp	5	0	1

Catelli	C	F	Cb
Meat Sauce, ½ cup	85	2.5	11
Garden Select 6, avg, ½ cup	80	2	14
Garden Select Pizza Sauce, 1 oz	15	0.5	2.5
Thick & Chunky Pasta Sauce, avg. all types, ½ cup	70	1.5	12
Cento: *Per Serving (½ Cup)*			
Sauces: Passata Tomatoes	40	0	8
Pasta, all natural	50	3	3
Pizza, fully prepared	25	0	5
Tomato: Arrabbiata; Vodka	70	3	6
Marinara; Puttanesca	115	9	6
White Clam	165	13	5
Classico: *Per ½ Cup Unless Indicated*			
Alfredo, ¼ cup	120	11	3
Classic Beef w. Onion	120	5	14
Florentine Spinach & Cheese	80	5	6
Four Cheese	95	5	10
Hearty Steak w. Wine	115	5	13
Italian Sausage w. Peppers	90	2	13
Roasted Garlic Alfredo, ¼ cup	100	9	3
Spicy Red Pepper	50	1.5	7
Spicy Tomato & Pesto	90	4	11
Sundried Tomato	80	3	11
Sundried Tomato Alfredo, ¼ cup	120	10	4
Traditional Basil Pesto, ¼ cup	230	21	6
Other varieties, avg.	60	1	11
Contadina			
Pasta Sauces: *Per ½ Cup*			
Alfredo Sauce	360	32	10
Lite	160	10	10
Garden Vegetable Sauce	40	0	9
Marinara Sauce	80	4	9
Mushroom Alfredo	200	14	12
Mushroom Marinara Sauce	70	2.5	11
Pesto w. Basil, Red. Fat	460	26	22
Pesto w. Sundried Tomato	380	30	20
Roasted Garlic Marinara	60	2	10
Pizza Squeeze Sce, ¼ cup	35	1.5	6
Del Monte			
Pasta Sauces: *Per ½ Cup*			
Chunky Sce, average all varieties	60	1.5	11
D'Italia Pasta: Four Cheese	60	2	8
Other varieties	50	1.5	9
Spaghetti Sauce: Traditional	60	0.5	15
Garlic & Onion	60	1.5	11
w. Mushroom/Meat	70	1.5	14
Sloppy Joe Sauce, ¼ cup, 67g	50	0	11

Brands (Cont)

	C	F	Cb
Dominick's: *Per ½ Cup*			
All Natural: Garl. & Onion; Marinara	80	4	10
Mushr. & Olive; Tomato & Basil	80	1	8
Italian Classics: Four Cheese	80	2.5	12
Portabella Mushroom	60	2	9
Puttanesca	70	3	8
Spicy Roasted Garlic	70	2	10
Sun Ripened Tomatoes	80	4	8
Tomato Basil	50	1	8
Estee			
Barbecue Sauce, 1 Tbsp	18	0.5	3
Spaghetti Sauce, ¼ cup, 4 oz	60	2	13
Steak Sauce, 1 Tbsp	14	0.5	3
Enrico's			
Tomato Basil, 3.5 oz	65	2	10
Traditional Italian Style, 3.5 oz	55	0.5	11
Mushroom Onion, ½ cup, 125g	70	1	12
Other varieties, ½ cup, 125g	70	2	12
Emiril's: *Per ½ Cup (123g)*			
Puttanesca	80	5	9
Roasted Red Pepper	60	3	7
Vodka Sauce	130	8	13
French's Grill & Glaze			
Honey Mustard, 2 Tbsp	90	1	18
Teriyaki, 2 Tbsp	60	0	13
Garden Valley: *Per ½ Cup*			
Chunky Vege. Primavera	35	0.5	12
Four Cheese	35	1	8
Millina's Finest; Roasted Garlic	50	0	12
Sundried Tomato; Tomato Mushr.	50	0	11
Sweet Tomato Basil	60	0	13
Green Giant			
Sloppy Joe S'wich Sce, ¼ c., 2.5 oz	50	0	11
Sloppy Joe Sauce & Meat	200	11	11
Healthy Choice: *Per Serving*			
Creamy Alfredo, ¼ cup	45	3	3
Garlic & Herbs, ½ cup	50	0	13
Garlic Lovers, ½ cup	45	0	10
Mushroom Alfredo	45	3	3
Roasted Garlic & Romano	60	1	11
Sundried Tomato & Herb	60	0.5	12
Traditional Pasta Sauce, ½ cup	50	0	13
Super Chunky: Vege Primavera, ½ c.	60	0	13
Tomato, Mushroom Garlic, ½ c.	50	0	10

Heinz: *Per 1 Tbsp (Approx. ½ oz)*	C	F	Cb
Barbecue Sauces, all flavors	35	0	9
Chili Sauce, 1 Tbsp	15	0	4
Horseradish Sauce	70	7	2
Mustard: Pourable/Mild, 1 Tbsp	8	0.5	0
Spicy Brown	13	1	1
Seafood Cocktail Sauce	20	0	3
Steak Sauce 57	15	0	4
Tartar Sauce, 1 Tbsp	70	7	2
Tomato Ketchup	16	0	4
Worcestershire Sauce, 1 Tbsp	8	0	1
Sloppy Joe Sauce, ½ cup, 125g	70	0.5	14
Hunt's			
BBQ Sauce: Original, 36g, 2 Tbsp	50	0	13
Hickory & Brown Sugar, 38g, 2 T.	70	0	18
Manwich Sloppy Joe Sce, ¼ c., 64g	30	0	6
KC Masterpiece: *Per Tablespoon*			
Marinades: Garlic & Herb	30	1.5	4
Honey & Teriyaki	35	0.5	7
Original BBQ	40	1.5	7
Knorr (Sauce Mix)			
Pasta Sauce: *Per 2 Tbsp (Makes ½ Cup)*			
Alfredo; Carbonara	65	3	7
Creamy Cheddar	60	3	7
Creamy Pesto	50	2	6
Four Cheese	65	3	7
Garlic Herb; Parma Rosa	65	3	8
Sundried Tomato Pesto Pasta, 0.8 oz	60	0	14
Pesto, 2 tsp	15	0	3
Classic Sauce: *Per 2 Tbsp (Prepared)*			
Bernaise	20	0	4
Hollandaise	20	0	4
Classic Gravy, avg., ¼ cup, prepared	25	0	4
Knudsen: Potato Toppings, 2 Tbsp	50	4.5	2
Kraft			
CarbWell Sauce, 2 Tbsp	15	0	3
Sauceworks: Cocktail, 2 Tbsp	30	0.3	6
Horseradish, 1 tsp	20	1.5	0
Sweet 'n Sour, 1 Tbsp	30	0	7
Tartar: 1 Tbsp	50	5	2
Lemon & Herb, 1 Tbsp	75	8	0
Nonfat Tartar, 1 Tbsp	12	0	5
Barbecue Sauces: Average, 2 T.	50	0.5	9
Other Sauces: Mustard, 1 Tbsp	10	0	0
Horseradish, Reg./Crm Style, 1 T.	10	0	0
Sandwich Spread & Burger, 1 T.	50	4	3
Sweet 'n Sour, 1 Tbsp	40	0.5	9

Brands (Cont)	C	F	Cb
Las Palmas			
Red Chile Sauce, ¼ cup, 2 oz	15	0.5	2
Enchilada Sauces: Green Chile	25	1.5	3
Hot/Original, ¼ cup, 2 oz	15	0.5	3
Salsa: Mexicana. Mild, 2 Tbsp, 1 oz	5	0	1
Mexicana Hot/Medium, 2 Tbsp	10	0	2
Lawry's 30 Minute Marinade: *Per Tbsp*			
Carribean Jerk; Teriyaki	25	0	6
Hawaiian; Dijon & Honey	20	0	3.5
Mediterranean; Lemon Pepper	10	0	2
Mesquite	5	0	1
Thai Ginger; Herb & Garlic	10	0	2
Packet Seasonings: *Per Tablespoon (Dry)*			
Fajitas; Taco	30	0	6
Average other flavors	40	0	8
Libby's			
Sloppy Joe Sauce, ⅓ cup, 78g	45	0	10
McCormick Sauce Mixes			
Grillmates: Marinade, avg., 2 tsp	15	0	2
Sauce Blend Seasoning Mixes:			
Lemon Herb Chicken, 1 Tbsp	30	0	5
Chicken Fried Rice, 1 Tbsp	35	0	6
Stir Fry Chicken, 1 Tbsp	20	0	4
Chicken Teriyaki, 1⅓ Tbsp	40	1	5
Mr Yoshida's			
Original Gourmet, 2 Tbsp, 30ml	90	0	20
Hawaiian Sweet & Sour, 2 Tbsp	35	0	9
Muir Glen: *Per ½ Cup (125g)*			
Organic Pasta Sauce:			
Mushr. Marinara; Portobello Mushr.	50	0	11
Other varieties, average	50	1	11
Newman's Own: *Per ½ Cup*			
Bombolina (Tomato & Basil)	100	5	15
Roasted Garlic & Peppers	100	5	15
Vodka	100	5	11
Old El Paso			
Salsa: Thick 'n Chunky, 2 T., 1 oz	10	0	2
Homestyle; Green Chili; Verde 2 Tbsp, 1 oz	10	0	2
Taco Sce, all varieties, 2 Tbsp, 1 oz	10	0	2
Enchilada Sce, all types, ¼ c., 2 oz	20	1	3
Grilling Sauces, all types, 2 Tbsp	60	0	14
Tom. & Gr. Chiles/Jalapenos, ¼ c., 2 oz	10	0	2
Old World: Traditional	70	3	8
Flavored w. Meat, ½ cup	80	4	7
Pace: Picante Sauce, ¼ cup, 2 oz	25	0	5
Chunky Salsa, avg. all types	10	0	2
Salsa Con Queso	45	3	4

Prego: *Per ½ Cup*	C	F	Cb
Extra Chunky: Garden Comb.	90	2	16
Garlic Supreme	120	3	23
Mushroom & Green Pepper	120	4.5	18
Mushroom Supreme	120	4.5	21
Pasta Bake: *Per Serving*			
Fresh Mushrooms, ½ cup	130	5	15
Hearty Meat Sauce, ⅛ jar	120	6	12
Italian & Garlic, ½ cup	120	5	16
Italian Sausage, ⅛ jar	90	3.5	12
Meatball Parmesan, ½ cup	160	7	15
Mushroom w. Garlic & Onion, ⅛ jar	90	3	13
3-Cheese Marinara, ⅛ jar	100	4.5	11
Tomato, Garlic & Basil, ⅛ jar	80	3.5	11
Premier Japan (Organic)			
Garlic/Ginger/Wasabi Tamari, 1 T.	10	0	2
Thai Soynut, 1 Tbsp	25	2	2
Ragu: *Per ½ Cup*			
Meat Flavored Sauce	80	4	7
Traditional	70	3	8
Cheese Creations:			
Double Cheddar	200	18	6
Mushroom Green Pepper	110	3	16
Roasted Garlic Parmesan	240	22	6
Chunky Garden Style:			
Gard. Combo; Mushr. Gr. Pepper	100	3	16
Other varieties, average	110	3	18
Rich & Meaty: Classic Italian Style	150	10	9
Beef, Onion & Garlic	100	5	9
Mama's Meat Sauce	130	8	8
Sausage, Peppers & Onions	160	11	9
Robusto!: Six Cheese	80	3	9
Italian Sausage & Cheese	100	4.5	11
Sauteed Onion & Mushr./Garlic	90	4	11
Tomato, Olive Oil, Garlic	90	4.5	9
Pizza Sauce: ¼ cup	30	1	4
Pizza Quick, average, ¼ cup	40	1.5	6
Rainforest Organic			
Ginger Curry, 1 Tbsp	15	1.5	1
Mango; Papaya Pepper, 1 Tbsp	5	0	1
Tamarind Spice, 1 Tbsp	5	0	1
Rinaldi: *Per ½ Cup*			
3-Cheese	90	2	15
Original; Meat/Mushroom	90	4	11
Tomato & Basil	80	2.5	11
Tomato, Garlic, Onion	80	2	12
Roberto's			
Salsa: Peach, 1 Tbsp, 15g	10	0	2
Black Bean & Corn, 2 Tbsp, 32g	10	0	2
Burrito Sce, ¼ cup, 60g	50	4	3
Enchilada Sauce, ¼ cup, 65g	95	5	10
Green Chile, Hot/Mild, 1 Tbsp, 15g	0	0	0

S & W: *Per Tablespoon*	C	F	Cb
Mesquite Marinated Cooking	10	0	3
Teriyaki, Light/Marinade	25	0	5
Seeds of Change: *Per ½ Cup*	50	0.5	9
Steel's Gourmet Sauce			
Barbeque Sce, Sweet & Spicy, 2 Tbsp	15	0	2
Cocktail Sce w. Dill & Lemon, 4 Tbsp	36	0	1
Hoisin, 2 Tbsp., 1 fl.oz	10	0	2
Rocky Mountain Ketchup, 1 oz	10	0	0
Spiced Cranberry Sce, 4 Tbsp	16	0	4
Sweet & Sour, 2 Tbsp, 1 oz	10	0	2
Sutter Home: *Per ½ Cup*			
Other varieties	80	2	12
Marinara Pasta Sauce	70	2	11
Taj: *Per ½ Cup*			
Bombay Curry Simmer Sauce	90	5	10
Calcutta Masala Simmer Sauce	100	5	13
Kashmir Tandoori Marinade Sce	50	3	5
Seasoning Mixes: Chili, 1 tsp	40	1	6
Meat Loaf; Sloppy Joe's, 1 tsp	30	0	4
Beef Stew, 1 tsp	15	0	3
Chicken/Taco Seasoning, 1 tsp	25	0	4
Spaghetti Sauce: Italian Style, 1 T.	25	0	5
The Wizard's (Organic)			
Hot Nutz, 1 Tbsp	30	2	2
Hot Stuff, 1 Teaspoon	0	0	0
Vegetarian Worcestershire, 1 Tbsp	10	0	2
Troy's Sauces (Organic)			
Ginger Sauce, 1 Tbsp	5	0	1
Peanut Sauce, 1 Tbsp	30	2	1
Timpone's: *Per ½ Cup*			
Spaghetti Sauce: Classic	50	2.5	8
Family Recipe	80	3	7
Mom's	70	3.5	8
Tomaso's: *Per ½ Cup*			
Basil & Fresh Garlic; Spicy Eggplant	60	3	7
Black Olive Fresh Basil	40	2	5
Extra Garlic	55	2	8
Fresh Mushroom & Artichoke	50	2	7
Sugo Rosa	105	7.5	8
Tree of Life: *Per ½ Cup*			
Pasta Sauce Plus, all varieties	45	0	9
Organic, average all varieties	35	0	8
Walnut Acres: *Per ½ Cup (125g)*			
Organic Pasta Sauce, average	50	1	9
Wild Oats: *Per 2 Tbsp (1 oz)*			
Wasabi; Seafood Marinade & Grilled	30	3	4
Korean Sesame Marinade & Grilled	30	0	8

Quick Guide

Mayonnaise	C	F	Cb
Regular			
Average All Brands, 1 Tbsp	100	11	0
Bestfoods, Kraft, 1 Tbsp	100	11	0
½ cup, 4 oz	800	88	0
Light/Reduced Fat			
Kraft, 1 Tbsp	50	5	1
Best Foods, 1 Tbsp	45	4	2
½ cup, 4 oz	360	32	4
Hain, Eggless, Tbsp	60	6	2
Hain, Safflower Oil, Tbsp	50	5	2
Hellman's, 1 Tbsp	50	5	1
Wild Oats Canola Oil, 1 Tbsp	100	12	0
Fat Free			
Kraft, 1 Tbsp	10	0	3
½ cup, 4 oz	80	0	16
Smart Beat, 1 Tbsp	10	0	3
Sugar Free: *Dukes* Mayo, 1 Tbsp	10	12	0
Mayonnaise Style Dressing			
BAMA Dressing, 1 Tbsp, 0.5 oz	50	4	3
Gourmayo (French's), 1 Tbsp, 0.5 oz	50	5	1
Miracle Whip Salad Dressing:			
Regular, 1 Tbsp, 0.5 oz	70	7	2
Light, 1 Tbsp, 0.5 oz	40	3	3
Free, 1 Tbsp, 0.5 oz	15	0	3
Nayonaise (Nasoya)			
(Tofu Base/Dairy Free/Eggless)			
Regular, 1 Tbsp, 0.5 oz	35	3	1
Fat-Free, 1 Tbsp, 0.5 oz	10	0	2

"Take two of these and call me in the morning"

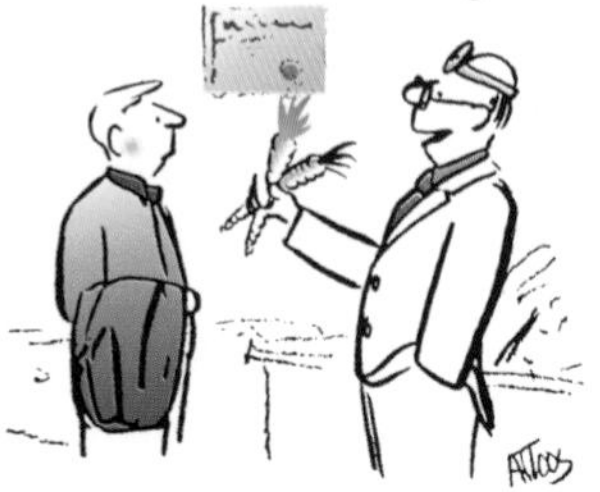

Quick Guide

Salad Dressings
Average All Brands
Per 2 Tbsp (Approx 1 fl.oz)

	C	F	Cb
Balsamic Vinaigrette: Reg., 1 oz	90	8	4
Light, 2 Tbsp, 1 oz	45	4	2
Fat Free, 2 Tbsp, 1 oz	5	0	1
Blue Cheese: Regular, 2 Tbsp, 1 oz	150	16	2
Regular, ¼ cup, 2 oz	300	32	4
Light, 2 Tbsp, 1 oz	80	8	1
Caesar: Regular, 2 Tbsp, 1 oz	140	14	2
Regular, ¼ cup, 2 oz	280	28	4
Light, 2 Tbsp, 1 oz	50	5	0.5
Coleslaw: Regular, 2 Tbsp, 1 oz	150	12	8
Regular, ¼ cup, 2 oz	300	24	16
Light, 2 Tbsp, 1 oz	90	7	7
French/Italian: Regular, 1 oz	120	11	5
Regular, ¼ cup, 2 oz	240	22	10
Light, 2 Tbsp, 1 oz	70	7	2
Fat/Oil-Free, 2 Tbsp, 1 oz	20	0	4
Ranch: Regular, 2 Tbsp, 1 oz	180	18	3
Regular, ¼ cup, 2 oz	360	36	6
Light, 2 Tbsp, 1 oz	90	8	3
Fat-Free, 2 Tbsp, 1 oz	50	0	2
Thousand Island: Regular, 1 oz	130	12	5
Regular, ¼ cup, 2 oz	260	24	10
Light, 2 Tbsp, 1 oz	50	4	3
Fat-Free, 2 Tbsp, 1 oz	35	0	3

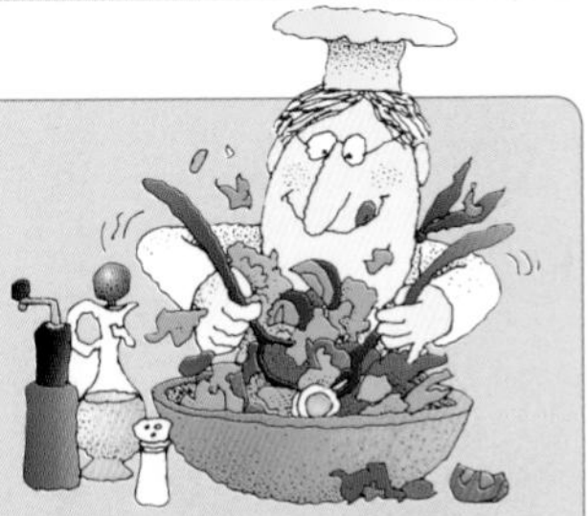

Enjoy a healthy salad but don't drown it in high-fat salad dressings.

Use 'light' dressing to halve the fat and calories.

Brands ~ Salad Dressings

Per 2 Tbsp (Approx 1 fl.oz)

	C	F	Cb
Annie's Naturals			
Cowgirl Ranch, 2 Tbsp	120	11	3
French; Goddess, avg.	90	9	3
Gardenstyle (vinegar free)	120	12	3
Organic: Buttermilk	70	7	1
No-Fat Yogurt	20	0	3
Red Wine & Olive Oil	160	17	1
Thousand Island	90	7	5
Tuscany Italian	80	7	5
Vinaigrette: Black Olives & Truffle	110	12	1
Balsamic; Cilantro & Lime, 2 T.	100	10	2
Low-Fat: Honey Mustard	45	2	6
Gingerly	40	2	4
Raspberry	35	1.5	5
Roasted Red Pepper	70	6	3
Shiitake & Sesame	120	13	1
Yellow Pepper & Tomato	70	7	2
Bernstein's			
Creamy Caesar, 2 Tbsp	120	13	1
Fat-Free Cheese & Garlic Italian	10	0	2
Italian	110	12	1
Olive Oil Vinaigrette	90	9	3
Restaurant Recipe Italian	130	13	1
Other varieties, avg., 2 Tbsp	110	11	2
Light Fantastic: Cheese Fantastico	25	1.5	3
Roasted Garlic Balsamic	45	3.5	3
Best Foods			
Dijonnaise, 1 tsp	5	0	1
Dippin' Sauce: Rockin' Ranch	110	12	1
Honey Mustard Madness, 2 Tbsp	90	6	8
Mayonnaise: Just 2 Good! 2 Tbsp	50	4	4
Light, average., all varieties	100	10	2
Real Mayonnaise, average	95	10	0
w. Lime Juice, 2 Tbsp	200	22	0
Bob's Famous			
Ranch Country, 2 Tbsp	150	15	1
Roquefort; Thousand Isld; Blue Chse	140	14	1
Tartar Sauce	170	16	2
Brianna's			
Blue Cheese; Zesty French	130	13	4
Blush Vintage	100	6	12
French Vinaigrette, 2 Tbsp	150	17	0
Honey Mustard; Poppy Seed	130	12	6
Lemon Tarragon	35	8	8
Rich Santa Fe Blend	15	0	3

Per 2 Tbsp (Approx 1 fl.oz)	C	F	Cb
Carb Options: Italian	70	8	0
Ranch	155	17	0
Whipped, 30g	90	10	0
Cardini's			
Caesar, 2 Tbsp	160	17	1
Fat-Free Caesar	40	0	9
Light Caesar	80	7	5
Extra Virgin Olive Oil Ital.; Zesty Garl.	120	13	1
Honey Mustard	140	13	5
Kalamata Olive w. Romano Cheese	120	13	2
Lemon Herb	120	13	1
Parmesan Ranch	150	15	2
Poppyseed w. Shallots	160	14	8
Vintage White Wine	110	12	1
El Torito: Cilantro Pepita Caesar	140	14	2
Emeril's: *Per 2 Tbsp*			
House Herb Viniagrette	140	14	2
Kicked Up Gaaalic	150	15	3
Girards: *Per 2 Tbsp*			
Balsamic Basil	90	7	3
Blue Cheese Vinaigrette	100	10	3
Caesar	150	16	1
Lite	80	7	2
Champagne	150	16	2
Lite Champagne	60	5	2
Greek Feta Vinaigrette	110	11	1
Honey Dijon Peppercorn	120	13	7
Olde Venice Italian	120	13	2
Oriental Chicken Salad	120	11	6
Original French	120	13	0
Raspberry	90	10	9
Romano Cheese	130	13	2
Shiitake Chardonnay	100	9	4
Spinach Salad	80	2	14
Fat-Free: Balsamic/Red Wine, avg.	25	0	6
Caesar	40	0	9
Raspberry	50	0	13
Good Seasons (Mix)			
Per 2 Tbsp (Prepared from 4g Dry Mix)			
Blue Cheese, Cheese Garlic	145	16	2
Cheese Italian, Garlic & Herbs	145	16	2
Classic Dill	30	0	5
Gourmet Caesar	150	16	3
Italian varieties	145	16	2
Lite Italian varieties	55	6	2
Ranch	115	12	2
Fat-Free: Italian; Roasted Garlic	10	0	2
Gourmet Caesar	15	0	2

Hidden Valley: *Per 2 Tbsp*	C	F	Cb
Light Ranch: B.L.T.	90	7	5
Light Ranch	80	7	3
Original Ranch: w. Sour Cream	145	7	6
w. Sundried Tomato	140	14	2
Regular Ranch: BBQ Ranch	120	12	3
B.L.T. Ranch; Coleslaw	150	15	5
Caesar w. Garlic	120	11	4
French w. Honey & Bacon	150	12	10
Old Fashioned Buttermilk	130	14	2
Original Ranch	140	14	1
Spicy	140	14	2
White Cheddar	130	13	1
w. Bacon	140	14	1
Fat-Free: Original Ranch	30	0	6
Honey & Bacon French	50	0	11
Original Ranch w. Bacon	40	0	5
Ken's Steak House Dressings: *Per 2 Tbsp*			
3 Cheese Italian	110	10	4
Balsamic & Basil Vinaigrette	110	12	1
Chunky Blue Cheese	140	15	1
Country French	130	11	9
Creamy Caesar	170	19	0
Peppercorn Ranch	180	19	2
Ranch	180	20	1
Italian w. Aged Romano	110	12	1
Thousand Island	130	13	4
Lite: Chunky Blue Cheese	80	7	4
Caesar/Olive Oil Vinaigrette	70	6	3
Creamy Parmesan	90	8	3
Ranch	100	9	4
Knott's Berry Farm: *Per 2 Tbsp (1 oz)*			
Honey Dijon, 2 Tbsp	130	13	4
Honey Poppyseed	120	9	10
Oriental Chicken Salad	130	11	5
Parmesan & Peppercorn	160	17	1
Sun Dried Tomato	100	10	3
Low-Fat: Raspberry	50	2	8
Tropical Fruit	45	1	9

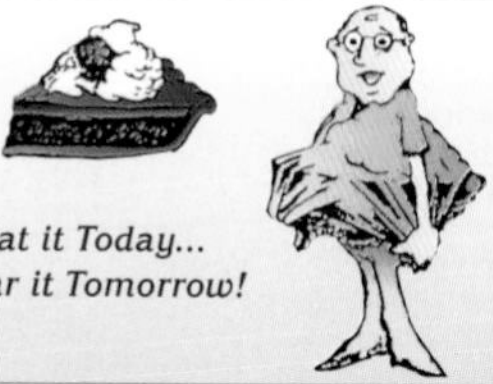

Eat it Today...
Wear it Tomorrow!

Salad Dressings (Cont)

Per 2 Tbsp (Approx 1 fl.oz)	C	F	Cb
Kraft			
Regular Dressings: *Per 2 Tbsp*			
3 Cheese Ranch	135	14	1
Honey Dijon	115	10	6
Classic Caesar	110	11	0.5
Coleslaw	150	12	8
Creamy Italian	105	11	3
Creamy French	155	15	5
Horseradish Sauce, 1 tsp	20	1.5	1
Roka Brand Blue Cheese	130	13	2
Thousand Island, avg.	105	10	5
Kraft Free (Fat-Free): Italian	15	0	4
Caesar Italian	25	0	4
Other varieties, avg.	45	0	11
Carb Well: Italian	70	8	0
Classic Caesar; Ranch	110	11	0
Roka Blue Cheese	120	13	0
Light Done Right!: Catalina	30	1	5.5
Italian; Ranch	75	7	3
Other varieties, avg.	70	6	3
Special Collection: Caesar Italian	100	10	2
Balsamic Vinaigrette	90	8	4
Sweet Honey Catalina; Poppyseed	130	11	8
Other varieties, avg.	55	4	4
Seven Seas, all varieties	90	9	2
Kroger: Cream Cucumber	155	16	3
Creamy French, 2 Tbsp	130	12	6
Honey French	145	12	9
Poppy Seed	160	14	8
Real Mayonnaise	100	11	0
Zesty Italian	95	9	3
Lite: Zesty Italian	35	2	4
3 Cheese Ranch	80	8	2
Ranch	65	6	3
Fat-Free, avg., 2 Tbsp	30	0	8
Litehouse: Caesar	140	14	1
Chunky Bleu Cheese	150	16	1
Coleslaw	90	7	7
Jalapeno Ranch	120	12	1
Lite Bleu Cheese	70	6	2
Other varieties, avg.	120	13	3
Maple Grove: *Per 2 Tbsp (1 fl.oz)*			
Balsamic Vinaigrette	50	3	6
Regular: Honey Mustard	120	9	9
Parmesan & Pepper	115	11	4
Sweet & Sour	110	7	12
Fat Free: Balsamic Vinaigrette	5	0	1
Caesar Vinaigrette; Greek	10	0	3
Dijon; Poppyseed	40	0	10
Other varieties, avg.	30	0	8

Maple Grove (Cont)	C	F	Cb
Low Carb: Dijon	80	8	1
Balsamic; Raspberry Vinaigrette	5	0	1
Lite: Caesar; Pesto Parmesan	65	5	5
Honey Mustard	80	5	9
Lemon & Dill	75	5	7
Romano	40	3.5	1
Marie's: *Per 2 Tbsp*			
1000 Island	190	20	2
Blue Cheese	170	18	0
Caesar	150	13	8
Poppy Seed	190	20	1
Ranch (8 fl.oz ctn), 2 Tbsp	160	16	4
(15.5 fl.oz ctn), 2 Tbsp	170	19	1
Light: Blue Cheese	70	7	2
Ranch	70	7	2
Nasoya: *Per 2 Tbsp*			
Vegi-Dressing (Tofu Base/Dairy Free):			
Thousand Island	60	4	6
Other flavors	60	5	3
Nayonaise: Regular, 2 Tbsp, 1 oz	70	6	2
Fat-Free, 2 Tbsp, 1 oz	20	0	4
Newman's Own: *Per 2 Tbsp*			
Balsamic Vinaigrette, 2 Tbsp	90	9	3
Caesar; Olive Oil & Vinegar	150	16	1
Creamy Caesar	170	18	1
Family Recipe Italian	120	13	1
Parmesan & Roasted Garlic	110	11	2
Parmesan Italiano	140	14	2
Ranch	180	18	2
Two Thousand Island	140	14	4
Lighten Up: Light Italian	60	6	1
Light Raspberry & Walnut	70	5	7
Light Balsamic Vinaigrette	45	4	2
Pritikin: Honey Dijon	45	0	11
Dijon Balsamic; Zesty Italian	30	0	6
Honey French Style	40	0	10
Raspberry	35	0	11
San-J: Tamari Peanut	60	2	9
Tamari Sesame	45	2	5
Tamari Vinaigrette	45	3	4
Fat-Free: Tamari Mustard	25	0	5
S & W: *Per 2 Tbsp (1 oz)*			
Light: Italian	35	0	8
Red/White Wine; Raspberry Blush	40	0	10
Seeds of Change: *Per 2 Tbsp (1 oz)*			
Balsamic/Greek Feta Vinaigrette	60	5	4
Italian Herb Vinaigrette	50	4	4

	C	F	Cb
Spike Splashes!			
Original, 2 Tbsp	100	11	1
Salt-Free	100	10	2
Fat-Free	10	0	2
Spectrum: *Per 2 Tbsp (Approx 1 fl.oz)*			
Fat Free: Creamy Dill/Garlic	20	0	4
Sweet On. & Garlic; Tstd Sesame	10	0	3
Low-fat: Honey Dijon	35	2	4
Zesty Italian	30	2	1
Organic: Greek Goddess, 2T.	110	11	2
Balsamic Vinaigrette	85	8	3
Provencal Garlic Lovers	55	5	2
Rocky Mountain Ranch	135	14	1
Steel's (Sugar-Free)			
Honey Mustard, 2 Tbsp	180	14	0
Sweet Ginger Lime, 2 Tbsp	140	14	2
Subway Select: *Per 2 Tbsp (1 oz)*			
Premium Collection: Caesar	170	16	1
Lite Blue Cheese; Lite Ranch	80	7	1
1000 Island	130	13	4
Jalapeno Ranch	100	10	1
The Spice Hunter: *Per 2 Tbsp (Mix Prepared)*			
Caesar Salad, 2 Tbsp	150	13	1
Chinese Salad; Garlic & Herb	140	13	2
T. Marzetti's: *Per 2 Tbsp (1 oz)*			
Regular: Balsam./Wild Berry Vinaig.	100	9	4
Buttermilk	180	19	1
Creamy Caesar	150	17	0
Caesar Lite	70	6	2
Italian	100	10	3
Original Slaw	170	16	6
Ranch	160	17	2
Red Wine Vinegar & Oil	130	14	2
Roasted Garlic	150	15	2
Roasted Garlic Vinaigrette	130	10	8
Sesame Oriental	110	9	8
Sour Cream Blue Cheese	170	16	0
Sun Dried Tomato Vinaigrette	130	11	6
Vinaigrette Blue Cheese	120	11	4
Light: Buttermilk Ranch	80	8	2
Chunky Blue Cheese	90	5	5
Original Slaw	100	7	10
Tree of Life: *Per 2 Tbsp (1 oz)*			
House Dressing: Cafe Venice	120	12	2
Maison Caesar	70	6	1
Shanghai Palace	80	7	3
Low-Fat: Blue Cheese	15	1	2
Fat-Free: Honey French	35	0	8
Italian Garlic	20	0	4
Oriental Ginger	15	0	3

	C	F	Cb
Walden Farms			
Fat-Free, Calorie Free Range, 2 Tbsp	0	0	0
Weight Watchers			
Salad Celebrations Dressings			
Fat Free: Caesar (Single), 0.75 oz	5	0	1
Caesar, 2 Tbsp	10	0	1
Creamy Italian (8 oz), 2 Tbsp	30	0	7
French Style, 2 Tbsp	40	0	9
Honey Dijon, 2 Tbsp	45	0	11
Italian (8 oz), 2 Tbsp	10	0	2
Ranch Style, 2 Tbsp	35	0	7
Ranch (Single), 0.75 oz	25	0	6
Wild Oats: *Per 2 Tbsp (1 oz)*			
Balsamic Vinaigrette; Thousand Isle	80	7	5
Caesar Style	120	12	1
Creamy Peppercorn	100	10	1
Honey Toasted Sesame Ginger	100	10	3
Ranch	120	11	3
Thousand Isle	90	7	5
Wishbone: *Per 2 Tbsp (1 oz)*			
Regular: 5 Cheese Italian	120	10	6
Chunky Blue Cheese	170	17	2
Classic Caesar	110	10	2
Creamy Caesar	180	18	1
French: Deluxe French	120	11	5
Sweet 'N Spicy	140	12	6
Italian: Regular	80	8	3
House Italian	110	10	3
Robusto Italian	90	8	4
Ranch: Original	160	17	1
w. Garlic/Spring Onion	150	15	2
Red Wine; Balsamic Vinaigrette	60	5	3
Russian, regular	110	6	15
Thousand Island	130	12	7
Fat-Free: Chunky Blue Cheese	35	0	7
Italian	15	0	2
Ranch	40	0	9
Dressing & Marinades: Asian	45	2	6
Balsamic Olive Oil & Herbs	40	2.5	4
Lemon Garlic & Herb	50	2.5	6
Tangy Honey Mustard	70	4	10
Ranch Up!	140	15	2
Just 2 Good!: Blue Cheese	45	2	6
Classic/Creamy Caesar; Ranch	40	2	5
Country Italian; Italian	30	2	5
Parmesan Peppercorn Ranch	45	2	6
Thousand Island	60	2	9

Breakfast Cereals

Quick Guide

Cooked Cereals	C	F	Cb
Buckwheat Groats, roasted:			
Dry, ½ cup, 3 oz	280	2	60
Cooked, 1 cup, 7 oz	180	1	39
Bulgar: Dry, ½ cup, 2½ oz	240	1	53
Cooked, 1 cup, 6½ oz	150	0.5	34
Corn/Hominy Grits:			
Dry, ¼ cup, 1.4 oz	145	0.5	33
3 Tbsp, 1 oz	110	0.5	25
Cooked, ¾ cup, 6½ oz	110	0.5	25
Instant, 1 pkt, 0.8 oz	80	0.5	18
w. Imitation Bacon Bits, 1 oz	100	0.5	22
Cream of Rice, ckd, ¾ c, 6 oz	90	0	20
Cream of Wheat:			
Regular, ckd, ¾ cup, 6 oz	180	0.5	37
Quick, ckd, ¾ cup, 6 oz	95	0.5	20
Instant, ckd, ¾ cup, 6 oz	110	0.5	23
Farina: Cooked, ¾ cup, 6 oz	85	0	18
Millet, dry, ¼ cup, 1 oz	100	0	20
Oat Bran: Raw, ⅓ cup, 1 oz	75	2	21
Cooked, ½ cup	40	1	11
Oatmeal: Dry, ⅓ cup, 1 oz	110	0	19
Regular, ckd, ¾ cup, 6 oz	110	2	19
1 cup, 8 oz	145	3	25
Instant: Regular, avg., 1 oz	100	2	18
Flavored, average	150	2	32
Wheat Hearts, 1 oz dry, ¾ c. ckd	110	1	21

Brans, Wheatgerm, Add-Ons

Bran: Wheat, unprocessed,			
1 Tbsp, 3g	10	0	3
Rice Bran, raw, 1 Tbsp, 5g	16	1	2.5
¼ cup, 1 oz	90	6	14
Oat Bran, 1 Tbsp, 5g	15	0.5	3
⅓ cup, 1 oz	75	2	15
Wheat Germ, 1 Tbsp, ¼ oz	25	1	3.5
¼ cup, 1 oz	105	3	15
Fruit: Dried, average, 1 oz	80	0	21
Banana, ½ medium	50	0	23
Prunes in Syrup, 5, 3 oz	90	0	24
Honey, 1 Tbsp, ¾ oz	65	0	17
Lecithin Granules, 1 Tbsp, 10g	50	5	1
Nuts, Almonds, 6 (¼ oz)	40	4	5
Bee Pollen Granules, 1 T., 8g	25	1	2
Psyllium Husks, 1 Tbsp, 5g	10	0	1

Hot/Cooked Cereals ~ Brands

Per Serving	C	F	Cb
Albers Grits, ¼ cup, 1.4 oz	140	0.5	31
Bobs Red Mil-10 Grain, ¼ c., 40g	180	2.5	35
CarbSense: MiniCarb Instant	170	6	17
Instant Cereal: Country Spice, ½ c.	170	7	15
Roasted Hazelnut, ½ cup	190	9	15
Country Choice Oats, ½ cup, 40g	150	3	27
Dr McDougall's			
Oatmeal: 4 Grains, 2.2 oz	220	2	44
Barley, all varieties, 2.5 oz	270	3	51
Wheat, 2.4 oz	220	2.5	44
Erewhon: Barley Plus, ¼ c., 1.7 oz	170	1	37
Brown Rice Crm, ¼ cup, 1.6 oz	170	1	36
Instant Oatmeal, 1.2 oz pkg	140	2	26
Oat Bran, ⅓ cup, 1.8 oz	170	2.5	31
Health Valley: Hot Cups,			
Apple; 10 Grain, 1 cup	220	2.5	42
Maple; Banana, 1 cup	240	2.5	46
McCann's Instant Irish Oatmeal			
Apple & Cinnamon, 1.23 oz	130	1.5	26
Maple & Brown Sugar, 1.5 oz	160	2	32
Original, 1 oz pkg	100	2	18
Steel Cut Oats, ¼ cup, 1.4 oz	150	2	26
Mothers Oat Bran, ½ cup, 1.4 oz	150	3	25
Nabisco: Cream of Rice, ¼ c., 46g	170	0	38
Cream of Wheat: Orig., 3T., 1 oz	120	0	25
Maple Brown Sugar, 1.2 oz pkg	120	0	27
Malto Meal: Orig., 3T., 1.2 oz	120	0.5	26
Maple Brown Sugar, ¼ cup	170	0	37
Natures Path: Apple Cinn.1.7 oz	190	2	38
Average other varieties	200	4	35
Quaker: Oatbran, ½ cup, 1.4 oz	150	3	25
Brown Sugar Bliss, 1 cup, 1.7 oz	190	2.5	39
Grits: Reg. all types, 1 pkg	130	0.5	31
Instant, all types, 1 pkg, 1 oz	100	1	22
Honey Nut Heaven, 1 cup, 1.7 oz	190	3.5	38
Multigrain, ½ cup	130	1.5	29
Old Fashioned Oats, ½ cup, 1.4 oz	150	3	27
Stone-Buhr Bran, ¼ cup, ½ oz	65	0	14
Sun Country Quick Oats, ½ c.,1.4 oz	130	1	30
Instant Oatmeal: *Per Package*			
Oatmeal Regular, 1 oz	100	2	19
Bakery Favorites, avg. all types	160	2	33
Breakfast Blast, avg. all flavors	155	2.5	32
Fruit and Cream, avg. all flavors	140	2.5	26
Low Sugar, avg. all flavors	115	2	23
Nutrition for Workers, avg. all flav.	165	2.5	33
Oatmeal Express, avg. all flavors	205	3	42
Supreme, avg. all flavors	160	3	32
Silver Palate Oatmeal, ⅓ c., 40g	160	2.5	28
Uncle Sam Oatmeal, 1.2 oz	145	3	24

Quick Guide

Cold Cereals

Average All Brands

	C	F	Cb
Bran Flakes, ¾ cup, 1 oz	**90**	0.5	21
Corn Flakes, 1 cup, 1 oz	**110**	0.5	24
Granola, ¼ cup, 1 oz	**130**	4	21
Oat Bran Cereal, ⅓ cup, 1 oz	**110**	1	22
Puffed Rice, 1 cup, ½ oz	**55**	0	12
Puffed Wheat, 1 cup, ½ oz	**55**	0	12
Raisin Bran, ½ cup, 1 oz	**85**	0.5	20
Rice Crisps, 1 cup, 1 oz	**110**	1	25
Shredded Wheat, 1 bisc., ¾ oz	**80**	0.5	18
Sugar-frosted Flakes, ¾ c, 1 oz	**110**	0.5	26
Wheat Flakes, 1 cup, 1 oz	**105**	0.5	23

Breakfast Bars: *See Page 137*

Ready-To-Eat Cereal

	C	F	Cb
Arrowhead Mills			
Amaranth, 1 c., 1.2 oz	**130**	1	23
Bran Flakes, 1 cup, 1 oz	**90**	1	18
Corn Flakes, 1 cup, 1.2 oz	**130**	0	30
Kamut Flakes, 1 cup, 1.1 oz	**110**	1	25
Maple Buckwheat Flake, 1 c., 1.5 oz	**160**	1	35
Multi Grain Flakes, 1 cup, 1.2 oz	**140**	1.5	29
Nature O's, 1 cup, 1.1 oz	**130**	2	24
Oat Bran Flakes, 1 cup, 1.2 oz	**140**	2.5	24
Perfect Harvest, 1 cup, 1.2 oz	**140**	2	25
Puffed Corn/Rice, avg., 1 c., 0.8 oz	**60**	0.5	12
Puffed Kamut, 1 cup, 0.6 oz	**50**	0	11
Puffed Millet/Wheat, 1 cup, 1 oz	**90**	0.5	19
Raisin Bran, 1 cup, 2 oz	**190**	1.5	40
Rice Flakes, 1 cup, 1.7 oz	**80**	1	19
Shredded Wheat, 1 cup, 2 oz	**200**	1	44
Spelt Flakes, 1 cup, 1.1 oz	**100**	1	22
Sweetened Nature O's, 1 c., 1.5 oz	**160**	2.5	31
Wild Wheat Flakes, 1 cup, 1.5 oz	**160**	0.5	37
Atkins			
Morning Start: Blueberry, ⅔ cup	**100**	2	10
Banana Nut Harvest, ⅔ c., 1 oz	**115**	2.5	11
Crunchy Almond Crisp, ⅔ cup	**105**	1.5	8
Back to Nature			
Flax and Fiber Crunch, 1 cup, 2.1 oz	**200**	3	41
Granola, ½ cup, 1.6 oz	**170**	3	34
Hi Fiber Multibran, ½ cup, 1 oz	**70**	0.5	22
Hi Protein Crunch, ½ cup, 1.6 oz	**150**	1	27
Muesli, ¾ cup, 2.3 oz	**230**	4	48
Barbara's Bakery			
Alpen Original, ⅔ cup, 1.9 oz	**200**	3	41
Breakfast O's, 1 ¼ cup	**130**	1.5	22
Brown Rice Crisps; Corn Flakes, 1 c.	**110**	0.5	25
Crispy Wheats/Soy Essence, ¾ cup	**115**	0.5	25
Fruity Punch; Puffins, ¾ cup, 1 oz	**120**	0.5	26
Grain Shop, ⅔ cup	**120**	1	24
Honey Crunch 'n Oats, ¾ cup, 1oz	**115**	1	24
Shredded Oats, 1¼ cup, 2 oz	**230**	2.5	46
Shred. Spoonfuls; Toasted O's, ¾ cup	**125**	1.5	24
Shredded Wheat, 2 bisc., 1.4 oz	**150**	1	31
Wild Puffs Caramel, ¾ cup, 1.1 oz	**110**	1	25
Breadshop			
Cranberry Crunch Muesli, 1 cup	**200**	3	44
Granola: Triple Berry Cr., ⅔ cup	**220**	7	36
Other varieties, avg., ½ cup	**220**	7.5	32
Bulk Cereal Nabisco - Malto Meal			
Apple Zings, 1 cup, 1.1 oz	**130**	1	30
Balance with Berries, 1 cup, 1.1 oz	**110**	0.5	26
Cocoa Roos/Dyno-Bites, ¾ c., 1 oz	**120**	1	27
Frosted Flakes, ¾ cup, 1.1 oz	**120**	0	28
Frosted Mini Spooners, 1 c., 1.9 oz	**190**	1	45
Golden Puffs, ¾ cup, 1 oz	**100**	0	25
Mateys/Toasty O's, 1 cup, 1 oz	**110**	1	25
Toasted Cinnamon Twists, ¾ c., 1 oz	**130**	3.5	24
CarbSense: *Per ½ Cup*			
MiniCarb Granola, Apple Cinnamon	**285**	15	29
Cascadian Farms			
Honey Nut O's, 1 cup, 1 oz	**120**	1.5	24
Multi-Grain Squares, ¾ c., 1 oz	**110**	0.5	25
Oats & Honey Granola, ⅔ c., 2 oz	**240**	6	42
Wheat Crunch, ¾ cup, 1 oz	**115**	0.5	25
Purely O's, 1 cup, 1.1oz	**110**	2	22
Hearty Morning, ¾ cup, 1.9 oz	**200**	2.5	43
Raisin Bran, 1 cup, 1.9 oz	**180**	1	43
Dr McDougall's: Muesli, 2.7 oz	**260**	3	51
Ener-G (Gluten-Free Cereals)			
Crisp Rice Cereal, 1 cup, 1.7 oz	**180**	2.5	40
Granola & Trail Mix, ½ cup, 1.8 oz	**260**	16	2
Rice Nuts, ½ cup, 50g	**190**	1	41
Erewhon			
Apple Stroodles, ¾ cup, 1 oz	**110**	0.5	25
Aztec, 1 cup, 1 oz	**110**	0	26
Banana O's, ¾ cup, 1 oz	**110**	0	26
Corn Flakes, 1¼ cups, 2 oz	**210**	2.5	45
Crispy Brown Rice, 1 cup, 1 oz	**110**	0	25
Fruit'n Wheat, ¾ cup, 1.9 oz	**170**	1.5	39
Kamut Flakes, ⅔ cup, 1.2 oz	**110**	0	25
Raisin Bran, 1 cup, 1.8 oz	**170**	1	40
Whole Wheat Flakes, 1 cup, 2 oz	**180**	1	42

Ready-To-Eat (Cont)

	C	F	Cb
General Mills (Big G)			
Basic 4, 1 cup, 1.9 oz	**200**	3	42
Boo Berry, 1 cup, 1 oz	**120**	1	27
Cheerios: Regular, 1 cup, 1 oz	**110**	1.5	21
Apple Cinnamon, ¾ c., 1 oz	**120**	2	25
Berry Burst, all types, 1 c., 1 oz	**110**	1.5	24
Frosted; Team, avg., 1 cup, 1 oz	**120**	1	25
Honey Nut, 1 cup, 1 oz	**120**	1.5	22
Multi-Grain, 1 cup, 1 oz	**110**	1	24
Chex: Corn, 1 cup, 1 oz	**105**	0.5	24
Frosted Mini Chex, ¾ cup, 1 oz	**110**	0	27
Honey Nut, 1 cup	**120**	1.5	22
Morning Mix, 1 pouch, 1.15 oz	**135**	3.5	24
Multi-Bran, 1 cup, 2 oz	**200**	1.5	49
Rice, 1¼ cup, 1 oz	**120**	0.5	24
Wheat, 1 cup, 2 oz	**180**	1	41
Cinnamon Grahams, ¾ cup, 1 oz	**120**	1	26
Cinnamon Tst Crunch, ¾ c., 1 oz	**130**	3.5	24
Cocoa Puffs, 1 cup, 1 oz	**120**	1	27
Cookie Crisp; Count Choc, 1 c., 1 oz	**120**	1	26
Fiber One, ½ cup, 1 oz	**60**	1	11
French Toast Crunch, ¾ c., 1 oz	**120**	1.5	25
Frosted Wheaties, 1 cup, 1.9 oz	**110**	0	27
Gold Medal Raisin Bran, 1 cup, 1.9oz	**180**	1	44
Golden Grahams, ¾ cup, 1 oz	**110**	1	24
Honey Nut Clusters, 1 cup, 2 oz	**210**	2	47
Kix: 1 cup, 1.9 oz	**120**	0.5	24
Berry Berry, ¾ cup, 1 oz	**120**	1.5	25
Lucky Charms, ¾ cup, 1 oz	**120**	1	23
Oatmeal Crisp Almond, 1 c., 2 oz	**220**	5	41
Raisin Nut Bran, ¾ cup, 2 oz	**200**	4	41
Reese's P'nut Butter Puffs, ¾ cup	**130**	3	24
Total: Brown Sugar & Oats, ¾ cup	**110**	0.5	23
Corn Flakes, 1⅓ cup, 1 oz	**110**	0	24
Protein, ¾ cup, 1 oz	**120**	3.5	11
Raisin Bran, 1 cup, 2 oz	**170**	1	41
Whole Grain, ¾ cup, 1 oz	**110**	1	23
Trix, avg., 1 cup, 1 oz	**120**	1	27
Wheaties: 1 cup, 1 oz	**110**	1	24
Energy Crunch, 1 cup, 1.95 oz	**210**	3	42
Hansen's Natural: *Per ½ Cup (2 oz)*			
Orange & Chocolate Cereal	**230**	9	35
Strawberry & Yogurt Cereal	**230**	9	30
Toasted Nut Crunch Cereal	**230**	6	39
Tropical Cluster Cereal	**210**	5	36

Health Valley	C	F	Cb
Corn Crunch-Ems!, 1 cup, 1 oz	**125**	0	27
Crunches & Flakes: Honey, ¾ cup	**135**	0	31
Other varieties, ¾ cup	**210**	3	41
Amaranth; Blue Corn Flakes, ¾ c.	**110**	0	24
Empower, 1 cup, 2 oz	**220**	3	42
Fiber 7 Flakes, ¾ cup	**110**	0	24
Granola, ⅔ cup	**200**	1	43
Golden Flax, ¾ cup	**205**	3	38
Healthy Fiber Flakes, ¾ cup	**105**	0	23
Heart Wise, 1 cup, 2 oz	**215**	3	36
Just Flakes, avg.	**110**	2	19
Oat Bran Flakes, avg., ¾ cup	**115**	0	26
Oat Bran O's, ¾ cup	**105**	0	23
Raisin Bran Flakes, 1 ¼ cup	**210**	0	47
Raisin Cinnamon Granola, ⅔ cup	**200**	1	43
Raisin Soy Flakes, 1 cup, 2 oz	**205**	1	39
Real Oat Bran Alm. Crunch, ½ cup	**185**	3	34
Rice Crunch-Ems!, 1 cup, 1 oz	**120**	0	26
Slender, 1 cup, 2 oz	**195**	1.5	35
Soy Flakes, 1¼ cup, 2 oz	**205**	1.5	35
Soy O's, 1 cup, 1.7 oz	**190**	2	31
Heartland Natural Cereal: *Per Cup*			
Granola Cereal: Original, ½ cup	**300**	11	41
Low-fat Raisin, ½ cup	**205**	3	4
Kashi: Breakfast Pilaf, ½ c., ckd	**170**	3	30
Cinna-Raisin Crunch, 1 c., 1.76 oz	**170**	1.5	41
GoLEAN Crunch!, 1 cup, 1.8 oz	**205**	3	36
Good Friends, 1 cup, 1.8 oz	**170**	2	43
Heart to Heart, ¾ cup, 1.2 oz	**110**	1.5	25
Honey Puffed Kashi, 1 cup, 1 oz	**120**	1	25
Kashi GoLEAN, 1 cup, 1.8 oz	**180**	1	30
Medley, ¾ cup, 1.1 oz	**100**	1	26
Organic Promise: Cranberry, 1 oz	**110**	1	26
Autumn Wheat, 1 cup, 1.9 oz	**190**	1	45
Strawberry Fields, 1 cup, 1.1 oz	**120**	0	28
Seven in the Morning, ½ cup, 2 oz	**210**	1.5	47
Puffed Kashi, 1 cup, 0.9 oz	**70**	0.5	13
Kellogg's: Apple Jacks, 1 c., 1 oz	**120**	0	30
All-Bran: ½ cup, 1 oz	**80**	1	24
Bran Buds, ⅓ cup, 1 oz	**80**	0.5	16
with Extra Fiber, ½ cup, 1 oz	**50**	1	20
Apple Cinn. Squares, ¾ c., 2 oz	**180**	1	44
Apple Raisin Crisp, ½ cup, 1 oz	**90**	0	23
Cinnamon Krunchers, ¾ cup	**130**	3.5	23
Cinn. M'mallow Scooby-Doo, ½ cup	**140**	4	25
Cinn. Mini Buns, ¾ cup	**120**	0.5	27

Kellogg's (Cont)	C	F	Cb
Complete Oatbran Flakes, ¾ cup	110	0.5	23
Wheatbran Flakes, ¾ cup	90	0.5	23
Cocoa Krispies, ¾ cup	120	1	27
Corn Flakes: 1 cup, 1 oz	110	0	24
Honey Crunch, ¾ cup, 1 oz	120	1	26
w. Real Bananas, ¾ cup	110	0	27
Corn Pops, 1 cup, 1 oz	120	0	28
Cracklin' Oat Bran, ¾ cup, 2 oz	190	7	35
Crispix: 1 cup, 1 oz	110	0	25
Cinnamon Crunch, ¾ cup, 1.1 oz	120	1	26
Finding Nemo, 1 cup, 1 oz	110	0.5	25
Froot Loops: 1 cup, 1.1 oz	120	0.5	27
Other types, avg., 1 cup, 1 oz	120	1	28
Frosted Flakes, ¾ cup, 1 oz	120	0	28
Fruit Harvest: Strawberry, ¾ c.	110	1.5	24
Apple Cinnamon, 1 cup, 1.8 oz	190	2.5	42
Hunny B's, 1 cup, 1 oz	110	1	25
Just Right, 1 cup, 2 oz	210	2	48
Low-fat Granola: ½ cup, 2 oz	190	3	39
w. Raisins, ⅔ cup, 2 oz	220	3	48
Mickey's Magix, 1 cup, 1 oz	110	0.5	25
Mini Wheats: Frosted, ¾ cup	180	1	41
Frosted Bite Size, 1 cup, 2 oz	200	1	48
Raisin Squares, ¾ cup, 1.8 oz	180	1	42
Strawberry Squares, ¾ c., 1.8 oz	170	1	40
Mud & Bugs, 1 cup, 1 oz	110	1	25
Müeslix, ¾ cup	200	5	39
Nutri-Grain, Golden Wheat, ¾ c.	100	1	23
Bars: *See Page 137*			
Product 19, 1 cup, 1 oz	100	0	25
Raisin Bran/Crunch, 1 cup, 2 oz	190	1.5	45
Rice Krispies: 1¼ cup	120	0	29
Fruity Marshmallow, ¾ cup	110	0	25
Treats, ¾ cup	120	1.5	26
Smacks, ¾ cup, 1 oz	100	0	24
Smart Start: Soy Protein, 1 cup	200	1.5	40
Original, 1 cup, 1.8 oz	180	0.5	43
Smorz, 1 cup, 1.1 oz	120	2	28
Special K: Regular, 1 cup, 1.1 oz	110	0	22
Red Berries, 1 cup, 1 oz	110	0	25
Vanilla Almond, ¾ cup, 1.1 oz	110	1.5	25
Low Carb Lifestyle, ¾ cup, 1.1 oz	100	3	14
Spider-Man, 1 cup, 1 oz	120	1	25
Sponge Bob Sq. Pants, 1 cup, 1 oz	120	1	26
Wheat Chex, 1 cup	170	1	38
Pop Tarts: Sponge Bob Sq. Pants	195	5	36
Fruit/Frosted, avg. all flavors	200	5	37
Low-fat, all flavors	190	3	39
Pastry Swirls, avg., 2.2 oz	260	11	37
Snak Stix, 1 pastry, 1.8 oz	200	5	36
Yogurt Blasts, 1 pastry	210	6	37
French Toast, 1 pastry	220	8	34

Mother's	C	F	Cb
Cinnamon Oat Crunch	245	3	48
Cocoa Bumpers, cup	130	0.5	29
Groovy Grahams; Round-Ups, ¾ cup	115	0.5	25
Peanut Butter Bumpers, cup	140	2.5	26
Toasted Oat Bran, ¾ cup	125	1.5	24
Nature's Path			
Corn Flakes, all types, ¾ cup, 1 oz	110	0	25
Eight Grain, ⅔ cup, 1 oz	100	1	23
Flax Plus, ¾ cup, 1 oz	100	1.5	22
Multigrain Oatbran, ⅔ cup, 1 oz	100	1	24
Pumpkin Flax Plus, ½ cup, 1 oz	140	6	19
Granola: Ginger Zing; Hemp, 1 oz	145	6	20
Avg. other varieties	125	3	22
Heritage, all types, ¾ cup, 1 oz	115	1	23
Heritage Muesli w. Raspberry, 1 oz	125	3	22
Honeyed Raisin Bran, ¾ cup, 1 oz	110	0.5	24
Optimum: Power Breakfast, 1 cup	190	2.5	40
Slim, 1 cup, 1.9 oz	180	2.5	38
Zen, ¾ cup, 1.9 oz	200	2.5	43
New England Natural Bakers			
Fat Free: Muesli, ½ cup	170	0	39
Granola: Almond Raisin Crisp, ½ c.	255	9	36
Apple Sunrise, ⅓ cup	195	6	30
Berry Good, ⅔ cup	255	6	44
Grateful Date, ½ cup	245	8	37
Honey Crunch; Pecan, ½ cup	295	13	37
Low-fat Granola, ½ cup	205	2.5	41
Marple Almond Date, ½ cup	285	11	39
Peachy Keen, ½ cup	215	7	33
Low-fat Granola, ½ cup	205	2.5	41
Save The Forest: Chocolate Mix	175	10	18
Fruit & Nut Mix	140	6	19
Nut Granola, ½ cup	275	12	35
Granola: Absolutely Nuts, ⅔ cup	225	9	30
Raspberry Razzmatazz, ½ c.	255	9	37
New Morning			
Cocoa Crispy Rice, ¾ cup, 1 oz	120	0.5	26
Cocomotion, ¾ cup, 1 oz	100	0.5	22
Kamutios, 1 cup, 1 oz	120	1	25
Oatios: Honey Almond, 1 cup, 1 oz	120	1	17
Original, 1 cup, 1 oz	120	1.5	24
Ultimate Oat Bran, ¾ cup, 1 oz	110	2	22
Nutritious Living			
Hi-Lo, all types, ½ cup, 1 oz	90	1.5	11
40-30-30 Honey Almd, ¾ c., 1.4 oz	150	5	17

Breakfast Cereals (Cont)

Post	C	F	Cb
100% Bran, ⅓ cup, 1 oz	**115**	1	22
Alpha Bits, cup, 1 oz	**135**	1.5	27
w. Marshmallows, cup, 1 oz	**120**	1	26
Bran Flakes, ¾ cup, 1 oz	**115**	0.5	24
Carb Well: Cinnamon Crunch, 1 oz	**120**	2	14
Golden Crunch, 1 oz	**110**	1	14
Cocoa Pebbles, ⅞ cup, 1 oz	**120**	1.5	25
Fruit & Bran, 1 cup, 2 oz	**210**	3	42
Fruity Pebbles, 1.25 cup, 1 oz	**110**	1	24
Golden Crisp, ½ cup, 1 oz	**110**	0	25
Grape-Nuts, ½ cup, 2 oz	**225**	1	47
Grape-Nuts Flakes, ½ cup, 1 oz	**115**	1	24
Grape-Nuts O's, cup, 1 oz	**120**	0	28
Honey Bunches of Oats, ¾ c., 1 oz	**120**	1.5	25
Honey-Comb Strawb. Blasted, c., 1 oz	**120**	1	26
Hulk w. Marshmallow Bits, cup, 1 oz	**110**	0	27
Oreo O's w. M'mallow Bits, ¾ c., 1 oz	**110**	2	22
Raisin Bran, ⅔ cup, 2 oz	**210**	1	46
Selects: Banana Nut Crunch, ½ c.	**250**	6	44
Blueberry Morning, cup, 2 oz	**240**	3.5	48
Cranberry Almond Crunch, c., 2 oz	**215**	3	43
Great Grains, Crunchy Pecan, ⅔ c.	**225**	6	38
Raisins Dates Pecans, ⅔ c.	**215**	4.5	39
Maple Pecan Crunch, ¾ cup, 2 oz	**225**	6	39
Shredded Wheat: Frosted, c., 1.8 oz	**195**	1	43
Honey Nut, cup, 1.8 oz	**205**	1.5	43
Original, cup, 1.7 oz	**195**	1	40
Shredded Wheat & Bran, 1.25 c.	**235**	1.5	48
Toasties Corn Flakes, cup, 1 oz	**105**	0	24
Waffle Crisp, cup, 1 oz	**130**	2.5	25
Quaker			
Ready to Eat Cereal:			
Oat Bran, 1¼ cup	**210**	3	41
100% Natural Granola: ½ cup	**220**	9	31
Low-fat, ⅔ cup	**210**	3	44
w. Raisins, ½ cup	**230**	9	34
Captain Crunch: Regular, ¾ c., 1 oz	**110**	2	23
Choco-Donuts, ¾ cup, 0.9 oz	**100**	1	23
Crunch Berries, ¾ cup, 1 oz	**110**	2	23
Peanut Butter Crunch, 1 oz	**110**	3	21
Crunchy Corn Bran, 1 cup, 1 oz	**90**	1	23
Honey Graham Oh's, ¾ cup	**110**	2	23
Life, all types, ¾ cup	**120**	1.5	26
Puffed Rice, 1 cup, ½ oz	**50**	0	12
Puffed Wheat, 1 ¼ cups, ½ oz	**50**	0	11
Shredded Wheat, 3 biscuits	**220**	1.5	50
Unprocessed Bran, ⅓ cup	**30**	0	11

Quaker (Cont)	C	F	Cb
Bagged Cereal: Cocoa Blasts, 1 cup	**130**	1	29
Apple Zaps; Fruitany O's, 1 cup	**120**	1	27
Frosted Flakers, ¾ cup	**120**	0	28
Frosted/Honey Nut Oats, 1 cup	**110**	1	24
Frosted Oats/ Sweet Crunch, 1 c.	**110**	1.5	23
Rice Crisps, 1 cup	**110**	0	26
Fruitangy Oh's, 1 cup	**120**	1	27
Honey Crisp Corn Flakes, ¾ cup	**110**	0	27
Honey Dipps, 1¼ cup	**130**	1.5	28
Instant Oatmeal: *See Page 94*			
Bars: *See Page 140*			
Sweet Home Farm			
Honey Nut Granola, ½ cup, 1.9 oz	**200**	7	34
Low-fat Granola, ½ cup, 1.9 oz	**180**	3	38
Maple Pecan Crisp, 1 cup, 1.9 oz	**220**	7	36
Trader Joe's			
10 & 10 Cereal, ¾ cup, 1.7 oz	**170**	3	31
Banana Nut Clusters, 1 cup, 1.9 oz	**220**	6	38
Blueberry Medley, ¾ cup, 1.7 oz	**200**	5	36
Corn Puffs Sweetened, 1 cup	**120**	0	28
Cornflakes, 1 cup, 1.1 oz	**110**	0	26
Cranberry Almd Clusters, 1 c., 2 oz	**220**	5	40
Crunch: Cherry Almond, 1 c., 2 oz	**210**	5	39
Van. Almd/Maple Pecan, 1 c., 2 oz	**220**	6	38
Essentials, 1 cup, 2 oz	**170**	3	37
Flakes n'Fruit, 1 cup, 1.1 oz	**120**	0.5	25
Frosted Flakes, ¾ cup, 1 oz	**110**	0	27
Golden Flax Cereal, ¾ cup, 1.7 oz	**190**	3	38
High Fiber Cereal, ⅔ cup, 1.1 oz	**90**	1	25
Honey Nut O's, ¾ cup, 1 oz	**120**	1.5	24
Joe's O's, 1 cup, 1 oz	**110**	2	22
More & Less Apple Cinn., ⅔ cup	**100**	1.5	12
Morning Lite, 1 cup, 1.4 oz	**140**	2	31
Muesli Cereal Blend, ¾ cup, 2 oz	**200**	1.5	42
Oat Bran Flakes, avg., 1 cup	**200**	1.5	45
Raisin Bran, 1 cup, 1.9 oz	**170**	1	44
Shred. Wheats, Bite Size, 1 c., 1.7 oz	**200**	1	42
Soy Granola, 1 cup, 1.9 oz	**220**	3	39
Touch of Honey, ⅔ cup, 1 oz	**120**	1.5	25
Triple Berry O's, ¾ cup, 1 oz	**110**	1	25
Toasted Oatmeal Flakes, ¾ c., 1.1 oz	**110**	1	23
Very Berry Clusters, 1 cup, 1.9 oz	**200**	4.5	36
Uncle Sam			
Cereal w. Real Mixed Berries, 55g	**230**	4.5	39
w. Flaxseed, 1 cup, 55g	**190**	5	38
Weetabix: 2 biscuits, 1.23 oz (35g)	**120**	1	28

Grains & Flours

Per ½ Cup (8 level Tbsp)	C	F	Cb
Amaranth, ½ cup, 3½ oz	350	6	60
Arrowroot, ½ cup, 2¼ oz	230	0	57
Atkins Bake Mix, low carb, 1 oz	115	2	6
Barley: Regular, ½ cup, 3¼ oz	325	2	56
Pearled, raw, 3½ oz	350	1	78
Flakes, ½ cup, 1½ oz	150	0.5	33
Buckwheat: Regular, ½ c., 3 oz	290	3	61
Groats, roasted, dry, 3 oz	285	2	60
Roasted, cooked, 3½ oz	90	0.5	19
Flour, whole-groat	200	2	42
Bulgur: Dry, ½ cup, 2½ oz	240	1	54
Cooked, ½ cup, 3¼ oz	75	0.5	17
Carob Flour, ½ cup, 1.8 oz	95	0.5	25
Corn Kernels (blue/yellow), 3 oz	300	4	66
Corn Bran, ½ cup, 1.4 oz	85	0.5	32
Corn Flour/Masa, 2 oz	210	2	44
Corn Grits: Dry, ½ cup, 2¾ oz	290	1	62
Cooked, ½ cup, 4¼ oz	75	0.5	16
Corn Germ, toasted	245	13	21
Cornmeal: Average All Types			
3 Tbsp, 1 oz	100	0.5	22
½ cup, 2.2 oz	220	2	46
Mixes: same as above	220	2	46
Cornstarch: 1 Tbsp, 8g	30	0	7
½ cup, 2¼ oz	230	0	57
Couscous: Dry, 3¼ oz	345	0	72
Cooked, 4.1 oz	60	0	12
Farina: Dry, 3 oz	325	0	70
Cooked, 4.1 oz	60	0	13
Flax Seeds: Seeds, 2 oz	280	20	22
Ground, 2 Tbsp	60	4.5	4
Flour: *See 'Wheat flour' Next Page*			
Garbanzo (Chick Pea), ½ c., 2 oz	200	3	35
Kuzu Root Starch, 1 Tbsp, 10g	35	0	8
Matzo Meal, ½ cup	260	1	55
Millet: Raw, ½ cup, 3½ oz	375	4	76
Cooked, ½ cup, 4¼ oz	145	1	29
Oat Bran: Raw, ⅓ cup	75	2	21
Cooked, ½ cup, 4 oz	40	1	11
Oats, rolled/oatmeal:			
Dry/Groats, ½ cup, 1.5 oz	155	3	28
Cooked, ½ cup, 4.2 oz	75	1	13
Polenta: *See Cornmeal*			
Made Up, ½ cup, 5 oz	220	2	24
Potato flour, ½ cup, 3.2 oz	315	0	72
Psyllium Husks, 1 Tbsp (5g)	10	0	2
Quinoa: Dry ½ cup, 3 oz	320	5	53
Cooked, ½ cup	105	1.5	17

Grains & Flours (Cont)

Per ½ Cup (8 level Tbsp)	C	F	Cb
Rice Bran, ⅓ cup, 1 oz	90	6	14
Rice Flour, ½ cup, 2¾ oz	290	2	63
Rice Polish, ½ cup	220	7	39
Rye Flour: Dark, 1 cup, 4½ oz	415	3.5	88
Medium, 1 cup, 3½ oz	360	2	79
Light, 1 cup, 3½ oz	375	1.5	82
Rye Grain: ½ cup, 3 oz	280	2	59
Flakes, ½ cup, 1½ oz	150	0.5	32
Semolina, ½ cup, 3 oz	305	1	61
Sorghum, ½ cup, 3.4 oz	325	3	72
Soybean Flakes, ½ cup, 1½ oz	190	8	14
Soy Bean Flour:			
Defatted, 1 cup, 3½ oz	330	1	34
Low-Fat, 1 cup, 3 oz	325	6	30
Full-Fat, 1 cup, 3 oz	370	18	27
Soy Meal, defatted, 1 cup, 4.3 oz	410	3	44
Spelt Flour, 1 cup	425	3.5	82
Tapioca, pearl, Dry: ½ c., 2.7 oz	260	0	67
3 Tbsp, 1 oz	100	0	26
Teff (Seed) Flour, 2 oz	200	0.5	41
Tortilla Flour Mix, ½ cup, 2 oz	225	12	37
Triticale: ½ cup, 3.4 oz	325	2	70
Flour, whole-grain, ½ cup	220	1	47
Wheat: Average, ½ cup, 3½ oz	320	2	28
Wheat Bran, unproc., ½ c., 1 oz	65	1	20
Wheat Flakes, ½ cup, 1½ oz	160	0.5	32
Wheat Germ: ¼ cup, 1 oz	105	3	15
Toasted, ¼ cup, 1 oz	108	3	14
Wheat Flour:			
White, All Purpose/Self-Rising,			
1 level Tbsp, 0.6 oz	55	0	12
½ cup, 2.1 oz	225	0.5	47
1 cup, 4.4 oz	450	1	95
Whole Wheat, 1 cup, 4.2 oz	410	2	87

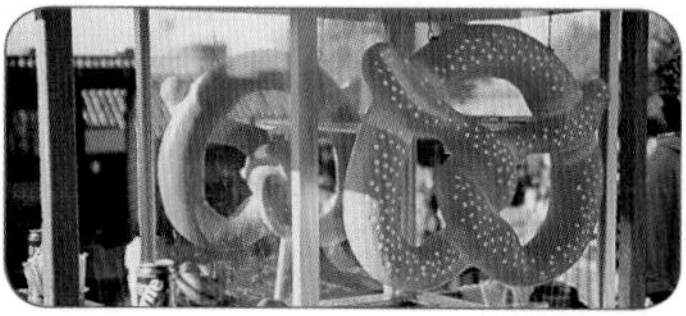

Rice

White Rice

	C	F	Cb
Raw: Short/Med. Grain, 1 c., 7 oz	**720**	1	156
Long Grain, 1 cup, 6½ oz	**670**	1	144
Glutinous, 1 cup, 6½ oz	**680**	1	150
Cooked Rice (Boiled/Steamed/Hot):			
Short/Medium Grain:			
½ cup, 3¼ oz	**120**	0	27
1 cup (½ Pint), 6½ oz	**240**	0.5	54
2 cups (1 Pint), 13 oz	**480**	1	108
Long Grain: ½ cup, 2¾ oz	**100**	0	22
1 cup, 5½ oz	**200**	0.5	44
Glutinous/Sticky, ckd, 1 c., 6 oz	**170**	0.5	36
Parboiled, cooked, ½ cup, 3 oz	**90**	0	20
Precook./Instant: Dry,½ c., 3½ oz	**370**	0	80
Cooked, ½ cup, 3 oz	**90**	0	20
Wild Rice: Raw, 1 cup, 5½ oz	**570**	13	120
Cooked, 1 cup, 5¾ oz	**165**	0.5	35

Brown Rice

	C	F	Cb
Average of Short or Long Grain			
Raw/Dry: ½ cup, 3½ oz	**350**	2.5	72
1 cup, 7 oz	**700**	5	144
Cooked: ½ cup, 3½ oz	**110**	0.5	23
1 cup, 7 oz	**220**	1.5	46

Rice Dishes

	C	F	Cb
Chinese Fried Rice:			
½ cup, 2½ oz	**160**	5	21
1 cup, 5 oz (½ Pint)	**320**	13	42
2 cups, 10 oz (1 Pint)	**640**	26	84
Mexican Rice: 1 cup	**500**	12	90
Taco John's, 1 serving (6 oz)	**250**	5	44
Taco Time, 1 serving (4 oz)	**150**	2	30
Rice-A-Roni: *See Page 74*			
Rice Pilaf: Restaurant, 1 cup	**270**	7.5	43
Boston Market, 1 cup	**140**	4	24
Rice w. Raisins/Pinenuts, 1 cup	**400**	11	70
Risotto, 1 cup	**420**	18	65
Saffron Rice, 1 cup	**370**	12	66
Spanish Rice: 1 cup	**390**	9	72
El Pollo Loco, small serving	**155**	1	33
Taco Cabana, 4 oz	**180**	5	30
Sticky Thai Rice, plain, 1 cup	**170**	0.5	36
Sushi Rice, 1 Tbsp	**25**	0	6
Uncle Ben's: *See Page 67*			

- Macaroni includes all shapes and sizes; (e.g. spaghetti, fettuccini, shells, tubes, ziti, twists, sheets, cannelloni, manicotti, elbows).
- All regular macaroni products have the same cals/fat/carb. on a weight basis.
- 1 oz Dry = approx. 2½ -3 oz cooked.

Dry Spaghetti/Macaroni

	C	F	Cb
1 oz quantity	105	0.5	21
1lb box/pkg., 16 oz	1680	7	336
Elbows, 1 cup, 3¾ oz	395	2	77
Shells, small, 1 cup, 3¼ oz	340	2	66
Spirals, 1 cup, 3 oz	315	2	61

Cooked Spaghetti/Macaroni

	C	F	Cb
Plain, All Types (no added fat):			
Firm/Al Dente (8-10 mins.), 1 oz	42	0.5	8.5
Medium (11-13 mins.), 1 oz	37	0.5	7.5
Tender (14-20 mins.), 1 oz	32	0.5	7
(Longer cooking increases water absorbed)			
Spaghetti, ½ cup, 2 ½ oz	90	0.5	18
Medium serving, 1 cup, 5 oz	185	1	37
Large (restaurant), 2 c., 10 oz	370	2	74
Elbows/Spirals, 1 cup, 5 oz	185	1	38
Small Shells, 1 cup, 4 oz	150	0.5	31
Protein-fortified: Dry, 1 oz	107	0.5	21
Cooked, 1 cup, 5 oz	230	0.5	44
Spinach/Vegetable: Dry, 1 oz	105	0.5	21
Cooked, 1 cup, 5 oz	180	0.5	37
Whole-wheat: Dry, 1 oz	100	0.5	21
Cooked, 1 cup, 5 oz	175	0.5	37

Fresh Pasta (Refrigerated)

	C	F	Cb
Plain/Spinach/Tomato, average:			
As purchased, 4 oz	325	2.5	64
Cooked, 1 cup, 5 oz	190	1	38
Home-made, without egg:			
Cooked, 1 cup, 5 oz	175	1	35
Buitoni			
Pasta: Angel Hair, 9 oz	230	2.5	43
Fettuccine/Linguini: 9 oz	240	2.5	45
Spinach, 9 oz	260	3	45

Buitoni (Cont):	C	F	Cb
Ravioli: Chicken Parmesan, 9 oz	310	8	45
Four Cheese, 9 oz	330	14	40
Light, 9 oz	230	4	37
Garden Vegetable, 9 oz	250	5	39
Beef Ravioletti, 7 oz	300	7	46
Roast Chicken & Garlic, 9 oz	340	11	47
Tortellini: Cheese & Rst Garlic, 9 oz	270	8	37
Chicken & Prosciutto, 9 oz	330	9	47
Herb Chicken, 9 oz	340	9	52
Mozzarella & Pepperoni, 9 oz	330	10	45
Mushroom & Cheese, 9 oz	270	6	46
Sundried Tomato, 9 oz	310	9	46
Sweet Italian Sausage, 9 oz	330	9	48
Three Cheese, 9 oz	320	7	50

Pasta Sauces: *See Page 86*

Noodles

	C	F	Cb
Plain/Egg: Dry, 1 oz	108	1	20
1 cup, 1⅓ oz	145	1.5	28
Cooked, 1 oz	38	0.5	7
½ cup, 2¾ oz	105	1	20
1 cup, 5½ oz	210	2	40
Stir-Fried: 1 cup, 5½ oz	270	9	40
2 cup serving, 11 oz	540	18	80
Yolk Free (Cooked): *Per Cup*			
'No Yolks' *(Foulds)*	210	2	40
Passover Gold *(Manischewitz)*	200	0	42
Chinese: Cellophane/Rice, dry, 1 oz	100	0	25
Chow Mein/hard, dry, 1 oz	150	5	17
Ramen Noodles: *See Page 74*			
Japanese: Soba, dry, 1 oz	95	0.5	21
cooked, 1 cup, 4 oz	110	0.5	24
Somen, dry, 1 oz	100	0.5	22
cooked, 1 cup, 6 oz	225	0.5	49
Japanese Style Pan Fried:			
Maruchan's Yaki-Sobu, 5.6 oz cup	260	3	50
Udon *(Chikara)*, avg., 7.5 oz pkt	250	1	52
Stir Fry *(Yakisoba)*, 3.5 oz serving	220	2	44
Thai Kitchen: *See Page 75, 83*			

Egg Roll Skins/Won Ton

	C	F	Cb
Egg Roll Skins:			
(Golden Dragon) 1 pce, 1 oz	80	0	18
(Wung Hung) 4 skins, 4 oz	300	0	64
Won Ton Wrappers:			
(Dynasty) 10 wrappers, 2.1 oz	170	1	36
Egg Roll/Spring Roll Wrapper:			
(Dynasty) 3 wrappers, 2.1 oz	170	1	36

Breads

Note: Most breads have similar calories on a weight basis. However, volume may vary.

For example, 1 oz of bread may equal 1 slice regular bread or 2 slices of a lighter bread.

It is best to weigh bread used and calculate on 1 oz bread = 70 calories.

Quick Guide

Bread

Average All Varieties:	C	F	Cb
Thin slice (¼") 1 oz	70	1	13
Extra thin slice ¾ oz	55	0.5	10
Light thin slice, 0.6 oz	40	0.5	7.5
Toasting slice, 1.2 oz	85	1	16
Thick slice (⅜"), 1.5 oz	105	1.5	20
Large thick (½"), 2 oz	140	2	26
1-lb Loaf, 16 oz	1120	6	208
Toast has same calories as bread used.			
1 Toasting Slice:			
w. 2 tsp fat spread	175	10	16
w. 2 tsp "light" spread	120	5	16
w. 1 Tbsp fat spread	185	12	16
w. 1 Tbsp "light" spread	135	7	16

Breads

	C	F	Cb
12-Grain, 1½ oz slice	120	1.5	23
Batard (8 oz), thick slice, 2 oz	140	0.5	28
Boule, ½" thick, 2 oz slice	130	0	29
Bran style/Dark, 1 oz slice	70	1	14
Bread w. Soy Isoflavones, 1.2 oz	80	2	11
Buttermilk, average, 1½ oz slice	120	1.5	24
Caraway Rye, 1 oz slice	70	0	15
Challah, 1 oz slice	85	2	14
Chapati, 2.2 oz	200	7.5	30
Ciabatta, 1 slice, 0.7 oz	50	0.5	10
Corn Bread, average, 1 pce, 3 oz	180	7	30
Cracked Wheat Sourdough, 1½ oz	130	0.5	27
Croissants: *See Page 113, 173*			
Crustless Bread, regular slice ¾ oz	40	0.5	8.5
Crusts Only, regular slice, ¼ oz	30	0	7
Date & Nut, 1 oz slice	90	1	14
'Enriched' Breads, average, 1 oz sl.	75	1	18
Flax & Sunflower Round, 1.2 oz	90	2	18
Foccacia: Plain, 2 oz portion	150	4	23
Cheese & Garlic; Pesto, 2 oz	170	8	21
Tomato & Olive, 2 oz	120	2	20
French Stick/Baguette, 1 oz slice	70	1	15

Breads (Cont)

	C	F	Cb
French Toast, 1 slice, 2¼ oz	160	7	18
Sticks *(Aunt Jemima)*, 1 pce, 1 oz	75	3	12
Garlic Bread/Toast:			
Small slice + 1 tsp spread, ¾ oz	80	5	7
Med. slice + 2 tsp spread, 1½ oz	160	10	14
Thick slice + 3 tsp spread, 1.8 oz	220	14	20
Pepperidge Farm, 1 slice, 1.4 oz	160	10	15
Hemp Bread, 1.2 oz	95	2	12
Italian Bread, 1 oz slice	75	1	15
Light Bread, avg., 0.8 oz slice	40	0.5	8
Lower Carb (higher Protein/fiber),			
average all brands, 1 oz	60	1	7
Melba Toast, 2 pces	25	0	6
MultiGrain: 1 slice, 1 oz	75	1	14
Nut/Health Nut, 1 oz slice	85	2	15
Oatmeal/Oatbran Bread, 1 oz sl.	70	1	13
Party Breads *(Pepp. Farm):* Rye, 1 sl.	15	0.5	3
Dijon; Pumpernickel, 1 sl.	18	0.5	3.5
Pita: Average all types,			
Small (4" diam) 1 oz	75	0.5	15
Large (6½" diam) 2 oz	150	1	30
Extra Large (9" diam) 4 oz	300	1.5	60
Popovers (1), no butter	90	2	14
Poppyseed (Vienna), 0.8 oz sl.	55	1	10
Pumpernickel, 1 oz slice	75	1	15
Cocktail size, 0.4 oz	30	0.5	6
Raisin Bread, 1 oz slice	80	1.5	15
Raisin Walnut, 2 oz slice	160	3.5	29
Roman Meal, 1 oz slice	70	1	14
Country Potato & Oat, 1½ oz	110	1.5	20
Rye: Average, 1 thin slice, 1 oz	75	1	13
1 thick slice, 2 oz	150	2	25
Cocktail size, 0.4 oz	25	0.5	4
Sandwich Bread, 1 oz slice	70	1	13
Sandwich Pockets, Reg., 2 oz	150	1	30
Sourdough, 1½ oz slice	100	1	20
Sourdough French, 1 oz	75	0	14
Spelt, 1.2 oz	90	3	14
Sprouted 7-Grain, 1.5 oz slice	110	1.5	18
Squaw, 1.1 oz slice	85	0.5	13
Tacos/Tortillas: *See Page 104*			
Turkish/Middle Eastern, 1 oz sl.	80	1.5	16
Wheat-Free Breads: Spelt, 1.2 oz	70	0	14
Healthseed Rye, 1.6 oz	90	1	20
Kamut, 1.2 oz	80	0	16
Millet, 1.5 oz	100	1	20

Bread Brands

	C	F	Cb
Ener-G: Gluten-Free Breads			
Brown Rice Bread, 1 slice, 38g	130	6	18
Light Brown Rice, 1 slice, 19g	70	4	9
Corn Loaf, 1 slice, 19g	40	2.5	8
Light Tapioca, 1 slice, 19g	70	3	10
Nature's Path: *Per Slice (2 oz)*			
Manna: Carrot Raisin	130	0	27
Cinnamon Date	150	0	29
Fruit & Nut	140	1	27
Millet Rice	130	0	28
Sun Seed	160	2	29
Whole Rye	150	0	32
Whole Wheat; Multigrain	125	0	26
Orowheat			
100% Whole Wheat, Light, 1 slice	48	0.5	9
Carb Counting, 1 slice, 1 oz	65	1.5	9
Pepperidge Farm: *Per Slice*			
100% Whole Wheat	85	1	15
Apple Walnut Swirl	80	2	14
Golden Swirl	95	2	15
Hearty 7-Grain	100	2	18
Light Style, average	45	0	9
Raisin w. Cinnamon	85	2	14
Pillsbury			
Popovers: Perfect (1), 1/10 container	95	2	14
Original, w. skim milk, butter & eggwhites (1), 1/6 container	95	0	18
Original, w. whole milk & whole eggs (1), 1/6 container	140	5	18
Sara Lee: *Per Slice*			
Delightful White, ¾ oz	50	0.5	9
Honey Wheat, 1 oz	60	0.5	11
Multi-Grain, 1.4 oz	100	1	19
Round Top, 1 oz	65	0.5	13
Sandwich, ¾ oz	60	0.5	11
Schwan's: *Per Serving*			
Cheese & Herb Biscuits (1), 34g	110	6	11
Chse Stuffed Bread w. Sauce, 56g	155	5	20
Five Chse Garlic French Bread (1), 96g	330	20	26
French Baguette Bread, ¼ loaf, 49g	120	0	25
French Dinner Rolls (1), 51g	130	1.5	24
Frozen Bread Dough, 1/8 loaf, 56g	140	1.5	27
Southern Style Biscuits (1), 62g	200	10	23
Wonder: Sandwich, 1 slice, 1.1 oz	80	1	15
Light (Low-Fat), 1 slice, ¾ oz	40	0	9

Bread Rolls & Buns

	C	F	Cb
Brown 'n Serve, average, 1 oz	80	2	15
Carb Monitor *(Pillsbury),* 1.1 oz roll	70	2	11
Ciabatta Roll, 3½ oz	230	4	41
Concha (Mexican Sweet Bread), 3 oz	400	19	50
Dinner Rolls: 1 small, 1 oz	85	2	15
1 medium (3" diam),1½ oz	130	3	23
English Muffins, avg., 2 oz	140	2	27
Frankfurter/Hot Dog: 1¼ oz	100	2	19
1½ oz size	120	2	23
French: 1 medium, 1.3 oz	110	1	24
1 large, 3 oz	240	2	52
Hamburger: Regular, 1½ oz	120	2	23
Large, 3 oz	240	4	46
Hoagie/Submarine, 4¾ oz	400	8	77
Hot Cross Bun, Medium, 2.3 oz	185	5	31
Kaiser Roll, 2 oz size	170	3	18
Onion Roll, 2 oz size	170	2	20
Parker House Roll, 0.7 oz size	65	1	12
Party Roll, 0.6 oz	55	1	10
Sandwich Roll, 1.6 oz size	120	2	23
Soft Pretzel Bun *(J & J),* 3 oz	235	3	50
Sourdough Roll, 1¼ oz	100	1	18
Sweet Rolls, 1 oz	100	2	20
w. Icing, average	160	6	20
Wheat Roll: Small, 1 oz	75	0.5	14
Medium, 1½ oz	110	1	20

Breadsticks, Croutons

	C	F	Cb
Breadsticks: *Boboli,* 1.75 oz	130	2	22
Stella D'oro: Sesame (1)	50	2	7
Plain/Onion/Wheat, 1 pce	40	1	7
Keebler/Lance, 2 sticks	30	0.5	6
Salt Sticks, plain, 1 oz	110	1	20
Fresh baked (1), 2 oz	180	2.5	34
Croutons: Seasoned, 2 Tbsp, ¼ oz	35	1.5	4
9 small or 6 large, ¼ oz	35	1.5	4
Fat-Free *(Pepp. Farm),* 2 Tbsp	30	0	5

Bread Products

	C	F	Cb
Bread Crumbs, dry:			
Plain or seasoned, 1 oz	110	1	20
1 rounded Tbsp, 10g	35	0.5	6
1 cup, 3½ oz	390	5	73
Corn Flake Crumbs, 1 oz	110	1	20
Graham Cracker Crumbs, 1 oz	115	1	21
Keebler, 1 cup, 4¼ oz	520	14	84
Bread Dough: Frozen, 1 slice	75	0.5	14
Refrigerated, French, 1" slice	60	1	13
Wheat/White, 1" slice	80	2	14
Coating Mixes: Average, 1 oz	110	3	20
Featherweight, 1.4 oz pkg	70	0.5	17
Stuffing: Average, dry mix, 1 oz	110	1	10
Made-up, ½ cup, 4 oz	180	9	11

Bagels • Tacos • Rice Cakes

Quick Guide

Bagels	C	F	Cb
Average All Brands			
Plain/Onion:			
1 mini/bagelette, 1 oz	**80**	1	15
1 small bagel, 2 oz	**160**	1.5	30
1 medium bagel, 3 oz	**240**	2	45
1 large bagel, 4 oz	**320**	3	60
Bagel Chips (New York Style),			
4 slices, ¾ oz	**90**	2	17
Pizza Bagel, 6 oz each	**380**	7	60
Bagel Bites *(Ore-Ida)*, 4 pces	**190**	7	25
Bagel Crisps *(Burns Ricker)*, 1 oz	**150**	9	28

Bagel Brands

Amy's Kitchen, average, 3½ oz	**235**	2	50
Awrey's, 2.7 oz each	**190**	0.5	42
Bruegger's Bagels: *See Fast-Foods Section*			
Cosco Bakery: Plain, 4 oz	**300**	1	61
Everything, 4 oz	**330**	3.5	62
Einstein Bros: *See Fast-Foods Section*			
Enjoy Life, all types, 3.2 oz	**270**	6	50
Lenders, all flavors, 3.6 oz	**280**	3	55
Oroweat: Oatmeal, 3.4 oz	**270**	4	49
Multi-Grain, 3.4 oz	**260**	1.5	51
Sara Lee: Mini, average, 1 oz	**70**	0	15
Toaster Size, all types, 2.2 oz	**165**	0.5	34
3.4 oz Size (95g): Plain	**255**	1	52
Other flavors, 3.4 oz	**260**	1	55
4 oz Size (113g): Honey	**310**	2	61
Apple Cinnamon	**310**	1.5	64
Banana Walnut	**350**	7	61
Cranberry Orange	**310**	1.5	64
Sun Dried Tomato Basil	**300**	1.5	61
Western: All flavors, avg., 3 oz	**230**	1	47
Bagel Sandwiches: *See Page 173*			

Bagel Spreads

Cream Cheese:			
Plain: 2 Tbsp, 1 oz	**80**	8	2
2 oz mini-tub	**160**	16	4
Reduced Fat: 2 Tbsp, 1 oz	**60**	5	2
2 oz mini-tub	**120**	10	4
Flavors: Lox, 1 oz	**75**	6	1
Raisin Walnut, 1 oz	**90**	6	8
Strawberry, 1 oz	**60**	3	7
Sundried Tomato, 1 oz	**80**	7	2
Vegetable, 1 oz	**60**	6	1

Rice Cakes

	C	F	Cb
Average All Types/Brands:			
Regular size, 1 cake, 9g	**35**	0	7.5
Hain, Mini, average, 3g each	**12**	0.5	2
Lundberg, all types, 15g each	**60**	0.5	14
Quaker: Large, all flavors, 13g each	**50**	0	11
Crispy Mini's, average, 15g	**70**	2	12
Westbrae, 1 cake, 7g	**25**	0	5

Taco Shells & Tortillas

Tacos: Mini Size (1)	**25**	1.5	2
Regular size, all types (1)	**55**	3	6
Super Size (1)	**90**	4	11
Salad Shell, flour *(Azteca)*, 1.4 oz	**180**	11	19
Tortilla (Soft Taco), each	**85**	2	15
Corn Tortilla: 6", 1.2 oz each	**45**	0.5	9
Flour Tortilla: each, 1.75 oz	**160**	3	28
Low-fat	**110**	1.5	22
Burritos, 1 tortilla, 2.3 oz	**190**	5	32
Low-fat	**110**	1.5	22
Tostada Shells, each	**55**	3	6
La Tortilla Factory			
Fat Free Flour Tortillas:			
Burrito size, 2.5 oz	**165**	0.5	34
Soft Taco, 1.8 oz	**110**	0	24
Low Carb Low-fat Tortillas:			
Large, 1.26 oz	**135**	3	19
Original; Flavors, 1.26 oz	**80**	2	11
Mission Foods			
Low Carb Flour Tortilla: 6"	**50**	2	5
8" Tortilla	**70**	2.5	7
Low Carb Whole Wheat Tortilla: 6"	**45**	2	4
10" Tortilla	**110**	4.5	10
Wraps, average, 10"	**205**	5	34

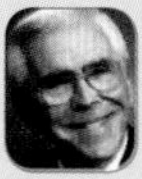

Rev. Dr Robert Schuller

'Inch by inch Life's a cinch'

'You'll never win If you don't begin!'

Crispbreads

Per Crispbread/Cracker	C	F	Cb
Ak-Mak: Sesame, 5 crackers, 1 oz	35	0	7
Finn Crisp: Original, rye,1	35	0	7
Other types,1	19	0	3
Kavli Norwegian: Thin,1	17	0	3
Thick,1	20	0	3
Malsovit Meal Wafers,1	75	4	7
New York Flatbread Crisps, 1	35	0	7
Ry-Krisp: Natural, 1 crispbread	20	0	3
Seasoned,1	30	0	5
Sesame,1	25	1	3
Ryvita: Dark/Light, 1 piece	26	0	4
WASA: Breakfast; Sesame	50	0	9
Extra Crisp; Light Rye	25	0	5
Fiber Plus	40	1	7.5
Hearty Rye	45	0	9
Organic Rye; Soya	25	0	7
Sourdough Flatbread, 3	50	0	11
Sourdough Rye	35	0	7
Westbrae Rice Wafers (7), 15g	50	0	11

Matzos

Manischewitz			
American Matzos, 1 board, 1 oz	115	2	22
Passover Matzos, 1 board, 1.1 oz	130	0	27
Passover Egg Matzos, 1.1 oz	130	2	27
Egg 'n Onion Matzo, 1 oz	112	1	23
Thin Salted Tea Matzos, 0.9 oz	100	0	21
Unsalted; Whole Wheat, 1 oz	110	0	24
Dietetic Matzo Thins, 0.83 oz	90	0	19
Crackers: Miniatures, 1 cracker	9	0	20
Passover Egg Matzo, 1 cracker	11	0	20
Matzo Meal, 1 cup, 4¾ oz	515	2	110
Matzo Farfel, 1 cup, 2.7 oz	180	0.5	60
Grape Matzo, 1 oz each	110	0	25

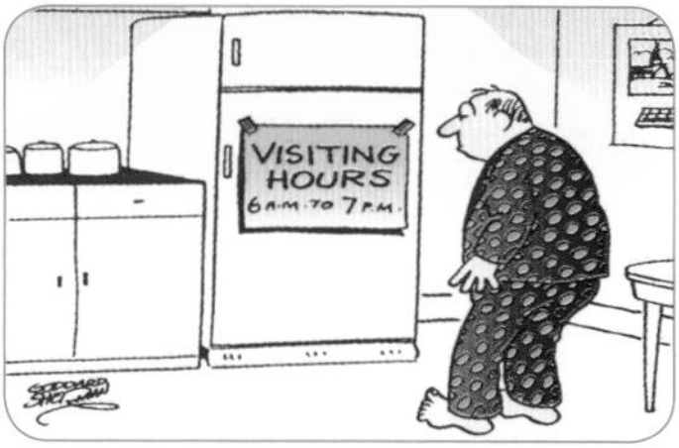

Quick Guide

Crackers

Average All Brands: Per Cracker	C	F	Cb
Cheese Crackers: Plain, 1" square	5	0	0.5
Small, octagonal	10	0	1
Round (2" diam.)	15	0	1.5
Sandwich (Peanut Butter)	35	1	4
Graham, 2½" square,1 cracker	30	0.5	5
Melba Toast, plain, 1 piece	20	0	4
Oyster & Soup Crackers, ¼ oz (40 small oysters/20 lge hexagons)	60	2	10
Rice Crackers: 1 small	9	0	2
Rice Snax *(Amsnack)*, ½ oz	60	1	12
Saltines, 2 crackers	25	1	4.5
Snack-type, 1 round cracker	15	0	3
Soda, 1 cracker, ½ oz	60	2	10
Water Cracker *(Carr's)*, regular, 1	32	0	7
Small, 1 cracker	14	0	4
Wheat, thin, 1 cracker	9	0	1
Zweiback Toast, 1 piece	30	0	5

Quick Guide

Cookies

Average All Brands: Per Cookie	C	F	Cb
Biscotti: Small, 0.5 oz	65	2.5	10
Regular, 1 oz	130	5	20
Chocolate Chip Cookies:			
Small/Thin 0.5 oz	55	3	7
Regular, 1 oz	110	6	15
Large, 2.3 oz *(Mrs Field's)*	280	13	38
Jumbo, 4 oz	450	22	64
Oatmeal/Oatmeal Raisin:			
Small/Thin 0.5 oz	50	1.5	8
Regular, 1 oz	95	3.5	15
Large, 2.3 oz *(Mrs Field's)*	280	12	39
Jumbo, 4 oz	380	14	62
Peanut Butter:			
Small/Thin 0.5 oz	60	3	7
Regular, 1 oz	125	6.5	14
Large, 2.3 oz (Mrs Field's)	310	16	34
Jumbo, 4 oz	500	25	54
Low-fat Cookies			
Choc Chip (Low-fat), 1 oz (1)	100	1	21
Oatmeal Raisin (Fat-free), 1 oz (1)	90	0	20
Peanut Butter (Low-fat), 1 oz (1)	105	2	14

Brands	C	F	Cb
Per Cookie/Cracker (Unless Indicated)			
Archway			
Coconut Macaroon	100	6	12
Apple/Date-filled Oatmeal	100	3	16
Apricot/Strawb.-filled Oatmeal	100	3.5	16
Frosty Lemon/Orange	110	4.5	17
Ginger Snaps: Regular/Iced (5)	150	5	23
Reduced Fat (5)	140	3.5	25
Lemon Snaps (5)	150	7	20
Molasses	100	3	18
Oatmeal: Regular; Raisin	110	3.5	17
Iced	120	5	19
Peanut Butter; Pecan Icebox	120	6	15
Peanut Butter Choc	150	7	17
Sugar Cookies (1)	100	3	16
Bed & Breakfast Crispy Classics:			
Chocolate Chunk Pecan	145	9	15
Coconut Macaroon	105	5	14
Dutch Cocoa; Oatmeal	110	3.5	18
Fruit Filled Apple Oatmeal	90	3	15
Pecan Shortbread	150	10	14
White Choc. & Macadamia	140	8	16
Windmill	90	3.5	14
Fat-Free: Oatmeal Raisin (1)	110	0	25
Devil's Food Cookie (1)	70	0	16
Atkins			
Cookies; Crackers, avg. all	140	9	10
Meringue Cookies, avg. all flav. (1)	5	0	1
Sesame; Whole Wheat, crackers (2)	45	3	4
Austin			
Crackers: *Per Package*			
50% More Peanut Butter S'wich	250	14	25
Cheddar/Peanut Butter Chse S'wich	200	10	24
Dolphins Snacks	120	5	16
Cheese w. Cheddar Jack S'wich	195	10	23
Sandwich Crackers: Grilled Cheese	195	10	23
PB & J	200	10	24
Toasty Crackers: Peanut Butter	200	10	23
Reduced Fat	175	7	25
Wheat Crackers: Cheddar	200	10	24
Reduced Fat	175	7	25
Zoo Animal Crackers (16)	125	2	25
Baker's: *Per Cookie (3.5 oz)*			
Peanut Butter	355	10	55
Peanut Butter & Jelly	345	8	60
Vegan Peanut But. Choc. Chunk	380	10	60
Other varieties, average	320	6	58
Barbara's Bakery			
Cookies: Fig Bars, avg. (1)	60	15	14
Animal Cookies, Vanilla (8)	120	4.5	18
Crisp Cookies; average (1)	75	4	9
Snackimals, avg. (10)	115	4	18
Crackers: Cheese Bites (22), 1 oz	120	3	20
Organic Go Go Grahams (8), 1 oz	130	4	22
Rite Lite Rounds, avg. (5)	65	2	11
Wheatines, average all varieties	55	1	11
Brent & Sam's			
Cookies: Chocolate Chip (2)	130	6	18
Chocolate Chip Pecan (2)	145	8	16
Key Lime White Chocolate (2)	135	6	19
Raspberry Chocolate (2)	125	6	17
White Choc. Macadamia (2)	145	8	17
Carr's			
Crackers: Table Water (5)	70	1.5	13
Monterey: Hearty Wheat (3)	60	2	9
Savory/Sesame (3)	70	3	9
Entertainer; Whole Wheat (2)	80	3.5	11
Cocktail, Croissant Orig. Gold (22)	140	3	21
Cookies: Bisc. for Tea (2)	140	6	20
Choccines (3)	150	9	16
Ginger Lemon Cremes (2)	140	7	19
Hob Nobs (2)	140	6	19
Imperials: Milk Chocolate (2)	140	7	18
Dark Choc (2)	150	7	19
Milk Choc & Creme	140	7	18
Petites Bijoux (4)	140	5	21
Cookies &			
M&M's (1)	170	9	20
Milky Way (1); Snickers (1)	180	11	21
Peanut Butter (1)	150	9	17
Twix (1)	180	10	21
Country Choice			
Cookies: Ginger Snaps, (5)	125	5	19
Sandwich Cremes, (2)	125	5	19
Soft Baked: Peanut Butter	105	5	13
Avg. other varieties	100	4	16
Vanilla Wafers, (7)	125	5	19
Dr Soy: Average (2)	85	2	5
Entenmann's			
Soft Baked: Milk/Choc Chip	100	5	13
Gourmet English Toffee	100	5	13
White Choc Macadamia Nut (1)	100	6	12
Estee			
Chocolate Chip; Fudge Cookies	40	2	5
Coconut Cookies, Oatmeal Raisin	35	1.5	5
Fig Bars, each	50	0.5	11
Sandwich Cookies	55	2	6
Shortbread; Vanilla; Lemon	35	1.5	5

Per Cookie/Cracker (Unless Indicated)

Famous Amos	C	F	Cb
Choc Chip (4)	**150**	7	20
Choc Chip & Pecan (4)	**150**	8	19
Chocolate Creme Sandwich (1)	**55**	2	8
Oatmeal Choc Chip & Walnut (4)	**150**	7	19
Oatmeal Raisin (4)	**140**	5	21
Low-fat: Gingersnaps	**205**	3	41
Lemonsnaps	**205**	2.5	42
Frookie			
Cookies, average all types	**45**	2	7
Animal Frackers	**10**	0.3	1.5
Frookwich, avg. all varieties (3)	**155**	6	23
Fruitins, Apple; Fig	**60**	1	12
Large Frooks, all types	**120**	4	18
Wafers, Fat Free (8)	**100**	0	24
Grandma's			
Peanut Butter Sandwich Creme (5)	**215**	10	28
Rich 'N Chewy, Choc Chip, pkg.	**270**	12	39
Sugar Wafers (3)	**160**	7	23
Vanilla Sandwich Creme (5)	**220**	10	30
Homestyle Big: Molasses (1)	**160**	4	29
Fudge Chocolate Chip (1)	**185**	7	28
Oatmeal Raisin (1)	**180**	6	30
Peanut Butter (1)	**200**	10	24
Chocolate Chip (1)	**200**	9	28
Mini S'wich: Reg./P'nut Butter (9)	**155**	7	21
Vanilla (9)	**160**	7	22
Tiny Bites: Animal Crackers (12)	**260**	9	42
Chocolate Chip; Sugar (12), avg.	**275**	12	38
Great American Cookies			
Doozies:			
Chewy Chocolate Supreme	**205**	8	30
Chewy Pecan Supreme	**210**	11	25
Chocolate Chip; Snickerdoodle	**240**	11	32
Cookie Monster; Sugar, avg.	**195**	9	27
Elmo Cookie	**200**	9	29
M&M; Triple Chocolate	**240**	11	32
Oatmeal; Double Fudge	**240**	10	34
Peanut Butter M&M	**280**	15	30
Peanut Butter Supreme	**260**	14	28
Pecan Supreme	**250**	13	30
White Chunk Macadamia	**225**	9	32
Double Doozies: Sugar	**490**	22	67
Chocolate Chip; M&M	**590**	28	79
Big Bites: Peanut Butter Supreme	**130**	7	14
White Chunk Macadamia	**140**	8	15
Other varieties, avg.	**130**	5	19

Great American Cookies (Cont)	C	F	Cb
Big Bite Doozies: Choc Chip	**355**	17	47
M&M varieties	**395**	19	53
Sugar varieties, avg.	**340**	15	48
Colossal: M&M	**510**	24	68
Cups: Original Cookie Cup	**275**	13	37
Peanut Butter	**255**	13	30
Cakes, avg. 1 slice, ⅛ cake	**670**	30	95
Brownies: Cheesecake Brownie	**400**	21	48
Cheesecake Chocolate Swirl	**485**	25	60
Fudge	**495**	22	67
Fudge Nut	**525**	27	63
Hain			
Cookies: Animal (9), 1 oz	**125**	2.5	23
98% Fat-Free, all types (11)	**110**	0	23
Crackers: Cheese Bites (22)	**120**	1.5	23
Cookie Jar Bits (Rice Cakes), (17)	**60**	0.5	12
Oyster Crackers, Fat-Free (36)	**60**	0	13
Veg/Rice/Sesame Crackers (11)	**140**	6	19
Harvest Bakery			
Crackers, average all types (2)	**75**	3.5	10
Health Valley			
Cookies: Fat Free, avg. all flavors (3)	**100**	0	24
Cafe Creations, Choc. Chip (1)	**100**	5	13
Choc./Dble Choc. Chunk (1)	**125**	7	15
Cookie Cremes, avg. (2)	**125**	5	19
Oatmeal: Raisin (1)	**95**	3.5	14
Avg. other varieties (1)	**100**	4	14
White Chocolate Chunk (1)	**135**	7	17
Low-fat, Biscotti/Amaretto (2)	**130**	3	23
Crackers: Corn Bread (1)	**15**	5	3
Graham: Amaranth; Oat Bran (1)	**15**	0	3
Original Amaranth/Oat Bran (1)	**20**	0.5	4
Healthy Pizza, all flavors (6)	**50**	0	11
Low-fat/Whole Wheat, all flavors (1)	**10**	0	2
Original Rice Bran (1)	**18**	0.5	3
Joseph's Cookies			
Lite Cookies: Almd; Choc Chip (2)	**80**	3	13
Choc Peach	**90**	4	12
Nut & Raisin (2)	**30**	1	7
Oatmeal Raisin (2)	**100**	2	18
Pecan Double Fudge (2)	**90**	3	14
Vanilla (2)	**25**	1	8
Sugarfree Cookies: Oatmeal (4)	**115**	5	15
Chocolate Walnut (4)	**115**	6	14
Lemon (4)	**100**	4	15
Other varieties, avg., (4)	**105**	5	14
Kalahari Rusks, avg. all types (1)	**110**	3	18

Keebler	C	F	Cb
Crackers: Sandwich, 1 pkt, 1.3 oz	**190**	10	23
Club: Orig.; 50% Red. Sodium (4)	**70**	3	9
33% Reduced Fat (5)	**70**	2	12
Grahams: Regular (8), 1 oz	**130**	3.5	22
Low-fat varieties (9), 1 oz	**115**	1.5	24
Munch'ems, average (40), 1 oz	**140**	5	20
Snax Stix, average (20)	**130**	5	18
Toasted: Reduced Fat (5)	**60**	2	10
Regular varieties (5)	**80**	3.5	10
Town House: Regular (2)	**80**	4.5	9
Reduced Fat (6)	**70**	2	11
Wheatables: Reduced Fat (13)	**130**	4	22
Other varieties, average (12)	**140**	6	20
Cookies:			
Chips Deluxe: Soft & Chewy (1)	**70**	3	10
Rainbow (1)	**80**	4.5	9
Chocolate Lovers; Coconut (1)	**90**	5	11
Chips Deluxe, avg. (1)	**90**	6	9
Mini's, all types (4)	**150**	8	19
Cookie Stix (5)	**140**	6	22
Country Style Oatmeal w. Rais. (2)	**140**	6	18
Danish Wedding (4)	**130**	6	19
E.L. Fudge Sandwich w. Fudge (2)	**120**	6	17
Butter w. Dble Fudge Creme (2)	**180**	9	23
Mini Butter S'wich w. Fudge (7)	**130**	6	21
Double Creme (2)	**180**	9	23
S'mores Blasted (2), avg.	**170**	9	23
Fudge Shoppe: S'mores (3)	**160**	8	22
Clusters, 1 pkg	**310**	17	36
Deluxe Grahams: Reg. (3)	**140**	7	19
Double Fudge 'n Caramel (1)	**80**	4	11
Fudge Sticks (3), avg.	**150**	8	20
Fudge Stripes (3), avg.	**160**	8	21
Mini, 1 pkg	**320**	16	42
Reduced Fat (3)	**140**	5	21
Grasshopper, 1 pkg	**220**	11	28
Mini's (4)	**150**	7	20
Mini Grahams (10)	**160**	8	22
Iced Animal (6)	**150**	5	24
Sandies Cookies: Red. Fat (1)	**80**	3.5	10
Cookies (1) avg. all flavors	**80**	5	9
Mini Pecan (4)	**160**	9	18
Soft Batch (1)	**80**	3.5	10
Vienna Fingers: Regular (2)	**150**	6	21
Reduced Fat (2)	**140**	4.5	23
Fudge Varieties (4)	**160**	7	22
Wafers: Vanilla Wafers (8)	**150**	6	22
Mini Vanilla (18)	**140**	6	21
Rainbow (8)	**130**	5	20
Sugar: Vanilla (3)	**130**	6	19
Peanut Butter (4)	**160**	9	18

Keto	C	F	Cb
Cookies (1), 1 oz	**160**	9	6
Ketogenics, avg., 1.76 oz	**250**	19	26
Kraft			
White Cheddar Chse Nips (27), 1 oz	**150**	7	19
Teddy Graham Bearwiches (1)	**150**	7	21
100 Calorie Pack, 4.4 oz	**100**	3	15
Kroger			
Cookies: *Per Serving*			
Fudgie Sticks Wafers (3)	**125**	7	16
Fudgie Stripes Shortbread (3)	**160**	8	21
Old Style Pecan Shortbread (2)	**150**	9	15
Crackers: Cheese Bits (31)	**135**	5	20
Socialites (12)	**150**	8	17
Lance: Big Town, 1 pkg	**250**	11	38
Chocolate Chip, Bite Size (1)	**130**	6	18
Dunking Sticks, each	**180**	10	22
Fig Cake (1)	**220**	4	2
Oatmeal Creme (1)	**240**	10	35
Peanut Butter Creme, 1 pkg.	**230**	12	26
Toastchee Poppers Pouch	**150**	8	15
Low Carb Enchantments			
Cookies: Sugar Free, avg. (1), 1 oz	**150**	9	11
Little Debbie: Apple Flips	**150**	5	24
Figaroos (1), 1.5 oz	**150**	3.5	31
Fudge Rounds (1)	**150**	6	23
German Choc Cookie Rings	**140**	8	18
Ginger Cookies	**90**	3	15
Marshmallow Pies, avg. (1)	**185**	7	28
Marshmallow Supremes (1)	**135**	5	22
Nutty Bar (2)	**310**	18	32
Oatmeal Creme Pies (1)	**140**	2	29
Peanut Butter & Jelly Sandwich	**140**	5	22
Peanut Clusters (1)	**205**	11	23
Raisin Creme Pies (1)	**140**	5	23
Star Crunch Comic Snacks (1)	**145**	6	22
Crackers: Chse w. P'nut Butter (4)	**140**	8	16
Toasty w. P'nut Butter (4)	**140**	7	16
Lu			
Cookies: Marie Lu (3)	**160**	6	25
Le Fondant Wafers (4)	**175**	10	19
Le Petit Beurre (4)	**150**	4	26
Le Petit Ecolier, avg. (2)	**130**	6	17
Pim's: Chocolatier (3)	**155**	9	17
Orange; Raspberry (2)	**95**	3	16
Manischewitz			
Matzo Boards: *See Page 105*			
Biscotti: Toffee Crunch Macaroons	**50**	2.5	7
Cappuccino Chip	**70**	2.5	10
Chocolate Macaroons, each	**45**	2	8
Matzo Cracker, Miniatures	**9**	0	2
Whole Wheat Crackers	**9**	0	2

Per Cookie/Cracker (Unless indicated)

	C	F	Cb
Miss Meringue			
Meringue Classiques: *Per 4 Pieces*			
Choc./Mint/Triple Choc Chip	**100**	1.5	20
Other varieties (4)	**85**	0	20
Meringue Minis: *Per 13 Pieces*			
Orange (13)	**110**	0	27
Toasted Coconut	**120**	1.5	26
Other varieties	**85**	0	20
Mrs Fields Cookies: *See Fast-Foods Section*			
Mother's			
ABC Cinnamon Grahams (1)	**12**	0.5	1.5
ABC Sugar Cookies (1)	**12**	0.5	1.5
Butter Cookies (6)	**165**	8	21
Candy Chip (4)	**150**	7	21
Checkerboard Wafers	**20**	1	3
Chocolate Creme (3)	**160**	7	23
Chocolate Chip: Cookies	**80**	4	10
Cookies (bag) (1)	**30**	1	5
Chocolate Chip Parade	**35**	1.5	5
Cocodas Coconut	**30**	2	4
Cookie Parade: Animal (8)	**140**	6	20
Cookie (4)	**140**	7	18
Circus Animal (1)	**25**	1	3
Fudge Circus (6)	**140**	7	20
Dinosaur Grrrahams	**65**	1.5	12
Double Fudge	**90**	4.5	12
English Tea/Taffy Sandwich	**90**	3.5	13
Flaky Flix Fudge/Vanilla	**70**	3.5	8
Fudge & Mint (2)	**150**	8	21
Fudge Gauchos (2)	**190**	8	26
Fudge & Peanut Butter (2)	**160**	8	20
Hawaiian Chocolate Chip (2)	**185**	11	20
Iced Chocolate (2)	**155**	7	22
Iced Lemonade (2)	**165**	8	22
Peanut Butter Gaucho	**95**	5	11
Iced Raisin (2)	**180**	8	24
Oatmeal Cookies: Regular	**55**	2.5	9
Butterscotch Chip	**60**	2.5	9
Iced; Chocolate Chip	**65**	2	11
Oatmeal Raisin Cookies	**30**	2	4
Oatmeal Walnut Choc. Chip	**65**	3	9
Oatmeal Cremes (2)	**195**	9	26
Peanut Butter	**75**	4.5	8
Shortbread (8)	**165**	8	21
Striped Shortbread Cookies	**55**	2.5	7
Sugar Cookies	**70**	3	10

	C	F	Cb
Mother's (Cont)			
Sugar Free Lemon Creme (3)	**160**	7	23
Sugared Lemon	**75**	4	9
Taffy	**90**	4	13
The Big Fig (1)	**80**	1.5	16
Vanilla Cremes (2)	**175**	7	26
Vanilla Wafers (8)	**135**	5	22
Murray SugarFree Cookies			
Choc Chip/& Pecan (3)	**160**	9	19
Double Fudge (3)	**140**	6	23
Fudge-Dipped Wafer: Vanilla (4)	**140**	10	19
Shortbread (5)	**150**	7	20
Gingersnaps (7)	**140**	4.5	23
Lemon/Choc Cremes (3)	**120**	7	18
Lemon Crisp (4)	**140**	4.5	22
Lemon Wafers (6)	**170**	10	19
Oatmeal (3)	**155**	7	21
Peanut Butter (3)	**150**	7	18
Shortbread (8)	**120**	4.5	20
Shortbread Pecan (3)	**180**	11	18
Vanilla Sugar Wafers (6)	**160**	9	21
Nabisco			
Crackers:			
Flavor Orig.: Bacon Flav. Thins (1)	**10**	0.5	1
Better Cheddars, avg. (1)	**5**	0.5	1
Cheese Nips, avg. (1)	**5**	0.2	0.5
Chicken in a Biskit (1)	**15**	1	1.5
Sociables Crisps (1)	**10**	0.5	1
Swiss Crisps/Cheese; Thins (1)	**10**	0.5	1.5
Vegetable Thins (1)	**10**	0.5	1
Barnum's Animal Cracker (1)	**15**	0.5	3
Honey Maid Graham, sticks (1)	**10**	0	2
Premium: Saltine, avg. (1), 1 oz	**10**	0.5	2
Fat Free (1)	**10**	0	2.5
Other varieties (1)	**15**	0.5	2.5
Royal Lunch (1)	**60**	2	8
Uneeda, Unsalted Tops	**30**	0.5	3
Wheat Thins: Orig., (8) ½ oz	**70**	3	10
Big Wheat Thins (10)	**140**	6	20
Ranch (14)	**150**	7	19
100 Calorie Packs, 4.4 oz	**100**	3	16
Wheatsworth (1)	**20**	1	10
Cookies:			
100 Calorie Packs: Cheese Nips	**100**	3	15
Chips Ahoy!, 1 pkg	**100**	3	18
FruitSnacks (Mixed Berry)	**100**	0	24
Oreo (Thin Crisps), 1 pkg	**100**	2	20
Wheat Thins, minis, 1 pkg	**100**	3	16
Biscos Sugar Wafers	**20**	1	2
Cameo Creme Sandwich	**65**	2.5	10

Per Cookie/Cracker (Unless Indicated)

Nabisco (Cont):	C	F	Cb
Chips Ahoy!: Candy Blasts (1)	**80**	4	10
Chocolate Chip (1)	**80**	4	10
Chewy Chocolate (1)	**50**	2.5	7
Chunky varieties; Cremewiches	**80**	4	10
Mini Chips Ahoy! (1)	**30**	1.5	4
Snack Saks, 1 oz (31)	**165**	8	21
Peanut Butter (1), 0.5 oz	**75**	4	9
Reduced Fat (1)	**45**	1.5	7
Warm 'n Chewy, avg. (2)	**240**	10	38
Famous Chocolate Wafers	**30**	1	5
Fig Newtons: 1 cookie, 31g	**110**	2.5	22
Snack Pack, 2 pces, 1 oz	**90**	0	22
Snackable Dessert, avg. (2)	**125**	3	25
Fat-Free Fig (1)	**90**	0	22
Apple/Fruit Newtons, avg. (2)	**90**	0	22
Cobblers, Apple/Peach (1)	**70**	0	17
Raspberry/Strawb. & Yogurt (1)	**130**	2.5	26
Grahams	**15**	0.5	3
Honey Maid: Grahams, all types (2)	**30**	0.5	6
Low-fat Cinnamon Grahams (2)	**30**	0.3	6
Imperio (1)	**85**	3.5	8
Lorna Doone Shortbread (1)	**70**	3.5	9
Mallomars (1)	**60**	2.5	8.5
Marshmallow Twirls (1)	**130**	6	20
Morelianas, 1 oz	**125**	5	19
Nilla Wafers: Original (1)	**15**	0.5	3
Reduced Fat	**15**	0.3	3
Chocolate	**15**	0.2	3
Nutter Butter: Bites, each	**15**	0.5	2
S'wich Cookie, 1 oz pkg	**135**	6	18
Real Peanut Butter, 1.9 oz	**265**	11	36
Ginger Snaps (1)	**30**	0.5	5
Oatmeal/Iced Oatmeal (1)	**80**	3	12
Oreo: Original, 3 cookies	**160**	7	23
Snack pkg, 2 oz	**270**	12	40
Cookie Barz, 1 bar	**180**	10	23
Reduced Fat, 3 cookies	**130**	3.5	25
Choc. Creme; Coffee 'n Creme (2)	**150**	7	20
Double Delight: Mint 'n Creme (2)	**140**	7	20
P'nut Butter & Choc Creme (2)	**140**	7	20
Double Stuf, 2 cookies	**140**	7	20
Fudge-Covered, 1 cookie	**90**	5	13
Mini Oreo: 9 pieces, 1 oz	**140**	3	21
Snack Pack, 1.5 oz (43g)	**200**	9	31
Uh-Oh!, 3 cookies	**165**	7	24
100 Calorie Packs (1) 4.8 oz	**100**	2	20
Pecanz (1)	**90**	5	9
Pinwheels, Choc./Marshmallow	**130**	5	21
Social Tea Biscuits (1)	**20**	0.5	3
Teddy Cheddy Crackers (23), 1.1 oz	**140**	6	19
Teddy Grahams Snacks, all types (1)	**5**	0.1	1

Newman's Own	C	F	Cb
Alphabet Cookies, avg. (10)	**125**	3	22
Champion Chip: Expresso Choc (4)	**160**	7.5	21
Double Choc Mint Chip (4)	**165**	8	21
Choc Creme Filled Choc. (2)	**130**	4.5	20
Chocolate Chip (4)	**155**	7	21
Chocolate Chocolate Chip (4)	**160**	8	20
Creme Filled Chocolate (2)	**130**	4.5	20
Fig Newman's: Fat Free, 2 bars	**120**	0	28
Low-fat, 2 bars	**140**	2	28
Ginger-O's, Creme Filled Ginger (2)	**120**	4.5	19
Orange Choc Chip (4)	**155**	7	21
Snack Pack, 46g bar	**135**	0	32
Tops & Bottoms Wafers (6)	**120**	3	21
Peak Freans: Assorted Creme (2)	**135**	6	19
Fruit Creme (2)	**130**	5	20
Arrowroot; Ginger Crisp (2)	**155**	4.5	27
Nice Biscuits (2)	**160**	6	25
Petit Beurre (2)	**130**	4	22
Shortcake (2)	**140**	7	18
Pepperidge Farm			
American Collection: Sante Fe	**120**	4.5	18
Sausalito, Choc Macadamia (1)	**155**	8	18
Average other flavors	**140**	7	16
Chocolate Chunk Big Cookies (1)	**140**	8	15
Dessert Bliss: Choc. Alm.; Mint Choc. (3)	**160**	8	22
Distinctive: Bordeaux	**45**	1.5	7
Brussels (3)	**150**	7	20
Brussels Mint; Milano (2)	**130**	7	16
Chantilly Raspberry (2)	**160**	6	23
Double Choc. Milano	**75**	4	9
Geneva	**55**	3	7
Milk Choc. Bordeaux/Milano	**60**	3	7
Mint/Orange Milano	**70**	4	8
Homestyle: Choc Chip; Gingerman	**45**	2.5	6
Lemon Nut Crunch; Shortbread	**70**	3.5	8
Mini: Chessmen (9)	**145**	6	21
Milano (6)	**150**	8	18
Mint Milano (6)	**170**	9	20
Nantucket: Choc Chunk Minis (4)	**150**	8	20
Double Choc Chunk (1)	**140**	7	18
Pirouette, avg. (2)	**135**	6	19
Soft Baked: Oatmeal Raisin (1), 31g	**135**	5	21
Other varieties	**130**	7	16
Vanilla Raspberry Tart	**60**	1.5	12
Goldfish Crackers: Plain (55)	**140**	6	19
Flavor Blasted (51)	**150**	8	17
Giant: Wheat (14)	**140**	5	21
Flavor Blasted, average (31)	**145**	7	19
Graham Snacks: Average (38)	**140**	5	22
Cookie varieties (4)	**20**	0	2

Per Cookie/Cracker (Unless Indicated)	C	F	Cb
Pirouline: 8 rolls, 1 oz	**130**	3.5	23
Ritz			
Crackers: Original Cracker, ½ oz	**80**	4	10
Flavor Assortment, ½ oz	**80**	4	10
Mini Ritz, Original Bite Size (33)	**155**	8	19
Ritz Bits Sandwiches: Cheese, 1.5 oz	**230**	14	23
Graham Cracker S'mores, 1.2 oz	**165**	7	25
Halloween, 1 oz	**140**	6	20
w. Jalapeno Cheddar (14)	**165**	10	17
w. Peanut Butter (14)	**155**	8	18
Peanut Butter Go-Pak, 1 oz	**155**	8	18
Cheese, 1.5 oz	**230**	14	23
Ritz Chips, all varieties (33), 1 oz	**140**	6	20
Smilin' Fun Shapes, all varieties	**20**	1	2.5
Snack Mix, Cheddar Baked Snacks	**205**	9	27
With Peanut Butter, 1.4 oz	**195**	9	24
With Real Cheese, 1.4 oz	**200**	11	22
Stay Fresh: Reduced Fat, 0.5 oz	**65**	2	11
Whole Wheat (5), 0.5 oz	**70**	2.5	11
Other varieties, avg., ½ oz	**85**	4	11
Salerno			
Almond Windmill (2)	**120**	4.5	17
Bonnie Shortbread (4)	**160**	7	22
Butter Cookies: Original (6)	**160**	7	22
Reduced Fat (6)	**150**	5	22
Coconut Bar (4)	**150**	8	18
Creme Wafer Sugar-free (5)	**190**	13	18
Farm Animal Crackers (13)	**140**	5	22
Iced Oatmeal (2)	**120**	5	18
Mini Butter: Flavored (25)	**150**	6	20
Angel/Chocolate Creme (9)	**140**	6	20
Mint Creme Patties (2)	**130**	7	16
Santa's Favorites, Aniseed (6)	**150**	5	22
Scooter Pie Choc Marshmallow	**140**	5	23
Sugar Wafers, assorted (5)	**180**	11	20
Vanilla Wafers (7)	**130**	5	21
Graham Crackers: Cinnamon (2)	**130**	3.5	22
Chocolate (2)	**130**	3	24
Oyster Crackers: Regular (42)	**60**	1.5	11
Fat-Free (42)	**60**	0	12
Saltine Crackers: Reg./Unsalted (5)	**60**	1.5	11
Fat-Free (5)	**50**	0	11
Santa Fe Farms			
Fat Free, average, 1 pkg	**120**	0	26

Snackwell's (Nabisco)	C	F	Cb
CarbWell: Grahams (2)	**120**	7	18
Shortbread (2)	**110**	6	16
Chocolate Chip: Bite Size (13)	**130**	4	22
Sugar Free (3)	**170**	8	23
Coconut Creme (1)	**55**	2	9
Creme Sandwich (2)	**110**	3	20
Devil's Food Cake, Fat Free (1)	**50**	0	12
Golden Devil's Food Cake (1)	**55**	0.5	11
Sugar Free: Fudge Brownie	**105**	3.5	17
Oatmeal (1)	**95**	2.5	17
Shortbread (3)	**140**	5	22
Sandwiches: Creme Packs 2 Go!	**205**	5	38
Chocolate (2)	**110**	3	20
Sugar Free varieties(3)	**160**	6	24
Crackers: Cracked Pepper (4)	**60**	1.5	10
Fat Free (4), 15g	**55**	0	12
French Onion; Zesty Cheese (5)	**125**	3	23
Wheat (5), 15g	**60**	1.5	11
Stella D'Oro			
Almond Delight, 1 oz	**150**	8	18
Almond Toast, 1 oz	**115**	2.5	21
Anginette, 1 oz	**130**	3.5	22
Biscotti, avg., 0.7 oz	**100**	4.5	13
Breakfast Treats: Mini, 1 oz	**125**	3.5	21
Choc.; Cinn.; Original, 0.8 oz	**90**	3	15
Coffee Treats: Angel Wings, 1 oz	**170**	12	14
Anisette Sponge (2)	**90**	1	18
Anisette Toast/Mini (3)	**125**	1	27
Toast, avg. all, 1 oz	**100**	2	19
Roman Egg Biscuits, 1.1 oz	**130**	4	21
Egg Jumbo, 1.1 oz	**125**	1.5	26
Lady Stella, Assorted, 1 oz	**125**	4.5	20
Margherite: Avg., (2)	**130**	4.5	20
Mini, 1.1 oz	**150**	5	24
Swiss Fudge (2)	**120**	6	15
Sunshine: Cheez-It Crackers (1)	**5**	0.5	0.5
Big Cheez-It (1)	**10**	1	1
Cheez-It Cheddar Jack (26), 1 oz	**165**	10	16
Cheez-It Juniors (44), 1 oz	**140**	7	13
Grab Bags Crackers (1)	**5**	0.5	0.5
Heads & Tails, 1 pkt, 1.5 oz	**210**	9	28
Hi-Ho Crackers, avg. (1)	**15**	0.5	2
Krispy: Original (1)	**10**	0.3	2
Oyster & Soup, 17 crackers	**60**	1.5	11
Reduced Fat (1)	**10**	0	2
Party Mix: 1 pkt, 1.7 oz	**230**	9	32
Reduced Fat, ½ cup, 1 oz	**130**	3	21
Snack Mix: Original, ½ cup	**130**	4.5	21
Get Nutty, ½ cup	**150**	9	16
Big Crunch; Dble Chse, avg.,½ c.	**170**	4	14

Per Cookie/Cracker Unless Indicated

Trader Joe's	C	F	Cb
All Butter Shortbread			
w. Apricot/Raspberry Filling (2)	145	8	17
w. Chocolate Filling (2)	125	7	15
Brownie Bites (3)	150	7	20
Chocolate: Almond Laceys (2)	155	10	13
Chip Dunkers (2)	145	6	21
Coated Choc. Chip Dunkers (2)	190	9	25
Cinnamon Butter Sticks (5)	145	7	18
Crispy Crunchy varieties (12)	145	7	19
Fat Free: Fig Bars (2)	130	0	31
Lemon (4)	100	0	24
Ginger Animal (7)	140	6	19
Lemon Crisp (5)	120	4	19
Low-fat varieties (15)	120	1.5	25
Meringues: Cappuccino (4)	85	0	20
Chocolate (4)	100	2	20
Fat Free (5)	105	0	25
Mint (5)	100	1.5	20
Milk Choc. Macadamia Laceys (2)	145	10	13
Southern Style Pecan (4)	150	9	15
Swiss Almond Crunch (6)	135	8	14
Teddies, Vanilla (12)	135	5	21
Triple Ginger Snaps (6)	135	5	21
Way More Chocolate Chips (3)	160	11	14
Triscuit			
Original (15), 1 oz	135	5	20
Baked Whole Wheat: Wafers (7)	145	5	22
Cheddar (6)	135	5	20
Reduced Fat (8)	125	3	21
Deli-Style Rye; Rsted Garlic (8)	145	5	22
Garden Herb, Whole Wheat (6)	135	4.5	20
Thin Crisps French Onion (15)	135	4.5	21
Wild Oats			
Ginger Snaps (1)	25	1	4
Crunchy Peanut Butter (1)	30	1.5	3
Oatmeal Raisin (1)	25	1	4
Sandwich cremes, avg., (3)	180	7	28
Water Crackers (1)	15	0.5	3
Zesta			
Saltine: Export Sodas (3)	60	1.5	10
Fat Free, 5 crackers	50	0	13
Original, 5 crackers	60	1.5	11
Red. Sodium; Unsalted tops (5)	70	1.5	11
Soup & Oyster, 45 crackers	70	3	9
Unsalted Tops, 5 crackers	70	1.5	11

Thaw, Bake & Serve	C	F	Cb
Cookietree: *Per Cookie*			
Buttersugar; Cinn. Apple Oatmeal	120	5	17
Choc. varieties; Pecan/Macadam.	130	7	17
Cookie w. M&M's; Dble Fudge	120	6	17
Fat Free varieties, average	125	0	28
Peanut Butter/Chocolate	130	7	17
Raisin Oatmeal	110	3.5	18
Grands! Biscuits: Extra Rich	220	12	25
Blueberry; Golden Corn	210	9	28
Butter Tastin'; Buttermilk	200	10	24
Reduced Fat	190	7	27
Cinn. Raisin; Extra Fluffy; Wheat	200	8	28
Flaky; Homestyle; Southern Style	200	10	24
Hungry Jack: Avg. all types (1)	100	4.5	14
Jewel: Biscuits (2)	100	1.5	20
Pillsbury Cookies: *Per 1 oz*			
Cookies: Peanut Butter (1)	125	6	16
Chocolate Chip, Reduced Fat (1)	105	3	19
Double Chocolate Chip Chunk (1)	135	7	17
Oatmeal Chocolate Chip (1)	125	6	17
Ready To Bake: P. Butter Cup (1)	185	9	24
Choc. Chip with Walnuts (1)	125	7	14
Sugar (1)	125	5	19
Refrigerated Dough: Sugar (1)	130	1.5	19
Choc Chip w. Walnuts (1)	130	2	16
Chocolate Chip (1)	140	7	17
Cookies w. M&Ms (1)	130	2	18
Double Choc Chip & Chunk (1)	140	2.5	17
Peanut Butter (1)	120	1.5	15
Toll House ***(Nestlé)***			
Cookies: Choc Chip Caramel (1)	110	4.5	16
Fudge (1)	110	5	15
Ultimates: Chocolate Chip			
& Chunks w. Pecans (1)	200	11	23
Choc. Chip Lover (1)	200	10	25
Peanut Butter Cup (1)	195	10	24
White Choc. Macadamia Nut (1)	200	11	23
Walnut Chocolate Chip (1)	115	6	14
Refrigerated Dough: Sugar (1)	120	5	18
Choc Chip Reduced Fat (1)	130	3.5	23
Choc Chip White Fudge (1)	150	6	21
Chocolate Chip (1)	140	6	20
Chocolate Chunk (1)	150	6	22
Peanut Butter Choc Chip (1)	150	7	19

Ready-to-Eat

	C	F	Cb
Angel Food: Plain, no oil, 2 oz	**120**	0	25
Plain with oil, 2 oz	**160**	1.5	25
w. Cream Frosting	**230**	7	37
Apple Fritters, 3 oz	**360**	22	38
Apple Pie: *See Pies/Tarts Page 116*			
Baklava, 1½" square, 1½ oz	**110**	6	13
Banana w. Butter Cream, 3 oz	**300**	13	40
Black Forest, 3 oz	**230**	10	34
Brownie, 3.5 oz	**420**	25	52
Bundt, 3 oz	**300**	17	35
Carrot Cake: Plain, 3 oz	**230**	8	41
w. Cream Cheese Frosting	**380**	21	42
Cheesecake: Small serving, 3 oz	**260**	18	24
Large serving, 5 oz	**430**	30	40
w. Low-fat Cheese/fruit, 3 oz	**150**	8	30
Cheesecake Factory: See Fast-Foods Section			
Denny's Cheesecake, 1 slice	**470**	27	48
Cherry Cobbler, 5 oz	**350**	10	62
Chocolate Cake: Plain, 2 oz	**220**	11	40
w. Chocolate Frosting, 3 oz	**320**	15	42
& Cream Filling, 3½ oz	**360**	21	43
Churros, 1 stick, 1½ oz	**150**	8	18
Cinnamon Crumb Cake, 4 oz	**450**	23	57
Cinnamon Roll, Large, 6 oz	**630**	27	87
Coffee Cake, 2½ oz	**230**	7	38
Concha: Small, 2½ oz	**250**	8	38
Large (5" diameter), 5½ oz	**550**	18	84
Cream Cheese Crumb, 4 oz	**410**	20	52
Cream Puff (custard fill), 4½ oz	**300**	18	26
Creme Horns, each	**190**	13	19
Croissants: *See Next Column*			
Cupcake: Plain, 1½ oz	**140**	6	25
w. Frosting	**170**	7	30
Danish Pastry: Small, 2 oz	**220**	10	25
Large, 4 oz	**440**	20	51
Date Nut Roll, ½" slice	**80**	2	12
Devil's Food, w. Frosting, 3 oz	**460**	25	55
Donut Holes, 1¼" balls, 2 oz (5)	**220**	10	30
Donuts: *See Page 115*			
Eclair, Choc., Cust. fill, 3½ oz	**240**	14	23
Fried Twinkie (1)	**420**	34	45
Fig Bars, average, each	**150**	3	30
Fig Cake, ½ piece	**110**	2	21
Fruit Cake, Dark/Light, 1½ oz	**165**	7	26
Fudge Nut Brownie, each	**340**	13	56
Funnel Cake (1), 9"	**390**	1	85
Gingerbread: From mix, 3" sq.	**200**	6	37
Honey Bun, each	**330**	13	47
Jelly Roll, 1/10 roll	**150**	2.5	29
Key Lime Pie, 4.5 oz	**440**	22	54
Kolacky, Apricot/Rasp., ½ oz (1)	**60**	3.5	8

Ready-to-Eat (Cont)

	C	F	Cb
Lemon Cake, 2½ oz piece	**220**	9	40
Lemon Poppy Seed Creme, 3 oz	**310**	15	40
Marble Cake, 1 slice, 4 oz	**380**	14	60
Mississippi Mud Pie, 4 oz	**380**	24	37
Mud Cake, 1 piece, 3½ oz	**350**	16	48
Muffins: *See Next Page*			
Orange Creme (Ring), 3 oz	**300**	15	40
Pineapple Upside Down, 2½ oz	**230**	9	37
Peach Melba, 3½ oz	**300**	8	52
Strawberry Creme, 3 oz	**290**	14	40
Strudel Bites, ¾ oz	**85**	4	12
Pecan Twirls, 1 piece	**110**	5	16
Pecan Pie, 3 oz	**330**	13	51
Pies & Tarts: *See Page 116*			
Pound Cake, 3 oz	**420**	27	42
Sponge: Plain, 2½ oz	**190**	3	36
w. Cream & Strawberry	**325**	8	38
w. Chocolate Icing	**300**	12	38
Raisin Bun, 1 bun, 2¼ oz	**180**	2	37
Strudel, fruit, average, 3 oz	**280**	8	45
Sweet Roll, average, 1½ oz	**155**	7	24
Swiss Rolls, each	**170**	9	23
Tarts: *See Page 116*			
Tiramisu, 1 piece, 5 oz	**400**	29	30
Toaster Strudel, 2 oz	**190**	10	26
Turnovers, fruit, average, 3 oz	**270**	12	36
Zeppole (Italian Donut), 1	**65**	1	12

Croissants

	C	F	Cb
Average All Brands			
Plain/All Butter:			
Petite, 1 oz	**120**	7	14
1 Medium, 1½ oz	**180**	10	21
1 Large, 2½ oz	**300**	18	35
Sweet: *Per Croissant (3½ oz)*			
Almond Croissant	**420**	25	39
Apple Croissant	**250**	10	30
Chocolate Croissant	**400**	24	36
Croissants Sandwiches: *See Page 173*			
Au Bon Pain: *See Page 187*			
Burger King: *Croissan'wich, See Page 194*			
Dunkin' Donuts: Plain Croissant	**330**	18	37
Sara Lee: All Butter, 1½ oz	**180**	9	19
All Butter Petite, 1 oz	**120**	6	13

Muffins, Sweet Rolls

Quick Guide

	C	F	Cb
Muffins: Ready-To-Eat			
Average All Types:			
Small, 1 oz	**80**	3	12
Medium, 2 oz	**160**	6	24
Large, 3 oz	**240**	9	36
Extra Large, 4 oz	**320**	12	48
Giant, 6 oz	**480**	18	60
Super Size, 8 oz	**640**	24	96
English Muffin, 2 oz	**150**	2	29

Brands ~ Ready-To-Eat

	C	F	Cb
Au Bon Pain: *See Fast-Foods Section*			
Awreys: Blueberry, 2.25 oz	**210**	9	29
Raisin Bran, 2.5 oz muffin	**190**	7	30
Carl's: Blueberry Muffin	**340**	14	49
Bran Raisin Muffin	**370**	14	61
Dunkin' Donuts: *See Fast-Foods Section*			
Hostess: Mini, average, each	**55**	3	7
Fruit Pie, avg., 4.5 oz	**480**	21	70
Krispy Kreme: *See Fast-Foods Section*			
McDonald's: Apple Bran, 4 oz	**300**	3	61
My Favorite Muffin: Plain, 6 oz	**600**	30	75
Chocolate, 6 oz	**510**	24	69
Fat Free, avg., 6 oz	**380**	0	88
Oroweat: Cinnamon Rais., 2.4 oz	**170**	1	35
Extra Crisp; Sourdough, 2 oz	**130**	0.5	26
Health Nut, 2.3 oz	**170**	3	30
Otis Spunkmeyer: *Per Whole Muffin (4 oz)*			
Banana Nut, 4 oz	**480**	24	60
Cheese Streudel	**440**	20	60
Wild Blueberry	**420**	22	48
Our Daily Muffin: Each, 3 oz	**120**	0	31
Pepperidge Farm: Average	**150**	3	28
Ralphs: Banana, 4.5 oz muffin	**470**	21	62
Blueberry, 4.5 oz	**410**	16	60
Bran & Raisin, 5 oz	**380**	8	78
Sara Lee: Blueberry	**220**	11	27
Corn	**260**	14	30
Snackwell's: Blueberry, 1/6 pkt	**120**	0	28
Starbucks: *See Fast-Foods Section*			
Uncle Wally's: Rich & Moist, 4 oz	**390**	20	48
All Natural; Gourmet, 2 oz	**140**	2	28
Fat Free Gourmet, 2 oz	**125**	0	28
Weight Watchers: *Per Muffin*			
Chocolate Chocolate Chip	**190**	2	39
English Muffin Sandwich	**210**	5	28
Fat Free, average, all flavors	**165**	0	39
Low-fat, average, all flavors	**175**	3	37
Winchell's: *See Fast-Foods Section*			

Muffin Mixes

	C	F	Cb
Prepared: Per Muffin			
Atkins: Muffins, average	**70**	1	8
Betty Crocker: Apple Streusel	**210**	8	33
Blueberry	**160**	6	25
Choc Chip; Cinn. Streusel	**170**	8	23
Fat Free, all flavors	**120**	0	26
CarbSense: Mini Carb, Apple	**225**	15	7
Mini Carb, Sweet Corn	**225**	16	8
Duncan Hines: Blueberry, reg.	**120**	3	21
Bakery Style: Pecan Crunch	**220**	11	27
Avg. all other flavors	**200**	7	32
Oat Bran Blueberry	**110**	4	17
Oatmeal & Apples/Walnuts	**210**	9	30
Entenmann's			
Little Bites Muffins: *Per Pouch*			
Fudge Brownies, 2.1 oz	**280**	15	34
Other varieties, avg., 1.8 oz	**210**	10	28
Gold Medal: Apple; Blueberry	**250**	8	41
Chocolate Chip w. Glaze	**330**	12	51
Cornbread varieties	**140**	3.5	25
Variety	**105**	7	9
Average other flavors	**280**	8	46
Sweet Rewards: Low-fat	**230**	1.5	51

Sweet Rolls & Buns

Note: Weigh for actual weight as can be 10-50% higher than label weight.

	C	F	Cb
Cinnabon: Classic	**815**	32	117
Caramel Pecanbon, 1 roll	**1090**	56	141
Minibon, 1 roll	**335**	13	49
CinnaPretzel	**755**	6	156
CinnaPoppers (3)	**370**	21	41
Cinnabon Stix (5)	**350**	11	54
Entenmann's: Cinn. Bun, 2.15 oz	**230**	10	32
Reduced Fat, 2.15 oz	**160**	3	32
Swirl Buns, average (1)	**330**	15	44
Pecan/Walnut Danish Ring, 2 oz	**250**	15	25
Twists: Raspberry, 1/8, 2 oz	**220**	11	27
Nonfat, 1/8, 2 oz	**140**	0	32
Cinnamon Danish, 1/8, 2 oz	**240**	13	29
Lemon Danish, 1/8, 2 oz	**210**	11	26
Hostess: Honey Bun, Glazed, 2.7 oz	**320**	19	34
Actual weight up to 3.9 oz	**460**	27	49
Iced/Frosted, 3.5 oz	**410**	24	42
Little Debbie: Pecan Spinwheels, 1 oz	**110**	4	16
Mickey: Cinnamon Pastry, 4 oz	**200**	5.5	35
Cinnamon Nut, 2½ oz	**230**	8	37
Raisin Cinnamon, 2½oz	**200**	4.5	35
Pillsbury: Cinnamon Roll, 1.5 oz	**150**	5	23
Reduced Fat, 1.5 oz	**140**	3.5	24
Svenhard's: Viking Size Cinn. Bun, 4 oz			
Actual weight up to 5.6 oz	**650**	35	79
Label data based on 4.8 oz	**560**	30	68

Quick Guide

Donuts	C	F	Cb
Average All Brands			
Plain, 1¾ oz	**210**	12	25
Sugared, 1¾ oz	**220**	11	27
Glazed, 2 oz	**250**	12	34
Chocolate Iced, 2 oz	**260**	14	29

Brands

	C	F	Cb
Buttercrumb			
Cinnamon, 1 cake, 1.6 oz	**170**	6	28
Dolly Madison			
Regular, 1¾ oz	**270**	12	40
Gem varieties, ½ oz each	**65**	3	8
Powdered Mini, ½ oz each	**60**	3	8
Dunkin' Donuts: *See Fast-Foods Section*			
Dutch Mill: Plain, 1¾ oz	**210**	12	25
Sugared, 1¾ oz	**220**	11	27
Glazed, 2 oz	**250**	12	34
Double-Dipped Chocolate, 2 oz	**280**	17	31
Entenmann's			
Powdered, 1¾ oz	**230**	14	25
Glazed Buttermilk, 2¼ oz	**270**	13	35
Iced Buttermilk, avg., 2.3 oz	**285**	16	34
Light, 2 oz	**190**	7	31
Light Fantastic Fudge, 2 oz	**210**	9	40
Milk Chocolate Frosted, 2.4 oz	**310**	19	35
Dark Choc. Frosted, 2 oz	**280**	19	27
Hostess			
Cinnamon Sweet Rolls, 2.3 oz	**210**	7	34
Regular: Plain, 1 oz	**140**	7	15
Chocolate Frosted, 1½ oz	**180**	11	19
Powdered, 1½ oz	**150**	8	19
Old Fashioned Glazed, 1½oz	**260**	13	33
Blueberry, 1½ oz	**210**	13	21
Hostess O's, Raspberry, 2 oz	**230**	10	34
Donettes: Plain, ½ oz	**70**	4	8
Frosted, 0.5 oz ea	**65**	4	7
Crumb, 0.7 oz ea	**80**	3.5	10
Powdered, ½ oz ea	**60**	3	8
Jewel: Cinnamon Spiced, 2 oz	**230**	15	24
Krispy Kreme: *See Fast-Foods Section*			
Little Debbie			
Donut Sticks, 1.6 oz pkg	**210**	13	21
3 oz pkg	**390**	23	39

Brands (Cont)

	C	F	Cb
Mickey			
Egg Fluff (2) 1.65 oz	**210**	11	25
French Twirl (2) 1.65 oz	**240**	16	21
Jumbo, avg. all types (1) 1.5 oz	**190**	11	21
Mini (2) 1 oz	**130**	8	15
Sara Lee			
Choc. Frosted Mini, ¾ oz each	**100**	5.5	13
Powdered Mini, ½ oz each	**85**	4.5	9
Glazed, ½ oz each	**110**	5	14
Reduced Fat, ½ oz each	**55**	2.5	8
Tastykake			
Plain, 1½ oz	**190**	10	22
Cinnamon, 1½ oz	**180**	8	26
Frosted Rich, 2 oz	**260**	16	28
Glazed, Mini (6) 2½ oz	**270**	12	38
Honey Wheat, 2 oz	**210**	8	32
Powdered Sugar, Mini (6) 2½ oz	**280**	13	38
Van De Kamp's			
Old Fashioned: Plain	**270**	11	40
Chocolate, 2.4 oz	**340**	22	34
Powdered, 2 oz	**240**	11	35
Assorted, 2¼ oz	**280**	17	32
Mini Donuts: Chocolate (4) 2 oz	**290**	17	32
Crumb (4)	**220**	8	35
Powdered (4)	**250**	12	33
Low-fat: Maple Buttermilk (1)	**200**	2	43
Chocolate Buttermilk (1)	**200**	2	43
Double Chocolate (1)	**190**	2.5	41
Powdered (1)	**150**	1.5	32
Zingers			
Devil's/Vanilla Food, 2 cakes	**280**	8	50

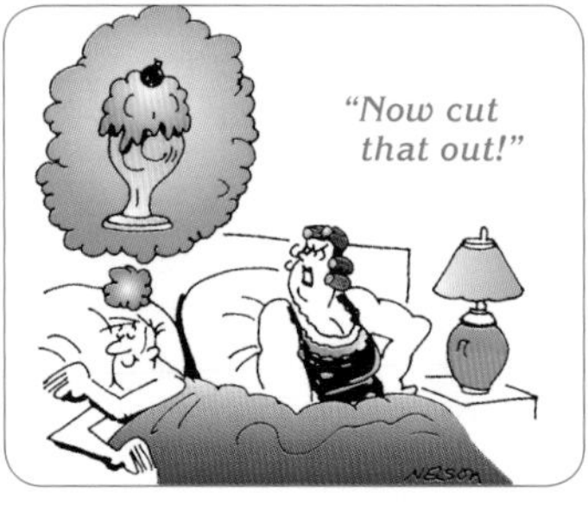

Quick Guide

Pies: *Average All Brands*	C	F	Cb
Apple; Blueberry; Cherry:			
Small Serving, 4 oz, 1/8 pie	290	13	46
Large Serving, 6 oz, 1/5 pie	440	19	69
Extra Large Serving, 8 oz, 1/4 pie	580	26	92
Other Pies: *Per Small Serving (1/8 of 9" Pie)*			
Chocolate Cream Pie	300	18	35
Custard; Coconut Custard	250	13	27
Lemon Chiffon Pie	360	14	50
Lemon Meringue	270	11	42
Pecan Pie	470	24	52
Pumpkin Pie	240	13	28
Strawberry Pie	230	9	37

Brands ~ *Per Serving*

	C	F	Cb
Denny's: Apple Pie	485	24	64
Chocolate Peanut Butter	665	39	64
Entenmann's			
Homestyle Apple, 1/6 pie, 4.3 oz	340	12	56
Hostess: Fruit; Cherry, 4.5 oz pie	470	22	65
Lemon, 4.5 oz pie	500	24	66
Long John Silver's: *Per Pie*			
Chocolate Cream Pie	310	22	24
Pecan Pie	370	15	55
Pineapple Cream Pie	290	13	39
Marie Callender's			
Per 1/5 Pie: Apple	865	49	92
Blueberry	885	57	76
Boysenberry	860	57	82
Cherry	900	58	87
Banana Cream	630	28	67
Chocolate Cream	535	29	66
Coconut Cream	650	32	64
Per 1/4 Pie: Fresh Strawberry	615	28	89
Mince	885	59	97
Lemon Meringue	550	23	76
Pumpkin	615	28	80
Tastykake: Fruit, average	310	11	50
French Apple	360	12	61
Coconut Creme	390	20	47
Lemon Pie	300	13	44

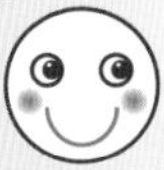

"Success is 1% Inspiration and 99% Perspiration."

Pastry & Pie Crusts

	C	F	Cb
Pie Crust: Baked, 9" diameter shell			
1 Pie Shell, 6½ oz	900	60	79
2-crust Pie, 9", 11¼ oz	1500	93	137
Piecrust Sticks, 8 oz	960	64	90
Choux Pastry, raw, 1 oz	60	4	3
Filo Pastry: 4 sheets, 2½ oz	210	2.5	40
Athens: 5 sheets, 2 oz	180	1	35
Mini Dough Shells, 2, 8g	45	2	1
Pepp. Farm, 2 sheets, 1½ oz	120	1	25
Flaky Pastry, 1 sheet, 6 oz	780	72	18
Puff *(Pepp.Farm)*, ½ sheet, 4.5 oz	510	33	42
1/6 sheet, 1½ oz	170	11	14
Bake & Fill Shell, 1.7 oz	190	13	16
Pizza Crust, 1/8 whole	90	1	16
Bisquick: Baking Mix,			
Original, 1/3 cup, 1½ oz	160	6	25
Reduced Fat, 1/3 cup, 1½ oz	140	3	27
Betty Crocker, 9", 1/8 shell	110	8	9
Boboli, thin Pizza Crust, 1/5, 2 oz	170	4	28
Hershey's Choc Crust, 1/8	110	5	14
Jewel, 1/8 of 9" crust	130	8	13
Keebler Graham Cracker, 1/8 of 9"	110	5	14
Reduced Fat, 1/8	90	3.5	14
Shortbread Crust, 1/8	110	5	14
Mrs Smith's Deep Dish, 9" (1/8)	110	7	11
Nabisco Oreo, 1/6 of 9" crust	140	7	18
Honey Maid Graham, 1/6, 1 oz	140	7	18
Nilla Pie Crust, 1/6, 1 oz	140	8	18
Pet-Ritz, all types, 1/8, ¾ oz	90	5	10
Pillsbury (All Ready), 1/8 pie, 1 oz	120	7	13

Pie Filling (Canned)

Average All Brands: *Per 4 oz*	C	F	Cb
Apple: 4 oz	120	0	28
21 oz Can	600	0	145
Apricot, 4 oz	150	0	36
Blackberry, Blueberry, Cherry, 4 oz	120	0	28
Chocolate, Coconut, 4 oz	140	3	33
Lemon, 4 oz	200	2	47
Mincemeat, 4 oz	190	1	45
Peach, Strawberry, 4 oz	120	0	28
Pumpkin, 4 oz	170	0	40
Raisin, 4 oz	130	0	30
Raspberry, Black/Red, 4 oz	190	0	45
Strawberry, 4 oz	120	0	28

Cakes & Pastries	C	F	Cb
Atkins			
Cheesecake, 3 oz slice	**250**	24	3
Dessert Cake Roll: *Per 1/6 Whole*			
Carrot, 2.6 oz slice	**220**	18	5
Chocolate, 2.6 oz slice	**240**	20	6
Mini Cheesecake. avg. all flavors	**250**	24	3
Banquet: Crm Pies, avg., 1/3 pie	**350**	21	42
CarbSense: *Per Serving (Prepared)*			
Brownie, 1/12 pk	**220**	17	11
Carrot Cake, 1/9 pkt	**280**	20	10
Chocolate Cake, 1/9 pkt	**230**	18	16
Cheesecake Factory: *See Fast-Foods Section*			
Dolly Madison: Honey Bun, 3.75 oz	**440**	25	49
Cinnamon Sweet Rolls (1)	**210**	7	34
Dunkin' Stix, 1 stix	**170**	9	20
Eli's Frozen *Cheesecakes: Per 1/8 Pkg (3 oz)*			
Cookies N Creme; Choc. Caramel	**320**	23	11
Keylime; Original, average	**320**	22	26
Entenmann's			
All Butter Loaf, 1/6 loaf, 2 oz	**210**	9	30
Banana Cake, 1/8 cake, 2.5 oz	**290**	15	39
Cheese-Topped Coffee, 1/8, 2 oz	**200**	9	26
Cheese-Filled Crumb Coffee, 2 oz	**210**	10	25
Chocolate Fudge, 1/6 cake, 3 oz	**280**	12	42
Chocolate Loaf, Light, 1/8, 2 oz	**120**	0	29
Creme-Filled: Choc Cupcakes, 1	**160**	0	39
Golden Cakes, 1 cake, 2.3 oz	**280**	15	34
Golden Loaf (Light) 1/8, 1.7 oz	**130**	0	28
Louisiana Crunch, 1/9, 3 oz	**330**	14	48
Mocha Cake, 1/6 cake, 3 oz	**340**	17	45
New York Crumb Coffee, 1/10, 2 oz	**250**	12	33
Ultimate Crumb, 1/10, 2 oz	**250**	13	33
Brownie: Ultimate Fudge, 1	**220**	13	27
Light: Fudge, 1/10 strip, 1.4 oz	**110**	0	27
Lemon; Coffee, 1/8 strip, 1.9 oz	**130**	0	29
Buns/Twists: *See Page 114*			
Glenny's Slim Carb Cheesecake: *Per 1/6 Cake*			
Natural New York, 3 oz	**210**	13	15
Other varieties, 3.5 oz	**135**	1	23
Grands!: Blueberry Biscuits, 2 oz	**210**	9	29
Cinnamon Rolls, 3.5 oz each	**300**	7	54
Hostess: *Per Cake Unless Indicated*			
Angel Food Cake, 1/8 cake	**160**	1.5	33
Brownie Bites, each	**57**	3	7
Caromel Ho Ho's, 2 cakes			
label weight, 2 oz	**250**	11	35
actual weight, up to 2.4 oz	**295**	13	42
Carrot Cake, 2 pces, 3.5 oz	**300**	7	55
Hostess (Cont)			
Chocodiles	**240**	11	33
Coconut Cakes, Creme (1) 1 oz	**260**	13	32
Crumb Coffee	**130**	5	19
Cup Cake, each	**160**	6	30
Dessert Cups, each	**100**	2	17
Ding Dongs	**190**	10	23
Fudge Brownie	**330**	11	54
Hearty Muffin, avg.	**620**	33	73
Ho Ho's, each	**125**	6	17
Honey Bun: Glazed, 2.7 oz	**320**	19	34
Actual weight up to 3.9 oz	**460**	27	49
Muffin Loaf, avg.	**440**	19	63
Mini Muffins (3)	**160**	9	16
Snoballs	**180**	5	31
Suzy Q's, 1 cake, 2 oz	**230**	9	35
Twinkies, 1 cake, 1.5 oz	**150**	5	25
Low-fat Cupcakes; Twinkies, avg.	**135**	1.5	28
Jewel Bake Shop			
Choc Mini Cupcakes, 1 cake	**100**	12	30
Cinnamon Swirl Bread, 1 oz slice	**160**	2.5	30
Creme Horns, 1 horn	**190**	13	19
Elephant Ears, 2.5 oz	**340**	22	34
Fancy Jelly Roll, 1/6 roll, 2.7 oz	**190**	2.5	38
French Torpedo Roll, 2.7 oz	**170**	1	35
Gourmet Cinn. Rolls, 6 oz roll	**640**	29	88
Key Lime Meringue Pie, 1/6, 5 oz	**340**	12	55
Little Debbie			
Cakes: Coffee (2) 2 oz	**230**	7	39
Choc Chip Snack (2), 2.4 oz	**290**	14	42
Creme-filled Strawb. Cupcake (1)	**200**	9	29
Devil Cremes, 1.65 oz cake	**190**	8	29
Devil Squares, 2 cakes, 2.2 oz	**270**	13	37
Frosted Fudge , 1.5 oz cake	**200**	10	25
Swiss Cake Rolls, 2 cakes	**260**	12	39
Zebra Cakes, 2 cakes, 2.6 oz	**330**	16	45
Honey Buns, 1.75 oz bun	**220**	13	24
Manischewitz: Cheesecake, 3 oz	**250**	19	16
Marie Callendar (Frozen)			
Apple Pie, 1 slice, 1/5 pie	**865**	49	92
Cherry Pie, 1 slice, 1/5 pie	**900**	58	87
Cobbler, all types, 1/4 pie, 4.25 oz	**390**	19	45
Pumpkin Pie, 1 slice, 1/5 pie	**615**	28	80
Mrs Smith's			
Cream Pies: Oreo, 1/6, 4.3 oz	**380**	17	54
Choc Chip Delight, 1/6, 4.9 oz	**410**	18	59
Moose Tracks, 1/6, 4.5 oz	**495**	29	51
Flip it Cake Frozen Desserts: *Per 1/2 Cake (5 oz)*			
Apple Caramel	**490**	13	90
Chocolate Caramel	**580**	25	84

Pepperidge Farm	C	F	Cb
Cakes Supreme: *Per 3 oz Slice*			
Lemon Mousse	**290**	12	35
Chocolate Mousse	**250**	10	35
Boston Creme	**260**	9	32
Cream Cakes Supreme:			
Cream Cheese Carrot, 1/9, 3 oz	**320**	20	38
Pineap./Strawb. Crm., 2.7 oz sl.	**240**	10	38
Old Fashioned Cakes: *Per 3 oz Slice*			
Butter Pound	**290**	13	39
Deluxe Carrot	**310**	16	39
Turnovers (Frozen): Apple, 3.2 oz	**290**	15	36
Raspberry, 3.2 oz	**290**	15	35
3-Layer Cakes: Coconut, 1/8, 2.5 oz	**250**	11	35
Golden, 1/8 cake, 2.5 oz	**250**	12	33
Fruit Squares: Apple/Blueb./Cherry	**210**	10	27
Rich's: Chocolate Eclairs (Frozen)	**190**	9	24

Sara Lee (Frozen)	C	F	Cb
Cakes: *Per Serving*			
All Butter Pound, 1/6, 2.7 oz	**320**	16	38
Reduced Fat, ¼, 2.7 oz	**280**	11	42
All Butter; Chocolate, ¼, 2.7 oz	**320**	16	40
Banana Sundae, 1/10, 3 oz	**270**	14	32
Butter Streusel Coffee, 1/6, 2 oz	**220**	12	25
Choc Layer, 1/8, 3 oz slice	**340**	17	46
Dble Choc Layer, 1/8, 2.8 oz	**260**	13	33
Free & Light, ¼, 2.7 oz	**200**	4	39
Golden Butter, ¼, 2.7 oz	**300**	13	41
Pecan Coffee, 1/6, 2 oz	**230**	12	24
Red, White, Blueb. 1/10, 3 oz	**210**	8	31
Strawberry, ¼, 2.7 oz	**290**	11	44
Dessert Cakes: Carrot, 1/6, 3.2 oz	**320**	17	39
Banana, 1/6, 2.3 oz	**230**	8	37
Layer Cakes: *Per 1/8 Whole*			
Strawberry Shortcake, 2.5 oz	**180**	7	27
Other flavors, average, 3 oz	**260**	13	32
Bars: 1 bar, 2.75 oz	**190**	14	14
Cheesecake: *Per Serving*			
Cherry/Strawberry, avg, 4.75 oz	**340**	12	53
Chocolate Chip, 4.3 oz	**410**	21	47
Peanut Butter Cup, 3.5 oz	**380**	22	34
New York Cheesecake: Classic, 1/6	**500**	30	50
Mixed Berry Swirl, 1/6	**490**	28	52
Choc Chip Cookie Crumble, 1/6	**520**	27	61
Cream Pies (9"): *Per Serving (5 oz)*			
Choc. Silk; Coconut Cream, 1/5	**500**	32	49
Lemon Meringue, 1/6	**350**	11	59

Sara Lee (Cont)	C	F	Cb
Classic Cheesecakes:			
Original Cream, ¼ cake, 4.3 oz	**340**	18	38
Orig. Strawb., ¼ cake, 4.8 oz	**330**	12	49
French, 1/5 cake, 4.7 oz	**410**	25	41
Cheesecake Singles: *Per Slice*			
Caramel Choc Pecan, 110g	**400**	25	37
Strawberry Drizzle, 113g	**380**	20	46
Bites: Carrot Cake Bites, 5 pces	**370**	25	32
Choc-Dipped Orig., 5 pces	**480**	33	40
Choc Praline Pecan, 5 pces	**470**	30	42
Toasted Almond, 5 pces	**450**	29	42
Triple Choc Fudge, 2 pces	**170**	8	24
Oven Fresh Pies (9"): *Per 4½ oz (1/8 of Pie)*			
Apple; Cherry, average	**340**	16	46
Blueberry; Dutch Apple	**355**	15	53
Mince/Raspberry, average	**380**	19	48
Pecan	**520**	24	70
Pumpkin	**260**	11	37
Southern Sweet Potato	**280**	10	45
Deep Dish Pies: *Per 1/10 Pie (4.7 oz)*			
Cinnamon French Apple	**360**	15	48
Golden Peach	**340**	16	46
Orchard Apple	**400**	24	43
Individual Slices: *Per Slice*			
Apple/Cherry Pie, 4 oz	**300**	11	47
Carrot; Cookies N Cream, 3.5 oz	**335**	20	40
Lemon Icebox Pie, 3.5 oz	**260**	10	41
Southern Pecan Pie, 4 oz	**470**	23	62
Strawberry Swirl Ch'cake, 3.5 oz	**300**	17	31
Round Danish: Cheese, 1/6 whole	**180**	6	28
Butter Streusel/Pecan, 1/6	**225**	12	24
Raspberry, 1/6 whole	**200**	8	27
Deluxe Cinnamon Roll, 1/6	**320**	15	41
TastyKake: Chocolate Jnr, 3.4 oz	**320**	12	52
Creme Filled Koffee Kakes, 3 oz	**360**	14	54
Koffee Kake Junior, 2½ oz	**250**	8	40

Weight Watchers: *Per Serving*	C	F	Cb
Brownie à la Mode	**190**	4	33
Chocolate Mousse	**190**	5	31
Chocolate Eclair	**150**	4	25
Choc. Chip Cookie Dough Sundae	**190**	4.5	35
Choc. Raspberry Royale	**190**	3	39
Double Fudge Brownie Parfait	**190**	2.5	39
Double Fudge Cake	**190**	4.5	36
French Style Cheesecake	**170**	4	28
Mississippi Mud Pie	**160**	5	24
New York Style Cheesecake	**150**	5	21
Strawberry Parfait Royale	**180**	2	35

Made As Directed	C	F	Cb
Arrowhead Mills: *Per Serving (Prep'd)*			
Cookie (1), avg. all types	**90**	2.5	**16**
Perfect Harvest Muffin, 1/12 pkg	**270**	12	**40**
Wheat Free Brownie, 1/20 pkg	**160**	7.5	**21**
Aunt Jemim			
Coffee Cake, 1/8 cake, prep.	**180**	6	**27**
Banquet			
Dessert Bakes: *Per Serving (Prep'd)*			
Apple Crisp, 1/6	**210**	3.5	**42**
Choc. Cherry Decadence, 1/6	**310**	5	**62**
Chocolate Lava Cake, 1/7	**370**	7	**73**
Peach/Cherry Cobbler, 1/6	**230**	3.5	**46**
Betty Crocker			
Cakes (Super Moist): *Per 1/12 Cake (Prep'd)*			
Butter Recipe Yellow	**260**	11	**36**
Chocolate Chip	**250**	11	**35**
Chocolate varieties	**270**	13	**36**
Cinnamon Swirl	**280**	11	**42**
Devil's Food	**270**	13	**35**
White	**230**	10	**34**
Other flavors, average	**250**	10	**35**
Per 1/10 Cake (Prepared): Carrot	**320**	15	**42**
Sour Cream	**280**	12	**43**
If using No Cholesterol Recipe, deduct 40 cals and 4g fat.			
Other Cakes: Pound Cake, 1/8	**260**	8	**35**
Angel Food Cake, 1/12 mix	**140**	0	**32**
Gingerbread Cake, 1/8	**230**	6	**39**
Pineapple Upside Down, 1/6	**400**	14	**64**
Sunkist Lemon Bar (1)	**140**	4.5	**24**
Brownie Mixes: *Per 1/20 Pkg (Prep'd)*			
Chocolate Chunk varieties	**180**	9	**25**
Dark Chocolate	**170**	7	**25**
Fudge	**170**	7	**24**
Original Supreme	**160**	6	**27**
Peanut Butter; Walnut	**180**	9	**24**
Turtle (Caramel & Pecan)	**170**	8	**23**
Cookie Mix: *Per 2 Cookies (Prep'd)*			
Rainbow Chocolate Candy	**150**	7	**33**
Other varieties, average	**160**	8	**21**

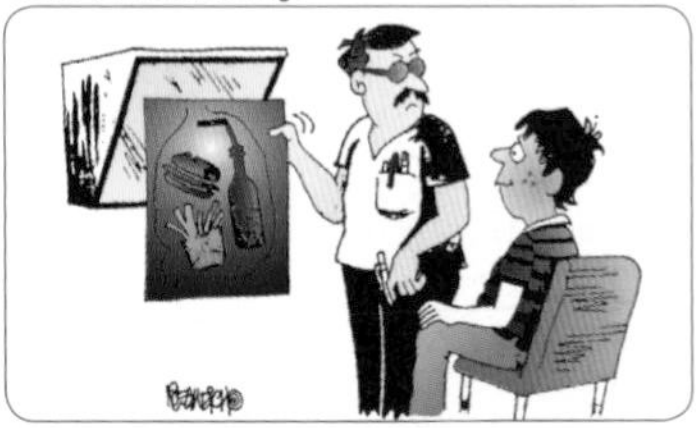

Betty Crocker (Cont)	C	F	Cb
Muffin Mix: *Per Muffin (6.5 oz)*			
Apple Streusel	**210**	8	**33**
Blueberry; Golden Corn	**160**	6	**25**
Triple Berry	**120**	3	**23**
Twice the Blueberries	**140**	4	**25**
Wild Blueberry	**170**	5	**28**
Other varieties, average	**175**	7	**24**
Snackin' Cake: *Per 1/9 Pkg*			
Banana Walnut	**180**	6	**31**
Cinnamon Swirl	**190**	5	**34**
Chocolate varieties	**180**	5	**32**
Carb Monitor: *Per Serving (Prep'd)*			
Brownie: Choc Chunk, 1/16 pkg	**150**	10	**20**
Walnut (1), 1/16 pkg	**160**	11	**20**
Cookie, 2 cookies, 1/14 pkg	**130**	7	**18**
Muffin (1), 1/12 pkg	**100**	9	**27**
Dr Oetker: *Per Serving (Prep'd)*			
Chocolate Chip Cookie Mix, 1/12	**170**	7.5	**24**
Muffin Mix, 1/12 pkg, average	**170**	2	**30**
Simple Organic Cake Mix, 1/12	**255**	11	**32**
Duncan Hines			
Angel Food, 1/12 whole	**140**	0	**30**
Brownie Mix (low-fat recipe)			
1/16 pkg, avg. all types	**140**	3.5	**22**
Cookies, all flavors, 1 cookie	**65**	3	**8**
Moist Deluxe Cake Mix:			
Average, 1/12 pkg, prepared	**250**	11	**36**
Lower Fat Recipe, 1/12 pkg, prep.	**200**	5	**36**
Estee: Brownie, 1 pce, 2"x 2"	**50**	2	**12**
All cakes, 1/5 cake	**200**	4	**38**
Choc. Chip Cookie, 1 cookie	**45**	2.5	**6**
Ghirardelli: *Per Serving (Prepared)*			
Brownie, 1/16 pkg	**200**	10	**27**
Chocolate Chip Cookie (1)	**280**	13	**38**
Dble Choc Muffin (1)	**250**	10	**37**
Jell-O-No Bake Cheesecakes: *Prep'd As Directed*			
Cherry/Strawberry, 1/9 pkg	**300**	13	**42**
Chips-Ahoy!, 1/16 pkg	**360**	17	**46**
Chocolate Silk Dessert, 1/6 pkg	**280**	15	**34**
Oreo, 1/6 pkg	**360**	16	**48**
Peanut Butter Cup, 1/8 pkg	**360**	23	**38**
Real, 1/6 pkg	**360**	17	**42**
Krusteaz: Cinn. Crumb Cake, 1"	**230**	7	**38**
Lemon/Key Lime Bar, 2" bar	**160**	4.5	**29**
Muffins: Blueberry (1)	**150**	4	**26**
Oat Bran (1)	**180**	4	**32**
Fat-Free varieties (1)	**140**	0	**33**

Cakes & Dessert Mixes (Cont)

Made As Directed

	C	F	Cb
No Pudge			
Fudge Brownie, 1/12 pkg, prep'd.	100	0	21
Pamela's			
Ultra Chocolate Brownie, 1/16 pkg	170	8	23
Oil Free, 1/16 pkg	110	1.5	24
Pillsbury			
Moist Supreme: *Per 1/12 Cake (Prepared)*			
Angel Food Cake	140	0	31
Devil's Food Cake	270	14	33
French Vanilla; German Choc.	250	11	34
Funfetti	250	9	36
Streusel Coffee, 1/16 cake	260	11	37
Other flavors, average 1/12 cake	255	12	35
Thick 'n Fudgy Deluxe Brownie *(Prepared)*			
Caramel Swirl, 1/20 pkg	190	8	27
Cheesecake Swirl, 1/18 pkg	150	8	19
Choc./Vanilla Frosted, 1/16 pkg	200	9	27
Double Choc, 1/16 pkg	160	7	23
Fudge, 1/20 pkg	170	8	33
Fudge Toffee, 1/20 pkg	170	8	23
White Chunk, 1/16 pkg	160	8	21
w. Walnuts, 1/12 pkg	200	11	24
Muffins, avg. all types (1)	185	6	30
Robin Hood: Yellow 1/5 cake	280	13	37
Devil's Food, 1/5 cake	310	17	36
Fudge Brownie (1)	170	7	24
Muffin, 1/6 pkg	150	6	25

Cake Frostings

	C	F	Cb
Betty Crocker			
Rich & Creamy, average, 2 Tbsp	130	5	24
Whipped, all flavors, 2 Tbsp	100	5	15
Easy Flow Icing, 1 Tbsp	25	1	4
Duncan Hines: *Per 2 Tbsp (1.2 oz)*			
Creamy Homestyle, avg all flavors	140	5	23
Pillsbury: *Per 2 Tbsp (approx. 1/12 Tub)*			
Caramel Pecan	150	8	19
Chocolate Cream Cheese	140	6	21
Chocolate Walnut	150	7	20
Coconut Pecan	160	10	17
Cream Cheese; Lemon	150	6	24
French Vanilla	160	6	26
Milk/Chocolate; Choc. Fudge	140	6	21
Rainbow Chip	140	5	23
All other flavors	150	6	23
Decorators, Choc., 1 Tbsp	70	2	11

Baking Ingredients

	C	F	Cb
Almond Paste:			
(Marzipan), 1 oz	125	7	12
Baking Powder: Regular, 1 tsp	3	0	0.5
Cream of Tartar, 1 tsp	2	0	0.5
Baking Mix *(Bisquick)*:			
Original, 1/3 cup, 1½ oz	170	6	25
Reduced Fat, 1/3 cup, 1½ oz	150	2.5	28
Butter/Margarine, ½ cup, 4 oz	820	91	0
Carob Flour, ½ cup	90	0.5	26
Chocolate Baking Bars: *Average All Brands*			
Unsweetened, 1 oz	150	15	8
Grated, 1 cup, 4 ½ oz	680	68	36
Semi-sweet, 1 oz	160	8	20
Bitter-sweet/White Baking 1 oz	160	8	20
Chocolate Baking Chips: *Average All Brands*			
Milk Choc./Semi Sweet 1 oz	160	9	18
¼ cup, 1½ oz	240	12	30
1 cup, 6 oz	960	48	120
Mini Kisses *(Hershey)*, 1 pce	5	0.5	1
Cocoa Powder, Baking: Nestle, 1 T.	15	1	3
1/3 cup, 1 oz	80	4	12
Hershey's, 1 Tbsp	20	0.5	3
1/3 cup, 1 oz	115	3.5	21
Coconut, dried: Unsweet., 1 oz	190	18	7
Sweetened/flaked, 1 oz	135	9	14
½ cup, 1.3 oz	175	12	18
Toasted *(Baker's)*, 1 oz	170	13	17
Coconut Cream/Milk: *See Page 39*			
Cornstarch, 1 Tbsp	30	0	7
Flour, white: 1 Tbsp, 0.6 oz	55	0	12
1 cup, 4.4 oz	450	1	95
Whole Wheat, 1 cup, 4.2 oz	410	2	87
Flavor Extracts: *Average All Brands*			
Imitation, 1 tsp	15	0	3.5
Pure Extract, 1 tsp	20	0	4
Almond, Vanilla, 1 tsp	10	0	3
Fruit Pectin: Swtnd, 1 Tbsp, ½ oz	35	0	10
Unsweetened, 1 Tbsp	2	0	0.5
Gelatin, dry, ¼ oz pkg	30	0	0
Lemon/Orange Peel, ¼ cup	30	0	4
Rennin, 1 pkg (11g)	12	0	3
Sprinkles: All types, 1 Tbsp, ½ oz	70	3	10
Vinegar, avg. all types, 1 oz	4	0	2
Whey, sweet, dry, 1 oz	90	0.5	20
Yeast: Active, dry, ¼ oz pkg	15	0	2
Bakers, compressed, 1 oz	25	0	3
Brewers; Torula, 1 oz	80	0.5	11
Fleischmann's, 0.6 oz pkg	15	0	2

Ready-To-Serve

	C	F	Cb
Instant Pudding, Reg., ½ cup	**170**	4	30
Reduced Calorie: *D-Zerta;* Estee	**70**	0	12
Jell-O, sugar-free, ½ cup	**80**	2	11
Royal, sugar-free, ½ cup	**100**	2	17
Del Monte Pudding Snacks	**130**	4	24
Fat-free Vanilla	**90**	0	20
Dr McDougall's Rice Pudd., 3 oz	**310**	1.5	69
Hershey's Portable Pud., 2.25 oz	**100**	3	16
Hunt's Snack Pack: *Per 3.5 oz Cup*			
Puddin' Cakes: Choc Brownie	**180**	7	27
German Choc Cake	**160**	3.5	30
Puddin Pie: Lemon Meringue	**130**	2.5	20
Apple; Choc Mud	**170**	7	26
Dessert Favorites, avg. all flavors	**140**	5	22
Jell-O: Pudding, Choc., ⅕ pkg	**190**	5	33
Pudding Bites, average 1 pouch	**90**	1.5	18
No Bake Mix: Oreo, ⅙ pkg	**270**	8	48
Peanut Butter Cup, ⅛ pkg	**290**	15	38
Real Cheesecake, ⅙ pkg	**220**	6	40
Other flavors, avg.	**200**	3	42
Pudding & Pie Filling: *Per ¼ Pkg*			
Cook & Serve, average	**150**	0	22
Instant, regular, avg.	**100**	0	25
Fat & Sugar Free, avg.	**30**	0	8
Pudding Snacks: Fat-Free, 4 oz	**100**	0	23
Cheesecake Snack; Oreo, avg.	**150**	4	26
Chocolate; Creme Savers, 4 oz	**160**	5	28
Smoothie Snacks, 4 oz	**100**	2.5	18
Jewel: Chef's Kitchen			
Rice Pudding, ½ cup, 4.5 oz	**230**	8	35
Tapioca Pudding, ½ cup, 4.5 oz	**170**	8	35
Jolly Rancher: Reg., 3.5 oz cup	**100**	0	25
Sugar-Free, all flavors, 3.5 oz cup	**10**	0	2
Kozy Shack: Avg. all types, 4 oz	**140**	4	25
Lite, 4 oz	**110**	1	22
Creme Caramel Flan, 1 cup, 4 oz	**160**	4	28
Kraft Handi Snacks: *Per Cup (3.5 oz)*			
"Doubles", avg. all flavors	**125**	3.5	22
Chocolate Pudding Fat-Free	**85**	0	21
Rice Pudding	**140**	6	19
Tapioca; Vanilla Pudding	**115**	3.5	20
Kroger: *Per Container*			
Peaches & Cream w. Natural Flav.	**180**	2.5	36
Whipped Varieties	**145**	2.5	27
Manischewitz: Choc., ½ cup	**110**	0.5	26
Passover Gold Noodle, ½ cup	**140**	2	28
President's Choice			
Key Lime Pie (36 oz) ⅛ pie, 4.5 oz	**440**	22	54
Mississippi Mud Pie (36 oz) ⅑, 4 oz	**380**	24	37
Swiss Miss Pudding Snacks			
Swirls, Choc. Pudd. Snacks, 3½ oz	**150**	5	23
Tapioca: 1 pudding cup, 3½ oz	**120**	3.5	21
Fat-Free varieties, 3½ oz	**90**	0	20
Weight Watchers (Frozen)			
Chocolate Mousse, 2¾ oz	**190**	5	31

Homemade Puddings

	C	F	Cb
Apple Tapioca, ½ cup	**150**	0	32
Bread Pudding, ½ cup	**250**	8	40
Blancmange, ½ cup	**140**	5	19
Chocolate, ½ cup	**190**	6	30
Corn Pudding, ½ cup	**135**	4	21
Crème Brûlée, ½ cup	**400**	35	16
Plum Pudding, 2 oz	**170**	3	32
Rice with Raisins, ½ cup	**200**	4	38
Sponge Pudding, 3½ oz	**340**	16	45
Tapioca Cream, ½ cup	**110**	4	15
Trifle, ½ cup	**180**	7	26

Custards

	C	F	Cb
Custard Mix			
Jell-O (Americana) Golden Egg:			
Dry, ⅙ pkg	**80**	0	19
Prep. w. 2% milk, ½ cup	**140**	2.5	19
Jello Flan, w. 2% milk, ½ cup	**140**	2.5	20
Royal-Flan: Prep. w. 2% milk, ½ c.	**130**	2.5	18
Homemade Custard			
Baked: Plain, ½ cup, 4½ oz	**150**	7	16
w. skim milk, artif. sweetened	**70**	3	4
Boiled, ½ cup	**165**	7	18

Meringues

	C	F	Cb
Meringue Swirl, ½ oz	**50**	0	8
Meringue Shell, 1 oz shell	**100**	0	16

(Add extra calories/fat/carbohydrate for fillings)

Jell-O • Cups • Parfait

	C	F	Cb
Gelatin Mix: *Jell-O, Royal ~ Made Up*			
Regular, all flavors, ½ cup	**80**	0	18
Sugar Free/Low Calorie, ½ cup	**8**	0	0
Creme Gelatin/Parfait: *Per ½ Cup*			
Ida Mae, ½ cup	**60**	2	10
Winky: Strawberry (109g)	**110**	1.5	22
Rainbow (130g)	**100**	0	24
Reser's, Dessert Parfait (110g)	**100**	2	19
Mrs Crockett's Kitchen, Str. Parfait	**160**	4	26
Gel Snacks (Jell-O): Regular, 3.5 oz	**70**	0	17
Sugar Free, 3.2 oz	**10**	0	1
X-Treme Cups, 2.5 oz	**100**	0	24
X-Treme Sticks, 2.2 oz	**60**	0	16

Pancakes & Waffles

Quick Guide

	C	F	Cb
Pancakes			
Plain: *Average All Types*			
Small (3" diam.), ¾ oz	**50**	2.5	6
Medium (4" diam.), 1¼ oz	**80**	3	11
Large (5" diam.), 2½ oz	**160**	6	21
Add Extra for Syrups/Butter			
Pancake Syrup: Regular, 1 Tbsp	**50**	0	13
¼ cup	**200**	0	52
Lite, 1 Tbsp	**25**	0	6
¼ cup	**100**	0	24
Butter/Margarine: Regular, 1 T.	**100**	11	0
Whipped, 1 Tbsp	**70**	7.5	0

Restaurant Style Pancakes

Denny's			
Buttermilk Hot Cakes: Plain, 3	**675**	23	47
w. Syrup & Margarine	**905**	33	83
Original Grand Slam Breakfast	**675**	49	33
w. Syrup & Margarine	**1030**	60	101
Maple Flavor Syrup, 1 serving	**145**	0	36
Whipped Margarine, ½ oz	**90**	10	0
Hardees: 3 Pancakes (no fat)	**280**	2	56
w. Sausage Pattie	**430**	16	56
w. 2 Bacon Strips	**350**	10	56
IHOP (International House of Pancakes)			
Pancakes (Syrup/Butter extra):			
Buttermilk, 1 (2 oz)	**110**	3	17
Short Stack, 3	**330**	9	51
Full Stack, 5	**550**	15	85
Buckwheat, 1 (2 oz)	**110**	4	15
Country Griddle, 1 (2 oz)	**120**	3.5	19
Harvest Grain 'N Nut, (2¼ oz)	**180**	9	20
Crepes (Egg Pancakes), 1 (2 oz)	**120**	6	14
Waffles (Plain): Regular, 1 (3 oz)	**310**	15	37
Belgian: Regular, 1 (4 oz)	**390**	19	48
McDonald's			
Hotcakes: Plain (3)	**340**	8	58
w. Marg. (2 pats) & Syrup (1)	**600**	17	104
Perkins: Buttermilk, 3, plain	**440**	12	70
Harvest Grain: Short Stack, Plain (3)	**270**	2	56
w. Low-Cal Syrup	**295**	2	63
5-Stack w. Low-Cal Syrup	**475**	3.5	93

Waffles

Homemade: 7" waffle, 2½ oz	**245**	13	26
From Mix: 7" waffle, 2½ oz	**205**	8	28

Pancake Brands

	C	F	Cb
Atkins: All-Purpose, 2 tsp. dry mix	**30**	0	5
Pancake & Waffle, ¼ cup dry mix	**90**	1.5	6
Aunt Jemima			
Syrup Dunkers, 13 mini	**520**	4	114
Pancake & Waffle Mix:			
Original, ⅓ cup, prepared	**155**	1	33
Complete, ⅓ cup	**160**	2	31
Mini Pancakes (13)	**240**	4	46
Buttermilk Pancake Batter:			
½ cup, 4 x 4" pancakes	**230**	2	46
Betty Crocker Pancake Mixes			
Complete Original/Buttermilk, 3	**200**	2.5	40
Bisquick (Shake 'N Pour), 3	**200**	3	38
CarbSense, ½ cup dry mix, 2 pancakes	**320**	2	7
Hungry Jack Pancakes			
Mixes: *Per ⅓ Cup (Prepared)*			
Buttermilk: Complete, ⅓ cup	**160**	1.5	32
Original, w. 2% Milk, Oil, Egg	**290**	13	32
w. Skim Milk, Oil, Egg Whites	**220**	6	32
Extra Lights: Complete	**150**	2	30
Microwave: Pancakes (3)	**270**	4.5	51
Northern Pines: Complete Gourmet 3 x 4" pancakes, 3.5 oz	**380**	7	71

Frozen Waffles

Aunt Jemima: Blueberry (1)	**95**	3	15
Buttermilk (1)	**100**	3	17
Syrup Dunkers, 8 sticks & Syrup	**370**	7	74
Eggo *(Kelloggs)*: Banana Bread (1)	**95**	3	16
Chocolate Chip, 1 waffle	**100**	3.5	16
Cinnamon Toast/Homestyle (1)	**95**	5	15
Nutri-Grain (1)	**85**	2.5	14
Special K (fat-free), 1	**65**	0	13
Waf-fulls, all types (1) 2 oz	**155**	5	25
GO-LEAN *(Kashi)*: Average, 1	**90**	1.5	16
Hungry Jack: Blueberry, 1 waffle	**105**	4	17
Buttermilk; Homestyle (1)	**95**	3	15
Mini Funfetti (1)	**65**	2	11
Lifestream, avg. (1)	**120**	4	17
Gorilla; Koala, avg.	**110**	3.5	16
Nature's Path: Optimum Power (1)	**190**	4	33
Average other types (1)	**125**	4	16
Pilsbury Waffle Sticks:			
6 sticks & syrup, avg.	**325**	6	62
Van's: Belgian Original (1)	**95**	2.5	15
97% Fat Free (1)	**80**	1	15
Mini Homestyle (4)	**115**	3.5	18
Carb Manager: Butter Pecan (1)	**50**	3	4
Other varieties (1)	**125**	6	10

Sugar

	C	F	Cb
White Sugar, granulated:			
1 level teaspoon, 4g	15	0	4
1 heaping teaspoon, 6g	25	0	6.5
1 cube, ½"	24	0	6.5
Single portion, 1 packet	25	0	6.5
1 Tablespoon, 12g	48	0	12
1 ounce, 1 oz	110	0	20
1 cup, 7 oz	770	0	203
1 pound	1760	0	464
Brown Sugar:			
1 Tbsp, 13g	50	0	13
1 ounce, 1 oz	109	0	28
1 cup, not packed, 5 oz	540	0	140
1 cup, packed, 7¾ oz	845	0	218
Powdered/Confectioners:			
Sifted, 1 cup, 3½ oz	385	0	98
Unsifted, 1 cup, 4¼ oz	460	0	117
Other Sugars: **Glucose,** 1 oz	110	0	27
Tablets *(Dex 4)*, 1	15	0	4
Barley/Wheat/Rye Malt,			
1 Tbsp, ¾ oz	60	0	14
Cinnamon Sugar, 1 tsp	15	0	4
Dextrose, 1 oz	110	0	27
Fructose: 1 tsp	15	0	4
3 Tbsp, 1 oz	110	0	27
Palm Sugar, 3 Tbsp, 12g	45	0	11
Piloncillo (Brown Sugar), 3oz Cone	325	0	81
Sorbitol, 1 oz	110	0	27
Turbinado Sugar, 2 Tbsp, 1 oz	110	0	27
Unrefined Cane Sugar, 1 oz	110	0	27
FruitSource, 1 oz (powder)	110	0	27

Sugar Substitutes

	C	F	Cb
DiabetiSweet, 1 teaspoon *(Carbohydrate as Sugar Alcohol)*	9	0	4
Equal: Tablet/Liquid	0	0	0
Granulated, 1 pkg	4	0	1
Powdered, sachet, 0.04 oz	0	0	0.5
NutraSweet Spoonful, 1 tsp	2	0	0.5
Nutra Taste; Sweet One, 1 pkt	0	0	0
PerfectSweet, 1 tsp	15	0.5	1
Splenda: Powder, cup	96	0	24
Sachet, sachet	0	0	0.5
Granular, 1 tsp	5	0	1
Sprinkle Sweet, 1 tsp	2	0	0.5
Stevia; Walgreens Wal-Sweet, 1 pkt	0	0	0
Sugar Delight, 1 pkt	8	0	2
Sugar Like (Bateman's), 1 tsp	4	0	1
Sugar Twin: 1 pkt	3	0	0
Sugar Substitute, 1 tsp	2	0	0
Sweet 'N Low, 1 pkt	0	0	1
Weight Watchers; Whey Low, 1 tsp	4	0	1

Honey, Jam, Preserves

Average All Brands	C	F	Cb
Honey: 1 tsp, ¼ oz	22	0	5.5
1 Tbsp, ¾ oz	65	0	17
1 ounce, 1 oz	86	0	23
1 cup, 12 oz	1030	0	269
Single Portion, ½ oz pkg	43	0	11
Jams/Jellies/Marmalade/Preserves			
Regular, 1 tsp, ¼ oz	18	0	5
1 Tbsp, ¾ oz	65	0	16
1 ounce	90	0	22
Single Portion, ½ oz pkg	38	0	11
Apple/Fruit Butters, 1 T., 0.6 oz	20	0	6
Fruit Spreads: Regular, 1 tsp	16	0	4
Low Sugar, 1 tsp	8	0	2
Low Cal. *(Featherweight)*, 1 tsp	4	0	1
Jelly: Regular, average, 1 tsp	18	0	4.5
Imitation, Low Calorie, 1 tsp	4	0	1

Syrups, Molasses

	C	F	Cb
Syrups: *Average All Brands* *(Corn/Rice/Maple/Pancake/Sundae/Waffle) Includes Aunt Jemima, Cary's, Karo, Hershey's, Hungry Jack, Log Cabin, Mrs Butterworth's*			
Regular/Dark/Light Color:			
1 Tbsp, ½ fl.oz	55	0	14
¼ cup (4 Tbsp)	220	0	55
Single Portion: 1½ oz pkg	170	0	42
Lite: 1Tbsp	25	0	6
¼ cup (4 Tbsp)	100	0	25
Sugar-Free: *Atkins*, all types	0	0	0
Cary's, 2 Tbsp, 1 oz	18	0	5
Cozy Cottage, 2 Tbsp	10	0	3
Da Vinci, 2 Tbsp, 1 oz	5	0	1
Molasses: Dark/Light: 1 T., ¾ oz	55	0	14
1 cup, 11½ oz	880	0	224
Blackstrap: 1 Tbsp, ¾ oz	47	0	13
1 cup, 11½ oz	750	0	208

Ice Cream Toppings

	C	F	Cb
Average All Types & Brands (Hershey's, Kraft, Smuckers)			
Butterscotch, Caramel, 2 Tbsp	140	1	30
Chocolate, Hot Fudge, 2 Tbsp	140	4	22
Fat Free Chocolate, 2 Tbsp	100	0	23
Pineapple, Strawberry, 2 Tbsp	110	0	28
Smuckers: Guilt-Free, all flavors	100	0	24
Magic Shell, 2 Tbsp	210	15	18
Milky Way, 2 Tbsp	130	3.5	24
Lite Hot Fudge, 2 Tbsp	90	0	23

Candy, Chocolate

Quick Guide

Chocolate *Average All Brands*	C	F	Cb
Milk Chocolate, regular:			
Plain/Nuts/Fruit, average, 1 oz	**150**	10	13
1½ oz Bar	**225**	15	23
2 oz Bar	**300**	20	30
4 oz Block	**600**	40	60
8 oz Block	**1200**	80	120
1 Pound, 16 oz	**2400**	160	240
Dark/White Chocolate, 1 oz	**150**	10	16
Sugar Free *(Hershey's)* 1 pce, 0.3 oz	**225**	14	23
Chocolate-coated:			
Almonds, 5-6, 1 oz	**160**	11	11
Clusters, nut, 2, 1 oz	**160**	11	15
Coffee Beans, 1.4 oz	**180**	10	23
Creme/Cordial Centers, 1 oz	**120**	4	21
Fudge, 1 oz	**125**	5	18
Macadamias, 2-3 pces, 1 oz	**180**	13	11
Mints, 1 med., 11g	**45**	1	9
Nougat & Caramel, 1 oz	**120**	4	21
Peanuts, 12 med., 1 oz	**160**	11	15
Raisins, 30 med., 1 oz	**120**	4	21
Cooking Chocolate:			
Sweet/Semi-sweet, 1 oz	**160**	8	20
Chips, ¼ cup, 2½ oz	**210**	12	24
Unsweetened, 1 oz	**150**	15	8
Dipping Choc *(Bakers)*, ½ oz, 1T.	**80**	5	9
Carob: Plain, 1 oz	**160**	11	9

Brands & Generic

Per Piece/Serving	C	F	Cb
Abba Zaba, 2 oz bar	**250**	5	48
Absolutely Almond, 2.5 oz bar	**380**	23	40
Aero Bar *(Nestlé),* 1.45 oz bar	**210**	13	26
After Dinner Mints, 1 small	**45**	1	9
After Eight Mint *(Nestlé),* each	**35**	1.2	6
Air Head, 2 bars, 1 oz	**120**	1	30
Allen Wertz: Simply Sugar Free			
Coffee Time (decaf), 4	**45**	1.5	8
Coffee Toffee, 6	**120**	3	23
Other types, 4	**120**	2.5	24
Almond Joy: 1.76 oz bar	**230**	13	28
King Size, 2 pces, 1.7 oz	**425**	24	53
Snack, 1, 0.68 oz bar	**90**	5	11
Bites (8)	**90**	6	9
Swoops, 1 cup, 1.26 oz	**200**	12	20
Almond Roca, 3 pces	**220**	15	19
Sugar Free, 3 pces	**205**	15	16
Almonds, sugar-coated, 7, 1 oz	**130**	5	20

Brands & Generic (Cont)

Per Piece/Serving	C	F	Cb
Almond Clusters *(Trader Joe's),* 2 pce, 1.2 oz	**210**	14	5
Altoids *(C & B),* each	**3**	0	1
Amazin' Fruit, 1 bag, 1.9 oz	**180**	0	41
Andes: Creme de Menthe; Cherry Jubilee			
Choc covered Patty, (3), 1½ oz	**180**	3	35
Thins, avg. all flav., (8), 1.4 oz	**210**	13	22
Anthon Berg: Cognac, each	**180**	8	25
After Dinner Sweet:			
Marzipan w. Madeira, 1.4 oz	**175**	7.5	26
Marzipan Brod	**120**	7	13
Asteroid *(Nestlé),* 1.9 oz	**260**	10	40
Baby Ruth: King Size, 3.7 oz bar	**480**	24	66
2.1 oz bar	**280**	13	34
Fun size, each	**100**	4.5	17
Snack, 1 bar, ¾ oz	**100**	5	12
Baci *(Perugino),* each	**85**	5	8
Bar, 1.58 oz	**230**	15	27
Bar None, 1.5 oz bar	**240**	14	23
Barley Sugar, 1 pce, 0.2 oz	**25**	0	6
Baskin-Robbins, 3 pce, 0.5 oz	**60**	1	13
Big Hunt, 2 oz	**230**	3	47
Bit-O-Honey, 1.7 oz	**200**	3.5	41
Chews, 6 pces, 1.4 oz	**170**	3	34
Blow Pops, each	**50**	0	14
Bon Bons (1)	**25**	0	6
Bonus Bar, 2.1 oz bar	**290**	16	34
Boston Baked Beans, 30 pces, 1 oz	**135**	5	20
Brach's: Almond Supremes (11)	**215**	13	22
Butterscotch Disks (3), 0.6 oz	**70**	0	16
Caramel Clusters (3), 1.5 oz	**225**	13	2
Choc Bridge Mix (16), 1.3 oz	**185**	8	26
Circus Peanuts, each	**25**	0.6	33
Double Dippers (15)	**215**	12	23
Golden Butter Toffee (3)	**80**	2	15
Malted Milk Balls (15), 1.3 oz	**190**	7	30
Milk Maid Caramel (18)	**170**	6	28
Orange Slices (2), 1.3 oz	**130**	0	32
Breath Savers, all types, each	**10**	0	2
Brite Crackers, 1 bag, 1.5 oz	**140**	0	32
Breath Savers, all types, each	**10**	0	2
Brite Crackers, 1 bag, 1.5 oz	**140**	0	32
Brock: Candy Corn (10) 0.7 oz	**75**	0	18
Gummy Bears; Sour Balls, each	**26**	0	6
Lemon Drops, each	**20**	0	5
Orange Slices, each	**35**	0	9
Spice Drops, each	**12**	0	3
Starlight Mints, each	**20**	0	5
Toffee, each	**25**	0.8	5

Brands & Generic (Cont)

Per Piece/Serving	C	F	Cb
Bubble Gum: *See 'Gum' Page 131*			
Buncha Crunch, ½ cup, 1.4 oz	200	10	26
Burnt Peanuts, 40 pces, 40g	190	8	32
Butterfinger: 2.1 oz bar	270	11	41
King Size, 3.7 oz bar	480	18	75
Fun size, each	100	4	15
Mini, each	45	1.5	7.5
Snack (2) 1.3 oz	170	7	27
Butterfinger B.B's, 1.7 oz bag	220	9	34
Buttermints, 18 pces, 1½ oz	160	0	40
Butterscotch: 5 pces	120	2.5	20
Buttons *(Walgreens)*, 3, 18g	70	0	16
Chips *(Hershey's)*, 1 oz	160	8	20
Discs *(Sathers)*, 3, 0.6 oz	110	0	16
Candy Apple, medium, 6.5 oz	260	4	54
Candy Cane, medium, 5", ½ oz	50	0	12
Candy Corn, 1 oz	110	0	27
4 oz Pkt: 24 pces, 1½ oz	150	0	37
Candy Jar Mix *(Jewel)*, 3, 17g	70	0	17
Candy Necklaces, 20g each	80	0.5	20
Caramels: each	30	1	6
Chocolate, each	25	0.3	6
Creams, 3 pces, 1¼ oz	130	3	23
2.75 oz pkt, 5 pces, 1½ oz	160	3.5	30
Hershey's Classic Caramels:			
Soft 'n Chewy, 3 pces	80	2.5	13
Choc Creme Filled, 3 pces	80	3	13
Caramel Nips, each	30	1	6
Caramel Popcorn, 1 cup, 1 oz	120	1.5	26
Caramel Truffles *(Godiva)*, 1 pce	110	6.5	11
Caramello *(Hershey's)*, 1.6 oz bar	220	10	28
Snack, 0.66 oz	90	4	12
Cadbury: 1.6 oz bar	210	9	29
Kingsize, 2.7 oz bar	360	16	49
Certs: Breath Mints, 1 pce	6	0	2
Sugar-free, 1 piece	7	0	2
Charleston Chew, 1 bar, 53g	230	7	40
Chews, all types, 1 oz	110	1	25
Chocolate Mints *(Hershey's)*, each	20	0.5	4
Chocolate Parfait Nips, each	30	1	5
Chuckles Jelly: each	35	0	9
Jujubes *(Hershey's)*, each	10	0	3
Chunky Bar *(Nestlé)*, 1.4 oz	210	11	24
Chupa Chups, 1 pce, 0.42 oz	50	0	11
Cinnamon Bears *(Walgreens)*, 5	150	0	38
Cinn. Buttons *(Walgreens)*, 3 pce	70	0	17
Cinnamon Drops *(Sathers)*, 19 pce	150	0	36

Per Piece/Serving	C	F	Cb
Coconut Stacks, 4, 41g	190	6	33
Coffee Go Coffee/Cappuccino, ea.	18	0.4	4
Coffee Rio-Gold, each	15	0.5	3
Collard & Bowser, Eng. Toffee (2)	80	4	12
Conversation Hearts *(Necco)*, 1 lge	16	0	4
Cote d'Or: Bouchee, each	130	8	12
Chokotoff, each	210	9	30
Nougatti	150	8	19
Bar & Nuts, 1.3 oz	220	18	12
Cotton Candy, 1 oz	70	0	17
Cough Drops: *See Page 131*			
Cracker Jack, 1.25 oz box	150	2.5	29
Creme Savers *(Sugar-Free)* 1 pce	10	0.5	2.5
Crisped Rice: Almond, 1 bar	130	6	18
Choc Chip, 1 bar	115	4	18
Crispy Rice Snacks *(Hershey's)*, 1 bar	60	2	9
Crows, 12 pieces, 1.5 oz	140	0	35
Crunch: 5 oz bar	725	38	90
King Munch, 2.75 oz bar	400	20	51
1.55 oz bar	230	12	29
Fun size, each	50	2.5	7
Snack (3), 1½ oz	220	11	28
Pieces, ¼ cup, 38g	190	10	25
White Bar, 1.4 oz bar	220	13	23
Crunch Berries Treats, 1.6 oz bar	190	4.5	36
Decadence *(NuBar)* Bar, 1.3 oz	140	2.5	30
Doctor's Carbrite, 12 pces	30	2	4
Dots, 12 dots, 1.5 oz	140	0	35
Double Dip Stick, 1 stick	16	0.5	3
Dove: Dark/Milk, 1.3 oz bar	200	12	22
Bar, 6 oz	920	56	104
Miniatures, each	30	2	3
Drops Candy *(Hershey's)*, 9 pces	100	0	24
Dum Dum Pops *(Spangler)*, 1 pop	25	0	6
Endulge *(Atkins)*: *Per Serving*			
Candy Bits, avg., 1 oz bag	150	8	16
Caramel Nut Chew Bar, 1.23 oz	175	9	17
Chocolate Almond Bar, 1.1 oz	180	13	14
Chocolate/Crunch Bar, 1.1 oz	130	12	3
Chocolate Peanut Bar, 1.1 oz	135	13	3
Peanut Butter Cups (3), 1.2 oz	195	13	17
Peanut Caramel Cluster, 1.23 oz	170	9	13
Wafer Crisp Bars (2), 1 oz	155	9	15
English Toffee, 1 pce	48	3	5
Eda's Sugar Free, all flav., 5, ½ oz	40	0	15

Brands & Generic (Cont)

Per Piece/Serving	C	F	Cb
Estee Dietetic Candies:			
Caramels, all flavors, 1 pce	30	1	5
Chocolate, Dark/ Mint, ½ bar	200	14	23
Gummy Bears; Gum Drops, 1 pce	7	0	1.5
Hard Candies: Butterscotch (2)	25	0	6
Peppermint (3)	30	0	7
Lollipops; Mint/Toffee (5)	60	0	15
Lollipop	30	0	8
Milk Chocolate, ½ bar, 4 oz	230	17	17
Peanut Butter Cups, 1 cup	40	3	3
Fructose Sweetened, 1 cup	40	2	3
Peanut Brittle, ⅓ box, 1.5 oz	240	9	28
5th Avenue: 2 oz bar	280	12	37
King Size bar	460	20	64
Snack Size, 0.58 oz	75	3.5	10
Fanny May: Single Wrapped Pieces			
Mint Meltaway Patty, 1.5 oz	250	17	22
Pixie, 1.5 oz	215	12	24
Trinidad, 1.5 oz	205	11	24
Fast Break *(Reese's)*, 2 oz	275	13	35
Ferrero Rocher: each	75	5	6
3 pces, 1.3 oz	220	15	17
Fifty 50 Snack Bars:			
Peanut Butter, 2	200	14	16
Almond Choc., 7 pce, 1½ oz	210	15	20
Crunch Choc., 7 pce, 1.1 oz	160	11	19
Fruit & Nut Choc., 7 pce, 1½ oz	200	14	21
Milk Choc., 3 pce, ½ bar, 43g	210	14	25
Mini Bars, 8 bars, 1 oz	140	9	16
Fluffy Stuff *(Charms)*, 0.6 oz bag	70	0	17
Fondant: Choc-coated, 1.2 oz	130	3	28
Mint, 1 oz	105	0	27
Franklin Crunch 'N Munch:			
all varieties, average, 1.25 oz	170	7	30
Fran's: Gold Bar, 1.75 oz	260	14	34
Gold Bites (Almonds), 1	130	7	17
Frootsies, 12 pces	145	3	29
Fruit Crystals *(Walgreens)*, 3 pces	70	0	17
Fruit Drops, each	6	0	1
Fruit Gems *(Sunkist)*, 3, 1.1 oz	105	0	26
Fruit Leathers, average, 0.5 oz	45	0	12
Fruit Pastilles, 1 roll, 1.4 oz	100	0	26
Fruit Rolls, 1 roll	80	0	20
Fruit Roll-Ups, ½ oz	50	0	12
Fruit Runts *(Walgreens)*, 1T., ¼ pkt	60	0	14
Fruit Shapes *(Fruitfield)*, 1 oz (10)	100	0.5	23
Fruit Waves, 0.5 oz	50	0	12
Fudge: Chocolate/Vanilla, 1 oz	115	3	20
with Nuts, 1 oz	120	4	21
Choco. Marshmallow, 1 oz	120	5	18
w. Nuts, 1 oz	125	5.5	18
Peanut Butter, 1 oz	105	2	21

Per Piece/Serving	C	F	Cb
Ghirardelli: Milk/Dark Chocolate,			
1.25 oz bar	185	12	20
w. almonds, 1.5 oz bar	220	14	25
Creme filling, 3 pces, 1.5 oz	220	12	26
Godiva: Hearts, each	45	2	4
Almond Butter Dome, 1 pce	80	6	6
Bouchee au Chocolate, 1 pce	220	13	23
Cordial Assortment, each	60	2.5	9
Gold Ballotin, 1 pce	70	3.5	9
Milk/Dark/Ivory Assortment, each	75	4	8
Nut & Caramel, each	75	4	6
Truffle Amaretto, 1 pce	110	6.5	12
Golden Almond Bar, 1 bar	520	34	40
Golden 111 Bar, 1 bar	500	30	52
Go Lightly: Box Candies, 4	60	0	15
Bags: Assorted Taffy, 6	140	3	36
Vanilla Caramels, 5	150	6	31
Super Free Choc Crunch (7) 1½ oz	180	13	23
Goobers Peanuts, 1 pkg, 1.4 oz	210	14	22
Good 'N Fruity: 1 box, 1.8 oz	140	1	35
Snack Size, 1 box, 17g	60	0	15
Good & Plenty *(Hershey's)*: 1.8 oz box	160	0	40
Snack Size, 1 box, 17g	60	0	14
GooGoo Cluster, 1 bar, 1.75 oz	240	11	32
Gubor Surprise (3) 1.5 oz	235	15	22
Gum Drops: 1 small	15	0	3
1 large, 0.4 oz	40	0	7
6 oz pkt: 4 pces, 1.4 oz	130	0	31
Gummi Bears: 8 bears, 1½ oz	140	0	32
Gummi Novelties *(Walgreens)*, 6	150	0	22
Gummi Savers, each	12	0	3
Gummi Sweet Tarts, 1 bug, 1.5 oz	150	0	34
Gummi Watch, 1, 2 oz	105	0	24
Gummi Worms, each	25	0	5
Guylian: Milk Choc., 8 squares, 1 oz	126	9	15
Dark Choc., 8 squares, 1 oz	117	9	14
Halvah *(Joyvah)*: Plain, ½ bar, 2 oz	390	25	18
Choc.coated Sesame, ½ bar, 2 oz	380	23	20
Hard Candy: All flavors, 1 oz	110	0	28
1 regular piece	18	0	5
Heath: Original, 1.4 oz bar	210	12	24
Bites, 1 piece	15	1	1.5
Snack, 0.33 oz	50	3	6

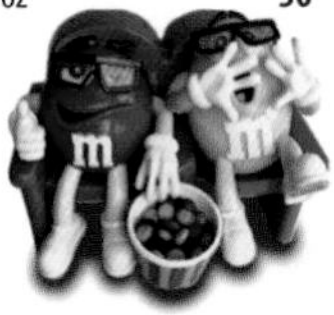

Brands & Generic (Cont)

Per Piece/Serving	C	F	Cb
Hershey's: Kisses, avg. all var. (1)	25	1.5	3
Bar: 1.55 oz bar	240	14	25
King Size bar, 2.6 oz	410	25	38
w. Almonds, 1.45 oz bar	230	14	20
Cookies 'n' Creme, 1.55oz bar	230	12	26
Bites: Almond Joy (8)	100	6	10
Cookies 'n' Creme (8)	90	5	10
York (9)	90	1.5	19
Milk Choc w. Almond (7)	90	6	8
Cookies 'N Mint: 1.55 oz bar	230	12	27
Snack, 0.6 oz	90	4.5	11
Crunchy Cookie Cups, 1.4 oz	210	12	23
Hugs: Regular (1), 4.5g	25	1.5	3
Regular (9), 40g	220	13	23
w. Almonds (9), 40g	230	13	22
Milk Chocolate: 1.55 oz bar	230	13	25
Eggs, candy coated (4)	90	4	12
Snack, 0.6 oz	90	5	10
Kingsize, 2.6 oz bar	400	23	42
7 oz bar, ⅓ bar	200	12	21
w. Almonds Snack, 0.6 oz	100	6	9
w. Almonds, 1.45 oz bar	235	15	20
Miniatures: 5 pces, 1.5 oz	230	13	25
Kisses, 1 bag	420	24	44
Nuggets: Snack, avg. all bars (1)	50	3	6
P'nut Butter Crispy Rice, (1)	230	13	25
Special Dark Choc., 1.45 oz bar	230	13	25
Sweet Escapes: 1.4 oz bar, avg.	180	7	27
Snack, avg. (1) 0.7 oz	80	3.5	12
Swoops, avg., 1 cup, 1.26 oz	190	11	20
Whoppers, 10 pieces	100	4	16
Candy-Coated Eggs:			
Milk Choc (4), 0.6 oz	90	4	12
w. Almonds (4) 0.6 oz	100	6	9
Sugar Free: Choc. Candy (3)	215	13	24
Dark Chocolate Candy (5)	220	13	24
Chocolate w. Almonds (5)	225	14	23
Peanut Butter Cups Minis (5)	210	12	23
1 gram Sugar Carb: Choc. Bar, 1 oz	130	11	18
w. Soy Crisps, 1 oz	120	10	16
w. Almonds, 1 oz	110	12	16
Honeycomb: Plain, 1 oz	115	0	27
Choc-coated, 1 oz	125	1	28
Hot Tamales: 1 box, 60g, 2.1 oz	220	0	55
Sathers, 19 pces, 1.4 oz	150	0	36
Ice Blue Mints *(Walgreens)*, 3, 17g	70	0	17
Jawbreakers *(Sathers)*, 3, 17g	70	0	17
Jellies, 3 medium, 1 oz	120	0	30

Per Piece/Serving	C	F	Cb
Jells Raspberry *(Joyva)*, each	70	1	8
Jelly Beans: Small, 22 beans, 1 oz	100	0	24
Regular, 12 beans, 1 oz	100	0	24
1 bean	8	0	2
Sugar Free	135	0	34
Jumbo, 1 bean	20	0	5
Jewel, 13 beans, 1.4 oz	140	0	36
Sathers/Walgreens, (17) 40g	150	0	37
Wonderbeans, 33 beans	100	0	24
Jelly Bellys: each	4	0	1
32 pces, 1.4 oz	150	0	37
1 tin, 2.5 oz	250	0	6
Jelly Rings *(Jewel)*, 3, 1.5 oz	160	0	39
Jolly Rancher: Candy (1)	40	0	9
Fruit Chews (6), 1.4 oz	150	1.5	33
Hard Candy (3), 18g	70	0	17
Jolly Jellies, 7 oz	120	0	30
Lollipops, 1 pce, 0.6 oz	60	0	16
Sugar Free, 4 pces, 0.5 oz	35	0	14
Junior Mints: 1.84 oz box	210	3.5	40
16 pces, 1.4 oz	160	2.5	34
Juicefuls: Red Raspb., (3), 0.6 oz	60	0	15
Assorted Fruits, 1 pce	20	0	5
Jujubes, all types (6), 1.4 oz	5	0	3
Juju Mix *(Sathers)*, 11 pce, 1½ oz	150	0	36
Juju Toys, 6 pce, 1.5 oz	150	0	37
Jujyfruits, 1 box, 0.2 oz	40	0	10
Kit Kat: 1.5 oz bar	235	11	29
2.8 oz bar	400	20	50
Big Kat, 1.94 oz	290	15	35
Bites (7), 1.4 oz	200	10	25
King Size, 3 oz bar	495	25	62
Miniature, 0.35 oz	50	2.5	6.5
Multipack/Snack Bar each	80	4	10
Krackel: 2.6 oz bar	330	18	38
Snack size, 0.6 oz	85	4	12
Kraft: Caramels, (5), 40g	160	3.5	30
Kudos: 1 oz bar, avg. all types	120	5	20
M&M's Milk Choc Minis, 0.8 oz	90	2.5	17
Snickers, 0.8 oz	100	3.5	16
Lance: Popscotch, 1.2 oz pkg	160	6	24
Chocolaty Peanut Bar, 2 oz bar	320	18	30
Peanut Bar, 1.8 oz pkg	260	14	24
Lemon Drops (3) ½ oz	50	0	12
Sugar Free *(Walgreens)*, 5, ½ oz	35	0	14
Lemonhead, 10, ½ oz	60	0	14

Brands & Generic (Cont)

Per Piece/Serving	C	F	Cb
Licorice: Average all types, 1oz	**100**	0	25
Bites *(Switzer)*, each	**10**	0	2
Chews *(Panda)*, each	**10**	0	1
Tid Bits, each	**5**	0	1
Twists: Black/Red, avg. 1 pce	**30**	0	7
American Licorice Co.: Laces, 1	**35**	0	8
Stick, (1) 0.5 oz	**45**	0	11
Choco Sticks, (4) 1.4 oz	**145**	0	35
Red Bites, 1.4 oz	**140**	0	34
Super Red Ropes, 1 rope, 2 oz	**200**	0	46
Vines, 1 pce	**70**	0	17
Lifesavers: Large size, 1 candy	**15**	0	4
Regular, all flavors, 1 candy	**10**	0	2
1 Roll (14 candies), 1.14 oz	**130**	0	32
Creme Savers (1)	**25**	0.5	4
Gummi Savers, 1.5 oz roll	**140**	0	32
Lollipops Fruit, 1 pce, 0.4 oz	**45**	0	11
Pepomint, 4 mints	**60**	0	15
Sugar-Free Delites: *Per Candy*			
Orchard Fruits; Summer Blend	**5**	0	2
Butter Toffee; European Collect.	**10**	0.5	3
Creme Savers (1)	**10**	0.5	2.5
Lik-m-aid *(Nestlé)*, 1.7 oz	**60**	0	15
Lindt: Lindor, Balls, average	**75**	6	5
Amaretto Balls	**65**	5	5
Milk Chocolate, 1.4 oz pce	**210**	12	23
Lollipops, each, 0.2 oz	**20**	0	5
Lollipops C Pops *(Glenny's)*, each	**35**	0	8
M & M's: Plain, 1.7 oz pkg	**235**	10	34
Milk Chocolate, 1 pce	**5**	0.2	0.5
20 pces, 0.6 oz	**80**	4	10
¼ cup, 1.8 oz	**255**	10	37
Almond Choc., 1.3 oz pkg	**200**	11	21
1.5 oz pkg	**230**	13	25
Crispy, 1.5 oz	**205**	8	31
Minis, Mega Tube, 1.1 oz tube	**150**	7	21
Peanut: 1.7 oz pkg	**255**	13	30
Fun Size, 0.7 oz pkg	**110**	5	13
Peanut Butter: 1.6 oz pkg	**250**	14	26
Fun Size, 0.7 oz pkg	**110**	6	12
Mamba, 9 pces, 1½ oz	**160**	2	36
Marathon *(Snickers)* Bar, 1.9 oz	**225**	7	32
M.Azing, 1 bar	**220**	12	29
Mars Bar: All varieties, 1.76 oz	**240**	13	31
Fun size, 1 bar	**95**	5	12
Marshmallow Egg, 1 egg	**110**	0	26

Per Piece/Serving	C	F	Cb
Marshmallows: Firm/Soft, 1 oz	**90**	0	23
Regular size, 6 pce, 33g	**110**	0	26
Mini-Marshmallow, ½ c., 30g	**100**	0	24
Choc-coat. Twists (Joyva), each	**95**	2	10
Fluff, 2 Tbsp, 18 g	**60**	0	15
Kraft: Mini, ½ cup	**80**	0	21
Creme, 2 Tbsp	**40**	0	10
Jet-Puffed, 5 pces	**90**	0	23
Funmallows, each	**25**	0	6
Miniature, ½ cup	**100**	0	25
Teddy Bear, ½ cup	**50**	0	12
Marzipan, 1 oz	**140**	7	16
Mauna Loa: Choc., 2.5 oz bar	**420**	29	36
Choc. coated Macadamias (9)	**230**	17	19
Mega Fruit Gummi, each	**10**	0	2
Mexican Hats (9)	**100**	0	24
Mentos, each	**10**	0	2
Mike & Ike: 1 pkg, 2.1 oz	**220**	0	55
19 pce, 1.4 oz	**150**	0	36
Milkfulls *(Storck)*, 6 pces, 1.4 oz	**170**	3	35
Milk Chocolate: *See Hershey's*			
Milk Choc. Crisp, 1.45 oz bar	**205**	11	22
Milk Duds *(Hershey's)*, 7 pces	**170**	6	28
Milk Shake Bar, 1.8 oz bar	**220**	7	37
Milky Way: Midnight Bar, 1.75 oz	**220**	8	36
Regular Bar, 2 oz	**270**	10	41
Fun size, 2 bars, 1.4 oz	**180**	7	28
King Size, 3.63 oz bar	**480**	18	72
Miniatures (5) 43g	**190**	7	30
Pop'ables (13) 39g	**200**	7	28
Choc. Covered Caramels, 2 oz	**200**	8	30
Milky Way Lite, 1.57 oz	**170**	5	34
Miniatures, 1.4 oz pkg (5)	**150**	4.5	29
Mints: Uncoated, 1 oz	**100**	0	23
1 small mint (¾" diam.)	**7**	0	2
1 large mint (1½" diam.)	**30**	0	7
Mon Cheri *(Ferrero)*, 4 pces, 45g	**260**	18	20
Mounds: 1.75 oz bar	**255**	13	31
Snack, 0.68 oz	**90**	5	11
Mr Goodbar: 1.75 oz bar	**280**	18	25
King Size, 2.6 oz bar	**420**	26	38
Snack, 0.6 oz	**100**	6	9
Miniatures (1)	**45**	2.5	5
Bites (9), 1.4 oz	**230**	14	21
Necco Candy Wafers (3) 57g	**15**	0	4
Neuhaus, average all types	**80**	5	7
Newman's Own, Pepp. Cups, 1 pkg	**170**	11	20
P'Nut B. Cups (Milk/Dark), 3, 1 pkg	**180**	12	17

Brands & Generic (Cont)

Per Piece/Serving	C	F	Cb
Nibs, all types, 1 pouch, 0.5 oz	45	0	10
Nips *(Pearson)*, all flavors, 2, 14g	60	2	10
Nite Bite *(Glucose Bar)*	100	3.5	15
Nothing But Nuts Butter Toffee			
3 Tbsp, 1 oz	200	15	9
Nougat, 2 pces, 1 oz	115	1	25
Chocolate Covered, 1 oz	120	4	20
Nougat Nut Cream, 3.5 oz	340	31	50
Now & Later *(Nabisco)*, 1 pkg	270	2.5	63
Nutrageous Bar *(Reese's)*, 1.8 oz	275	16	27
Snack, 0.6 oz	90	5	9
Oh Henry! 1.8 oz bar	240	10	32
100 Grand, 1.5 oz bar	190	8	30
Orange *(Lindt)*, 6 block, 40g	190	10	24
Orange Slices: *Jewel*, 3, 41g	140	0	36
Walgreens, 3, 43g	150	0	36
Pastel Mints *(Walgreens)*, 33 pce	150	0	38
Patteez *(Sweet n' Low)*, ½ ctn, 5	120	2.5	32
PayDay Bar: 1.85 oz bar	260	14	27
King Size, 3.4 oz	480	26	50
Snack, 0.7 oz	100	5.5	10
Peanut Bar, 1.6 oz bar	210	14	20
Peanut Butter Bars, 3 pces, 18g	80	1.5	15
Peanut Butter Cups: *See Reese's; Newman's Own*			
Peanut Brittle, 1 oz	130	5	20
Sugar Free *(Judy's)*, ¾ cup, 1 oz	75	6	2
Peanut Riesen (5), 41g	190	7	28
Peanuts, choc-covered, each	25	1.5	2
Pearson's Mint Patties, (5), 38g	150	2.5	31
Pecan Roll, ⅓ bar, 40g	200	10	26
Peppermints, 7 small, 0.5 oz	50	0	12
Hershey's, 3 pces	60	0	15
Peppermint Twists (2), 13g	60	0	12
Pez, 1 roll	30	0	6
Planters: Choc. Peanuts (25) 7 oz	220	13	20
Orig. Peanut Bar, 1.6 oz	230	14	22
Pop'ables: Average, 13 pces, 1½ oz	200	8	28
12 oz Package	1600	64	224
Positively Pecan, 2.5 oz bar	390	24	38
Pralines: Small, 0.3 oz	38	2	5
1 large piece, 1.4 oz	180	10	24
Pretzels: Choc-covered,			
3 minisize, 1.15 oz	150	5.5	23
1 regular, 1 oz	130	4.5	20
Pretzel Flipz *(Nestlé)*, 8 pces, 1 oz	130	5	19
Raisinets, 1 pkg, 1.7 oz	210	8	33

Per Piece/Serving	C	F	Cb
Raspberry Cream, each	80	2.5	5
Reception Sticks (4)	70	2	12
Red Hot Dollars, 7 pces	100	0	24
Reese's: Chocolate Bar, 2.8 oz	420	24	43
Candy (Multipack), each	95	5.5	9
Miniatures, each	40	2.5	4
Peanut Butter Bites (7)	90	5	10
Mini, 1 pce	40	2.5	5
Peanut Butter Cups: 1.6 oz pkg	250	14	25
Kingsize, 2.8 oz	420	24	43
Mini, 1 pce, 0.27 oz	45	2.5	4
Peanut Butter Eggs (1), 0.6 oz	90	5	9
Reese's Pieces (25), 1.6 oz	225	10	26
ReeseSticks, Kingsize, (2), 1.5 oz	230	13	23
Snack Size, (2), 1.2 oz (34g)	190	11	19
Swoops, 1 cup, 1.26 oz	180	10	17
Fast Break, 2 oz	120	13	35
Rice Krispies Treats *(Kellogg's):*			
Average all varieties	110	3.5	19
Rice Crunchy Bars, 19g bar	60	0	14
Riesen Choc. Chew, (5) 1.4 oz	180	7	29
Peanut & Milk Choc, (5)	190	7	28
Ritter Sport: Plain Choc, 50g	260	16	26
w. Hazelnuts, ½ pkg, 50g	290	19	24
Rocky Road, 1.8 oz bar	240	11	34
Robin Eggs: Large (2); Mini (10)	70	2	14
Medium, 4 pces	90	2.5	16
Rolo, all types (3), 0.64 oz	90	2.5	12
Root Beer Barrels (3) 0.5 oz	65	0	16
Ross Chocolate Bar: White, 1.2 oz	130	13	3
Almond; Crunchy, 1.2 oz	140	13	4
Russell Stover Candy: Creams (1)	60	2	10
Almond Delight, 2 oz	290	17	32
Caramel Bar, 46g	230	11	20
Jelly Cups (P/Nut Butter), 2, 34g	140	9	14
Mint Dream	160	8	19
Pecan Roll, 50g	260	18	23
Low Carb: Pecan Delight (2), 1.4 oz	180	13	24
Cups (3), 1.3 oz	170	11	23
Mint Patties, 1.4 oz	190	11	27
Sugar Free Dark Choc., 5 pces	220	15	21
Salt Water Taffy *(Sathers)*, 5, 43g	150	2.5	34
Scooby-Doo! *(Fruit Snacks)*, 10 pces	100	0	24
Seashells *(Guylian)*, 1 shell	65	4	6
See's Candies: *Average all Flavors*			
Brittles (2), 1.3 oz	220	15	18
Caramels & Chews, 2 pieces	175	10	19
Creams, 2 pieces	180	9	24
Little Pops, 4 pieces	60	2	11
Lollypops (1)	80	2.5	14
Nut Clusters, 3 pieces	225	16	16

Brands & Generic (Cont)

Per Piece/Serving	C	F	Cb
Sesame Crunch, 3 pces	**80**	4	7
Signature Treasures *(Nestlé):*			
Choc. Creme, 3 pieces, 1.2 oz	**210**	13	21
Creamy Caramel, 3 pieces, 1.3 oz	**175**	9	23
Dark Choc Mint, 4 pieces, 1.5 oz	**220**	10	30
Peanut Butter, 4 pieces, 1.6 oz	**260**	17	23
Strawberries & Creme, 3 pces	**195**	12	21
Simply Lite, ½ ctn, 36 pieces	**130**	5	18
Simply Sugar Free: *See Allen Wertz*			
Sixlets *(Hershey)*, 24 pces	**90**	3.5	14
Skittles: Sour, 1.8 oz bag	**200**	2	44
Orig./Trop./Wild Berry, 2.17 oz	**240**	2.5	54
Fun Size, 1 bag, 0.7 oz (20g)	**80**	1	18
King Size, 4 oz bag	**440**	4.5	100
Large bag (16 oz), ¼ cup, 1.5 oz	**170**	2	37
Mint (Pepp./Sprmint), 1.6 oz pkg	**180**	2	40
Skor Toffee Bar, 1.4 oz	**220**	13	24
Smarties Candy Rolls, 1 roll	**25**	0	5
Snackwell's Raisin Dips, 5 oz	**160**	5	34
Snickers: 2.07 oz bar	**280**	14	35
3.7 oz bar	**510**	24	63
Creme Egg, each	**170**	10	19
Cruncher, 2.54 oz	**370**	21	41
King Size, ½ bar, 1.2 oz	**170**	8	21
Marathon Bar, avg., 1.9 oz	**225**	7	32
Miniatures, each	**40**	2.5	5
Munch Bar, 1.4 oz bar	**230**	15	17
Pop'ables, 13 pieces, 1½ oz	**190**	9	24
Snack (2), 40g	**190**	10	24
Sno Caps, 2.3 oz pkg	**300**	13	48
Soft Chews *(Maalox)*, 1 chew	**20**	0.5	4
Soft 'N Chewy Butter Toffee, ea.	**30**	0.5	7
Soft Drops (9)	**100**	0	24
Soft Hot Dollars (11)	**90**	0	23
Sonic Boom Pops *(Walgreens)*, ea.	**60**	0	14
Sour Brite Crawlers, 13 pces	**140**	0	31
Sour Punch: All types, 2 oz	**190**	1	45
1 straw	**20**	0	5
Spearmint Leaves: *Jewel*, 5, 40g	**140**	0	35
Walgreens, 5, 1½ oz	**150**	0	38
Spice Drops, 10 pces, 1½ oz	**130**	0	33
Spree Candies: Original, 8 pces	**60**	0	14
Chewy Spree, 8 pces	**50**	0	12
Starburst: Candy Canes, 0.5 oz	**70**	0	18
Fruit Chews, each	**20**	0.4	4
2 oz pkg	**240**	4.5	48
Fruit Twist, each	**35**	0	8
Fruit Twist, 2 oz pkg	**190**	1	45

Per Piece/Serving	C	F	Cb
Starburst (Cont)			
Jellybeans, 1.5 oz	**150**	0	38
Jellybean Egg, 2 oz	**200**	0	51
Tropical Fruit, 2.07 oz pack	**240**	4.5	48
Starlight Mints, 3 pces, ½ oz	**55**	0	14
Suckers *(Walgreens)*, 1 sucker, 11g	**45**	0	11
Sugar Babies, 1.7 oz bag	**190**	2	43
Sugar Coated Peanuts, 1 oz	**120**	8	10
Sweet 'N Low: Chews, each	**14**	0	3
Coffee Cremes (1)	**70**	5	10
Sugar-Free Hard Candy, each	**8**	0	2
Wafer Bars, avg. (1)	**55**	3	7
Mint Patteez (1)	**25**	0.5	7.5
Sweet Escapes: *See Hershey's*			
Sweet Success Bars, 1 bar	**120**	4	23
Sweet Tarts *(Nestlé)*, 7 pces, ½ oz	**50**	0	13
Symphony: 1.5 oz bar	**240**	15	22
Snack: Chocolate (1), 0.6 oz	**90**	5	10
w. Almds & Toffee (1), 0.5 oz	**80**	5	7
Taffy, 1 pce, ½ oz	**55**	0.5	12
3 Musketeers: 2.13 oz bar	**260**	8	46
Fun size, each	**70**	2	13
Miniatures, each	**25**	0.5	5
Pop'ables (10), 41g	**180**	6	31
Tang-a-Roos: 1 roll	**25**	0	6
Tarts *(Walgreens)*, 4 pce, 15g	**60**	0	15
Tails *(Walgreens)*, 8 pce, 15g	**60**	0	15
Tastetations *(Hershey's)*, 3	**60**	1.5	12
Terry's Choc Orange, (5), 1.5 oz	**230**	12	27
Tic Tac, all varieties, each	**1.5**	0	0
Toblerone: 50g (1.76 oz) bar	**270**	15	32
1 bar, 100g (3.5 oz)	**540**	30	63
⅓ bar, 33g	**180**	10	21
Toffees, Regular, 1 oz	**150**	9	15
Toll House Bars, 2 pieces, 2 oz	**130**	6	18
Tongue Torchers *(Walgreens)*, 3	**70**	0	17
Tootsie Pops, Mini (3)	**50**	0	13
Tootsie Roll, 2.25 oz roll	**230**	5	26
Trolli Gumm Candy, avg., 5 pces	**120**	0	29
Truffles: Regular, 1 pce, 0.4 oz	**60**	4	5
Large *(Godiva)*, 0.75 oz	**110**	6.5	12
Extra Large *(J.Schmidt)*, 1½ oz	**220**	13	24
Turtles *(Nestlé)*, avg., each	**85**	4.5	10
Twists (Sugar Free): Licorice; Strawberry,			
6 twists, 40g	**140**	0	32
Twix: Caramel 2 oz pkg	**280**	14	37
King Size, 3 oz pkg	**405**	20	52
Fun Size: 0.5 oz	**80**	4	10
2 oz pkg, 2 bars	**280**	14	37
Peanut Butter, 1.8 oz	**280**	17	28
Snack, 1 cookie, 0.5 oz	**80**	5	8

Brands & Generic (Cont)

Per Piece/Serving	C	F	Cb
Twizzlers: Twists, 4 pieces, 1.6 oz	**160**	1	36
Pull 'n' Peel Cherry (1), 1 oz	**100**	0	25
Velamints Sugar Free, 2 pce	**5**	0	1
Werther's: Original, 3 pce, 15g	**60**	1	13
Chocolates (5), 20g	**110**	6	13
Whatchamacallit Bar, 1.6 oz	**230**	11	28
Snack (1), 0.57 oz	**80**	4	10
Whitman's: Pecan Roll, 2 oz roll	**300**	20	26
Sampler, 3 pces, 1.4 oz	**200**	11	25
Assorted; Dark Chocolate, 1 pce	**65**	3	9
Snoopy Treats, 2 pces	**190**	10	24
Sucratrol Mint Pattie, 1 oz	**120**	7	17
Whoppers, 9 pce	**100**	3.5	15
Yogurt Candy: Plain, 1 oz	**120**	6	15
Coated Raisins, 1 oz	**120**	4	21
York Mints: 1.5 oz patty	**145**	5	34
Snack size, 0.5 oz	**50**	1	11
Peppermint Patties, 3	**150**	2.5	30
Swoops, 1 cup, 1.26 oz	**190**	11	21
Zachary Old Fash. Creme Drops (3)	**170**	3	36
Zagnut: 1.75 oz bar	**230**	10	31
Snack size (1), 0.5 oz	**70**	3	9
Zero Bar, 1 pce, 0.6 oz	**70**	2.5	12
Zingos, 3 pce, 2g	**5**	0	2

Gum

Gum: *Per Piece*	C	F	Cb
Bazooka, each	**30**	0	7
Beechies	**6**	0	2
Big League Chew	**10**	0	2
Bubble Gum Balls *(Hershey's)*	**10**	0	2
Bubble Yum	**25**	0	6
Sugarless	**10**	0	3
Candilicious	**30**	0	2
Carefree (Sugarless/Regular)	**5**	0	2
Chiclets	**5**	0	1
Clorets, stick	**10**	0	2
Dentyne	**6**	0	2
Estee, bubble/regular	**5**	0	2
Extra *(Wrigley's)*, Sugar-Free (1)	**5**	0	2
Freshen-Up	**13**	0	2
Hubba Bubba: Regular	**23**	0	6
Sugar-free, average	**14**	0	0.5
Ice Breakers, 1 stick	**5**	0	2
Sonic Boom Bubble Gum	**15**	0	3
Sticklets	**7**	0	2
Super Bubble	**15**	0	4
Trident: Slab	**5**	0	1
Soft Bubble Gum	**9**	0	1
Wrigley's, all flavors	**10**	0	2

Carob Candy

Per Piece/Serving	C	F	Cb
Carob: Plain/Natural, 1 oz	**160**	11	9
Carob Coated: Raisins, 1 oz	**130**	8	15
Almonds/Peanuts, 1 oz	**150**	10	14
Malt Balls, 1 oz	**135**	8	15
Caramels, 1 oz	**110**	4	18
Dates, 1 oz	**125**	5	20
Soybeans	**145**	9	16
Trail/Party Mix, 1 oz	**140**	9	15
Carob Chips, unsweetened, 1 oz	**140**	7	19
Carob Bars: Plain/Nut, 1 oz	**160**	11	13
Fruit & Nut, 1 oz	**155**	10	13
Mint/Orange, 1 oz	**160**	11	14
Carafection: Cashew Coconut Crunch, ½ Bar, (42g) 1.5 oz	**250**	14	5
Caroby Natural Touch, 3 oz	**450**	27	36

Cough Drops

	C	F	Cb
Beech Nut, 1 drop	**10**	0	2
Diabetic Tussin, 1 drop	**0**	0	0
Halls Defense Vit. C, 1 drop	**15**	0	4
Halls Fruit Breezers, 1 drop	**15**	0	4
Halls Menthol Drops, 1 drop	**15**	0	4
Sugar Free, 1 drop	**5**	0	4
Halls Plus, 1 drop	**20**	0	5
Helps Cough, all flavors, 1	**15**	0	3
Listerine Lozenge (Amer. Chicle)	**10**	0	2
Luden's Throat Drops, all flavors, 1	**10**	0	2
Sugar Free, 1 drop	**0**	0	0
Pine Bros, 1 cough drop	**10**	0	2
Ricola: Cough Drops, 1 drop	**10**	0	3
Sugar-Free Lemon Mint, 2 mints	**0**	0	1
Rite Aid, Menthol Cough, 1 drop	**10**	0	3
Robitussin: Regular, 1 drop	**15**	0	3
Honey Cough, 1 drop	**40**	0	10
Sugar Free Throat, 1 drop	**10**	0	3
Sunny Orange Vit. C, 1 drop	**10**	0	3
Rolaids/Sodium Free, 1	**5**	0	1
Sathers Peppermint Lozenges, 1	**15**	0	3
Squibb Cough/Throat Loz.'s, 1	**15**	0	4
Sucrets *(Beecham)* Lozenges, 1	**10**	0	2
Wintergreen Loz. *(Walgreens)*, 1	**15**	0	3

Cough Suppresant Liquids: *See Page 142*

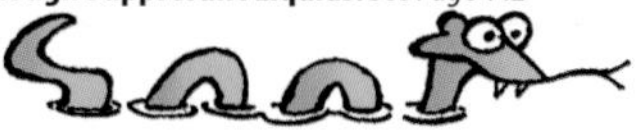

Popcorn

Home-Popped Popcorn

	C	F	Cb
Popping Corn Kernels:			
2 Tbsp, 1 oz (makes approx. 3½ cups)	100	1	22
Air-popped (no oil), plain, 1 oz	100	0	22
1 cup (6g)	20	0	4
Oil-popped, plain, 1 oz	140	8	10
1 cup (11g)	55	3	4
Popcorn Oil, 1 Tbsp	120	14	0

Microwave Popcorn

	C	F	Cb
Average All Brands (Popped)			
Butter: Regular, 1 cup	35	2	4
Light, 1 cup	25	1	4
Act II Popcorn:			
Butter, 1 cup, 0.3 oz	35	2	4
4 cups, popped, 1 oz	140	8	16
Light Butter, 1 cup, 0.2 oz	25	1	4
5 cups, popped, 1 oz	125	4	20
Butter Lovers,1 cup, 0.3 oz	45	3	4
3.5 cups, 1 oz	160	10	14
Butter Lovers (Reduced Fat), 1 c.	30	1.5	4.5
4.5 cups, 1 oz	130	6	20
American Fare (K-Mart):			
Butter, 1 cup, 0.3 oz	35	2.5	4
3.5 cups, 1 oz	130	9	14
Light Butter, 1 cup, 0.3 oz	30	1	5
3.5 cups, 1 oz	100	4	17
Healthy Choice: Butter, 6 cups	100	2.5	22
Natural, 6 cups, 1 oz	100	2	22
Jolly Time: America's Best, 1 cup	20	0	5
Blast O Butter: Regular, 1 cup	45	3	5
Light, 1 cup	30	1.5	4
Healthy Pop, 1 cup	20	0	4
Kettle Mania, 1 cup	50	4	5
Newman's Own: Butter, 1 oz	170	11	16
Light Butter Flavor, 3½ cups	110	3	20
Orville Redenbacher's: *Popped*			
Movie Theater Butter, 1 cup	40	3	4
4 cups, popped, 1 oz	170	12	16
Light Movie Theater Butter, 1 cup	25	1	4
5 cups, 1 oz	125	5	20
Smart Pop!: Butter, 7½ cups	120	0	30
Mini Bags, 6 cups	100	0	24
Tender White, 3½ cups	155	11	14
Pop Secret Popcorn: *Popped*			
94% Fat Free, 6 cups	125	2	23
Jumbo Pop Butter, all types, 3 ½ cups	140	9	14
Other varieties, avg., 4 cups	160	10	16
Light Butter, 6 cups	135	5	20
Movie Theater Butter, 4 cups	165	12	12

Bagged Popcorn

	C	F	Cb
Average All Brands (Ready-to-Eat)			
Regular: Plain, ½ oz pkg	80	5	7
1 oz pkg	160	10	14
4 oz pkg	640	40	56
Box (store/airport), 2 oz	320	20	28
Bag (9" high x 5" wide), 3 oz	480	30	42

Brands ~ Bagged Popcorn

	C	F	Cb
Act II Popcorn: Supreme, ¾ cup	130	5	22
Butter Toffee: ¾ cup, 1 oz	110	1	27
w. Peanuts, ¾ cup, 1 oz	120	2.5	24
Boston's: Fat Free, ⅔ cup, 1 oz	100	0	23
Lite, 2 cup, 1 oz	140	6	19
Gourmet Super Prem., 2 c., 1 oz	160	11	13
40% Less Fat, 2¾ cup, 1 oz	140	6	17
Cracker Jack: Original, ½ c., 1 oz	120	2	23
Fat Free varieties, ¾ cup, 1 oz	110	0	26
Crunch 'N Munch: ½ cup, 1 oz	140	5	22
Buttery Toffee, ⅔ cup, 1 oz	150	6	22
Caramel w. P'nuts, ⅔ cup, 1.2 oz	140	3.5	25
Fiddle Faddle: Skippy ¾ c., 1 oz	130	3	23
Honey Nut, ½ cup, 1 oz	130	3.5	24
w. Real Planters Peanuts, ⅔ cup	130	3	24
Hixon's: Caramel Corn, 1 oz	125	4.5	20
Cheese Corn, 1 oz	160	11	15
Jay's: Fat Free Caramel Corn, ¾ cup	110	0	26
Korn Krunch: *(Kornfections Treasures):*			
Almond Pecan (Sugar Free), 1 oz	150	8	19
Orville Redenbacher:			
Popcorn Cakes, avg. (8) ½ oz	65	1	12
Pre-Popped: Clusters, ½ cup, 1 oz	135	5	22
Drizzles, avg., ⅔ cup, 1 oz	160	6	24
Savory, avg., 2¾ cups, 1 oz	165	10	16
Pizza Hut Cheese Pizza, 2 oz bag	360	26	26
Poppycock: Pecan Delight, 1 cup	300	14	40
Just Be Nuts!, ¼ cup, 1.3 oz	205	15	13
Slimmons (Fat Free): ¾ c., 1 oz	110	0	25
Weight Watchers Butter, ⅔ oz	90	2.5	14
Wild Oats, all types, 2.5 cup, 1 oz	160	10	15

Movie Theater Popcorn

	C	F	Cb
Small (7 cups): Plain	400	27	30
with Butter	580	47	30
Medium (16 cups): Plain	900	60	70
with Butter	1170	90	70
Large (20 cups): Plain	1150	76	90
with Butter	1500	116	90

Potato Chips/Crisps

Average All Brands	C	F	Cb
Regular:			
Plain or flavored, 1 chip	9	1	1
17 chips, 1 oz pkg	150	10	15
4 oz quantity	600	40	60
Lay's Stax, avg. all, 1 oz	150	10	15
Pringles: 14 crisps, 1 oz	160	11	15
Large, 5.75 oz can	920	63	86
Snack Stack, 23g tub	140	9	12
Ruffles, 14 chips, 1 oz	160	10	14
Reduced Fat: *Pringles,* 1 oz	140	7	20
Crunch Tators, 1 oz	140	7	19
Sun Chips, 1 oz	140	6	19
Terra, average, 1 oz	140	7	19
Lowfat/Baked: Average, 1 oz	115	1.5	23
Kettle, 1 oz	115	1.5	22
Fat Free: *Childer's/Louise's,* 1oz	100	0	22
Pringles, 1 oz	70	0	15
Lay's Wow!, 20 chips, 1 oz	75	0	17
Ruffles Wow!: 17 chips, 1 oz	70	0	17
Cheddar Sour Crm (15) 1 oz	70	0	16
Low Carb: *Atkins* Crunchers, 1 oz	110	3	8
Carb Solutions, 1 oz	135	5	3
Tastemorr, average, 1 oz	130	5	8

Corn & Tortilla Chips

Average All Brands	C	F	Cb
Corn Chips: Avg. all types, 1 oz	160	10	15
8 oz bag	1280	80	120
Doritos: (12), 1 oz	150	7	20
Nachos; 4-Cheese, 1 oz	140	8	17
3D's Nacho Cheesier (32) 1 oz	130	5	19
Rollitos (17) 1 oz	160	10	16
Fritos *(Sabrositas),* 1 oz	155	9	17
Pringles, Torengos (13), 1 oz	140	9	15
Tortilla Chips: Average, 1 oz	150	8	22
(1 oz = approx. 12 chips or 13 strips)			
Boston, Baked, 13 chips, 1 oz	110	1.5	23
Doritos: 18 chips, 1 oz	140	6	20
Light, 13 chips, 1 oz	130	5	20
Wow! Nacho Cheesier, 1 oz	90	1	18
Edge *(Doritos/Tostitos),* 1 oz	140	8	9
CarbSense Soy Chips (15) 1 oz	140	8	12
Frito-Lay, Baked, (15) 1 oz	120	3.5	21
Garden of Eatin', 1 oz	145	7	18
Keebler Suncheros Light, 1 oz	150	8	18
Kettle, average, 1 oz	140	6	18
Munchies Mix, ¾ cup, 1 oz	135	6	18
Padrino Reduced Fat, 1 oz	130	4	22
Torengos, 13 chips, 1 oz	150	9	16
Utz Lowfat Baked, 8 chips, 1 oz	120	1.5	23
Wild Oats, 14 chips, 1 oz	150	7	18

Pretzels

Average All Brands	C	F	Cb
Hard Baked Pretzels: *Per Pretzel*			
1 oz	110	2	22
Sticks, thin, 2¼" (9/oz), each	12	0	3
Twists, thin, ¼" thick, (5/oz), 1	25	0.2	5
Dutch (2¾"x 2⅝") ½ oz, 1	55	1	11
Sourdough *(Shultz),* ¾ oz, each	80	0	17
Fat Free Pretzels:			
Snyders (1), 1 oz	100	0	22
Mini (20), 1 oz	110	0	25
Utz Wheels/Nuggets, 1 oz	100	0	22
Rold Gold: Sticks (48), 1 oz	100	0	23
Sourdough Nuggets (12), 1 oz	100	0	23
Sourdough Hards (1), ¾ oz	80	0	17
Thins (12), 1 oz	110	0	24
Twists (16), 1 oz	110	1	22
Tiny Twists/Sticks (18), 1 oz	100	0	23
Low Fat Pretzels:			
American Fare Mini Twists, 1oz	120	1	23
Frito-Lay, Rold Gold:			
Butter Checkers 20 pcs., 1 oz	110	1.5	22
Braided Twists (8), 1 oz	110	1	23
Choc-coated *(Nestlé),* 1 oz	130	6	20
White Fudge covered *(Nestlé),* 1 oz, 7 pieces	140	6	19
Yogurt *(Wild Oats)* 8 pcs., 1.4 oz	210	10	27
Soft Pretzels (Twists) average:			
Plain: Regular, 2.5 oz	190	0	41
King Size, 5 oz	390	0	83
Big Cheese, 5 oz	380	7	61
Peanut Butter filled *(Tr. Joe's)* 1 oz	160	7	18
Auntie Anne's: *See Fast-Foods Section*			
CarbSense, Soy Pretzels (15)	115	3	12
Frito-Lay Pretzels			
Flavor Twists, 23 pces, 1 oz	160	10	16
Braided Twists, 8 sticks, 1 oz	110	1	23
Rold Gold Flavor Rush, ⅓ c. 1 oz	150	7	20
Snyder's of Hanover Pretzels			
Logs (7), 1 oz	120	1	21
Homestyle (15), 1 oz	120	1	25
Mini (20), 1 oz	110	0	25
Super Pretzel: Soft Pretzels (1)	175	1	36
Softstix (2)	145	3.5	23
Soft Pretzel Bites (5)	140	0.5	29
Pretzelfils: Onion Veggie (2)	150	4	24
Pepperjack; Pizza (2)	140	3.5	22

Snacks

Note: Actual weight of packaged snacks is usually 5-10% more than label Net Wt. For accuracy, weigh snack and allow extra calories for any extra weight.

Snacks	C	F	Cb
Bacon Cheese Crackers, 1 oz	140	6	14
Baja Bob's Soy Munchables, 1 oz	120	4	7
Banana Chips, ¼ cup, 1 oz	150	8	20
Beef Jerky, average, 1 oz	70	1	3
Beef Sticks *(Frito-Lay's)* 0.3 oz	50	4	1
Bugles: Original, 1⅓ cup, 1 oz	160	9	18
Baked Bugles, 1½ cup, 1.1 oz	130	3.5	23
Carb Slim, Low Carb Bites, 1 oz	155	9	14
Cajun Jerky, 1½ oz	150	6	6
Carrot Chips *(Hain)*	160	9	26
Cheddar Lites *(Health Valley)* 1 oz	120	3	21
Cheese Crackers, 1 oz	130	6	18
Cheese Filled *(Frito-Lay's)*	210	11	24
Cheese Curls: 1¼ cup, 1 oz	160	9	19
Reduced Fat *(Utz)*, 1 oz	140	6	21
American Fare, 1¼ cup, 1 oz	140	5	22
Cheese Nips *(Nabisco)*, 38, 1 oz	190	7.5	19
Cheese Puffs: Average, 1 oz	150	10	15
Lowfat, 1 oz	140	5	20
Health Valley, 1½ cup	110	3	21
No Fries, 1 oz	110	0	23
Cheese Straws, 4 pieces	110	7	8
Cheese Twists, 23 twists, 1 oz	150	8	19
Cheetos: Regular all flavors, 1 oz	160	10	15
Light, cheese flavored, 1 oz	140	6	19
Cheez Balls: 45 balls, 1 oz	150	10	15
Reduced Fat, 45 balls, 0.73 oz	100	4.5	13
Cheez Bopps *(Boston's)*, (28) 1 oz	130	6	17
Cheez Curls/Doodles, 1 oz	160	12	15
Cheez Mania *(Planters)*, 35, 1 oz	160	10	15
Cheez It: White Cheddar, 1 pkt	145	7	18
Original	150	8	16
Reduced Fat	135	4.5	20
Chex Mix *(General Mills)*:			
Bold Blend (40% less fat), ½ c.	140	6	20
Chedder; Traditional, ⅔ cup	130	4	22
Chip's Chips: Snackers, avg., 1 oz	135	7	2
Cheese Thins, avg., 1 0z	135	8	0
Churros *(Mex. Pastry)* 10", 1.2 oz	140	9	12
Cinna Chips *(T.J. Cinn.)* 3, 1 oz	110	4	19
Combos *(Oven Baked)*:			
Crackers, ⅓ cup, 1 oz	140	7	18
1 cup, 3 oz	420	21	54
Pretzels, ⅓ cup, 1 oz	130	4.5	19
1 cup, 3 oz	390	14	57
Cookies: *See Pages 105-112*			
Corn Chips: *See Page 133*			

Snacks (Cont)

Snacks (Cont)	C	F	Cb
Corn Crunchies/Spirals, 1 oz	160	10	15
Corn Crisps *(Pringle)*, 1 oz	140	7	18
Corn Nuts: ⅓ cup, 1 oz	130	4	20
1.7 oz bag	220	7	34
Corn Puffs: *Health Valley,* 2 c., 1 oz	120	1.5	25
Pirate's Booty, 1 oz	130	5	18
Wotsits *(Walker)*, 21g pkg	110	6.5	11
Dunkaroos, 1 tray, 1 oz	130	4.5	20
Flavor Twists *(Fritos)*, 1 oz	160	10	16
French's Potato Sticks ¾ c., 1 oz	180	12	16
Funyun's: Onion flavor, 1 oz	140	7	18
Mini, 2 oz	270	13	35
Girlfriend's Booty, 1 oz	120	4.5	8
Goldfish *(Pepperidge Farm)*: 1 oz	140	7	18
2 oz pkg	280	14	36
Gold-N-Chees *(Lance)*, 1⅜ oz	180	7	25
Handi Snacks *(Kraft)*, Bearwiches	150	7	21
Honey Mustard Onion Pieces			
(Snyder's) 1 pkg, 2 oz	280	12	38
Hot Peanuts *(Lays)*, 1¾ oz pkg	310	25	10
Jerky (Beef), 1 oz stick	70	1	3
Keebler: Wheatables Snack Mix,			
Toasted Honey, ½ cup, 1 oz	130	5	20
Peanut Butter Crunch, ½ c., 1 oz	160	7	20
Chse & P'nut Butter			
Sandwich Cookies, 1 pkg	250	12	30
Koolstuf, all flavors, 1.3 oz bar	130	3	27
Lance Sandwich: Bonnie, 1 pkg	160	7	23
Capt. Wafers; Choc-O-Mint, pkg	190	10	23
Sour Dough w. Cheddar, 1 pkg	240	15	23
Other varieties, average, 1 pkg	200	10	22
Lunchables: Fudge Brownie	250	9	42
'S'Mores	200	6	35
Munchos, 16 pieces, 1 oz	160	10	16
Nabisco: Chips Ahoy, 1.3 oz	165	8	21
Chips Ahoy! Cookie Barz, 35g	180	10	23
Nutter Butter Bites (10)	150	6	20
Oreo, 1.3 oz	160	7	23
Oreo Cookie Barz, 1 bar	180	10	21
S'Mores	200	6	35
Sportz, Cheese Nips (38), 1 oz	190	7.5	19
Sweet Crisps (18), 1 oz	180	5	15
Nibblers *(Snyder's)*: Regular (13)	130	3	23
Fat Free (16)	110	0	25
Onion Rings *(Lance)*, 1 pkg	120	6	16
Oriental Mix *(Rice Snacks)*, 1 oz	155	7.5	15
Rice Snacks *(Wild Oats)* ⅔ c. 1 oz	110	0	25
Oyster Crackers *(Bradshaw's)*, 1 oz	140	5	14
Party Mix *(Flavor Tree)* ¼ c., 1 oz	160	11	14

Snacks (Cont)

Snacks (Cont)	C	F	Cb
Peanut Butter Nuggets (8), 1 oz	150	8	14
Pirate's Booty w. White Ched., 1 oz	130	5	18
Pita Snax, avg., (34) 1 oz	115	1.5	22
Popcorn: *See Page 136*			
Pork Skins/Rind: *Baken-ets,* 1 oz	160	10	0
Gram's Crunchies, avg., 1 oz	150	10	4
Grande, ⅔ cup	80	5	0
Lance, 1 pkg	65	4	1
Potato Chips: *See Page 133*			
Potato Puffs *(Health Valley),* 1 oz	110	3	21
Potato Skins *(TGI Friday's),* 1 oz	150	9	17
Potato Sticks *(French's),* ¾ c., 1.1oz	180	12	16
Puffs: 1⅔ cups, 1 oz	140	8	17
8 oz pkg	1120	64	136
Quakes: Corn Rings (25)	135	4.5	21
Mini Rice Snacks: Apple Cinn. (8)	65	0	15
BBQ (10); Ranch (10)	75	2.5	12
Caramel Corn (7)	55	0	13
Nacho/Cheddar Cheese (9)	70	2.5	11
Chocolate (7)	65	1	13
Sour Cream & Onion (10)	75	2.5	12
Ranch Puffs *(No Fries),* 1 oz	110	0	23
Rice Chips, Bar-B-Q/Onion, ½ oz	70	3	9
Santitas *(Frito-Lay),* 1 oz	140	6	20
Sesame Sticks *(Cityfarm),* 1 oz	160	11	13
Snack Crackers *(No Fries),* 1 oz	110	0	24
Soy Crisps, avg. 1 oz	130	2	18
Soy Nuts: Dry Roasted, ¼ cup, 1 oz	140	7	10
Choc-coated, 1 oz	140	8	14
Dr Soy Soy Nuts BBQ, 1 oz	180	8	8
Spicers Wheat Snacks, 1½ oz	150	7.5	18
Sun Chips *(Frito-Lay),* 1 oz pkg	140	6	19
TastyKake: Koffee Kake Jnr	250	8	40
Chocolate Jnr	320	12	50
Creme Filled Koffee Kakes	360	14	54
Toast/Cheese Crackers, 1 pkg	205	10	23
Tortilla Chips: *See Pages 133*			
Tostitos: Regular, average, 1 oz	140	8	18
Fat Free, 1 oz	90	0	20
Trail Mix (Nuts/Seeds/Dried Fruit):			
Regular, 3 Tbsp, 1 oz	130	8	13
Tropical, 3 Tbsp, 1 oz	120	5	19
w. Chocolate Chips, 1 oz	140	9	13
Dr Soy Trail Mix, 1 oz	110	4	12
Turkey Jerky Teriyaki *(Oberto)*	80	0.5	0
Vegetable Snacks/Chips, 1 oz	130	4	24
Veggie Chips, 1 oz	130	5	18
Veggie Stix, 1 oz	140	7	15
Wahoos, 1 oz, 23 pces	140	8	18
Weight Watchers: Chse Curls, ½ oz	70	2.5	10
Apple Chips, ¾ oz pkg	70	0	18
Yogurt Raisins, 1 oz	130	6	20

Fruit Snacks	C	F	Cb
Betty Crocker: *Per Serving*			
String Things, 1 pouch, 0.75 oz	80	1	17
Lucky Charms Fruit Shapes, 1 pouch, 0.9 oz (25g)	80	0	20
Squeezit, average, 1 bottle	100	0	25
Kellogg's Disney Fruit Snacks (25g)	80	0	20
Nabisco: Rugrats; Wacky Faces (1)	80	0	18
Blues Clues; Dora the Explorer (1)	60	0	14
Fruit Rolls, 1 roll, 0.74 oz	80	2	16
100 Calorie Fruit Snacks, 1.1 oz	100	0	24
Sunkist: All flavors, 1 pch, 0.9 oz	80	0	21
Fruit Snack Cups: *See Page 146*			

Vending Machines	C	F	Cb
Brownie, frosted	180	9	24
Cheese Balls, 1 oz	150	8	16
Choc Chip Cookies, 4	130	7	19
Choc Milk, 8 fl.oz	225	9	26
Coca-Cola Classic, 12 fl.oz	140	0	35
Diet Coke, 12 fl.oz	1	0	0
Corn Chips, 1 oz	160	10	15
Danish Pastry, 2 oz	220	10	25
Donut, plain, 1¾ oz	210	12	25
Fruit Pie, 4 oz	290	13	46
Granola/Cereal Bars	130	3	26
Hershey's, 1.55 oz bar	240	14	25
Hot Fries, 1 oz	140	10	11
Kellogg's Rice Krispies Treat	120	1.5	26
Lance: Captain's Wafers, 1 pkg	230	12	26
Big Town, 1 pkg	250	11	38
M & M's: Plain, 1.7 oz	240	10	34
Peanuts, 1.7 oz	250	13	30
Milk: Whole, 8 fl.oz	150	8	12
Reduced Fat, 2%, 8 fl.oz	120	5	12
Milky Way, 2 oz	270	10	41
Onion Rings, 1 oz	120	6	16
Orange Juice, 8.75 fl.oz	120	0	28
Peanuts, roasted, 1 oz	165	14	6
Popcorn, plain, 1 oz	160	10	14
Pork Skins, 1 oz	160	10	0
Potato Chips: 1 oz	150	10	15
Reduced Fat, 1 oz	140	7	20
Pretzels, 1 oz	110	2	22
Raisins, ½ oz pkg	40	0	9
Reece's Peanut Butter Cups, 1.8 oz	280	17	28
Snickers, 2.1 oz bar	280	14	35
Tortilla Chips, 1 oz	150	8	22

Breakfast Bars • Sports & Diet Bars

Note: Actual weight of bars is usually 5-10% more than label Net Wt. Weigh bar and allow extra calories.

Breakfast Bars

	C	F	Cb
Atkins, Morning Starts (1)	**175**	9	13
Barbara's Bakery: Multigrain, 1.3 oz	**120**	1.5	25
Puffins Cereal & Milk Bars, avg.	**135**	2	24
Carborite Cereal Bar, all types (1)	**50**	2.5	4
Carnation Breakfast Bars: *Per 1.2 oz Bar*			
Granola (Honey/Choc), average	**130**	2.5	26
Choc Chip/P.nut Butter, chewy	**150**	5	24
Entenmann's Multi-Grain, 1.3 oz	**140**	3	25
General Mills: Milk 'n Cereal Bars			
Chex; Cheerios, Cocoa Puffs 1.4 oz	**160**	4	26
Cinnamon Toast Crunch, 1.6 oz	**180**	4	31
Fruit & Cereal Bars, avg., 1 oz	**150**	2	31
Health Valley Cereal Bars (1)	**135**	2	27
Kellogg's: Cereal Bars, 1.3 oz	**145**	3	27
Cereal & Milk Bars, avg., 0.8 oz	**105**	3	16
Nature's Path: Crispy Rice, avg.	**115**	3	20
Flax Plus; Hemp Plus, average	**175**	5	29
Granola: Apricot 'n Nut	**185**	7	28
Cranberry Soy	**175**	5	28
New England Natural Bakers,			
Save the Forest Bars (1)	**125**	4	19
Nutri-Grain Bars: Twists Bar	**140**	3	28
Cereal Yogurt Bars, 1.3 oz	**140**	3	27
Granola Bar: 0.9 oz bar	**110**	3	18
Mini's, 1.5 oz pouch	**165**	3	32
Muffin Bars	**170**	4	30
Chewy Bars, avg., 1 oz	**110**	3.5	18
Chewy Bites, avg., 1 pouch	**130**	6	20
Post Carb Well Bars, 1.2 oz	**140**	5	15
Quaker: Fruit & Oatmeal Bites (3)	**140**	2.5	27
Oatmeal On The Go Bars, 1.6 oz	**205**	6	34
Fruit & Oatmeal Bars, avg.	**135**	3	26
Chewy Fruit 'N' Crunch Bars	**165**	3.5	31
Q Smart Bar, 1 oz	**120**	6	8
Toastables (1), 1.76 oz	**190**	4.5	36
Special K Cereal Bars, avg., 0.8 oz	**95**	1.5	18

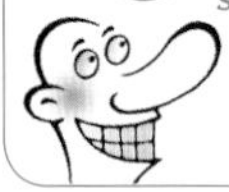

"In eating, one third of the stomach should be filled with food, one third with drink, and the rest left empty."
~ Gitten, the Talmud

Other Bars

	C	F	Cb
Per Bar			
AdvantEdge: Morning Bar	**170**	6	22
Carb Control Crisp Bar	**230**	7	27
Carb Control Nutrition Bar	**200**	5	21
Complete Nutrition Bar	**210**	5	27
Morning Bar	**170**	6	22
Perfection Bars	**120**	10	8
SoNutty Bars	**210**	8	18
All Goode Organics: *Per 1.73 oz Bar*			
Cashew Almond Passion	**190**	8	24
Chocolate flavors, average	**200**	8	29
Honey Nut Harvest	**160**	3.5	32
Nutty Choc Apricot	**200**	10	26
Alpen			
Cereal Bars: *Per 3.5 oz Bar*			
Apple & Blackberry w. Yogurt	**420**	12	73
Fruit & Nut	**395**	9	71
Fruit & Nut w. Chocolate	**430**	15	68
Strawberry w. Yogurt	**425**	12	74
ABB Rivets, 45g pkt	**200**	7	18
Animal Parade, 30g bar	**110**	3	15
Arbonne Balanced Nutr., 1 bar	**190**	4.5	24
Atkins: Endulge *(See Page 128)*			
Advantage Bar: Smores	**260**	10	26
Average other varieties	**230**	11	22
Balance: Balance Bars, 1.7 oz	**200**	6	23
Balance Plus Bars, 1.76 oz	**200**	6	22
Carb Well: Caramel 'n Choc., 1.7 oz	**210**	7	23
Chocolate Fudge, 1.7 oz	**200**	6	23
Chocolate Peanut Butter, 1.7 oz	**215**	8	22
GoMix, 1.5 oz bag	**205**	7	21
Gold Crunch Bars, avg., 1.7 oz	**210**	6	23
Gold Bars, avg., 1.7 oz	**210**	7	22
Outdoor Bars, 1.7 oz	**200**	6	21
Barbara's Bakery Granola, ¾ oz	**80**	2	14
Bariatrix Proti-Bar (15g Protein):			
Caramel Nut, 40g	**150**	5	10
Blueberry; CookitCrunch, 35g	**130**	4	6
Bear Valley: Meal Pack, 3.75 oz	**410**	12	56
Bumble Bar, avg. (1)	**210**	12	26
Biochem: Strive, avg.	**190**	9	24
Protein Bar, Caramel Nougat	**250**	9	26
Ultimate Protein Bar, 78g	**290**	4.5	19
Ideal For Her, avg., 1.7 oz	**200**	7	20
Bio-Tech, Bio-Protein, 81g	**300**	7	39
Body Smarts: Choc. P'nut Crunch	**210**	6	34
Yogurt Berry Crunch	**200**	5	35
Boost, Choc./Strawb. Crunch	**190**	6	30

Note: Actual weight of bars is usually 5-10% more than label Net Wt. Weigh bar and allow extra calories.

Other Bars (Cont)

Per Bar	C	F	Cb
Boulder Bar Endurance, 2.5 oz	220	4	13
Bumble Bar, 1.6 oz	150	12	21
Burn-IT, 50g bar	180	3	13
Carb Options, 1.76 oz bar	205	8	17
Carb Sense Soy Energy:			
Blueberry Crisp, 2 oz	235	6	33
Mocha Cappuccino Crisp, 2 oz	255	9	31
Peanut Butter Crisp, 2 oz	230	8	21
Carb Solutions: Sugar Free, 1 oz	170	7	14
Good Mornings, 1 oz bar	170	7	14
Taste Sensations: *Per Bar (60g)*			
Chocolate Toffee Hazelnut	260	13	15
Other varieties, avg.	250	10	16
Carb Watchers Lean Body, 2.5 oz	260	8	18
Carbolite: Choc Almond, 1.75 oz	230	17	25
Choc Crisp Bar, 1.75 oz	250	17	27
Milk/Dairy Choc, avg., 1.75 oz	250	19	28
CarboRite Bars, 1.06 oz	120	5	13
CarbRite Diet *(Doctor's)*, 2 oz	180	3	25
Champion Nutrition: SnacBar	180	3	25
UltraProtein Bar, 78g	300	4.5	32
Cheetah *(NutraFig)*, 2.25 oz bar	210	2	43
Choice, all types, 1.23 oz bar	140	4.5	19
Clif Bars: Luna Bar, average, 1.5 oz	180	4.5	27
Builders Bars, 2.5 oz	270	8	30
Luna Glow, 1.23 oz	155	7	15
Mojo Bar, average, 1.5 oz	200	8	23
Nutrition Sustained Energy (68g):			
Apricot; Cranb. Apple Cherry	250	3	48
Designer Whey Gourmet Bars: *Per Bar (2.7 oz)*			
Choc Malted Muscles	250	5	7
Choc Triplement/Espresso	250	7	7
Dble Chocolats; Lemon Crunches	260	4.5	7
Peanut Better Body	270	7	6
Perfect Absberry	260	6	9
Detour, 2.8 oz bar	310	10	25
Dexatrim All in One, 1.76 oz	180	5	21
Dr Phil's Shape Up! Bars, avg.	240	7	29
Dr Soy: Protein Bar, Lemon, 1.76 oz	180	2.5	28
Chocolate/Peanut, 1.76 oz	185	4	27
Healthy Snacker, avg., 1.7 oz bar	190	6	23

Per Bar	C	F	Cb
EAS Advantage Edge:			
Carb Control, average, 2.12 oz	200	5	21
HP Energy bar, avg., 2.46 oz	260	5	37
Extreme Outdoor, avg., 2.5 oz	250	6	42
Complete Nutrition, 2.12 oz Bar:			
Choc Caramel	240	7	32
Iced Oatmeal Raisin Crisp	220	5	31
EAS Myoplex:			
Deluxe Bar, average, 3.2 oz	340	7	44
Lite Bar, average, 1.97 oz	190	4	28
Carb Sense, average, 2.5 oz	250	7	20
EAS Results for Women:			
Weight Management Bar, 1.94 oz	190	5	17
Complete Energy Bar, 1.67 oz	200	6	28
Eclipse 2000 Deluxe Protein, 78g	290	6	29
ELEV8 Protein & Fruit Trail:			
All Fruit Blend, 66g bar	250	4.5	34
Cocoa & Coconut, 66g	255	7	29
Ensure Chewy Choc P'nut, 2.12 oz	230	6	35
Extreme Body, 3 oz bar	340	8	24
Extreme Ripped Force, 45g	160	3	33
Fi-Bar Nectar Granola Bars, 1 oz	100	0	22
Chewy & Nutty Bar, 1.2 oz	140	4.5	23
Figurines Diet Bar, avg., 1 bar	110	6	12
Fit! *(Medifast)*, 1.5 oz bar	160	4	20
Fruitein Energy Bar, 1.3 oz	130	3	18
General Mills Momentum Bars, 1.4 oz	150	3.5	17
GeniSoy			
Soy Protein Bars, avg., 2.2 oz	235	4.5	33
Low Carb Crunch, avg., 1.5 oz	185	6	18
Xtreme, avg., 1.5 oz	200	8	23
Xtreme Crunch, avg.. 1.5 oz	170	3.5	27
Glenny's			
Slim Carb: Double Fudge, 1.3 oz	160	4	19
Other varieties, 1.3 oz	90	4	2
Glucerna Meal Replacement, 2 oz	220	7	32
GNC ProCruncher, 2.3 oz	250	4	37
Gouinda's: Hemp Bar, 1.5 oz	170	9	22
Bliss Bar (1)	230	13	29
Greens + Bar: Avg., 2 oz	170	6	20
Hempower Bars, 1.6 oz	170	6	22
Grove Organic Energy Bars, 2 oz	250	10	30
Hansen's (1.4 oz): Active Nutr., avg.	140	3.5	20
Natural Crunch, avg. all flavors	185	3	37
Natural Functional, avg. all flav.	190	5	25
Health Valley Fruit/Granola Bars	140	0	34
Healthy Recipes *(Novartis)*	150	4	21
Healthy Shape n Slim, 1.7 oz	150	2	28
HeartBar, Orig., Cranberry, 50g	190	3	27

Per Bar	C	F	Cb
Henry's Top of the Vine:			
Roundup, 1.4 oz	170	5	26
Honey Peanutty, 1.4 oz	230	17	10
High Protein: Peanut Butter, 4 oz	420	16	45
Other varieties, average	335	8	36
HMR Benefit Bar, 1.1 oz	160	5	22
Iron-Tek, Vanilla Fudge, 2.73 oz	290	5	21
Jay Bar, average, 2 oz	230	10	27
Jenny Craig: Choc/Yogurt, 1.97 oz	220	5	33
Oatmeal Raisin, 1.97 oz	210	3	35
Milk Choc; Lemon Meringue	210	5	32
Jewel Granola Bars: Cereal	140	3	27
Choc Chip/P'nut Butter	130	4.5	20
Low-fat varieties	110	2	22
Joyva Sesame Crunch, 1.1 oz	190	8	15
Kashi Golean: Bars, avg., 2.7 oz	290	5	53
Crunchy!, avg., 1.76 oz bar	160	3	32
Kellogg's Krave: Bars, 1.7 oz avg.	200	7	29
Minis, Pouch, 44g	165	3	32
Keto Bar: Chocolate types, 65g	270	8	24
Average other flavors	250	7	24
Mini Bar, 32g, avg. all flavors	130	4	12
Kid Sport Bars, avg, 1.76 oz	200	6	29
Kudos: Bars, avg. (1)	90	2.5	17
Granola: M&M's; Snickers	105	4	16
Snack: M&M's	90	2.5	17
Snickers	100	3.5	16
Avg., other varieties	125	4.5	19
Larabar: Apple Pie, 1.6 oz	200	9	22
Banana Cookie Dough, 1.8 oz	210	15	24
Cherry Pie, 1.7 oz	190	9	24
Lean Body, 76g	300	6	15
Luna Bars, average, 1.5 oz	180	4.5	27
Marathon *(Snickers)*, avg. all flav.	220	7	32
Medifast Fit! 1.5 oz bar	160	4	20
Metabolife, average, 2 oz bar	230	6	36
Met-Rx: "Big 100", avg., 100g	340	3.5	52
Protein Plus, 3 oz bar	310	8	25
MLO Bio Protein, 2.85 oz	300	7	39
MRM Response, 2.1 oz	210	8	20
Muscle Tech: Nitro-Tech, average	290	6	33
Meso-Tech, avg., 3.11 oz	340	8	44
Meso-Tech Lite, avg., 2.12 oz	220	6	16
Myoplex: *See EAS*			
Natrol Prolab, 1.76 oz bar	190	6	12
Naturade, Total Soy, 2.1 oz	250	8	32
Nature Valley: Chewy, average	155	6	24
Crunchy, average	190	7	28

Per Bar	C	F	Cb
Nature's Best: Solid Protein, 2.75 oz			
Choc./Peanut Butter; S'Mores	290	7	12
Cookie Dough Chip; Dble Choc	270	4	10
Other varieties, average	290	4	11
Nature's Plus: Energy Bar, 1.45 oz	140	4.5	24
Chi Chinese Herbal, 1.5 oz	150	4	20
Calcium Almond Blitz, 1.5 oz	150	2.5	29
Spiru-tein, all flavors, 1.4 oz	150	4	20
New You: Peanut Butter, 1.65 oz	185	5	25
Choc Chip; Lemon Crisp, 1.65 oz	170	3	26
Next Proteins: Designer Whey, 78g	290	9	23
Detour, 2.8 oz	310	10	25
U-Turn Protein, 2.8 oz	300	8	26
NiteBite (Time-release Glucose Bar)			
Choc. Fudge; P'nut Butter, 25g	100	3.5	15
NuBar Decadence, 1.3 oz	140	2.5	30
NuSkin *(Pharmanex)* Body Design			
Meal Replacement Bars	250	6	34
Nutiva: Hempseed, 1.4 oz	210	14	11
Flax Chocolate, 1.4 oz	200	12	19
NutriSystem Sweet Success, 2.1 oz	220	3	33
Nutrilite: Protein Bars, average	250	9	22
Meal Replacements, average	230	8	30
Odwalla Energy Bars: Chocolate	240	6	40
Choc. Chip Peanut/Crunch, avg.	250	7	39
Carrot; Cranberry C Monster	225	2.5	47
Super Protein	235	5	31
Superfood	225	5	41
Perfect Rx Nutrition Bar, 100g	340	3	50
Perfect Solid Protein, avg., 2.7 oz	290	7	28
PR Bar Ironman, 49.6g	200	6	22
Power Bar: Harvest Dip'd, avg., 2.3 oz	255	5	45
Energy Bites, avg., 1.76 oz bag	210	5	33
Harvest; Performance, avg, 2.3 oz	240	3	45
Power Crunch, average, 1.3 oz	190	9	13
Premier: Protein Eight, 2.4 oz	250	6	22
Protein Meal Replacement, 2.5 oz	280	8	20
Complete Nutrition, 48g	190	4.5	28
Odyssey Protein, 80g	310	11	29
Pria *(Power Bar)*: Bars, 1 oz	115	3	16
Carb Select, avg., 1.7 oz	195	8	21
Pro 42, average, 3.7 oz bar	380	8	33
Promax, average, 2.7 oz bar	290	6	40
Protein Complete, avg., 1.97 oz	220	6	28
Protein Plus: Average, 2.75 oz	290	5	38
Layered: Strawberry Creme	220	5	30
Choc Caramel Nut	220	6	26
Sugar Free, average	170	4	20
Prozone Nutrition Bar, 50g	195	6	18
Pure Protein High Protein, 1.76 oz	180	4.5	18
Pure Fit, average, 2 oz bar	235	6	27

Other Bars (Cont)

Per Bar	C	F	Cb
Quaker Granola Bars: *Per Bar*			
Chewy Dipps: Caramel Nut	145	6	21
Chocolate Fudge	165	8	21
Peanut Butter	155	8	19
Chewy: Low Fat	110	2	22
Peanut Butter	110	3.5	18
Other varieties, average	120	3.5	20
Rapunzel: *Per Bar (1.4 oz)*			
Coco; Rio; Tango, avg.	230	17	16
Crisp	120	7	11
Real Protein, 2.75 oz bar	290	5	28
Resource, OptiSource Mini Bar	90	2.5	10
Restart: Peanut Butter, 1.25 oz	140	4	10
Strawb. Banana; Chocolate	130	2.5	21
Revival Soy Bars *(Direct)*: *Per Bar*			
Cool Krispy Protein:			
Choc. Temptation	220	3.5	30
Apple Cinnamon; Marsh.Krunch	220	3	33
Peanut Butter/Choc Pal, avg.	240	6	32
Low Carb, average all flavors	200	5	28
Russell Stover: Pecan Delight, 2 pieces	240	16	22
Pecan Delight Sugar Free, 2 pces	210	16	25
Diabetx : Toffee Square, 1 oz	100	7	14
Pecan Delights, 1 oz	130	9	16
SCAN Diet, 45g	160	2.5	26
Slim-Fast Bars: High Protein, avg.	215	6	25
Breakfast and Lunch Bars, avg.	150	6	19
Chewy; Meal On-the-Go, avg.	220	5	36
Snack Bar, avg. all flavors	120	4	21
Low Carb: Meal Bars, 50g	205	8	17
Snack Bars (1)	125	5	18
Skippy: Snack Bars, average, 1.2 oz	185	11	18
Snackwell's: Cereal Bars	120	0	29
Other varieties	130	3	26
Solid Protein Meal, 2.75 oz	270	6	28
Spiru-tein Energy Bar, 1.4 oz	150	4	20
Steel Bar (ABB), 65g	330	6	52

Per Bar	C	F	Cb
Steel Pro, 85g	330	6	15
Strive *(Biochem)*, avg., 2.1 oz	190	8	25
The Sports Club/LA:			
Caramel Cr./Choc P'nut (16g prot.)	190	5	22
P'nut Butter Fudge (13g prot.)	190	9	13
Think Protein Bar, 2.3 oz	280	9	18
Think Thin! Low Carb Diet, avg. all bars, 2.1 oz	250	10	22
Thunder Bar, all flavors	220	2	44
Tiger's Milk: 35g Bar	130	2.5	24
Peanut Butter varieties	150	7	18
Protein Rich	145	5	18
Tiger Sport, 65g	230	2	43
Tri-O-Plex, Peanut Butter, 4.2 oz	360	11	34
Ultimate Lo Carb: Honey Almd	245	7	24
Amaretto Irish Cream	140	6	1
Choc Brownie Nut	165	7	2
Creamy Peanut Butter	270	9	24
Ultimate Lo Carb 2: Choc Peanut	170	8	3
Choc S'Mores; Black Forest, avg.	150	7	3
Other varieties, avg.	250	8	25
Ultimate Protein Bar, 78g	290	4.5	19
Universal Muscle, 56.7g	280	5	35
Usana: Nutribar, 41g	150	4	20
Fibergy Bar	100	1.5	23
Verve *(Wholefoods Mkt)*, 2.4 oz	240	5	41
Viactive *(Mead Johnson)*, 1.6 oz	180	4.5	29
Vyo-Pro *(AST)* Chocolate, 2.2 oz	210	7	17
Weider Body Shaper: Diet Protein	200	4.5	18
Protein Layered, avg., 60g	220	7	27
Whole Foods: Everyday Bars, avg.	190	4.5	18
Choc Fudge/Raspberry	172	4	17
Honey Peanut Yogurt	200	4.5	18
Worldwide Sport Nutrition:			
Pure Protein Bars, 2.75 oz			
Peanut Butter	310	10	24
Honey Nut; Maple Pecan	310	9	26
Other varieties, average	290	7	27
Xetalean *(Nature's Bounty)*, 40g	140	4.5	21
You Are What You Eat, 56g	220	5	39
Zoe Flax & Soy, Choc., 1.8 oz	200	6	33
Zone Perfect, average, 1.76 oz	210	7	24

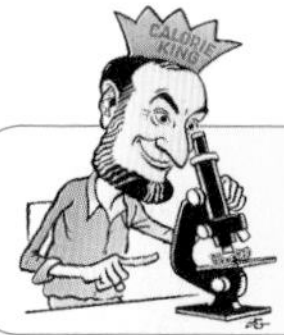

For full nutritional data and product updates check the food database of the author's website www.CalorieKing.com

Nuts

Per 1 oz Unless Indicated	C	F	Cb
Acorns, raw 1 oz	**105**	7	12
Almonds, Dried/Dry Roasted:			
Whole, 24-28 med., 1 oz	**170**	15	7
½ cup, 2½ oz	**420**	37	17
Chopped,½ cup, 2¼ oz	**380**	34	16
Sliced, ½ cup, 1⅔ oz	**280**	25	12
Choc. coated (5-6), 1 oz	**160**	11	14
Oil Rstd *(Blue Diamond)*, 1 oz	**175**	17	3.5
Almond Meal (partially defattened)			
1 cup (not packed), 2¼ oz	**260**	11	11
Honey Roasted, 1 oz	**170**	13	8
Brazil Nuts, 8 medium, 1 oz	**185**	19	3.5
Cashews, Dry or Oil Roasted:			
14 large/18 med./26 small, 1 oz	**165**	14	10
½ cup, 2.4 oz	**400**	33	23
Honey Roasted, 1 oz	**160**	12	11
Chestnuts, avg. all: Dried, 1 oz	**105**	1	22
Raw/Fresh, 5-6 nuts, 1 oz	**60**	0	13
Canned, water chestnuts			
sliced/whole/drained, 1 oz	**23**	0	5
Coconut: Flesh, 1 oz	**100**	10	4
Raw: 1 pce. (2"x2"x½"), 1.6 oz	**160**	15	7
½ medium (4½" diam.)	**650**	62	30
Dried (Desiccated):			
Unsweetened, 1 oz	**187**	18	17
Sweetened: Shredded, 1 oz	**140**	9	13
Grated, ½ cup, 1.3 oz	**185**	12	18
Cream (canned), ½ cup, 5.2 oz	**285**	26	12
Milk (canned), ½ cup, 4 oz	**225**	24	3
Water (center liq.), ½ c., 4¼ oz	**23**	0	4.5
Filberts or Hazelnuts:			
Shelled, 18-20 nuts	**180**	18	4.5
Chopped, ¼ cup	**180**	18	4.5
Ground, ¼ cup	**120**	12	3
Ginko Nuts, can., 14 med., 1 oz	**32**	0	6
Hickory, 30 small nuts	**190**	18	5
Macadamia Nuts, shelled:			
Raw, 7 med./14 small, 1 oz	**200**	21	4
½ cup, 2.3 oz	**460**	48	10
Oil roasted, 1 oz	**205**	22	3.5
½ cup, 2.4 oz	**490**	52	8
Choc. coated, 2-3 pces, 1 oz	**180**	13	15
Mixed Nuts: 18-22 nuts, 1 oz	**175**	13	7
Planters: Dry Roasted/Honey	**170**	15	7
Oil Roasted, all types	**180**	16	7
Sweet Roasts, 26 pces, 1 oz	**160**	12	10
Kettle: Choc Lover's Mix, 1 oz	**140**	7	16

Per 1 oz Unless Indicated	C	F	Cb
Nut Toppings:			
Chopped, 1 Tbsp, ¼ oz	**40**	4	1.5
Peanuts:			
Raw/Dried: In shell, 1 oz	**117**	10	3
Shelled, 1 oz	**160**	14	4.5
Boiled: ½ cup, 1.1 oz	**102**	7	7
Roasted, 30 lge./60 sml., 1 oz	**165**	14	6
1 cup, 5.1 oz	**840**	71	31
Chopped, 3 Tbsp, 1 oz	**165**	14	6
Planters: Oil Roasted, 1 oz	**170**	15	5
Beer Nuts, 1 oz pkg	**170**	14	7
Choc-coated, ½ cup, 2½ oz	**380**	25	36
Cocktail, oil roasted, 1 oz	**170**	14	5
Dry Roasted, 1 oz	**160**	14	6
Honey Roasted, 1 oz	**150**	11	10
Honey/Dry Roasted, 1 oz	**160**	13	7
Spanish Oil Roasted, 1 oz	**170**	14	5
Sweet 'n Crunchy, 1 oz	**140**	8	16
Pecans: Kernel halves, 1 oz	**190**	19	5
(20 Jumbo or 31 large halves)			
1 cup halves, 3.8 oz	**720**	73	20
Chopped, ½ cup, 2 oz	**380**	30	10
Oil Roasted, 1 oz	**195**	20	4.5
Honey Roasted, 1 oz	**200**	18	5
Pilinuts, dried, ¼ cup, 1 oz	**205**	23	1
Pinenuts, dried, 1 Tbsp, 10g	**50**	5	1.5
Pistachios:			
Unshelled, ½ cup, 2 oz	**165**	14	7
Shelled, ¼ cup, 45 nuts, 1 oz	**165**	14	7
Lance, 1⅛ oz package	**180**	14	8
Planters: Dry Roasted, 1oz	**170**	15	6
Fruit 'n Nut Mix, 1 oz	**150**	9	13
Nut Topping, 1 oz	**180**	16	6
Tavern Nuts, 1 oz	**170**	15	6
Trail Mix, 3 Tbsp, 1 oz	**140**	9	15
Sesame Nut Mix: Planters, 1 oz	**160**	12	8
Soy Nuts: Dry Roasted, 1 oz	**130**	6	9
½ cup, 3 oz	**390**	18	28
Dr Soy: Choc coated, 1 oz pkg	**130**	4.5	18
Honey Roasted, 1 oz pkg	**140**	6	21
Flavors, average, 1 oz	**150**	7	8
Walnuts:			
Black: 15-20 halves, 1 oz	**175**	16	3.5
Chopped, ¼ cup	**190**	18	4
Ground, ¼ cup	**120**	12	2.5
English/Persian:			
14 halves, 1 oz	**185**	18	5
Chopped, ¼ cup	**195**	19	5

Seeds

Seeds	C	F	Cb
Alfalfa Seeds, sprouted, ½ c., ½ oz	5	0	1
Caraway, Fennel, 1 tsp	10	0.5	1
Cottonseed Kernels, rst., 1 Tbsp	50	4	2
Flax Seeds, 3 Tbsp, 1 oz	150	10	11
Lotus Seeds, dried, ½ c., ½ oz	50	0.5	10
Poppy Seeds, 1 tsp	15	1	1
Pumpkin & Squash Seeds, whole:			
Roasted/Tamari, 1 oz	125	5.5	3
½ cup (32g)	140	6	3.5
Dried, 1 oz	155	13	5
Safflower Kernels, dried, 1 oz	150	11	10
Sesame Seeds: Dried, 1 Tbsp, 9g	50	4.5	2
Roasted/Toasted, 1 oz	160	14	7
Sunflower Kernels/Seed:			
Dry Roasted, 1 Tbsp, 8g	45	4	1.5
¼ cup, 1 oz	160	14	6
Oil Roasted, ¼ cup, 1 oz	180	17	6
Watermelon, dried, ¼ cup, 1 oz	160	14	4.5

Quick Guide

Peanut Butter: *Average All Brands*	C	F	Cb
1 teaspoon, 6g	35	3	1.5
1 Tbsp, 0.6 oz, (17g)	105	8.5	3.5
2 Tbsp, 1.2 oz, (34g)	210	17	7
1 oz Quantity (28g)	170	14	6
½ cup, 5 oz	850	70	30
Jif: Reduced Fat, 1 Tbsp	100	6	7.5
Creamy; Crunchy; Simply, 1 Tbsp	105	8	3.5
Peanut Wonder, 1 Tbsp	45	1.5	6
Smucker's: Honey Swtnd., 1 Tbsp	100	8	4
Goober Grape/Strawb., 1 Tbsp	90	5	4
Skippy: Carb Options, 1 Tbsp	100	8.5	5
Reduced Fat, 1 Tbsp	100	6	7.5
Squeez'it, 1 Tbsp, ½ oz	105	8.5	3.5

Other Nut & Seed Butters

Other Nut & Seed Butters	C	F	Cb
Almond Butter, 1 Tbsp, ½ oz	105	8	3
Almond Butter Honey Roasted	90	7	5.5
Beanut Butter, 1 Tbsp, ½ oz	90	5.5	7
Cashew Butter, 1 Tbsp, ½ oz	90	7	4.5
Cashew Peanut Date Butter	95	7	4
Hazelnut Butter, 1 Tbsp	100	10	2.5
Nutella, 1 Tbsp	100	5.5	12
Pecan Butter, 1 Tbsp	110	11	3.5
Pistachio Butter, 1 Tbsp	100	8.5	5
Sesame Butter/Tahini, 1 tsp	30	3	1
1 Tbsp, ½ oz	90	8.5	2
Soy Nut Butter, 1 Tbsp	85	6	2.5
Sunflower Seed Butter, 1 Tbsp	95	8	4

Supplements

Supplements	C	F	Cb
Aloe Vera Juice, undiluted, 2 fl.oz	5	0	1
Barlean's Flax Oil, 3 capsules	27	3	0
Cod Liver Oil, 1 Tbsp	120	13	0
Evening Primrose Oil, capsules, 1	5	0.5	0
Fiber Supplements: Tabs, 1	1	0	0
Bios Life 2, 1 packet	10	0	2
Metamucil, 1 packet	5	0	1
Regular, 1 rounded Tbsp	34	0	8
Sugar-Free, 1 Tbsp	6	0	1
Fish Oil Capsules, average, 1	10	1	0
Flax Oil Capsules, 2	10	1	0
Garlic Tablets/Capsules, each	3	0	0
Lecithin Granules, 1 Tbsp, 10g	50	5	1
Protein; Powders, average, 1 oz	100	0.5	0
Tablets, 20 tabs, ½ oz	70	0	0
Seaweed: Dried, 1 oz	85	0.5	22
Soaked, drained, 1 oz	15	0.5	3
Spirulina, 1 tablet	2	0	0.5
Vitamins/Minerals: Tabs/Caps, 1	2	0	0
Vitamin E Capsules, each	5	0.5	0
Yeast: Tablets, 2 tabs	4	0	0.5
Flakes, 1 heaping Tbsp, ⅓ oz	30	0.5	4
Powder, 1 heaping Tbsp, ½ oz	50	0.5	6

Cough & Pharmaceutical

Cough & Pharmaceutical	C	F	Cb
Cough/Cold Syrups: *Per Tablespoon*			
Regular: w. sugar, 1 Tbsp	35	0	9
w. alcohol, 1 Tbsp	46	0	9
Sugar-Free *(Diabetic Tussin)*, 1 T.	0	0	0
Cough Drops/Lozenges: *See Page 131*			
Antacids: Average, 1 tablet	4	0	1
Liquid, 1 Tbsp	6	0	1
Sudafed Syrup, 1 tsp	14	0	3
Tylenol Liquid: Child, 1 tsp	17	0	4
Extra Strength, 1 tsp	11	0	3

Nut eaters are healthier and live longer say medical researchers.

Nuts are a nutritious source of protein, antioxidants, vitamins, minerals, healthy fats and fiber.

Their fat and fiber content can help to lower blood cholesterol, but watch the quantity if overweight.

Weights As Purchased	C	F	Cb
Acerola, 1 cup, 20 pcs, 3½ oz	30	0	7.5
Apples: whole, average all varieties:			
1 small (4 per lb), 4 oz	55	0	14
1 medium (3 per lb), 5½ oz	70	0	17
1 large (2 per lb), 8 oz	110	0	28
1 extra large, 11 oz	150	0	37
without skin, 1 medium	60	0	15
Candy/Caramel Apple, 1 med.	170	0	42
Nut Coated, 1 medium	230	5	46
Apricots: 1 small (12 per lb)	17	0	4
1 medium (8 per lb), 2 oz	25	0	6
1 large (5-6 per lb), 3 oz	35	0	8
Avocado (w/out seed/skin):			
Average, ½ medium, 3½ oz	160	15	6
1 salad slice, ½ oz	25	2	1
Mashed/Puree, 2 Tbsp, 1 oz	50	4.5	2
¼ cup, 2 oz	90	9	4
Californian, ½ medium, 3 oz	160	14	8
Mashed/Puree, ½ c., 4 oz	210	18	12
Florida, ½ medium, 5½ oz	170	13	14
Mashed/Puree, ½ c., 4 oz	125	10	9
½ cup cubed, 3 oz	105	8	8

Note: Avocados are nutritious and contain no cholesterol. Fat is mainly monounsaturated and benefits blood cholesterol. Excellent substitute for butter or margarine.

	C	F	Cb
Banana: 1 small (4 per lb), 4 oz	90	0	23
1 medium (3 per lb), 5 oz	105	0	27
1 large (2½ per lb), 7 oz	120	0	30
w/out skin, 1 medium, 3¼ oz	80	0	20
½ cup, mashed, 4 oz	100	0	25
Berries: (Blueberries/Black/Boysenberries)			
½ cup, 2.5 oz	40	0	10
1 pint, 14 oz	225	1	56
Breadfruit, ½ cup, 4 oz	115	0	28
Cactus Pear, 1 fruit, 3½ oz	40	0	9
Cantaloupe: Flesh/no rind, 1 oz	8	0	2
½ small, 20 oz (w. rind/seeds)	125	1	30
½ medium, 28 oz (w. rind/seeds)	175	1.5	42
1 slice, 2.5 oz (w/out rind)	20	0	6
1 cup pieces/balls, 5.5 oz	25	0	13
Carambola (Star Fruit), 1 med	50	0	4
Cassava, ⅓ cup, 2½ oz	120	0	27
Cherimoya (Custard Apple), 4 oz	80	1	18
Cherries: Sweet, 8 fruit, 2 oz	30	0	7
½ lb (30 cherries)	110	0	27
Sour, 8 fruit, 2 oz	30	0	7
½ lb (30 cherries)	110	0	7
Clementine, 1 med., 3 oz	50	0	15

Weights As Purchased	C	F	Cb
Coconut: Fresh,			
1 piece, 2"x2"x ½", 1 oz	100	10	3
Shredded, fresh, ½ cup	140	13	6
Sweetened, dried, ½ cup	235	16	22
Crabapples, ½ cup slices, 2 oz	40	0	9
Cranberries, ½ cup, 2 oz	20	0	5
Currants: *Per ½ Cup*			
European Black, raw, 2 oz	35	0	8
Red & White, raw, 2 oz	30	0	7
Custard Apple, raw, 4 oz	110	1	27
Dates: *See Dried Fruits*			
Dragon Pearl Fruit, med., 11.6 oz	100	0.5	23
Durian, flesh, 4 oz	165	6	28
Elderberries, ½ cup, 2½ oz	55	0	13
Feijoas, 1 medium, 2½ oz	35	0	7
Figs, green/black: 1 med., 2 oz	40	0	10
1 large, 3 oz	60	0	15
Fruit Salad, fresh, average,			
½ cup, 3½ oz	60	0	15
1 cup, 7 oz	120	0	30
Gooseberries, raw, ½ c., 2½ oz	30	0	7
Grapefruit: Average all types,			
½ fruit, 10 oz (6 oz flesh)	50	0	12
1 cup sections w. juice, 8 oz	75	0	18
Grapes: Average, 1 cup, 5½ oz	105	0	25
1 small bunch, 4 oz	75	0	18
1 medium bunch, 7 oz	130	0	32
1 large bunch, 16 oz	305	0	75
Granadilla, flesh, 3½ oz	95	0	23
Groundcherries, ½ cup, 2½ oz	35	0	8
Guava: 1 fruit, 4 oz	80	0	15
½ cup, 3 oz	55	0	12
Honeydew, 1 wedge (⅛ of 7" diam.),			
8 oz (with skin)	50	0	12
1 cup cubes/balls, 6 oz	60	0	14
Honey Murcots, 1 only, 5 oz	45	0	11
Jaboticaba, flesh, 4 oz	75	2	15
Jackfruit, flesh, ⅛ average, 4 oz	105	0	25
Jambos (Brazil Cherry), flesh, 4 oz	35	0	8
Java-Plum, 4 plums, ½ oz	25	0	6
Jujube, 3 oz	65	0	16
Kiwifruit, 1 medium, 3 oz	45	0	11
1 large, 4 oz	60	0	15
Kumquats, 5 medium, 3½ oz	60	0	15
Kiwano, ½ medium, 5 oz	35	0	8
Langsat, Duku, 1 medium, 2 oz	25	0	5
Lemon: 1 medium, 4 oz	20	0	5
1 wedge, 1 oz	5	0	1.5
Peel, 1 Tbsp	4	0	1
Limes, 1 medium (2" diam.), 2 oz	20	0	5
Loganberries, froz., ½ cup, 2½ oz	40	0	9

Weights As Purchased	C	F	Cb
Longans, 5 fruit, ½ oz	**10**	0	2.5
Loquats, 4 fruit, 2¼ oz	**30**	0	7
Lychees, 4 fruit, 2¼ oz	**32**	0	7
Mamey Apple: 1 whole, 3 lb	**430**	4	100
¼ fruit (1 cup flesh), 7 oz	**100**	1	23
Mandarin: 1 small, 3 oz	**35**	0	9
1 medium, 4 oz	**45**	0	11
1 large, 6 oz	**50**	0	12
Mango: flesh, ½ cup sl., 3 oz	**55**	0	14
1 whole, medium, 11 oz	**135**	0	34
Melon, avg, 1 cup, cubes/balls, 6 oz	**60**	0	14
Monstera Deliciosa (Taxonia),			
Edible part, 4 oz	**50**	0	11
Mulberries, 20 fruit, 1 oz	**15**	0	3
Nashi Fruit (Asian Pear), 1 med., 7 oz	**85**	0	21
Nectarines: 1 medium, 4 oz	**50**	0	12
1 large, 5½ oz	**60**	0	14
Oheloberries, ½ cup, 2½ oz	**20**	0	5
Olives (Pickled): Green, 10 lrg, 1½ oz	**45**	5	0.5
Ripe, Greek Style, 10 med., 1 oz	**70**	7	2
Ripe (Black) Californian:			
1 small/medium	**5**	0.5	0.3
1 large/extra large	**6**	0.5	0.5
1 jumbo	**7**	0.5	0.5
1 colossal	**11**	1	0.5
1 super colossal	**13**	1	1
Oranges: Average all varieties,			
1 small, 5 oz (with skin)	**45**	0	11
1 medium (3" diam.), 7 oz	**60**	0	15
1 large, 10 oz	**85**	0	21
Flesh only, 1 cup, 6 oz	**80**	0	19
Californian Valencia,			
1 medium (2¾" diam.), 6 oz	**60**	0	15
Californ. Navels (3" diam.), 7 oz	**70**	0	17
Sunkist Navel, 14 oz	**130**	0	30
Florida Orange, 1 medium, 7 oz	**70**	0	17
Peel, 1 Tbsp	**0**	0	0
Papaya: ½ cup, cubed, 2½ oz	**30**	0	7
1 medium, (5"x3" diam.), 16 oz	**120**	0	28
Green (unripe), ½ cup, 3½ oz	**20**	0	5
Passionfruit, 1 medium, 1¼ oz	**20**	0	4.5
PawPaw (see Papaya)			
Peaches: 1 small/donut, 3 oz	**30**	0	7
1 medium (4 per lb), 4 oz	**40**	0	10
1 large, 6 oz	**60**	0	15
1 extra large, 10 oz	**90**	0	22

Weights As Purchased	C	F	Cb
Pears: Bartlett, 1 small, 4 oz	**80**	0	20
1 medium, 6.5 oz	**95**	0	24
1 large, 8 oz	**120**	0	30
1 cup slices, 6 oz	**95**	0.5	24
Asian, 1 medium, 7 oz	**85**	0	21
Bosc, 6 oz	**95**	0	24
D'Anjou, 1 medium, 8 oz	**120**	0	30
Forelle, 1 medium, 7 oz	**90**	0	22
Red Pear, 5 oz	**85**	0	20
Seckel (Wash'ton), 2¼ oz	**35**	0	9
Pepino, ½ medium, 4 oz	**20**	0	4
Persimmons: Native, 1 oz	**30**	0	7
Japan (2½"d. x 2½"h), 7 oz	**120**	0	30
Seedless (Maui), 1 md., 5 oz	**100**	0	25
Pineapple (no skin):			
1 thin slice, (½"), 2 oz	**28**	0	7
1 thick slice, (¾"), 3 oz	**40**	0	10
1 cup, diced, 5½ oz	**75**	0	19
1 medium, 1½ lb (peeled)	**325**	0	82
Wedges *(Del Monte),* 12 oz pkg	**168**	0	42
Canned: *See Page 146*			
Pitanga, 3 fruit, 1 oz	**6**	0	1
Plaintains, ½ cup slices, 2½ oz	**90**	0	22
Plums: Average all types,			
Mini/Damson, (1" diam.), ½ oz	**8**	0	2
Small (1¾" diam.), 2 oz	**30**	0	7
Medium (2¼" diam.), 3 oz	**45**	0	10
Large (2½" diam.), 4 oz	**65**	0	15
Pluot (plum-apricot), 1 med., 5 oz	**80**	0	19
Pomegranates, ½ fruit, 5 oz	**55**	0	13
Pummelo, flesh, ½ cup, 4 oz	**35**	0	8
Prickly Pears, 1 fruit, 5 oz	**50**	0	11
Quince, 1 medium, 3½ oz	**55**	0	14
Rambutan (Rambotang),			
Red/Yellow, 1 medium, 2 oz	**15**	0	4
Raspberries, ½ cup, 2 oz	**30**	0	7
Rhubarb, raw, ½ cup, 2 oz	**15**	0	3
Sapodilla (Chico), 1 md., 7½ oz	**140**	2	33
Sapotes, ½ medium, 5.5 oz	**150**	0	37
Satsuma Tangerine, 1 med., 3 oz	**50**	0	15
Soursop, 1 cup pulp, 8 oz	**150**	0	38
Strawberries: 1 cup, 5½ oz	**45**	0	10
6 medium/3 large, 2 oz	**15**	0	3
1 pint, 14 oz	**115**	0	28
Chocolate Dipped, 2 medium	**45**	2.5	6
Sugar Apples, ½ cup pulp, 4 oz	**120**	0	30
Tamarillo, 1 medium, 3 oz	**20**	0	3
Tamarind, 1 fruit, ¼ oz	**5**	0	0

Weights As Purchased	C	F	Cb
Tangelo: 1 small, 4 oz	30	0	7
1 medium, 5 oz	40	0	9
1 large, 7 oz	55	0	12
Tangerine, 1 medium, (2½" diam.), 4 oz	45	0	11
Tangor, 1 medium, 4 oz	35	0	7
Tomatillos, (3) 3 oz	20	0	5
Tomato: 1 small, 3 oz	15	0	4
1 medium, 5 oz	20	0	5
1 large, 7 oz	30	0.5	7
1 jumbo (salad/steak), 10 oz	50	1	11
Grape, 3 medium	8	0	2
Yellow Tear Drop, 4 medium, 1 oz	8	0	2
Cherry: 1 medium, ¾ oz	5	0	1
1 cup, 5¼ oz	27	0	6
Slices: (Medium Tomato):			
Thin slice, ½ oz	3	0	1
Medium (¼" thick), ¾ oz	4	0	1
Thick (3/8"), 1 oz	5	0	1
Fried Green Tomato, 1 slice (36g)	70	5.5	4.5
Canned Tomatoes/Products: *See Page 85*			
Tree Tomato (Tamarillo), 3 oz	20	0	5
Ugli Fruit, Tangelo type, 5 oz	40	0	8
Watermelon: Flesh only/no rind, 1 oz	9	0	2
1 cup cubes or balls, 5½ oz	45	0	11
Regular Long Shape:			
1 thick (1") slice (¼ circle, 4½" radius)			
9 oz w. rind (5½ oz no rind)	50	0	12
1 thin (½") slice (¼ circle)	25	0	6
1 thick (1") slice (½ circle)			
18 oz w. rind	100	1	24
1 whole melon (15" long, 7½" diam.)			
20 lb w. rind/10lb no rind	1360	7	340
Seedless Round Shape:			
Medium Size (13 lbs, 8¼" diam.)			
Edible Weight (no rind), 4 lbs	550	3	137
Wedge (⅛ whole melon),			
26 oz (with rind)	70	0.5	17
Flesh only (no rind), 8 oz	70	0.5	17
Wax Jambu (Rose Apple), 2 oz	10	0	2

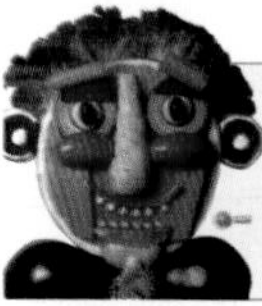

Eat at least 5 servings of fruit and vegetables every day . . . and Enjoy Better Health!

Dried Fruit

	C	F	Cb
Apples, 5 rings, 1 oz	75	0	18
Apricots, 8 halves, 1 oz	65	0	15
Banana Chips, ½ cup, 1½ oz	160	5	18
Banana Flakes, 4 Tbsp, 1 oz	80	0	20
Cranberries, swtn, dr., ⅓ c., 1.4 oz	130	0	33
Currants, ¼ cup, 1¼ oz	100	0	24
Dates: 5 medium dates, 1½ oz	120	0	28
Large Calif., 3 dates, 2 oz	160	0	37
½ cup, chopped, 3 oz	240	0	57
Date Crumbles *(Bob's Redmill),*			
1 oz, ¼ cup	90	0	23
Figs, 3 medium figs, 2 oz	145	0	34
Longans; Lychees, 1 oz	80	0	19
Mango Slices, 4 strips, 1 oz	70	0	15
Mixed Fruit, 1 oz	70	0	16
Papaya Spears, 1 oz	75	0	17
Peaches, 2 halves, 1 oz	60	0	14
Pears, 3 halves, 2 oz	75	0	17
Pineapple, 1 oz	80	0	18
Prunes (dried Plums): w. pits, 1 oz	60	0	14
1 Medium (60/lb)	16	0	4
1 Large (50/lb)	22	0	5
1 Extra Large (40/lb)	27	0	6
Without pits, 4 med., 1 oz	70	0	17
Cooked: w. sugar, ½ c, 5 oz	200	0	47
w/out sugar, ½ c, 4½ oz	125	0	30
Raisins: 2 Tbsp, 1 oz package	90	0	22
½ cup, 2.8 oz	260	0	62
CinnaRaisins, 1.4 oz pkg	135	0.5	32
Sunsweet: Fruitlings, ⅓ c., 1.5 oz	130	0	31
Plums (5) 1.4 oz	100	0	24

Candied Glacé Fruit

	C	F	Cb
Apricot, 1 medium, 1 oz	100	0	25
Cherry, 3 large, ½ oz	50	0	12
Citron/Fruit Peel, 1 oz	90	0	21
Fig, 1 piece, 1 oz	90	0	21
Ginger, 1 oz	95	0	23
Pineapple, 1 slice, 1¼ oz	120	0	30

Fruit Leather/Rolls

	C	F	Cb
Average All Brands, 1 oz	100	0	24
Fruit By The Foot, 1 roll, ¾ oz	80	0	17
Fruit Gushers, 1 pouch, 1 oz	90	1	20
Fruit Roll-Ups, 1 roll, ½ oz	50	0	12
Stretch Is. Leathers, 2 pces, 1 oz	90	0	21
Sunkist Fruit Roll, 1 roll	75	0	18

Other Fruit Confectionery/Snacks/Bars: *Page 137*

Canned/Bottled Fruit

Solids & Liquids: *Per ½ Cup (Approx. 4 ½ oz)*	C	F	Cb
Apples, sweetened	70	0	17
Apricots: In water/diet	35	0	9
In juice/lite	60	0	15
In syrup	105	0	27
Black/Blueberries: Heavy syrup	115	0	30
In light syrup	110	0	26
Cherries, pitted, in water	55	0	14
In light syrup	85	0	21
In heavy syrup	110	0	28
In extra heavy syrup	130	0	33
Maraschino, 5, 1 oz	50	0	12
Pie, ⅔ cup, 5 oz	60	0	14
Fruit Salad: In water/diet	35	0	9
In juice/Light	60	0	16
In heavy syrup	95	0	25
Gooseberries, Light syrup	90	0	23
Grapefruit: Juice pack	45	0	15
In light syrup	75	0	20
Lychees, ½ cup, 4.5 oz	105	0	26
Mixed Fruit: In water/diet	40	0	10
In fruit juices/light syrup	60	0	15
In heavy syrup	100	0	25
Peaches (halves/slices): In water/diet	30	0	8
In juice/light	50	0	14
In light syrup	70	0	20
drained, ½ peach	40	0	11
In heavy syrup	100	0	26
Pears: In water/diet	35	0	10
In juice/light	60	0	16
In heavy syrup	100	0	26
Pineapple: All types			
In own juice	70	0	17
In heavy syrup	90	0	22
Slices, drained, 2 slices			
In own juice, drained	30	0	7
In heavy syrup, drained	45	0	11
Plums: In water	50	0	14
In juice	75	0	20
In light syrup, 3 plums	85	0	21
In heavy syrup, ½ cup	160	0	41
Prunes: In heavy syrup	120	0	32
In Liqueur, ½ cup, 125g	280	0	70
In Water, ½ cup	135	0	32
Raspberries, in heavy syrup	120	0	30
Strawberries: In water	25	0	7
In heavy syrup	120	0	31
Tropical Fruit Salad: In light syrup	80	0	18
In heavy syrup	95	0	21

Fruit Snack Cups

	C	F	Cb
Mott's: Healthy Harvest, 4 oz cup	50	0	13
Blues Clues; Fruitsations, 4 oz c.	90	0	22
Del Monte Fruit Cups: *Per 4 oz Cup*			
Fruit Cocktail: In water/diet	40	0	11
In juice/light	55	0	15
In light syrup	80	0	21
In heavy syrup	95	0	25
Mandarin Orange cup	70	0	17
Mandarin Oranges: In water	40	0	10
In light syrup	80	0	20
Peach/Pear/Lite	50	0	13
Fruit Rageous cup	90	0	22
Fruit to Go, 4 oz cup	70	0	18
Pop Top Snack Cans:			
Fruit Cocktail, 8½ oz can	190	0	47
Lite Sliced Peaches, 8¼ oz can	115	0	28
Dole Fruit Bowls			
4 oz Bowls: Peaches/Mandarin Or.	70	0	17
Mixed Fruit	80	0	19
Pineapple/Tropical Fruit	65	0	15
Fruit n Gel Bowls 4.3 oz: Reg.	90	0	22
Reduced Sugar	50	0	13
Tree Top: Fruit Rocketz, 1 tube	45	0	11
Natural Apple, 1 Pkg., 4 oz	50	0	12
Vons: Mixed Fruit,			
In heavy syrup, 1 cup, 4.5 oz	90	0	22
In lite syrup, 1 cup, 4.5 oz	60	0	13

Apple & Fruit Sauces

	C	F	Cb
Apple Sauce:			
Regular/sweetened, 2 Tbsp, 1.1 oz	23	0	5
4 oz package cup	80	0	20
½ cup, 4.5 oz	90	0	22
Mott's Cinnamon, ½ cup, 4.5 oz	110	0	27
Cranberry Sauce: Whole Berry, 1 T.	15	0	3
¼ cup, 2½ oz	110	0	27
Jellied Cranberry, ¼ cup	110	0	27
Fruit Sauces & Purees:			
Average all fruit types, 2 Tbsp, 1 oz	25	0	6
½ cup, 4 oz	100	0	24

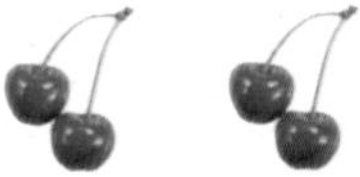

Vegetables	C	F	Cb
Alfalfa Sprouts, ½ cup, ½ oz	5	0	1
Artichokes, Globe/French:			
1 medium, 4½ oz	60	0	14
1 large, 7 oz	95	0	21
Artichoke Heart: Plain, 1 piece	8	0	2
Marinated, 1 piece	15	2	2
Asparagus, raw/froz.: 4 med. spears	12	0	3
Cuts & Tips, ½ cup, 3 oz	17	0	4
Bamboo Shoots, ckd, ½ c, 2 oz	7	0	1
Beans: Green/Snap, ½ c, 2 oz	17	0	4
10 beans (4" long), 2 oz	17	0	4
Dried Beans, *average all types: (Kidney, Brown, Haricot, Lima, Mung, Navy, Pinto, Red, White)*			
Raw: 2 Tbsp, 1 oz	95	0.5	18
1 cup, 7 oz	665	3	126
Cooked: 1 oz	35	0	7
½ cup, 3 oz	105	0	21
Bean Sprouts, avg., ½ cup, 2 oz	17	0	3
Beets: Raw, 1 beet (2" diam), 3 oz	35	0	8
Cooked, ½ cup, slices, 3 oz	37	0	8
1 beet, 2" diam., 1¾ oz	20	0	5
Beet Greens, ckd, ½ c., 2½ oz	20	0	4
Bell Pepper: *See Peppers*			
Bitter Melon/Gourd, 1 c. pces, 4 oz	15	0	2
Black Eyed Peas, ckd, ½ c., 2 oz	100	0.5	18
Bok Choy (Chinese Chard), 3 oz	13	0	3
Breadfruit, ¼ small fruit	100	0	25
Broadbeans (Fava Beans):			
Green (in pod), raw: 4 pods			
(3½ oz w. shell; 1.2 oz beans)	30	0	6
1 cup beans (no shell), 4½ oz	110	1	22
Mature Seeds: Raw, 1 c., 5.3 oz	510	2	87
Cooked, ½ cup, 3 oz	95	0	17
Broccoli: Raw, chopped,1 cup, 3 oz	30	0	6
3 Florets, 2½ oz	23	0	4
1 Spear (5" long) 1.1oz	11	0	2
1 Whole: Medium size, 14 oz	130	1	26
Large, 21 oz	200	2	39
1 Head (no stalk), 11 oz	105	1	21
1 Stalk, small (5" long), 5 oz	50	0.5	10
BroccoSprouts, ½ cup, 1 oz	16	0	2
Brussel Sprouts: ckd, ½ cup, 3 oz	30	0	6
2 Sprouts, 1½ oz	16	0	3
Butterbeans, cooked, ½ cup, 3 oz	90	0	20
Cabbage, All types/colors, average:			
Raw: 1 Leaf, large, 1.2 oz	8	0	2
Shredded, 1 cup, 2½ oz	17	0	4
½ Large Head (7" diam), 22 oz	150	1	35
Cooked, shredded, ½ cup, 2½ oz	15	0	3
Cactus (Nopal), sliced, 1 cup, 3 oz	15	0	3

Vegetables (Cont)	C	F	Cb
Carrots: Regular thick variety			
1 small, 4 oz	40	0	9
1 medium, 6 oz	65	0	15
1 large, 8 oz	85	0	19
Chopped, 1 cup, 4½ oz	50	0	12
Grated, 1 cup, 4 oz	45	0	11
Slices, 1 cup, 4¼ oz	48	0	11
Sticks (4"), 4, 1½ oz	16	0	4
Long thin variety, 1 medium, 2.2 oz	25	0	6
Baby, snack size, 5 medium, 1 oz	11	0	2
Snack Pack, 3 oz	35	0	7
Cauliflower, Raw: 1 cup (pces), 3½ oz	25	0	5
½ medium head, 10 oz	70	0	15
Cooked, 3 florets, 2 oz	12	0	2
Celeriac, ½ cup, raw, 2¾ oz	30	0	7
Celery: 1 large stalk, 11", 2 oz	8	0	2
1 small stalk, 5", ½ oz	2	0	0.5
4 Strips/sticks, ½ oz	2	0	0.5
Chopped, 1 cup, 3½ oz	14	0	3
Chard (Swiss), ½ cup, ckd, 3 oz	20	0	4
Chayote Squash, 1 cup, 1" pces, 4½ oz	22	0	5
Chick Peas (Garbanzo Beans):			
Dry, 1 cup, 6 oz	550	10	92
Cooked, 1 cup, 6 oz	270	4	45
Chicory, Greens, ½ cup, 3 oz	20	0	4
Chicory/Witloof: *See Endive*			
Chili Peppers: *See Peppers*			
Chinese Long Bean, sliced, 1 c., 3.2 oz	45	0	8
Chives, chopped, 1 Tbsp	1	0	0
Choy Sum, 3 oz	13	0	3
Cilantro (Coriander), 1 Cup	10	0	2
Collards, ½ cup, 3 oz	15	0	4
Corn, yellow/white:			
Raw, kernels, ½ c., 2¾ oz	65	1	14
Ear (5"x 1¾"), 5½ oz	80	1	17
Trimmed to 3½" long	65	1	14
Cooked, kernels, ¼ c., 1½ oz	35	0.5	7
(Also see Frozen & Canned Corn Page 149-150)			
Courgette: *See Zucchini*			
Cress, Garden, ½ cup, 1 oz	10	0	2
Cucumber: 1 whole, 11 oz	40	0	12
½ cup slices, 2 oz	5	0	1
Mini/Lebanese (1), 3 oz	10	0	3
Daikon Radish, 3 oz	18	0	4
Dandelion Greens, ½ cup, 1 oz	15	0	3
Edamame *(Immature green soybeans):*			
Shelled, ½ cup, 2.6 oz	120	5	11
With shells, 10 pods, 1¼ oz	30	1	3
Eggplant: ¼ medium, 4 oz	35	0	8
½ cup, 1" pieces, 1½ oz	10	0	2
1 slice, fried, 1 oz	75	4	10
Endive, Belgian/French:			
1 med. head (6"), 2½ oz	12	0	3

Vegetables (Cont)

	C	F	Cb
Fiddleheads, 3.5 oz	35	0.5	4
Fava Beans: *See Broadbeans*			
Fennel, 1 cup, sliced, 3 oz	27	0	6
Gai Choy Cabbage, ckd, 1 cup	20	0	5
Gai Lan (Chinese Kale), 3 oz	35	0	7
Garlic, 1 clove	4	0	1
Ginger: ¼ cup slices, 1 oz	20	0	4
Crystallized (sugared), 1 oz	95	0	20
Horseradish, 1 pod, ¾ oz	4	0	1
Jerusalem Artichoke, ½ cup	60	0	14
Jicama, raw, sliced, ½ cup, 2¼ oz	25	0	5
Kale, 1 cup, chopped	34	0	7
Kohlrabi, ½ cup, cooked, 3 oz	25	0	6
Lambsquarters, boiled, 3 oz	30	0.5	3
Leeks, cooked, 1 whole, 4½ oz	40	0	9
Lentils, green/brown: Dry, 1 oz	95	0.5	16
Dry, 1 cup, 6¾ oz	650	2	109
Cooked, ½ cup, 3½ oz	115	0.5	20
Lettuce: 1 c., chop./shred., 1½ oz	5	0	1
Butterhead, 2 leaves, ½ oz	2	0	0.5
Cos/Romaine, ½., shred., 2½ oz	4	0	1
Iceberg: 1 outer leaf, ¾ oz	3	0	1
1 medium head, 15-16 oz	60	0	15
Lamb's Lettuce, 2 ½ oz	15	0	1.5
Lima Beans, baby, ckd,½ c., 3 oz	90	0	17
Lotus Root, 10 slices, ckd, 3 oz	60	0	15
Mung Bean Sprouts, ½ cup, 2 oz	15	0	3
Mushrooms, Raw: 1 medium, 0.6 oz	4	0	1
1 large, sliced, ¾ oz	5	0	1
½ cup pieces, 1¼ oz	8	0	1
Cooked: ½ cup pieces, 2½ oz	20	0	4
Mustard Greens, ½ cup, 1 oz	7	0	1
Nopal (Cactus), 1 leaf, 4½ oz	22	0	5
sliced, 1 cup, 3 oz	15	0	3
Okra, cooked, ½ cup, slices, 2¾ oz	18	0	4
Onions, Raw: 1 small, 2 oz	22	0	5
1 medium, 4 oz	45	0	10
1 large, 8 oz	90	0	20
1 jumbo, 16 oz	180	0	40
Chopped, ½ cup, 3 oz	35	0	8
1 Tbsp, 0.3 oz	4	0	1
Slices: 1 cup, 4 oz	50	0	11
1 thin slice, small, 0.3 oz	4	0	1
⅛" slice, medium, ½ oz	6	0	1
¼" slice, large, 1.3 oz	16	0	4
Dehydrated flakes, ¼ c, ½ oz	45	0	11
Rings, breaded/fried, 2 rings	80	5	9
Scallions, ½ cup, 2 oz	15	0	4
Spring, ¼ cup, chopped, 1 oz	6	0	1
Blossom/Blooming: *See Fast-Foods (Chili's/Outback)*			

	C	F	Cb
Parsley, chopped, ½ cup, 1 oz	10	0	2
Parsnips: 1 medium, 4 oz	80	0	20
Cooked, ½ cup slices, 2¾ oz	65	0	16
Peas: Green, ¼ cup, 1½ oz	35	0	6
Raw, with pods, ½ lb	70	0	13
Snow Peas (8-9 pods), 1 oz	10	0	2
Split, dry, hulled, 1 oz	50	0	10
cooked, 1 cup, 7 oz	230	1	41
Peppers: Sweet, 1 medium, 5 oz	35	0	9
Bell: 1 medium, 5 oz	25	0	6
½ cup, chopped, raw, 1¾ oz	12	0	3
1 ring (3" diam. x ¼" thick)	2	0	0
Chile: Green/Red, 1½ oz	18	0	4
Habanero, 1 only, 8g	11	0	2
Pigeon Peas, cooked, ½ cup	85	1	16
Pimientos, 3 medium, 3½ oz	25	0	5
Poi, ½ cup, 4.2 oz	135	0	33
Pumpkin, mashed, ½ cup, 4 oz	25	0	6
Raw, 1" cubes, 1 cup, 4 oz	30	0	7
Pumpkin Flowers, 1 cup, 1.2 oz	5	0	1
Purslane, cooked, ½ c., 2 oz	10	0	2
Raw, 1" cubes, 1 cup, 4 oz	30	0	7
Potatoes: Raw (with skin)			
1 Baby, Gourmet, 2 oz	45	0	11
1 Small, 3 oz	65	0	15
1 Medium, 5 oz	110	0	26
1 Peeled, 4 oz	90	0	22
1 Large, 8 oz	180	0	44
1 Extra large (Russet), 12 oz	270	0	65
1 Jumbo (Russet), 16 oz	360	0	88
Baked (no fat); large, 10 oz raw:			
Plain, with skin, 7 oz	220	0	51
without skin, 5½ oz	145	0	34
With Toppings: + 2 tsp fat	290	8	51
+ Sour Cr./Chives, 2 Tbsp	270	6	53
+ Plain Yogurt, 2 Tbsp	240	1	55
+ Grated Cheese, 1 oz	330	9	56
+ Cottage Cheese, 2 oz	280	2	56
Mashed w. milk and fat, ½ c.	110	4	14
Roasted (w. fat), 1 small	155	8	21
Garlic Potatoes, 4 oz	120	2	22
Hash Browns: w. Butt. Sce, 2½ oz	125	6	10
Homemade, ½ cup, 2½ oz	165	10	10
Potato Skins: (w. Cheese topping),			
½ whole (8 oz baking), 4 oz	240	13	22
French Fries: Small serve, 2½ oz	220	12	14
Medium serve, 4 oz	350	20	22
Froz., uncooked, 18 fries, 4 oz	185	7	22
Oven-heated, 18 fries, 4 oz	185	7	22
Take-Out, 1 cup, 5 oz	440	25	28
McDonald's: Small, 2.6 oz	225	11	28
Medium, 4 oz	345	17	43

Vegetables (Cont)

	C	F	Cb
Potatoes (Cont)			
Fried, 18 fries, 3 oz	**275**	15	16
Au Gratin, ½ cup, 4.3 oz	**160**	9	22
Pancakes, 1 only, 5 oz	**90**	5	9
Kugel, 5 oz	**300**	20	26
Puffs, fried, 4 puffs, 1 oz	**65**	3	37
Scalloped, ½ cup, 4¼ oz	**105**	4	13
Ore-Ida Frozen Potatoes: *See Page 150*			
Potato Salad, ½ cup, 4½ oz	**180**	10	14
Radicchio, 2 leaves, ½ oz	**4**	0	1
Shredded, 1 cup, 1½ oz	**10**	0	2
Radish: Avg., 10 only, 1½ oz	**10**	0	2
Oriental, ½ c. slices, 1½ oz	**10**	0	2
Rutabagas, ckd., ½ c. cubes, 3 oz	**30**	0	7
Salsify, ckd, ½ c. slices, 2½ oz	**45**	0	11
Sauerkraut, ½ cup, 4 oz	**25**	0	5
Seaweed: Average, dried, 1 oz	**50**	0	13
Soaked, drained, 1 oz	**15**	0	4
Nori/Laver, dried, 6 sheets, ½ oz	**35**	0	5
Shallots, chopped, 1 Tbsp	**7**	0	1
Sorrel, raw, ½ cup, 4 oz	**23**	0.5	4
Soybeans: Mature, dry, 1 oz	**110**	5	7
Dry, ½ cup, 3½ oz	**385**	18	22
Cooked, ½ cup, 3 oz	**105**	5	6
(Soy Products/Tofu/Tempeh: See Page 77)			
Spinach, cooked, ½ cup, 3 oz	**20**	0	4
Creamed, ½ cup, 4½ oz	**140**	12	8
Raw: 3 leaves/1 cup, 1 oz	**20**	0	1
1 Bunch, 12 oz	**80**	0	12
Squash: Summer, raw, ½ c., 2¼ oz	**13**	0	3
cooked, ½ cup slices, 3 oz	**18**	0	4
Winter, cooked,			
Acorn, ½ cup cubes, 3½ oz	**55**	0	14
½ medium (10 oz raw wt.)	**85**	0	22
Butternut, ½ c. cubes, 3½ oz	**40**	0	10
¼ medium (9 oz raw wt.)	**95**	0	23
Spaghetti, ½ cup, 2¾ oz	**23**	0	5
Succotash, ckd, ½ cup, 3 1/3 oz	**110**	1	23
Sweetcorn: *See Corn*			
Sweet Potatoes: Cooked with Skin (no fat)			
1 medium, 4 oz	**120**	0	28
No skin, mashed, ½ c., 5½ oz	**170**	0	40
Swedes, ½ cup, 3 oz	**45**	0	10
Swiss Chard, ckd, chopped, 1 c., 6 oz	**35**	0	7
Taro, cooked, ½ cup, 2 oz	**95**	0	23

Vegetables (Cont)

	C	F	Cb
Tomatoes: 1 small, 3 oz	**20**	0	5
1 medium, 5 oz	**35**	0	8
1 large, 7 oz	**45**	0	10
Cooked, ½ cup, 4¼ oz	**30**	0	7
Fried, 1 small, 3 oz	**60**	4	5
Also See Fruit: *Page 145*			
Tomatillo, 1 medium, 1.2 oz	**10**	0	2
Turnips, White, cooked, ½ cup, 3 oz	**15**	0	4
Greens, cooked, ½ cup, 2½ oz	**15**	0	3
Water Chestnuts: 4 nuts	**40**	0	10
½ cup slices, 2¼ oz	**65**	0	15
Watercress, 10 sprigs, 1 oz	**4**	0	1
Yam: Cooked, ½ cup, 2½ oz	**80**	0	20
Baked, 1 medium (6") 8 oz	**260**	0	62
1 large (9") 12 oz	**390**	0	93
Yardlong Bean, 1 pod, ½ oz	**7**	0	1
Yucca Root, ½ cup, 2.5 oz	**60**	0	14
Zucchini: 1 medium, 10 oz	**45**	0	10
½ cup slices, cooked, 3 oz	**13**	0	3

Frozen Vegetables

	C	F	Cb
Birds Eye			
Broccoli/Corn/Red Peppers, ¾ cup	**50**	0.5	11
Carrots/Corn/Green Beans, 2/3 cup	**60**	0.5	11
Chopped Spinach, 1/3 cup	**20**	0	2
Other varieties, average, 1 cup	**30**	0	6
Baby: Bean & Carrot Blend, 1 cup	**30**	0	5
Broccoli Florets, 1 cup	**25**	0	4
Corn & Bean Blend, ¾ cup	**60**	0.5	12
Pea Blend, ¾ cup	**40**	0	7
Sweet Peas, 2/3 cup	**70**	0.5	12
White Corn, 2/3 cup	**110**	1	22
Pasta Secrets: Ranch, 1 c., 6.6 oz	**300**	15	29
Other varieties, average, 1 cup	**240**	10	31
Stir Fry: *Prepared (Includes Pasta)*			
Asparagus, 2 cup	**90**	0.5	16
Green Bean, 1¾ cup	**100**	0.5	19
Voila! Meals: *See Page 62*			
Green Giant			
Vegetables: Asparagus Cuts, 2/3 c.	**25**	0	4
Corn: Nibblers, 1 ear	**70**	0.5	14
Extra Sweet Niblets, 2/3 cup	**70**	1	13
S/Western & Rst Peppers, ¾ c.	**90**	1	18
Green Bean Casserole, 2/3 cup	**100**	5	11
Honey Glazed Carrots, 1 cup	**90**	3.5	13
Le Sueur Baby Sweet Peas, 2/3 cup	**60**	0.5	11
Spinach, ½ cup	**25**	0	3

Frozen Vegetables (Cont)

	C	F	Cb
Green Giant (Cont)			
Veges In Cheese & Cream Sauce: *Prepared*			
Alfredo Vegetables, ¾ cup	**80**	3	9
Broccoli, Cauliflower, Carrots, ⅔ c.	**70**	2.5	10
Cauliflower & Cheese Sce, ½ cup	**60**	2.5	8
Creamed Spinach, ½ cup	**80**	3	9
Cream Style Corn, ½ cup	**110**	1	23
Green Bean Casserole, ⅔ cup	**90**	5	9
Rice & Vegetables: *Prepared*			
Cheesy Rice & Brocc., 1 pkt, 10 oz	**300**	5	56
Oriental Rice, 1 pkt, 10 oz	**340**	12	52
Rice Medley, 1 pkt, 10 oz	**280**	4	52
Rice Pilaf, 1 pkt, 10 oz	**230**	3.5	44
White & Wild Rice, 1 pkt, 10 oz	**280**	6	51
French Fries: Country, 18 fries, 3 oz	**120**	4	19
Crispers 17 pces, 3 oz	**210**	12	23
Crispy Crunchies, 13 fries, 3 oz	**160**	8	20
Fast Food Fries, 35 fries, 3 oz	**160**	7	22
Ore-Ida (As Purchased):			
Pasta Accents: *Per Cup (Cooked)*			
Alfredo Broccoli	**105**	4	14
Crmy Cheddar w. Broc./Carrots	**125**	4	18
Garlic Seas. w. Broc./Corn/Carrots	**130**	5	18
Primavera	**140**	4.5	19
Three Cheese	**150**	4.5	21
White Cheddar	**135**	4	18
Funky Fries: Cinna-Stiks (17) 3 oz	**300**	17	27
Crunchy Rings, 11 pces, 3 oz	**230**	11	26
Fast-Food; Waffle Fries, 9 fries, 3 oz	**155**	7	21
Golden Crinkles, 13 pces, 3 oz	**150**	8	18
Golden Fries, 17 pces, 3 oz	**120**	4	20
Oven Chips, 7 pces, 3 oz	**160**	7	22
Shoestrings, 40 pces, 3 oz	**150**	6	22
Steak Fries, 9 fries, 3 oz	**110**	3.3	19
Zesties, 12 pces, 3 oz	**150**	7	20
Hash Browns: Toaster, 2 patties	**220**	12	25
Potatoes O'Brien, ¾ c., 2 oz	**60**	0	14
Onion Rings: Gourmet, 4 pces, 3 oz	**210**	10	28
Onion Ringers, 6 pces, 3.2 oz	**220**	12	25
Sweet Potatoes: 4 oz	**80**	0	18
Tater Tots: 9 pces, 3 oz	**170**	8	21
Mini, 19 pces, 3 oz	**180**	10	18
Onion 9 pces, 3 oz	**150**	7	21
Extra Crispy, 3 oz	**145**	7	19
Twiced Baked: Potatoes, 1, 5 oz	**190**	7	26
TGI Friday's			
Potato Skins, 3 pces, 3½ oz	**210**	11	19
Wild Oats: Oven Fries, (18) 3 oz	**130**	4	24
Potato Poppers (Bites), (10) 3 oz	**130**	8	14

Canned/Bottled

	C	F	Cb
Solids & Liquid			
Artichoke Hearts: Plain, 1 oz (1)	**30**	0	8
Marinated, 1 oz	**60**	5	2
Asparagus, ½ cup, 4½ oz	**20**	0	3
Bamboo Shoots, 1 cup, 4½ oz	**25**	0	4
Bean Salad, ½ cup, 3 oz	**90**	0	23
Bean Sprouts, ⅔ cup	**10**	0	2
Beans: Green, ½ cup, 4¼ oz	**20**	0	4
Baked Beans, ½ cup, 4½ oz	**120**	0.5	18
Butter Beans, ½ cup, 4½ oz	**90**	0	20
Italian, cut, ½ cup, 4½ oz	**30**	0	7
Kidney Beans, ½ cup, 4½ oz	**105**	0.5	20
Lima Beans, ½ cup, 4½ oz	**80**	0	15
Pinto Beans, ½ cup, 4½ oz	**100**	0.5	20
Beets: Sliced/Whole, ½ c., 4½ oz	**35**	0	7
Crinkle/Pickled *(Del Monte)* ½ c.	**80**	0	20
Carrots: Sliced, ½ cup	**35**	0	8
Honey Glazed *(Green Giant)* ½ c.	**45**	3.5	13
Corn: Kernels, ½ cup, 4½ oz	**90**	1	14
Drained Solids, ½ cup, 3oz	**65**	0.5	15
Creamed style, ½ cup, 4½ oz	**100**	0.5	24
Garbanzo/Chick Peas, 3 oz	**100**	2	20
Green Chilies: diced, 2 Tbsp, 1 oz	**5**	0	1
Hearts of Palm (1), 1.2 oz	**9**	0	2
Mushrooms: ½ cup, 2½ oz	**20**	0	4
in Butter Sauce, 2 oz	**30**	1	3
Onions: Pickled, 1 med., ¾ oz	**10**	0	2
Cocktail, 1 onion	**2**	0	0.5
Peas, ½ cup, 3 oz	**60**	0	10
Peppers: Hot Chilli, 1 only, 1 oz	**8**	0	2
Sweet, undrained, 2½ oz	**15**	0	3
Jalapeno, w. liq., ½ c. chopped	**17**	0	3
Fried, drain, 2 Tbsp, 1 oz	**60**	5	3
Salsa, average all types, 2 Tbsp	**15**	0	3.5
Sauerkraut, undrained, ½ c., 4 oz	**25**	0	6
Spinach, ½ cup, 3½ oz	**25**	0	3.5
Succotash: w. Cr. Style Corn,½ c.	**100**	1	23
w. whole kernels, undrained	**80**	1	17
Sweetcorn: *See Corn*			
Sweet Potato: ½ cup, 3½ oz	**105**	0	24
Candied *(Green Giant)* ¾ cup	**240**	7	41
Tomatoes, Sundr.: Natural, 5-6 pce	**22**	0	5
In Oil, drained, 6 pces, ½ oz	**60**	4	6
Tomato Products: *See Page 85*			
Vegetables, mixed, ½ cup, 4 oz	**45**	0	8
Yams: in Light Syrup, ½ cup, 4 oz	**105**	0	25
Candied, ½ cup, 5 oz	**170**	0	46
Zucchini in Tom. Sce., ½ c., 4 oz	**30**	0	8

Take-Out Salads & Vegetables

Avg. All Outlets: Per Serving	C	F	Cb
Antipasto Salad, 1 cup	**140**	10	2
Bean Salad, ½ cup	**110**	4	17
Bulgur Salad, ½ cup	**70**	2	12
Caesar Salad, Classic, 1 cup	**200**	14	15
Side Salad, no Dressing	**25**	0	6
Carrot Raisin: No Dressing, ½ cup	**20**	0	5
with Dressing, ½ cup	**65**	5	5
Chef Salad: Regular, no Dressing	**620**	37	8
w. 2 oz 1000 Island	**860**	61	8
Chicken Salad Platter, 6 oz	**200**	8	12
Coleslaw: Traditional, ½ cup	**150**	8	18
w. Low Cal Dressing	**60**	1	12
Corn, Mexican, ½ cup	**240**	12	33
Cucumber: Non-Oil Dressing, ½ c.	**60**	0	14
w. Oil Dressing, ½ cup	**140**	12	8
Eggplant Salad, ½ cup	**75**	5	7
Fettucini w. veges, ½ cup	**110**	5	15
Garden Salad, no Dressing	**35**	0	8
Greek Salad, 1 cup	**120**	10	7
Greek Vegetables, ½ cup	**140**	12	7
Lettuce, hearts, ¼ head	**20**	0	4
Lobster Salad Platter, 6 oz	**200**	8	12
Macaroni Salad, ½ cup, 4 oz	**180**	13	13
Nicoise, 1 cup	**450**	32	18
Pasta Salad, ½ cup	**160**	8	16
Pineapple Coconut Slaw, ½ cup	**150**	10	14
Potato Salad: Dijon	**140**	7	17
w. Mayonnaise, ½ cup	**170**	10	17
Lowfat, ½ cup	**110**	1.5	21
Rice Salad, ½ cup	**150**	10	13
Saffron Rice, ½ cup	**130**	3	24
Spinach Salad, 1 cup	**180**	13	13
Tomato & Mozzarella, ½ cup	**180**	14	10
Tabouli, ½ cup	**150**	6	22
Three Bean Salad, ½ cup	**80**	5	9
Tortelini w. Basil Pesto, ½ cup	**170**	10	19
Waldorf w. Mayo, ½ cup	**160**	12	12
Signature Salads: *Per Serving (6 oz)* *(Supplied to Deli's and Institutions)*			
Antipasto Salad, 6 oz	**510**	50	4
Artichoke Salad, marinated	**400**	41	8
California Medley	**120**	7	15
Cheese Agnolotti	**250**	8	23
Chicken Salad	**420**	33	11
Crabmeat Flavored	**450**	38	20

Take-Out Salads (Cont)

Signature Salads (Cont)	C	F	Cb
Egg Salad	**300**	23	14
Fresh Button Mushroom	**190**	16	6
Garden Olive	**630**	67	3
Ham Salad	**400**	32	14
Prima Pasta Salad	**360**	30	18
Seafood Pasta Del Mar	**170**	10	21
Seafood with Crab & Shrimp	**420**	34	20
Shrimp Salad	**360**	32	8
Tuna Salad	**450**	36	14

Fast-Food Restaurants: *See Page 183*

Fresh Salad Packs

Pre-Packaged (Supermarkets)	C	F	Cb
Dole: Complete Caesar, 3½ oz	**170**	13	8
Complete Oriental, 3½ oz	**120**	6	13
Complete Romano, 3½ oz	**150**	12	9
Complete Spinach Bacon, 3½ oz	**170**	10	18
Complete Sunflower Ranch, 3½ oz	**160**	16	5
Special Blends (no added dressing),			
avg. all varieties, 2 cups, 3 oz	**15**	0	3
Regular Salad Packs (no added dressing):			
Classic Coleslaw, 3 oz	**25**	0	5
Classic Iceberg, 3 oz	**15**	0	4
Zesty Italian, 7 oz	**110**	0	4
Fresh Express: *Per Package*			
Chicken Caesar, 1 pkg, 183g	**240**	16	13
Chick. Crmy. Ranch, 1pkg. 194g	**230**	14	15
Chicken Teriyaki 1pkg, 193g	**250**	15	17
Salad Kits: *Per Serving (Prepared)*			
Caesar, 2 cups	**160**	14	7
Caesar w. Light Dress., 2 cups	**100**	7	8
Caesar Supreme, 2 cups	**150**	12	7
Oriental, 1½ cups	**140**	9	13
European, 2½ cups	**15**	0	3
Ready Pac: Average all types	**15**	0	2

Salad Toppings

	C	F	Cb
Bacon Bits, average, 1 Tbsp	**30**	1.5	2
Chow Mein Noodles, dry, ½ cup	**120**	5	13
Croutons, 2 Tbsp, 10g	**35**	1	6
Olives, 5 medium	**25**	2	0
Potato Chips, 1 oz	**150**	10	15
Sunflower Seeds, 1 Tbsp, 8 g	**45**	4	1.5
Tortilla Chips, 1 oz	**150**	8	16

Fruit & Vegetable Juices/Smoothies

Quick Guide

	C	F	Cb
Orange Juice			
Average ~ Fresh or Sweetened:			
½ Cup, 4 fl.oz	55	0	13
Small Glass, 6 fl.oz	82	0	20
Regular Glass, 8 fl.oz	110	0	26
8¾ fl.oz Box	120	0	28
10 fl.oz Bottle	140	0	32
11½ fl.oz Can	160	0	36
16 fl.oz Bottle	220	0	52
20 fl.oz Bottle	280	0	72
64 fl.oz/½ Gallon	890	0	230

Juices ~ Generic

Average All Brands: Per 8 fl.oz Unless Indicated	C	F	Cb
Aloe Vera Juice, unsweet., 2 oz	5	0	1
Apple Juice: 8 fl.oz	120	0	30
10 fl.oz Bottle	150	0	38
16 fl.oz	240	0	60
Carrot Juice: Fresh, 6 fl.oz	60	0	14
Sweetened, 6 fl.oz	75	0	17
Cranberry Juice, Cocktail/Blend	120	0	34
Fruit Blends, average, 8 fl.oz	120	0	31
Fruit Nectars, average, 8 fl.oz	140	0	35
Grape Juice, 8 fl.oz	160	0	40
Grapefruit Juice, 8 fl.oz	100	0	23
Lemon/Lime Juice: 1 Tbsp	4	0	1.5
1 cup, 8 fl.oz	60	0	21
Concentrate, 1 tsp	0	0	0
Noni Juice: *Tahitian*, 2 Tbsp, 1 fl.oz	10	0	2
Southern Cross Botanicals, 1 fl.oz	6	0	2
Tahiti Traders, 1 fl.oz	20	0	5
Orange Juice, 8 fl.oz	110	0	26
Passion Fruit Juice (Fresh):			
Purple, 1 cup, 8 fl.oz	125	0	34
Yellow, 1 cup, 8 fl.oz	150	0	36
Papaya/Peach Nectar, 8 fl.oz	140	0	35
Pear Nectar, 8 fl.oz	150	0	40
Pineapple Juice, 8 fl.oz	110	0	27
Prune Juice, 8 fl.oz	180	0	43
Strawb./Raspberry Juice, 8 fl.oz	100	0	23
Tangerine Juice, 8 fl.oz	100	0	25
Tomato Juice, 8 fl.oz	50	0	12
Vegetable Juice, 8 fl.oz	50	0	12
Wheat Grass Juice: 1 fl.oz 'Shot'	5	0	1
2 fl.oz 'Shot'	10	0	2

Quick Guide

	C	F	Cb
Fruit Smoothies			
Average All Brands:			
Fruit Only: 8 fl.oz	105	0	25
12 fl.oz	160	0	38
16 fl.oz	210	0	50
24 fl.oz	320	0.5	76
Fruit + Nonfat Milk/Soy:			
12 fl.oz	190	0.5	40
16 fl.oz	250	0.5	53
24 fl.oz	380	1	80
Fruit + Nonfat Frozen Yogurt/Sherbet:			
12 fl.oz	210	0.5	47
16 fl.oz	280	0.5	62
24 fl.oz	420	1	94

Juice Brands

Per 8 fl.oz Unless Indicated	C	F	Cb
100% Fruit Juice Boxes: *Per Box (4.2 fl.oz)*			
White Grape	90	0	22
Average other flavors	60	0	15
Ame			
Sparkling Fruit Juice: *Per 8 fl.oz*			
Ame Dry	60	0	15
Ame Red/Rose	80	0	20
Ame White	90	0	23
Apple & Eve			
Naturally Cranberry	120	0	30
Cranberry/Raspberry Apple	120	0	30
Cranberry Grape	140	0	34
Bright & Early			
Orange Juice (Chilled/Frozen)	120	0	30
Grape Juice (Frozen)	140	0	33
Campbell's			
Tomato Juice: 5.5 fl.oz can	35	0	7
10.5 fl.oz	60	0	12
Capri Sun			
Sport, all flavors, 8 fl.oz	120	0	31
Big Pouch: *Per 11.2 oz Pouch*			
Raspberry Lemonade; Wild Cherry	200	0	50
Average other flavors	170	0	42
Carb Countdown *(Hood): Per 8 fl.oz*			
Lemonade	20	0	4
Juice Beverages	25	0	5

Juice Brands (Cont)

Per 8 fl.oz Unless Indicated	C	F	Cb
Clamato			
Tomato Cocktails, average, 8 fl.oz	60	0	13
Crystal Geyser			
Juice Squeeze: *Per Bottle (12 fl.oz)*			
Blackberry Pomegranate	170	0	43
Orange Lime	160	0	40
Ruby Grapefruit	150	0	36
Average other flavors	140	0	32
Dole			
100% Fruit Juice Blends, 8 fl.oz	120	0	30
Donald Duck			
100% Orange Jce (+Calcium), 8 fl.oz	120	0	29
Eden: Organic Apple, 8 fl.oz	80	0	23
Five Alive: Frozen Concentrate, made up, 8 fl.oz	120	0	30
Florida's Natural			
Cranberry Apple, 8 fl.oz	120	0	30
Orange Juice, 8 fl.oz	110	0	26
Ruby Red Grapefruit Juice, 8 fl.oz	100	0	24
Fresh Samantha: *Per 8 fl.oz*			
Apple	120	0	30
Banana Strawberry Smoothie	150	1	36
Carrot/Orange; The Big Bang	100	0	25
Crazy Cranberry	130	0	32
Desperately Seeking C	130	0	31
Grapefruit	90	0	24
Mango Mama; Get Smart	130	0	33
Raspberry Dream	120	1	29
Soy Shake, 16 fl.oz	320	8	33
Super Juice w. Echinacea	140	1	33
Fruit Whips: *Per 8 fl.oz Bottle*			
Smoothies, 236ml (8 oz)	125	0	29
Fruitopia			
All flavors, average, 8 fl.oz	115	0	29
20 fl.oz Bottle	290	0	72
Frulatte Smoothies: *Per Bottle (10.5 fl.oz)*			
Orange Mango	230	0	47
Strawberry Kiwi	220	0	45
Avg. other flavors	240	0	50
Frusia *(Cinnabon)*, 12 fl.oz	170	0	38
Fuze: *Per 8 fl.oz*			
Focus (11% Juice), Mojo Mango	100	0	25
Lemonaid	70	0	18
Vitamin Tea	60	0	16
Average other varieties	90	0	22

Per 8 fl.oz Unless Indicated	C	F	Cb
Good Day: Fruit Juice, 8 fl.oz	110	0	28
Goya Nectar			
Apricot Nectar, 12 fl.oz	130	0	31
Pear Nectar, 12 fl.oz can	240	0	59
Hain: Carrot Juice w. Lutein	75	0.5	16
Veggie Juice w. Lutein, 8 fl.oz	55	0.5	11
Hansen's: Natural Juice Cocktail			
Regular, all flavors, 8 fl.oz	110	0	28
Low Calorie Peach Mango	10	0	4
Apple Varieties, 8 fl.oz	120	0	28
Junior Juice, 4.32 fl.oz box	60	0	15
Juice Slam: *Per Box (8.45 fl.oz)*			
Apple; Paradise Punch	120	0	28
Strawb. Banana; Wildberry	110	0	28
Smoothies: *Per Can (10.8 fl.oz)*			
Fruit Flavors, regular	170	0	43
Lite Cranberry Raspberry	50	0	13
Energy Smoothies: *See Page 158*			
Hawaiian Punch			
Fruit Juicy, Red, 6 fl.oz	90	0	22
Box, 8.45 fl.oz	120	0	30
Hawaii's Own			
Frozen Concentrate: *Per 8 fl.oz (Prep'd)*			
Average all varieties	105	0	28
Hi-C Juice Drinks: Average, 8 fl.oz	130	0	32
6.75 fl.oz box, average	100	0	27
11.5 fl.oz can	180	0	45
Hood: Apple, 8 fl.oz	125	0	31
Fruit Punch	130	0	32
Orange	120	0	30
Jamba Juice (California): *See Fast-Foods Section*			
Jera's Juice (Boston): *Per 24 fl.oz*			
Berry Blitz	440	2	105
Cape Codder	335	0.5	80
Citrus Burst	320	1.5	75
Mango Passion	290	0	68
Orange Bite; Flu Fighter, avg.	280	1.5	65
Razzle Dazzle	380	1	94
Soy Smoothie (7g protein)	320	3.5	68
Strawberry Smile	345	0.5	84
Triathlete (15g protein)	300	1.5	71
Whey-Out Protein (27g protein)	325	1.5	56
Juicy Juice (Libby's): *Per Box (6.75 fl.oz)*			
Grape	110	0	26
Average other flavors	100	0	25
4.23 fl.oz box, average	60	0	15

Juice Brands (Cont)

Per 8 fl.oz Unless Indicated

	C	F	Cb
Kerns All Nectars			
Canned Juice: *Per Can (11.5 fl.oz)*			
Pear	220	0	54
Pineapple Coconut	280	8	53
Other flavors, average	210	0	52
Kool Aid			
Jammers: Lemonade, 1 pouch	110	0	29
Other varieties, 6.75 fl.oz pouch	90	0	24
Knudsen: *Per 8 fl.oz*			
Fruit Juices: Apple	120	0	30
Cranberry Raspberry	140	0	36
Creamed Papaya	40	0	10
Grapefruit; Just Blueberry	100	0	23
Guava Strawberry	110	0	27
Hibiscus Cooler; Just Boysenberry	90	0	23
Just Concord	160	0	40
Prune	180	0	43
Tomato	60	0	14
Other varieties, average	125	0	32
Sparkling Juice, 8 fl.oz	105	0	29
Nectars: Coconut	140	5	26
Peach	120	0	30
Boysenberry, average	130	0	36
Floats: Orange	140	0	33
Very Veggie, 8 fl.oz	50	0	10
Simply Nutritious:			
Blackberry Hibiscus Mist	100	0	24
Mega C	130	0	31
Average other varieties	120	0	30

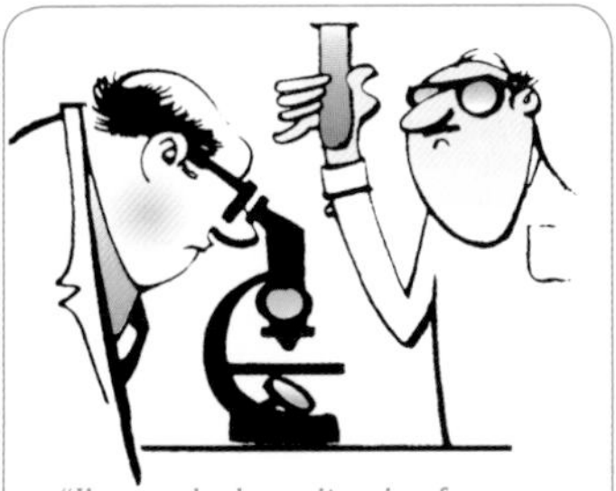

"I've worked on vitamins for years and I've discovered that the three most important elements necessary to life are breakfast, lunch and dinner."

Per 8 fl.oz Unless Indicated

	C	F	Cb
Krasdale: Cranberry Apple	170	0	42
Cranberry Juice Cocktail	130	0	32
Cranberry Raspberry	150	0	37
L & A: Black Cherry, 8 fl.oz	180	0	45
Grape Juice	160	0	40
Mixed Berry	120	0	30
Prime Juice	180	0	41
Average other varieties	140	0	32
Lakewood Organic			
Carrot Pineapple, 6 fl.oz	85	0	19
Coconut, 6 fl.oz	90	1.5	20
Cranberry/Lemonade, 8 fl.oz	85	0	21
Mango, 6 fl.oz	90	0	22
Papaya; Pure Carrot, 6 fl.oz	75	0	18
Pure Cranberry, 6 fl.oz	50	0	12
Pure Pineapple, 6 fl.oz	95	0	23
Pure Pine, 8 fl.oz	165	0	40
Pure Pink Grapefruit, 8 fl.oz	90	0	22
Red Tart Cherry, 8 fl.oz	110	0	19
Super Veggie, 6 fl.oz	40	0	9
Average other varieties	105	0	26
Langers: *Per 8 fl.oz*			
Apple Juice; White Cranberry avg.	120	0	28
Cranberry/100 Varieties, avg	140	0	35
Cranberry Berry	135	0	34
Cranberry Grape; White Grape	165	0	41
Cranberry Raspberry	150	0	36
Diet Apple Juice	60	0	40
Diet Cranberry	30	0	8
Diet Cranberry Grape	120	0	28
Frozen Concentrate: *Per 8 fl.oz (Prepared)*			
Cranberry	140	0	29
Avg. other flavors	120	0	29
Luzianne: *Per 8 fl.oz (Prepared)*			
Smoothies: Mixed Berry	90	0.5	19
Peach Mango	90	0	19
Strawberry Banana	80	0.5	18
Malibu Beach: *Per 8 fl.oz*			
Teas: Tropical Tea	10	0	3
Beach Peach; Oceanside	10	0	3
Juices: Malibu Mango	10	0	3
Sunset Strawberry; Redondo	10	0	3
Martinellis			
Sparkling Juice: *Per 8 fl.oz*			
Apple-Cranberry	110	0	27
Apple-Grape	120	0	31
Cider	140	0	35

Juice Brands (Cont)	C	F	Cb
Per 8 fl.oz Unless Indicated			
Mauna La'i Hawaiian: 8 fl.oz	140	0	32
Mistic (Mega 24 fl.oz)			
Average All flavors, 8 fl.oz	120	0	30
24 fl.oz	360	0	90
Minute Maid			
Orange Juice, Premium	115	0	27
Light Orange Juice	50	0	13
Heart Wise; Kids Plus	110	0	27
Lemonade, all flavors	110	0	28
Premium Blends, avg. all flavors	110	0	27
Simply Orange	105	0	26
Tropical Punches	110	0	30
Juices to Go: Avg. all flav., 10 fl.oz	160	0	40
Boxed Juices: Average, 6.75 fl.oz	100	0	25
Coolers, average, 6.75 fl.oz	110	0	28
Disney, 6.75 fl.oz box	100	0	25
Soft Frozen Lemonade, 12 fl.oz	300	0	78
Frozen Concentrates, 8 fl.oz (Prep'd),			
Average all varieties	105	0	28
Mott's			
Apple Juice, 8 fl.oz	120	0	29
Apple Raspb., Fruit Punch, 10 fl.oz	145	0	36
Apple Cranb., Grape Apple, 10 fl.oz	180	0	42
Fruitsations, all flavors, 4 oz	85	0	22
Juice Paks: All flavors, 8.45 fl.oz	120	0	30
Mini Motts, 4.23 oz	60	0	14
Naked Juice: *Per ½ Bottle (8 fl.oz)*			
Antioxidants: Orangecarrotbanana	115	0	27
Pomegranaberry-blue	140	0.5	33
Pomegranalicious	155	0	38
Strawberry Banana	120	0	28
Immunity: Berry Blast	136	0	33
Mighty Mango-Go; Power-C	125	0	30
Well Being	130	0	32
Just Juices: Carrot-o-copia	60	0	13
Just Apple	125	0	30
Just Grapefruit	95	0	23
Just O-J	110	0	25
Tangerine Scream	105	0	25
Organics: Organic Apple	115	0	29
Organic Carrot	60	0	13
Organic Orange	110	0	25
Proteins: Protein Zone	210	3.5	27

Naked Juice (Cont)	C	F	Cb
Quenchers: Just Made Lemonade	130	0	32
Raspberry-ade	145	0	35
Smoothies: Blue-nanas	150	1	34
Very Berry	130	0	30
Vanilla Soy Shake	175	1	33
Superfoods, average	225	3	42
Superfoods, all varieties	135	0	33
Nantucket Nectars			
Juice Cocktails: *Per 8 fl.oz*			
Carrot Orange Mango	130	0	30
Cranberry	140	0	34
Fruit Punch	130	0	32
Grapeade Guava; Orange Mango	130	0	33
Maine Berry Punch	110	0	27
Other varieties, avg.	120	0	30
100% Juice: *Per 8 fl.oz*			
Cranberry Raspberry Grape	150	0	38
Grape Juice	160	0	39
Peach Orange	130	0	31
Pineapple Orange Banana	140	0	35
Premium Orange Juice	120	0	27
Other varieties, avg.	100	0	25
Fruit Juice: Apple Cider	100	0	25
Squeezed Nectar Teas: *Per Bottle (16 fl.oz)*			
Diet Lemon Tea	0	0	2
Original Lemon Tea	180	0	46
NectarFizz, all other varieties, avg.	90	0	23
Nectar Lemonades, avg., 8 fl.oz	130	0	32
Newman's Own			
Lemonade (Reg./Pink), 8 fl.oz	110	0	27
Northland			
100% Juice: *Per 8 fl.oz*			
Cranberry/Peach/Blackberry	140	0	35
Cranberry Grape/Raspberry	150	0	38
Ocean Spray: *Per 8 fl.oz*			
Cranberry Cherry	150	0	39
Cranapple	160	0	41
Fruit Punch; Tangerine	130	0	32
Lite Cranberry varieties, avg.	40	0	30
Grapefruit: 100% Juice	100	0	24
Kiwi Strawb.; Summer Cooler	120	0	31
Lemonade flavors, average	130	0	32
Pink Grapefruit	110	0	28
Ruby Red & Strawberry	140	0	34
Ruby Red & Mango/Tangerine	130	0	33
Ruby Red; White Cranberry varieties	120	0	29
White Grapefruit	100	0	24

Fruit & Vegetable Drinks & Juices (Cont)

Juice Brands (Cont)	C	F	Cb
Ocean Spray (Cont): *Per 8 fl.oz*			
Cranberrry: Cranberry Grape	170	0	41
Cranberry Juice Cocktail	140	0	34
Light Style (Low Calorie)	40	0	10
Other Cranberry flavors, avg	150	0	35
Cravin' Less Sugar: Kiwi Strawb.	70	0	17
Tropical; Cranberry Wildberry	60	0	15
Odwalla			
AntioxiDance; Grapefruit, avg	90	0	23
B Berrier; Quencher	120	0	30
Carrot Juice	70	0	15
Carrot, Orange, Apple	110	0	25
C Monster	150	0.5	34
Blackberry Fruitshake	160	0	40
Glorious Morning; B Monster	140	0	33
Mango Tango	150	0	31
Mo'Beta	140	0	35
Strawberry Lemonade	120	0	28
Vegetable Blend	100	0	23
Wellness Echinacea	150	0	33
Old Orchard: Apple Juice, 8 fl.oz	120	0	29
Frozen Concentrate: *Per 8 fl.oz (Prep'd)*			
Apple	120	0	29
Other flavors	130	0	31
Orange Julius: Original (Orange, Strawberry),			
16 fl.oz	225	0	55
20 fl.oz	280	0	68
32 fl.oz	450	0	109
Other Drinks: *See Fast-Foods, Page 226*			
PS - Private Selection (Ralphs)			
Lemonade (Premium Juice), 8 fl.oz	110	0	29
Orange Juice, 8 fl.oz	110	0	27
Mango Nectar, 8 fl.oz	140	0	35
Realemon - Realime (Borden)			
Lemon/Lime Juice (from concentrate)			
1 teaspoon	0	0	0
2 Tbsp, 1 fl.oz	6	0	2
Pom Wonderful			
100% Juice: *Per 8 fl.oz*			
Pomegranate	145	0	35
Blueberry; Mango	140	0	34
Cherry	135	0	33
Tangerine	150	0	37
S&W			
Apple Juice, 8 fl.oz	120	0	30
Orange Juice, 6 fl.oz can	90	0	22
Grapefruit Juice, unswt'd, 8 fl.oz	105	0	25
Tomato Juice, 8 fl.oz	30	0	7

Per 8 fl.oz Unless Indicated	C	F	Cb
Santa Cruz			
Apple Juice; Cider & Spice	120	0	30
Concord Grape; White Grape	160	0	40
Orange Mango	130	0	31
Tropical Blend	140	0	33
Average other varieties	100	0	24
Nectars: Apricot; Cranberry	110	0	27
Berry	110	0	30
Average other varieites	120	0	30
Snapple			
Fruit Drink Blends, 8 fl.oz	120	0	30
Grapeade; Orangeade 8 fl.oz	120	0	30
Lemonade, all types	110	0	28
Vitamin Supreme	175	0	44
Diet: Snapple Apple	15	0	4
Kiwi Strawberry	20	0	5
Avg. other flavors	10	0	2
Snap.E Tom			
Tom. & Chile Cocktail, 11.5 oz can	70	0	15
Squeezit			
Average all flavors, 6.75 fl.oz	90	0	23
Stonyfield Farm: *Per Bottle (10 fl.oz)*			
Peach Smoothie	250	3	49
Wildberry; Strawberry Smoothie	250	3	45
Sunny Delight			
Florida Citrus, 6 fl.oz	90	0	22
Calcium Rich, 6 fl.oz	150	0	37
Mango Citrus	130	0	31
Smooth (California Style)	130	0	32
Sunny Delight Lite, 6 fl.oz	20	0	5
Tangy Original (Florida Style)	120	0	29
Tropical Fruit Punch, 6 fl.oz	90	0	22
Sunsweet			
Prune Juice/w. Pulp, 8 fl.oz	170	0	42
Superfood: Juice, 8 fl.oz	140	1	32
Tampico: Citrus Punch, 1 cup	100	0	25
Mango/Trop. Frt. Punch, 1 cup	110	0	28
Tang			
Pouches, average all flavors (1)	100	0	26
Mix: *Made Up, 6 fl.oz*			
Regular (2 Tbsp dry)	90	0	22

Juice Brands (Cont) *Per 8 fl.oz Unless Indicated*	C	F	Cb
Trader Joes: *Per 8 fl.oz*			
Carrot Juice	60	0	13
Ginger Lemonade	150	0	37
Organic Carrots & Greens	80	0	19
Strawberry Lemonade	160	0	41
Strawberry Smoothie	140	2	30
Avg. other varieties	110	0	25
Trader Darwin's (100%):			
Dairy Free Protein w. Pzazz	170	0.5	35
Very Green Juice Blend	110	0	27
Avg. other varieties	130	0	31
100% Juice: *Per 8 fl.oz*			
Apple Cranberry Blend	130	0	30
Original Lemonade	110	0	27
Other Apple varieties	140	0	33
All Natural Pasteurized: *Per 8 fl.oz*			
Combat; Lemon Ginger	110	0	26
Cranberry Harvest	135	0	35
Cranberry; White Grape	140	0	36
Garden Patch; Vege -10	50	0	12
Hawaiian Pineapple	110	0	29
Just Pomegranate; Concord Grape	160	0	40
Mango Lemonade	135	0	35
Mango Passion Fruit Blend	130	0	33
Rio Red Grapefruit	140	0	35
Average other varieties	125	0	30
Tree of Life			
Black Cherry	180	0	43
Concord Grape	160	0	40
Cranberry Nectar	150	0	38
Other varieties, average	130	0	33
Tree Top: *Per 6 fl.oz*			
Apple Cranberry/Grape	130	0	32
Avg. other varieties	120	0	30
Frozen Concentrates: *Per 8 fl.oz (Prep'd)*			
Apple Juice	120	0	29
Tropicana: *Per 8 fl.oz*			
Blends: Berry; P'apple, 8 fl.oz	130	0	32
Essentials: Light 'n Healthy	50	0	13
Healthy Heart/Kids	110	0	26
Immunity Defense; Low Acid	110	0	26
Pure Premium: Orange-Strawb.	130	0	30
Lemonade, 8 fl.oz	190	0	47
Average other varieties	120	0	26
Twister: Average, 8 fl.oz	120	0	32
10 fl.oz bottle	150	0	40
11.5 fl.oz can	160	0	40
Light: Average, 8 fl.oz	35	0	10
10 fl.oz bottle	50	0	11

Per 8 fl.oz Unless Indicated	C	F	Cb
Tropicana (Cont)			
100% Juice Blends: *Per 8 fl.oz*			
Pineapple Orange	120	0	30
Average other flavors	140	0	33
V8® Juices & Drinks			
V8 100% Vegetable Juice, 8 fl.oz	50	0	10
1 Can, 12 fl.oz	70	0	15
V-8 Splash, all flavors, 8 fl.oz	110	0	28
V-8 Splash Smoothies, 8 fl.oz	125	0	27
Diet V-8 Splash, all flavors, 8 fl.oz	10	0	3
Veryfine			
Grape Juice (100%)	150	0	37
Grapefruit Juice (100%)	90	0	20
Pink	120	0	30
Papaya Punch (100%)	120	0	30
Walnut Acres: *Per 8 fl.oz*			
Organic: Apple	115	0	29
Apricot; Raspberry	130	0	32
Blueberry; Concorde Grape	125	0	31
Cherry	135	0	34
Cranberry	105	0	26
Incredible Vegetable	55	0	12
Peach; Pineapple	130	0	32
Welch's: *Per 8 fl.oz*			
100% Grape Juice	170	0	42
100% Red Grape Juice	170	0	44
100% White Grape Juice	160	0	39
Mountain Berry; Guava Pineapple	140	0	34
Tomato Juice, 8 fl.oz	50	0	10
Concentrate: *Per 8 fl.oz Made Up*			
Apple	120	0	29
Grape	170	0	41
Fruit Fantastic	130	0	32
Wild Berry	140	0	36
Fruit Juice Cocktails: *Per 8 fl.oz*			
Grape; Strawberry Breeze	130	0	33
Country Pear; Wild Raspberry	145	0	35
Frozen Concentrates: *Per 8 fl.oz (Prep'd)*			
Grape	150	0	38
100% Grape	165	0	41
Strawberry Breeze	130	0	33
Orange Pineapple Apple	140	0	36
Sparkling Juice	160	0	40
Wild Oats			
Down to Earth, average, 8 fl.oz	140	0	34
Beautiful Juices, average, 8 fl.oz	120	0	27

Nutrition/Energy Shakes & Drinks

Nutritional Shakes/Drinks

Per 8 fl.oz Unless Indicated	C	F	Cb
180 High Energy, 8.2 fl.oz	120	0	33
ABB			
Performance: Power Drinks, 22 fl.oz	310	0	43
Mass Recovery	380	0	60
Avg., other varieties, 18 fl.oz	100	0	23
Weight Gain: Pure Pro, 22 fl.oz	180	0	2
Extreme XXL, 24 fl.oz	1025	0.5	215
Pure Pro Shake: Choc., 12 fl.oz	175	1	6
Vanilla, 12 fl.oz	160	0.5	4
AdvantEdge: *Per Container*			
Carb Control Fruit Flav'd Drink, 11 oz	60	0	2
Carb Control Ready-to-Drink	110	0	2
Coffee House Ready-to-Drink	110	3	3
Complete Nutrition Ready-to-Drink	210	4.5	27
Smoothie	240	2	43
Smoothie Lite	160	0	28
AllSport, all flavors, 8 fl.oz	70	0	18
AMP Energy Drink, 8.4 fl.oz can	120	0	30
Amway Positrim Drink Mix, 1 pkt	160	4	27
Fat Free Mix, 1 pkt, 65g	230	0	50
Appeal, avg. all flavors, 1 pkt	210	2	33
Arizona: Rx Energy, 16 fl.oz	240	0	60
Rx Health/Stress, avg.	75	0	19
Rx Power, 16 fl.oz	210	0	52
Rx Total Trim, 8 fl.oz	5	0	1
Atkins: Shake Mix, avg., 2 scoops	170	8	1.5
Shake Pwdr, avg. all flav., 1 scp	85	4	1
Advantage Shakes, 11 oz can	170	9	5
Balanced: Diet, avg., 11 fl.oz	180	2	35
Choc., Strawb.; Van., 11 fl.oz	230	3	36
Kids Chocolate, 8 fl.oz can	160	3	30
Bariatrix Shakes, 1 serving	100	2	6
Proti-Max Meal, 67g	250	3	20
Bawls Guarana, 10 fl.oz	120	0	32
Guaranexx Sugar Free, 10 fl.oz	0	0	0
Big Bang/Energy, 12 fl.oz	180	0	44
Blue Ox Energy: Citrus, 8.4 fl.oz	120	0	29
Black Cherry; Orange Rush, 8.4 fl.oz	110	0	26
Blue Sky Blue Energy, 8.3 fl.oz	110	0	27
Blue Thunder, 22 fl.oz	300	0	43
Body Design Shakes: 2 scoops	250	3.5	36
Lite, average, 2 scoops	170	4	16
Body Fuel *(w. NutraSweet)*, 8 fl.oz	4	0	1
Bong Water: Chronic Tonic 12 fl.oz	145	0	36
Green Dreams/Purple Haze, 12 fl.oz	165	0	42
Boost: Nutritional Energy, 8 fl.oz	240	4	41
Boost High Protein, 8 fl.oz can	240	6	33
Boost Plus, 8 fl.oz can	360	14	45
Boost w. Fiber, 8 fl.oz can	240	4	42
Breeze Juice Drink, 8 fl.oz can	160	0	31
Brain Wash, 12 fl.oz	140	0	35

Per 8 fl.oz Unless Indicated	C	F	Cb
Carb Solutions Shakes, avg. all types, 2 scoops	120	2.5	3
Carbolite At Last! Shake, 11 oz can	170	9	10
Carboplex *(Unipro)* mix, ½ cup, 2 oz	210	0	52
Carborite At Last! Shake, 11 oz can	170	9	7
Carnation Instant Breakfast			
Powder: 1 envelope, 1.3 oz	130	1	27
Carb Conscious, 1 envel., 21g	80	0.5	12
Ready-To-Drink, avg, 11 fl.oz	250	5	37
CeraSport: 27 Liquid, 11 fl.oz	70	0	17
34g package (makes 16 fl.oz)	110	0	32
Champion Nutrition:			
Heavywt Gainer 900, 4 sc., 5.4 oz	630	10	101
Lean Gainer, 3 scoops, 2.7 oz	280	4	11
Super H. Wt Gainer, 4 scoops	900	29	108
Choice dm, 8 fl.oz	220	10	24
Sugar-Free Shake, 12 fl.oz can	100	2.5	7
Crunk!!! Energy Drink, 8.2 fl.oz	120	0	29
Curves Protein Drink (mix): *Per 8 oz Glass*			
Chocolate; Vanilla, 2 scoops	100	1.5	8
made with skim milk	190	2	23
Cytomax: 8 fl.oz	65	0	13
Powdered Mix, 1 scoop	95	0	20
Designer Whey Prot. Blast, 16 fl.oz	170	1	1
Dr Phil's Shape Up!: Shake, 325ml	215	3	21
Mix + Drink, 40g pkt. prep.	150	2.5	14
Elements: Avg., all varieties	125	0	31
Diet Air/Ice, 8 fl.oz	10	0	2
Endura *(Unipro)*, 2 scoops, 1.3 oz	120	0	29
Perfect Protein Shake, 8.3 fl.oz	110	0	28
Ensure: High Protein, 8 oz bottle	230	6	31
Enlive! 8.1 fl.oz	300	0	65
Ensure Fiber, 8 fl.oz can	250	6	42
Ensure Light, 8 fl.oz can	200	3	33
Ensure Plus, 8 fl.oz bottle	350	11	50
Ensure Regular, 8 fl.oz can	250	6	40
Glucernos, 8 fl.oz can	220	11	22
Powder, made up, ½ cup	250	9	34
Enterex Diabetic (w/fiber), 8 fl.oz (Carbohydrates as Maltodextrin)	237	9	27
4Kick Energy, 8.3 fl.oz can	120	0	29
Fruit2O *(Veryfine)*, 8/16/20 fl.oz	0	0	0
G-Up, 8.4 fl.oz can	220	0.5	55
Gatorade: Energy Drink, 12 fl.oz	310	0	78
ThirstQuencher, 8 fl.oz	50	0	14
Nutrition Shake, 325ml can	370	6	62

Nutritional Shakes/Drinks (Cont)

Per 8 fl.oz Unless Indicated	C	F	Cb
Genisoy: Shake, 1 scoop, 1.4 oz	120	0	17
Protein Powder, 1 scoop, 1 oz	100	0	0
Glaceau: Vitamin Water, 20 fl.oz	110	0	28
Smart Water	0	0	0
Glucerna Wt Loss Shakes, 11 oz	290	11	39
HMR: 70 Plus, 1 package	110	0.5	13
500	100	0	17
Hansen's: *Per Can (8.3 fl.oz)*			
Energy Original	130	0	32
Power	120	0	30
Slim Down	0	0	0
D-Stress; B-Well; Stamina	125	0	31
Diet Red Energy	10	0	3
Energade, 8 fl.oz	65	0	16
Smoothies: *See Page 153*			
Health Source Soy, 2 scps, 1 oz	100	1	4
Hollywood Celebrity Diet, ½ cup	100	0	25
Hydra Fuel *(Tury Labs)*	65	0	16
Impulse Energy Drink, 8.3 oz	110	0	28
invigor8, all types, 8 oz	110	0	27
Isopure Perfect, 1 pkg (88g)	100	0	25
Jarrow: Whey Protein, 1 scoop	90	1	1
Muscle Optimal, 1½ scoops	155	2.5	10
Jones, avg., 1 can/8 fl.oz	120	0	30
Kashi GoLEAN Shakes: Vanilla	220	2.5	36
Chocolate, 325ml can	240	3	38
Powdered, avg., 2 scoops	220	1	32
Keto Nutritional Shake, 8 fl.oz	160	8	2
Knudsen: ReCharge, all flavors	80	0	18
Simply Nutritious, ½ bot., 16 fl.oz	60	0	14
Kombucha: Vit. Enriched, 8 fl.oz	30	0	7
Wonder Drink, 8.5 fl.oz	65	0	16
Lipovitan EB3, 8.2 fl.oz	110	0	29
Lost Energy Drink, 8.3 fl.oz can	105	0	27
Met-Rx: Original, 1 pkt	250	2.5	19
Lite, 1 pkt	175	1.5	15
Ultra, 1 pkt	265	2.5	20
Ultra Pure Protein, 11 fl.oz can	170	1	2
RTD 40, 15 fl.oz can	200	3	15
Metabolol: Endurance, 2 scp, 52g	200	5	24
Metabolol II, 2 scoops, 66g	260	3	40
Met Max, mix, 2 scoops	230	2	11
Monster Entergy (Low Carb), 12 fl.oz	15	0	4
MRM: Low Carb Protein, 1 scoop	120	2.5	4
Whey Protein Isolate, 1 scoop	115	1.5	1
Whey Pumped, 1 scoop	100	1	5

Per 8 fl.oz Unless Indicated	C	F	Cb
Myoplex: Original Shake, 17 fl.oz	300	0.5	20
Carb Sense Shake, 11 fl.oz	150	3.5	5
Low Carb Sense Shake, 11 fl.oz	120	3.5	2
Light Nutritional Shake, 11 fl.oz	190	2.5	20
Powder, 1 pkt, 2.7 oz	280	2	24
Lite Powder, 1 pkt, 2 oz	190	1.5	20
Naturade: Power Shake, 1 scoop	105	1	10
Protein Booster, avg. ⅓ c. dry	110	1	9
Pure Soy, 2 Scoops (1.3 oz), dry	170	5	21
Ribo-tein, avg., 1 oz scoop	105	1	10
Total Soy: Plus, 1 scoop, 1.3 oz	140	1.5	14
Calcium Shake, Chocolate, 1.2 oz	120	2.5	15
Menopause Relief, 1.1 oz	120	1.5	16
Ready to Drink: 10 fl oz	205	3	31
Other flavors, avg., 1.4 oz	150	1.5	21
Nature's Best: Isopure			
Zero Carb, 2 scoops, 2.1 oz	200	0	0
Low Carb, 2 scoops, 2.3 oz	210	0	3
Perfect Whey, 1 scoop, 0.7 oz	90	1.5	1
Nitro Speed, all flavors, 18 fl.oz	110	0	7
Noni: Tahiti/Pacific, 2 Tbsp	5	0	1
Noni Juice, 1 fl.oz	20	0	5
Liquid Hawaiian/Tahitian, 1 Tbsp	30	0	8
Nutrament *(Mead Johnson)*, 12 fl.oz	360	10	52
Ny-Tro Pro 40, average	260	1	23
Optifast 800: Powder, 1 serving	160	3	20
Ready-To-Drink, Chocolate	160	3	20
Optimum Pro Complex, 2 scoops	245	2	4
Pedialyte *(Abbott)*	25	0	6
Pimp Juice Energy, 250ml	140	0	35
Piranha Energy *(EAS)*, 8.4 oz	140	0	35
Pitbull Energy Drink, 1 can	110	0	28
Power Dream *(Imagine Foods)*:			
Java Jolt, 11 fl.oz	240	4.5	42
Mango Passion, 11 fl.oz	320	4.5	65
X-Treme Choc, 11 fl.oz	280	5	48
Vanilla Blast, 11 fl.oz	240	5	39
Powerade: Regular, 8 fl.oz	70	0	19
20 fl.oz bottle	175	0	48
Light, 8 fl.oz	25	0	7
20 fl.oz bottle	65	0	17
Rev-up, all flavors, 20 fl.oz	70	0	18
PowerBar: Performance, 1 scoop	90	0	20
Endurance, 1 scoop, 0.7 oz	70	0	17
Power Gel: Chocolate, 1.5 oz	120	1.5	26
Other flavors avg., 1.5 oz	110	0	26

Nutritional Shakes/Drinks (Cont)

Per 8 fl.oz Unless Indicated	C	F	Cb
ProBalance, 8.45 fl.oz	300	10	39
Pro-Cal 100 *(R-Kane)*, 1 pkt	105	2	7
Red Bull Energy Drink, 8.3 fl.oz	113	0	28
Sugar-Free, 1 can	10	0	3
Red Devil Energy Drink, 12 fl.oz	120	0	31
Red Tiger Energy Drink, 8.2 fl.oz	115	0	28
Resource *(Novartis)*: Plus, 8 fl.oz	360	11	52
Bene Protein, 1 scoop	25	0	0
Health Shake, 4 fl.oz	200	4	35
Shake, 6 fl.oz	270	6	45
Standard 8 fl.oz pak	250	6	40
Diabetic, 8 fl.oz pak	250	11	23
Revenge Pro *(Champ. Nutr.)*, 1 oz	100	0	20
Pro-Score 100, 2 scoops	160	2	1.5
Revival Soy Mix: Plain Soy, 1 pkg	110	1.5	2
Chocolate Day Dream, 1 pkg	240	2.5	36
Other varieties, avg., 1 pkg	225	2	33
Rhino's Energy Drink, 250ml can	125	0	31
Rite Aid: Nutritional Suppl., 8 oz	250	6	40
Rite Aid Plus, 8 oz	360	11	50
Rockstar: Energy Drink, 8 fl.oz	130	0	32
Diet Energy Drink, 8 fl.oz	10	0	2
Sav-on Nut'l: 8 fl.oz can	360	13	47
Light, 8 fl.oz can	200	3	33
Scan Diet (Soy-base), 1 scoop	160	3	21
Shark Energy Drink, 1 can	140	0	35
Slim-Fast:			
Shakes: Original, 325 ml can	220	1	42
Low Carb Diet, 340 ml can	180	9	4
Optima, all flavors, 325 ml can	180	5	24
Soy Protein (Orange P/apple), 1 can	220	1	46
Ultra Slim-Fast Mixes: Reg.flavors, avg.,			
1 scoop, 3 Tbsp, 33g	120	1	25
w. 8 oz fat free milk	200	1.5	36
Choc Delite w. Soy Protein,			
2 scoops, ½ cup, 48g	170	2	25
w. Fruit Juice Mix,			
1 scoop, ¼ cup, 31g	100	1	17
w. 8 oz fruit juice	220	1	42
Snapple: Low Carb, 11.3 fl.oz	90	0	16
Meal Replacement, 11.3 fl.oz	200	0	43
SoBe: Power, avg., 8 fl.oz	140	0	35
Juice Elixers, 8 fl.oz	90	0	24
Lean, all flavors, 8 fl.oz	5	0	1
Lizard, avg. all types, 8 fl.oz	130	0	33
Love Bus Brew, 8 fl.oz	140	1	28
No Fear, 8 fl.oz	145	0	36
Sports System, 591ml	190	0	45

Per 8 fl.oz Unless Indicated	C	F	Cb
Solaray Soytein *(Protein Energy Meal)*,			
Natural, 1 heaping scoop, 24g	70	0.5	5
Flav., avg., 1 heaping scoop, 32g	115	1	13
Sport Pharma Biomax, 2 scoops	250	3.5	6
Spiru-Tein: 8 fl.oz can	220	5	23
Powder, 1 scoop, avg., 35g	100	0	10
Sweet Success *(Nestlé)*:			
Healthy Shake, 10 fl.oz can	200	3	32
Fruit Flavors, 10 fl.oz	200	0.5	39
Powder, 2 scoops, 32g (1.1 oz)	100	1	25
Synergy: Mystic Mango, 16 fl.oz	100	0	24
Other flavors, 16 fl.oz	70	0	16
The Sports Club/LA, PTS Protein Powder,			
Choc/Mocha/Van., 2 scoops, 1 oz	112	3	5
Total Balance, 9.5 oz can	230	7	25
Drink Mix, avg., 2 scoops	190	6	20
Twin Lab: Ultra Fuel, 16 fl.oz	400	0	100
RxFuel, 1 pkt	250	0	62
Energy Fuel, 250ml can	0	0	0
Usana: Nutrimeal, 2 scoops, 43g	150	4	20
Fiergy Drink, 2 scoops	120	1.5	31
SoyaMax, 2 scoops	110	1	1
Vital Cal Shake, 7.5 fl.oz can	290	9	43
Walgreens Nutritional Drinks:			
Nutritional Drink, 8 oz can	250	6	40
Plus, 8 oz can	355	13	47
Slim for Less, 8 oz can	220	3	40
Weider (Powders):			
Body Shaper Powder, 1 pkt	140	1	8
Body Shaper Shake, 1 can	160	1	5
Celt Recovery Stack, 1 scoops	200	0	25
Creatine ATP, ½ cup, 1.7 oz	210	0	37
Mass 1000, 1⅓ cups	740	4	146
Ultra Whey Pro, ⅓ cup, 1 oz	110	1	4
Dynamic:			
Muscle Builder, 2 scoops, 45g	190	0	27
Weight Gainer, 4 scoops, 85g	330	0.5	62
Worldwide: Carbo Rush, 20 fl.oz	280	0	60
Fat Shredder, 20 fl.oz bottle	0	0	0
Pure Protein, 22 fl.oz bottle	170	0	0
Rapid Recovery, 20 fl.oz	280	0	25
Thermo 525, 20 fl.oz bottle	5	0	1
XS Energy Citrus/Energy, 8.4 fl.oz	8	0	0
Zone Perfect: Shake Mix, 2 scps	225	7	23
Protein Powder, 1 scoop	30	0	0
Nutritional Drinks, avg., 8 fl.oz	270	8	30

Quick Guide

Cola Soda Drinks

Average All Brands	C	F	Cb
Includes *Coca-Cola* and *Pepsi*			
8 fl.oz Cup	100	0	25
12 fl.oz Can	150	0	37
16 fl.oz Bottle	200	0	50
20 fl.oz Bottle	250	0	63
24 fl.oz (Pepsi)	300	0	75
1 Liter Bottle	400	0	100
2 Liter Bottle	800	0	200

Other Soda Drinks *(Average All Brands)*

	C	F	Cb
Club Soda, 12 fl.oz	0	0	0
Club Soda Cream, 12 fl.oz	170	0	42
Diet Soft Drinks, avg., 12 fl.oz	0	0	0
Ginger Ale, 12 fl.oz	120	0	30
Lemon Lime, 12 fl.oz	220	0	55
Orange, 12 fl.oz	180	0	45
Root Beer, 12 fl.oz	165	0	41
Tonic Water, 12 fl.oz	135	0	34
Mineral Water: Plain, 12 fl.oz	0	0	0
Sweetened/flavored, 12 fl.oz	150	0	37
w. Fruit Juice, 12 fl.oz	120	0	30
Seltzers: Plain/Diet, 12 fl.oz	0	0	0
Sweetened/flavored, 12 fl.oz	150	0	37
w. Fruit Juice, 12 fl.oz	120	0	30
Soft Frozen Lemonade, 12 fl.oz	300	0	78

Fountain, Movie Theater & Take-Out

Average All Flavors	C	F	Cb
Small Cup, 12 fl.oz: No Ice	160	0	40
With ⅓ Ice	120	0	30
Regular, 16 fl.oz: No Ice	210	0	53
With ⅓ Ice	160	0	40
Medium, 22 fl.oz: No Ice	290	0	73
With ⅓ Ice	220	0	55
Large, 32 fl.oz: No Ice	420	0	105
With ⅓ Ice	320	0	80

(Note: ⅓ Cup of Ice = ¼ Cup Liquid)

Soda Brands

Per 12 fl.oz Unless Indicated	C	F	Cb
A&W: Cream Soda	165	0	41
Diet Cream Soda/Root Beer	1	0	0
Root Beer	180	0	45
Albertson's: Cola	160	0	43
Lemon Lime	140	0	38
Other flavors, average	170	0	47

Soda Brands (Cont)

Per 12 fl.oz Unless Indicated	C	F	Cb
Barq's: Root Beer	165	0	41
Floatz, 12 fl.oz	190	0	48
Barrelhead, Rootbeer	165	0	41
Big Red, 12 fl.oz	150	0	38
Blue Sky: Cola; Orange Cream	160	0	44
Cherry; Raspberry; Root Beer	180	0	45
Grape; Lemon Lime; Dr Becker	140	0	36
Organic, all flavors	170	0	43
Other varieties, average	150	0	39
Bubble Up, 12 fl.oz	160	0	42
Cactus Cooler, 12 fl.oz	150	0	40
Canada Dry: Club Soda	0	0	0
Ginger Ale, all flavors	135	0	37
Tonic Water/Twist Lime	150	0	37
Diet, 12 fl.oz	0	0	0
Clearly Canadian, avg., 11 fl.oz	90	0	33
Coca-Cola: Classic/Caffeine Free	140	0	39
Diet Coke, all flavors	0	0	0
Cherry Coke/Vanilla Coke	150	0	40
C2: 12 fl.oz can	70	0	18
20 fl.oz bottle	115	0	29
Cragmont: Cola	165	0	41
Cherry	180	0	45
Diet, all flavors	0	0	0
Crush, all flavors	210	0	52
Crystal Light, all flavors	8	0	2
Diet Rite, all flavors	1	0	0
Dr Diablo, Cola	140	0	35
Dr Nehi, 12 fl.oz	150	0	41
Dr Pepper: Reg./Red Fusion	150	0	40
Diet (Reg.; Caffeine Free)	3	0	0.5
Fanta: Orange; Grape	180	0	45
Strawberry; Pineapple	180	0	48
Fresca, 12 fl.oz	4	0	1
Frutopia: *See Page 153*			
GuS, avg. all flavors	100	0	25
Hansen's: Diet Soda	0	0	0
Natural Orange Mango, 8 fl.oz	170	0	46
Other flavors, avg.	150	0	44
Hawaiian Punch, all flavors	180	0	45
Health Valley			
Ginger Ale; Sarsp. Root Beer	150	0	41
Rootbeer Old Fashioned	120	0	30
Hires: Cream; Root Beer	180	0	45
IBC: Root Beer	110	0	29
Cream Soda; Black Cherry	180	0	48
Diet Root Beer	0	0	0

Soft Drinks (Cont)

Per 12 fl.oz Unless Indicated	C	F	Cb
Icee: Coca-Cola, 12 fl.oz	105	0	27
Barq's; Minute Maid, 12 fl.oz	195	0	48
Smoothee Lemonade, 12 fl.oz	255	0	64
Jolt Cola, 12 fl.oz	150	0	41
Knudsen, Spritzers, average	170	0	43
Lucozade, 7 fl.oz	136	0	34
Mello Yello: Regular	180	0	45
Diet, 12 fl.oz	5	0	0
Minute Maid: Lemonade	160	0	40
Fruit Punch; Grape; Strawberry	180	0	45
Lemonade	160	0	40
Valencia Orange; Mixed Berry	180	0	50
Other regular flavors	165	0	41
Light Valencia Orange	10	0	2
Soft Frozen Lemonade, 12 fl.oz	300	0	78
Mistic: Punch, 16 fl.oz	230	0	57
'N Juice, average	155	0	38
Sparkling, average, 11.1 fl.oz	115	0	28
Mountain Dew: Live Wire; Code Red	170	0	45
Diet flavors	0	0	0
Moxie: Original Elixir	150	0	37
Mr Pibb, Regular	150	0	37
Mug Root Beer	160	0	43
Natural Brew: Vanilla, Cream	170	0	43
Ginseng Cola, Ginger Ale	170	0	43
Orange; Grapefruit, avg.	155	0	39
Nehi (Royal Crown): Cream	180	0	45
Ginger Ale, Quinine Water	135	0	45
Other flavors, average	195	0	45
Orangina: 10 fl.oz bottle	120	0	45
Rouge, 8 fl.oz	90	0	22
Pepsi: Regular/Blue/Caffeine Free	165	0	41
Diet Pepsi	0	0	0
One, 12 fl.oz	1	0	0.5
Pepsi Edge, 12 fl.oz	70	0	18
Twist	160	0	40
Wild Cherry; Vanilla	165	0	43
Perrier, Regular or flavors	0	0	0
Qibla-Gold, 330ml can	185	0	46
Ramblin' Root Beer, 12 fl.oz	180	0	45
RC Cola: Regular; Cherry	160	0	40
Diet Cola	1	0	0
Reed's: Spiced Apple Brew	160	0	41
Ginger Brew, avg. all varieties	145	0	38
7•UP: Regular	140	0	38
Cherry, Gold	155	0	38
Caffeinated	170	0	46
Diet varieties, 12 fl.oz	0	0	0
7•UP Plus, 12 fl.oz	12	0	3
Santa Cruz, Sparkling, all types	150	0	37
Schweppes: Bitter Lemon/Sour	165	0	41
Seltzer	0	0	0
Tonic Water; Ginger Ale	120	0	30

Per 12 fl.oz Unless Indicated	C	F	Cb
Shasta: Black Cherry	170	0	46
Cherry Cola; Doc Shasta	160	0	40
Club Soda; Diet, all flavors	0	0	0
Cola, regular	170	0	46
Caffeine Free	160	0	40
Cream Soda	190	0	47
Fruit Punch, Pineapple	200	0	50
French Vanilla Cola	180	0	45
Ginger Ale	130	0	33
Orange	200	0	49
Root Beer	170	0	42
Sierra Mist, Lemon Lime	150	0	39
Slice: Lemon Lime	150	0	38
Diet Lemon Lime	0	0	0
Orange	190	0	50
Diet Orange	0	0	0
Sprite: Regular	150	0	37
Diet, 12 fl.oz	4	0	1
Tropical Remix	140	0	38
Squirt: Citrus Burst	150	0	40
Diet Citrus Burst	0	0	0
Ruby Red Soda	170	0	46
Star Ruby: Dry Valencia Orange	100	0	26
Other flavors	95	0	24
Sunkist: Average all flavors	210	0	52
Diet Citrus	0	0	0
Diet Orange	7	0	1.5
Surge, Citrus	170	0	46
TAB, 12 fl.oz	0	0	0
Think!: Root Beer, 8.4 fl.oz	118	0	27
Sparkling Citrus, 8.4 fl.oz	130	0	31
Cola, 8.4 fl.oz	112	0	29
Upper 10 (RC): Regular	150	0	37
Diet, 12 fl.oz	4	0	1
Vernor's: Ginger Ale	150	0	37
Diet, 10 fl.oz	0	0	0
Welch's Sparkling, average	180	0	45
Wild Oats: Down to Earth	150	0	37
Wink, 12 fl.oz	195	0	48

Powdered Soft Drink Mix

Per 8 fl.oz (Prep'd)	C	F	Cb
Country Time: Lemonade	60	0	16
Other flavors, avg.	85	0	22
Crystal Light, 8 fl.oz	5	0	1
Flavoraid: 1/8 pkg	2	0	0.5
Sugar-Free, 6 fl.oz	5	0	1
Kool-Aid: All flavors	70	0	17
Unsweetened, 6 fl.oz	2	0	0.5
Tang, 8 fl.oz	100	0	24

Instant Coffee

	C	F	Cb
Powder/Granules: Regular or Decaffeinated,			
1 level tsp	2	0	0.5
1 rounded tsp	4	0	1
Ground, 1 Tbsp	5	0	1
Brewed/Percolated, 1 cup, 8 fl.oz	5	0	1
Coffee With Milk/Cream/Creamers:			
Per Cup Coffee (8 fl.oz):			
w. Whole Milk: Dash, 1 Tbsp	10	0.5	1
2 Tbsp, 1 fl.oz	20	1	1.5
w. 2% Milk, 2 Tbsp	15	0.5	1.5
w. 1% Milk, 2 Tbsp	12	0.3	1.5
w. Fat Free Milk, 2 Tbsp	10	0	1.5
w. Half & Half, 2 Tbsp	45	4	1
w. Cream (light coffee), 2 Tbsp	65	6	1
w. *Coffee Mate:* Liquid, reg., 1T.	40	2	5
Liquid Fat Free, 1 Tbsp	15	0	2
Powder, 1 heaping tsp	20	1	2
Sugar ~ Add Extra: 1 heaping tsp	25	0	6
Single portion, 1 package	25	0	6

Flavored Coffee Mixes

	C	F	Cb
Chicory: Instant Coffee, 1 tsp	6	0	1
Coffee Essence, 1 tsp	16	0	4
Caffé D'Vita: Mixes, ½ oz	65	2.5	9
Chai Mixes, ½ oz	125	3.5	21
Sugar Free Mixes, ½ oz	35	2	3
General Foods: Average, ½ oz	60	3	10
Sugar-free, average, 1 tsp	30	1.5	3
Cappuccino Coolers, ½ oz	60	0	15
Maxwell House: Mocha, 1 envelope	100	2.5	17
Mocha, sugar-free, 1 envelope	60	3	7
Van., Irish Cream, 1 envelope	90	1	20
Nescafé: Frothé, all flavors, average	90	1.5	19
Ice Java, 2 Tbsp	80	0	19

Coffee Substitute Mixes

	C	F	Cb
Roasted Cereal Beverages: (No Caffeine)			
Cafix Instant Beverage, 1 tsp	6	0	1
Kaffree Roma *(Natural Touch)*, 1 tsp	6	0	1
Postum, Instant Hot Beverage, 1 tsp	12	0	3
Revival Soy "Coffee", 1 Tbsp	5	0	1
Teeccino Caffe, 1 tsp	10	0	2

Vending Machine

	C	F	Cb
Cappuccino, 1 cup, 8 fl.oz	70	4	6

Coffee Shops/Restaurants

Per 8 fl.oz Cup (Unless Indicated)	C	F	Cb
Coffee (Regular/Percolated/Filtered)	5	0	1
Americano Drip Coffee, 1 cup	5	0	1
Cafe Au Lait: 1 cup, 8 fl.oz	65	2.5	6
Nonfat Milk, 1 cup	45	0	7
Caffe Latté:			
8 fl.oz cup: w. Whole Milk	100	5	8
w. 2% Milk	80	2.5	8
w. Nonfat Milk	60	0	8
12 fl.oz: w. Whole Milk	180	10	14
w. Nonfat Milk	110	0.5	15
16 fl.oz: w. Whole Milk	200	10	16
w. Nonfat Milk	120	0	16
Cafe Mocha (Mochaccino): 1 cup	120	3	15
12 fl.oz	180	4.5	15
16 fl.oz	240	6	15
Cappuccino:			
8 fl.oz cup: w. Whole Milk	70	4	6
w. 2% Milk	60	2	6
w. Nonfat Milk	40	0	6
12 fl.oz: w. Whole Milk	110	6	9
w. 2% Milk	80	3	9
w. Nonfat Milk	60	0	9
16 fl.oz: w. Whole Milk	140	7	12
w. Nonfat Milk	80	0	12
Mocha (with cream):			
8 fl.oz: w. Whole Milk	180	12	16
w. Nonfat Milk	150	8	16
Tall, 12 fl.oz: Whole Milk	290	18	25
w. Nonfat Milk	230	11	26
Iced Mocha (no cream):			
Tall, 12 fl.oz: w. Whole Milk	190	9	24
w. Nonfat Milk	140	2	24
Espresso: Regular	4	0	1
Doppio (Double)	8	0	2
Espresso Con Panna,			
(w. dollop whipped cream)	30	3	1
Espresso Macchiato, regular	15	0.5	2
Frappuccino: Tall, 12 fl.oz	200	3	39
Grande, 16 fl.oz	270	4	52
Frappuccino Mocha:			
Large/Tall, 12 fl.oz	230	3	44
Grande, 16 fl.oz	310	4.5	59
Iced Latte: *Similar to Caffe Latte*			
Intellicino: 12 fl.oz	150	7	15
Lowfat (2% Milk)	120	3.5	5

Starbucks: *See Fast-Foods Section*

Irish & Liqueur Coffees

	C	F	Cb
Irish Coffee (no sugar)	**175**	10	0
Liqueur Coffee, avg. all types	**200**	10	16

Cocoa & Hot Chocolate

Cocoa (8 fl.oz cup): w. Whole Milk	**210**	14	19
w. Nonfat Milk	**80**	8	2
Tall (12 fl.oz): w. Whole Milk	**300**	20	26
w. Nonfat Milk	**120**	11	5
Hot Chocolate:			
8 fl.oz cup: w. Whole Milk	**200**	10	25
w. Nonfat Milk	**140**	2	25
Tall (12 fl.oz): w. Whole Milk	**300**	15	38
w. Nonfat Milk	**210**	3	38
Cinnabon, Mocholatta Chill, 16 oz	**410**	18	54

Coffee Extras

Chocolate (Cocoa) Topping, ½ tsp	**10**	0	2
Flavored Syrups: Regular, 2 Tbsp	**80**	0	20
Sugar-free, 2 Tbsp	**0**	0	0
Half & Half Cream, 2 Tbsp	**40**	3	3
Light Whipped Cream, 2 Tbsp	**30**	2	2
Marshmallows, miniature, 2	**20**	0	5
Hershey's Chocolate Syrup, 2 Tbsp	**100**	0	24

Bottled Coffee (Chilled)

Ready-To-Drink: *Per Bottle*			
AdvantEdge Coffee House, 11 fl.oz	**110**	3	3
Arizona Mocha Latte 10½ fl.oz	**130**	2	24
Blue Luna: Cafe Latte 12½ fl.oz	**195**	3	36
Lite Cafe Mocha, 12½ fl.oz	**114**	3	15
Jakada *(Folgers)* Coffee Latte:			
French Roast, 10½ fl.oz	**170**	3.5	31
Mocha; Vanilla, 10½ fl.oz	**180**	3.5	33
Jaradelic *(Planet Java)*, 9½ fl.oz	**180**	3	34
Kahlúa Cappuccino Shake 15½ fl.oz	**195**	3	36
Main St Cafe:			
French Vanilla Ice Latte, 12 fl.oz	**190**	3	31
Meadow Gold Mocha Latte	**450**	16	61
Nescafe: Caffe Latte	**140**	3.5	23
Mocha	**140**	3	26
Royal Mills: *Per Can*			
Hawaiian Kona; Iced, 10.8 oz	**125**	2	27
Iced Cappuccino, 10.8 oz	**165**	3	32
Island Mocha, 10.8 oz	**220**	3.5	42
Kona Blend, 11.5 oz	**90**	1.5	18
Starbucks: *Per 9.5 fl.oz Bottle*			
Frappuccino: Caramel	**200**	3	37
Coffee	**190**	3.5	35
Hazelnut; Mocha	**200**	3.5	37
DoubleShot, 6.5 fl.oz can	**140**	6	18

Caffeine Counter

Moderate caffeine intake is not harmful to healthy adults. However, frequent large amounts (over 350mg/day) may cause dependency ('caffeinism') and adversely affect health. To be safe, limit caffeine to 200mg/day. Avoid if pregnant; breast feeding; a child under 8; or have heart arrhythmias.

	Caffeine (mg)
Coffee: Instant, Weak, 1 level teaspoon	45
Medium, 1 rounded teaspoon	70
Strong, 1 heaping teaspoon	100
Decaffeinated, 1 round teaspoon	2
Bags *(Folgers)*, 1 bag (6-8 fl.oz)	115
Ground, 1 Tbsp, 6g	60
Bottled (Ready-To-Drink), 9.5 fl.oz	70
Coffee Shop: Brewed, 8 fl.oz	110 - 150
Cappuccino: 1 cup, 8 fl.oz	80
Tall, 12 fl.oz	120
Large, 16 fl.oz	160
Decappuccino (decaffeinated)	5
Espresso: Regular/Solo	80
Double (Doppio) Espresso	160
Iced Coffee, 12 fl.oz	80
Latte, 1 cup, 8 fl.oz	80
Mocha, 8 fl.oz	90
Hot Chocolate, 8 fl.oz	10
Tea (Black/Green): Weak, 1 cup	20
Medium Strength, 1 cup	40
Strong, 1 cup	70
Herbal Tea	0
Iced Tea, Tall Glass/Can, 12 fl.oz	25
Soda Drinks: *Per 12 fl.oz Can*	
Coca-Cola (Classic/Van./Cherry); *Pepsi* (Reg./Diet)	35
Diet Coke; TAB; RC Cola (Regular)	45
Dr. Pepper (Reg./Diet)	40
Sunkist Orange Soda; *Mr PiBB*	40
Jolt Cola; *SunDrop*	65 - 70
Pepsi One; Mtn Dew; Mellow Yellow; Surge	55
Energy Drinks (w. caffeine), avg., 8 fl.oz	80
Red Bull (Regular/Sugar Free), 8.3 fl.oz	80
Chocolate Bars: Milk Chocolate, 2 oz	12
Dark Chocolate, 2 oz	30
Cocoa/Hot Choc. Mix, 1 oz pkt	5
Chocolate Milk, 1 cup, 8 fl.oz	3
Choc Chip Cookies, 1 medium, 1 oz	3
Chocolate Cake, 3 oz	5
Chocolate Icecream, ½ cup	2
Chocolate Syrup, 2 Tbsp, 1.4 oz	7

Extensive Caffeine Counter ~ www.CalorieKing.com

Quick Guide

Teas	C	F	Cb
Regular: Bag, Loose or Instant			
Brewed, 1 cup, 8 fl.oz	1	0	0
(Add extra for sugar/milk)			
Herbal: Average all varieties, 1 cup	1	0	0
Bigelow: Apple Orchard, 1 cup	5	0	1
Other Varieties	2	0	0.5
Celestial Seasonings:			
Bengal Spice; Spearmint	5	0	0.5
Lemon Zinger	4	0	1
Roastaroma	10	0	2
Other varieties	2	0	0.5
Bubble Tea, average, 12 fl.oz	240	0	55
Chai Tea *(Starbucks): See Fast-Foods Section*			
Tazo Tea *(Starbucks): See Fast-Foods Section*			

Iced Tea	C	F	Cb
Average All Brands			
Pre-Sweetened: 8 fl.oz	100	0	25
12 fl.oz	150	0	38
16 fl.oz	200	0	50
Unsweetened: 8 fl.oz	2	0	0

Iced Tea Mixes

Per Serving (1 Cup, Made-Up)			
4C Instant	90	0	22
Bigelow Nice Over Ice	1	0	0.5
Carb Options, 1 cup	0	0	0
Celestial Seasonings Iced Delight	4	0	1
Crystal Light Sugar Free	3	0	0
Kool-Aid Fruit T's	70	0	17
Lipton: Instant	0	0	0
Instant Lemon/Raspberry	3	0	1
Lemon	55	0	14
Peach/Raspb, Sugar Free	5	0	1
Nestea: 100% Instant	2	0	0
Decaffeinated	6	0	1
Ice Teasers, all flavors	6	0	1
Peach, Raspberry	90	0	22

"A woman is like a teabag. You never know her strength until she's in hot water."

~ Eleanor Roosevelt

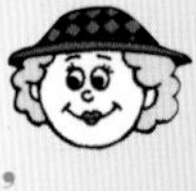

Bottled & Canned Teas

Per 8 fl.oz Unless Indicated	C	F	Cb
Arizona: Sweet Tea	90	0	23
Green Tea(s)/Asian Plum; Herb	70	0	18
Diet Green/Lemon	0	0	0
Ginseng Tea	60	0	15
Peach/Raspberry	100	0	25
No Carb, all flavors	5	0	2
Brisk: Raspberry, 1 can	95	0	24
Diet	5	0	1
Lemon: 8 fl.oz can	90	0	23
24 fl.oz Bottle	80	0	22
Hansen's: Natural Iced Tea, 8 fl.oz	70	0	21
Low Calorie Blueberry/Raspberry	10	0	3
Honest Tea: Green Dragon, 16 fl.oz	60	0	18
Lori's Lemon Tea	0	0	0
Knudsen Coolers, all flavors	90	0	23
Lipton (16 fl.oz Bottle): *Per 8 fl.oz*			
No Lemon	70	0	18
Lemon	90	0	21
Peach; Raspberry	110	0	26
Mistic Tropical Cooler, 8 fl.oz	45	0	12
Nantucket: Blueberry Tea, 8 fl.oz	80	0	20
Original Lemon Tea; Half & Half	90	0	23
Diet Lemon Tea	10	0	2
Nestea Iced Tea: Diet Lemon	3	0	0.5
Cool from Nestea, 1 cup, 8 fl.oz	80	0	20
Diet Cool from Nestea	2	0	0.5
Lemon/Peach/Raspberry	90	0	22
Sweetened Ice Tea	90	0	23
Oregon Chai: Herbal Bliss, ½ cup	70	0	18
Nirvana/Kashmir Green, ½ cup	80	0	20
Royal Mistic: Regular, 12 fl.oz	145	0	36
Diet, 12 fl.oz	8	0	2
Schweppes, 8 fl.oz	90	0	22
Shasta, 8 fl.oz	80	0	20
Snapple: Reg., sweetened, avg.	105	0	26
Diet/Unsweetened	0	0	0
SoBe: Green/Lemon Tea, 8 fl.oz	90	0	23
20 fl.oz bottle	225	0	57
Ssips *(Johanna Farms)*, 8.45 fl.oz	100	0	25
Tazo: Iced Teas, 8 fl.oz	70	0	17
Juiced Teas, 8 fl.oz	85	0	21
Organic Iced Teas, 8 fl.oz	35	0	9
Tropicana: Lemonfruit	100	0	25
Diet Lemon Fruit	15	0	4
Peach/Rasp./Tangerine, 8 fl.oz	120	0	28
11.5 fl.oz can	160	0	40
Twister: Apple Berry, 8 fl.oz	100	0	28
Turkey Hill: Regular	90	0	22
Raspberry Cooler	110	0	28

Alcohol Guide

- **Health Hazards: Excessive alcohol intake** contributes to obesity, high blood pressure, stroke, heart and liver disease, some cancers, and even impotence. **Concentration and short-term memory** are reduced as well as sporting performance.

  Other alcohol hazards include stomach upsets, menstrual problems, anxiety, headaches, insomnia, work absenteeism, risky behaviors, and social problems.
- **Alcohol contributes to obesity** through its high calories and by lessening the body's ability to burn fat. Fat storage is promoted, particularly in the belly - a health danger zone. Alcohol can also stimulate the appetite.
- **Alcohol is potentially more harmful while dieting.** Blood sugar levels may drop with resultant tiredness and further impairment of concentration, reflexes and driving skills - and maybe even the dieter's resolve!

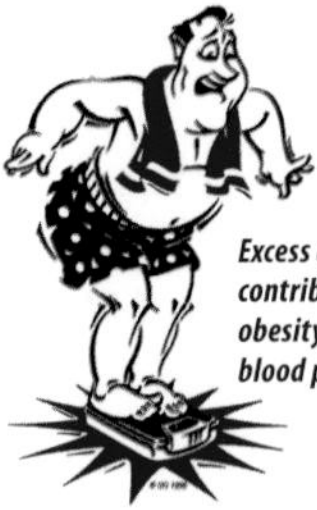

Excess alcohol contributes to obesity and high blood pressure

SAFE ALCOHOL LIMITS

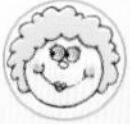

WOMEN: No more than **1 drink** per day.

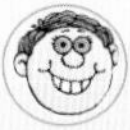

MEN: No more than **2 drinks** per day.

(At least 2 days a week should be alcohol-free.)

1 DRINK CONTAINS 14 GRAMS ALCOHOL →
- **12 fl.oz Regular Beer** (5% Alc.)
- **OR 14 fl.oz Light Beer** (4.2% Alc.)
- **OR 5 fl.oz Wine** (12% Alc.)
- **OR 1½ fl.oz Spirits** (80 Proof)

Note: You cannot save daily drinks for one occasion.
Binge drinking is particularly harmful ~
4 drinks 'in a row' for males or 3 drinks for females.

For some people, **safe drinking** will mean no alcohol drinks at all. (Even one drink may impair driving skills, particularly if tired; and 3-4 drinks daily has been linked to brain shrinkage in some social drinkers).

- **It is advisable not to drink at all if you are:**
  - pregnant or trying to conceive
  - taking medication or have liver or heart disease (unless approved by your doctor or pharmacist)
  - planning to drive, use machinery or play sport
  - studying or needing to concentrate
  - a child or adolescent

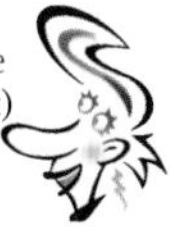

Note: Women and adolescents are more prone to alcohol's ill-effects due to their lower body weight, smaller livers and lesser capacity to metabolize alcohol.

- **Ten Hints to Avoid Harmful Drinking:** *See Page 172*

HOW TO CALCULATE ALCOHOL CONTENT

Percent alcohol on label refers to alcohol volume (ml alcohol/100ml).

100ml = 3½ fl. oz

To convert to grams (weight) of alcohol, multiply the percent volume by 0.8 - since 1 ml of alcohol weighs only 0.8 grams.

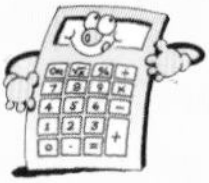

EXAMPLE
12 fl.oz Can Beer (5% alcohol)
5% alc.volume = 5% of 12 fl.oz
= 0.6 fl.oz
= 18ml alcohol
(1 fl.oz = 30ml)

Weight (18ml x 0.8) = 14.4g alc.

GOVERNMENT WARNINGS!

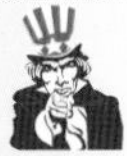

(1) According to the Surgeon General, women should not drink alcoholic beverages during pregnancy because of the risk of birth defects.

(2) Consumption of alcoholic beverages impairs your ability to drive a car or operate machinery, and may cause health problems.

Quick Guide

Alc ~ Alcohol (Grams)
Cb ~ Carbohydrate

Beer

Beer Contains Zero Fat

	C	Alc	Cb
Regular Beer (5% Alc. Vol.)			
7 fl.oz Glass	**80**	8.5	4
12 fl.oz Bottle/Can/Glass	**140**	14	10
16 fl.oz Bottle/Can	**185**	19	13
22 fl.oz Bottle	**260**	25	20
24 fl.oz Can	**280**	28	20
32 fl.oz Bottle	**370**	35	28
40 fl.oz Bottle	**470**	46	35
50 fl.oz Football	**590**	57	50
Light Beer (4.2% Alc. Vol.)			
7 fl.oz Glass	**65**	7	4
12 fl.oz Bottle/Can/Glass	**110**	12	7
16 fl.oz Bottle/Can	**145**	16	9
22 fl.oz Bottle	**200**	22	13
24 fl.oz Can	**220**	24	14
Non-Alcoholic/Near Beer (Less than 0.5% alcohol by volume)			
Average All Brands, 12 fl.oz	**80**	1	70

Beer Brands

Per 12 fl.oz Serving
Alc ~ Alcohol (Grams)
Percentage alcohol listed below is by volume - not by weight.

	C	Alc	Cb
Amber Ice (5.3% alcohol)	**130**	15	6
Amstel Light (3.5%)	**100**	10	5
Anheuser World Select (5%)	**165**	15	15
Anchor Steam (4.6%)	**155**	13	16
Arrogant Bastard Ale (7.2%)	**190**	20	12
Artic Ice (5.3%)	**150**	15	8
Artic Ice Light (3.9%)	**100**	11	6
Asahi Super Dry (5.2%)	**150**	15	11
Aspen Edge Low Carb (4.1%)	**95**	12	3
Augsburger Bock (4.9%)	**170**	14	17
Bass (5.51%)	**140**	16	13
Beck's (5%)	**145**	14	10
Beck's Light (3.8%)	**105**	11	6
Big Sky (4.8%)	**150**	14	12
Big Sky Light (4.5%)	**105**	13	5
Black Label (5.6%)	**155**	15	11
Blackhook Porter (4.9%)	**160**	14	14
Blatz (4.6%)	**145**	13	13
Blatz LA (2.3%)	**75**	7	6
Blatz Light (3.9%)	**110**	11	8
Blonde (4.3%)	**140**	12	10
Blue Moon: Belgian (5.4%)	**170**	15	14
Pumpkin Ale (5.8%)	**185**	16	18
Bud Dry (5%)	**130**	14	8

Brands (Cont)

Alc ~ Alcohol (Grams)

Beer Contains Zero Fat	C	Alc	Cb
Bud Light (4.2%)	**110**	12	7
Bud Ice (5.5%)	**150**	15	9
Bud Ice Light (4.2%)	**110**	12	7
Budweiser (5%)	**145**	14	11
Busch (4.6%)	**135**	13	10
Busch Ice (5.9%)	**170**	16	13
Busch Light (4.2%)	**110**	12	7
Carling (4.4%)	**140**	13	10
Carlsberg (5%)	**135**	13	10
Carta Blanca (4.0%)	**125**	11	11
Castlemaine XXXX (4.7%)	**140**	13	9
Colt 45 Malt (5.6%)	**160**	15	11
Coors Original (5%)	**140**	14	11
Coors Extra Gold (5%)	**145**	14	11
Coors Light (4.2%)	**105**	12	5
Coors Winter Fest (5.6%)	**190**	16	17
Corona Extra (4.6%)	**150**	13	13
Corona Light (4.1%)	**105**	12	5
Dos Equis Lager (5%)	**130**	14	9
Drop Top Amber Ale (4.8%)	**165**	13	15
Fosters Lager (4.9%)	**135**	14	9
George Killian's: Irish Brown (5.2%)	**185**	15	15
Irish Red (5%)	**160**	14	13
Goebel (4.1%)	**130**	11	12
Goebel Light (3.9%)	**110**	11	8
Grolsch Premium (5%)	**140**	14	10
Guinness Draught (4.2%)	**125**	12	10
Guinness Extra Stout (5.8%)	**175**	17	14
Hamm's (4.7%)	**145**	13	12
Special Light (4.1%)	**110**	12	7
Harp (4.5%)	**150**	12	13
Heineken (5%)	**150**	14	12
Heineken Special Dark (5.2%)	**175**	15	16
Hop Jack Pale Ale (5%)	**185**	14	14
Hurricane (5.8%)	**160**	16	10
Icehouse (5.0%)	**135**	14	8
Icehouse (5.5%)	**150**	15	9
Jacob Best Ice (5.8%)	**160**	16	11
Keystone: Premium (4.4%)	**110**	12	5
Ice (5.9%)	**145**	16	7
Light (4.2%)	**100**	12	5
Killarney's Red Larger (5%)	**200**	14	23
Killain's Irish Red (4.9%)	**165**	14	14
King Cobra (5.9%)	**170**	16	12
Kirin Lager (4.9%)	**145**	14	11
Kirin Light (3.2%)	**95**	9	7
Labatt's Blue (5%)	**145**	14	9

Brands (Cont)

Beer Contains Zero Fat
Per 12 fl.oz Serving

	C	Alc	Cb
Leinenkugel's: Original (4.6%)	**150**	13	14
Light (4.1%)	**105**	11	6
Lone Star: Regular (4.7%)	**140**	13	12
Light (3.9%)	**110**	11	8
Lowenbrau Dark/Special (4.9%)	**160**	14	15
Magic Hat #9 (4.8%)	**140**	14	12
Magnum Malt Liquor (5.6%)	**155**	16	10
Meister Brau (4.5%)	**130**	13	12
Memphis Brown (4.6%)	**120**	13	6
Michelob: Regular (5%)	**155**	14	13
Light (4.3%)	**135**	12	12
Amber Bock (5.2%)	**165**	15	15
Golden Draft (4.7%)	**150**	13	14
Golden Draft Light (4.1%)	**110**	11	7
Honey Larger (4.9%)	**175**	14	18
Michelob ULTRA (4.1%)	**95**	12	3
Mickey's Malt Liquor (5.6%)	**160**	16	11
MGD (5%)	**145**	14	13
MGD Light (4.5%)	**110**	13	7
Miller High Life (5%)	**145**	14	13
Miller High Life Light (4.5%)	**110**	13	6
Miller Lite (4.5%)	**100**	13	4
Milwaukee's Best (4.5%)	**130**	13	12
Milwaukee's Best Ice (5.9%)	**145**	16	6
Milwaukee's Best Light (4.5%)	**100**	13	4
Minnesota's Best (4.9%)	**140**	14	10
Molson Canadian (5%)	**150**	14	12
Molson Ice (5.6%)	**160**	16	12
Molson Special Dry (5%)	**145**	14	10
Moosehead (5%)	**125**	14	14
Natural Light (4.2%)	**95**	12	3
Negra Modela (5%)	**155**	14	14
Newcastle Brown Ale (4.5%)	**140**	12	13
Northstone Amber Ale (4.9%)	**150**	14	8
Olde English "800" (5.9%)	**160**	16	11
Old Milwaukee (4.6%)	**145**	13	13
Light (3.9%)	**110**	11	8
Ice (5.9%)	**180**	16	15
Old Style (4.7%)	**140**	13	12
Old Style Light (4.2%)	**115**	12	7
Olympia Gold Light (2.2 %)	**70**	6	6
Pabst (4.3%)	**145**	13	12
Pabst Blue Ribbon (4.7%)	**145**	14	12

Alc ~ Alcohol (Grams)
Cb ~ Carbohydrate

	C	Alc	Cb
Pabst Light (3.9%)	**110**	11	8
Pabst Extra Light (2.2%)	**70**	6	6
Pearl Light (2.2%)	**70**	6	6
Pete's Wicked Ale (5.3%)	**175**	15	17
Piels (4.3%)	**125**	12	9
Pilsner Urquell (4.4%)	**155**	13	16
Red Dog (5%)	**150**	14	14
Red Hook ESB (5.7%)	**180**	17	16
Red Hook India Pale Ale (4.7%)	**180**	13	19
Red Stripe Jamaican Ale (5.0%)	**155**	14	14
Red Wolf (5.4%)	**150**	15	10
Rolling Rock (4.5%)	**120**	13	7
Sam Adams Light (4%)	**130**	11	10
Samuel Adams (4.6%)	**170**	13	17
Samuel Adams Lager (4.7%)	**180**	13	19
Sapporo Draft (3.9%)	**135**	11	14
Schaefer (4.6%)	**145**	13	12
Schaefer Light (3.9%)	**110**	11	8
Schlitz (4.6%)	**145**	13	12
Schlitz Light (3.9%)	**110**	11	8
Schmidt's (4.6%)	**145**	13	13
Schmidt's Light (3.9%)	**110**	11	8
Sheaf Stout, 5.7%	**180**	16	17
Sierra Nevada: Pale Ale (5.6%)	**200**	16	12
Big Foot (9.6%)	**295**	28	25
Porter (5.6%)	**200**	16	16
Wheat Beer (4.4%)	**150**	12	12
Silver Thunder (5.9%)	**165**	17	11
Skyy Sport (5%)	**160**	14	15
Sol Cerveza Especial (4%)	**125**	11	11
Southpaw Light (5%)	**125**	14	7
St Pauli Girl (5%)	**135**	14	9
Stella Artois, 5%, 330ml	**135**	14	9
Stroh's (4.6%)	**145**	13	12
Stroh's Light (4.0%)	**130**	12	10
Tecate (4.7%)	**155**	13	16
Tequiza (4.5%)	**130**	13	9
The Governator (5.2%)	**150**	15	11
Warsteiner Verum/Dunkel (5%)	**155**	14	13
Weinhard's: Pale Ale (4/6%)	**150**	13	13
Hefewéizen (4.9%)	**155**	14	12
Wheat Hook (4.8%)	**150**	14	12
Widmer: Hefeweizen (4.7%)	**155**	13	16
Zeigenbock Amber (4.4%)	**145**	12	13

Home-Brewed Beer: Similar to regular beers, according to alcohol content.

Alc ~ Alcohol (Grams) Cb ~ Carbohydrate

Non-Alcoholic Brews

	C	Alc	Cb
Less Than 0.5% Alcohol			
Average All Brands (Busch NA, Coors NA, Kaliber, Kingsbury, O'Douls, Old Milwaukee NA, Pabst NA, Stroh's NA, Sharp's, Haake Beck, Texas Select)			
12 fl.oz Can/Bottle	**70**	1	14
O'Doul's Amber, 12 fl.oz	**90**	1	18

Cider

Alcoholic Cider: Average, 6% alcohol,			
Dry, 12 fl.oz	**130**	17	12
Sweet, 12 fl.oz	**170**	17	15
Hardcore Crisp Hard Cider (6%)	**190**	17	19
Hornsby's: Draft Cider (6%)	**170**	17	16
Hard Apple Cider (5.5%)	**200**	16	27
Woodchuck (5%) Amber, 12 fl.oz	**200**	15	21
Dark & Dry, 12 fl.oz	**180**	15	17
Granny Smith, 12 fl.oz	**165**	15	11
Wyder's: Raspb. (4%), 11.5 fl.oz	**140**	11	15
Peach (5%) 11.5 fl.oz	**150**	13	16
Pear (5%), 11.5 fl.oz	**130**	13	14
22 fl.oz bottle	**250**	25	28

Quick Guide

Table Wines

Average All Varieties (11.5% Alcohol)	C	Alc	Cb
4 fl.oz 1 small wine glass OR ½ large wine glass	**90**	11	3
6 fl.oz (¾ large wine glass)	**135**	16	4
8 fl.oz (1 large wine glass)	**180**	22	6
½ Carafe/Bottle, 375ml	**290**	34	10
1 Bottle, 750ml	**580**	68	20

Table Wines

	C	Alc	Cb
Red: Claret/Burgundy/Chianti, 4 fl.oz	**80**	11	2
Sparkling Reds, 4 fl.oz	**90**	11	3
Rose: Medium, 4 fl.oz	**80**	11	2
White: *Per 4 fl.oz*			
Dry (Chablis/Hock/Riesling)	**75**	11	1
Zinfandel Sweet (Moselle/Sauterne), 4 fl.oz	**85**	11	2
Sparkling, 4 fl.oz	**95**	11	4

Table Wines (Cont)

Champagne: *Per 4 fl.oz Serving*	C	Alc	Cb
Average 1 glass, 4 fl.oz	**85**	11	2
w. Orange Jce (3:1 orange)	**75**	8	4
w. Orange Jce (1:1 orange)	**65**	5	7
Cold Duck, 4 fl. oz	**108**	11	8
Mulled Wine *(Gluhwein)*, 4 fl.oz	**180**	14	20
Non-Alcoholic Wine, avg., 4 fl.oz	**50**	0	12
Reduced Alcohol Wine (6%):			
Average all types, 4 fl.oz	**50**	0	12
Sake: Rice Wine (16% alc.), 4 oz	**125**	15	5

Flavored Wine

Average All Brands (6% alcohol) *(Examples: Arbor Mist, Wild Vines, Boones)*			
1 small wine glass, 4 fl.oz	**80**	6	11
1 large wine glass, 8 fl.oz	**160**	11	21
1 bottle, 750 ml (25.4 fl.oz)	**510**	36	67

Dessert Wines

Madeira (18% alc), 2 oz	**85**	9	5
Marsala (18%), 2 oz	**110**	9	11
Port, Muscatel, (18%), 2 oz	**85**	9	5
Sherry (18%), 2 oz			
Dry, 1 Sherry glass	**65**	9	0.5
Sweet/Cream, average	**85**	9	5
Vermouth: Dry (18%), 2 oz	**65**	9	0.5
Sweet (15%), 2 oz	**85**	7	8

Cooking Wine

Average All Brands			
Red/White: 2 Tbsp, 1 oz	**20**	3	1
1 cup, 8 fl.oz	**160**	22	12
Marsala, 2 Tbsp, 1 oz	**35**	4	2
Sherry, 2 Tbsp, 1 oz	**40**	4	2

Cooking with Wine:

For alcohol to evaporate, sufficient heat and cooking time (at least 30 minutes) is required.

Red and white table wines would then contain negligible residual calories.

Sweetened wines (marsala/sherry) would contain 10 calories per 1 fl.oz.

Flambé Desserts: Only surface alcohol is burnt off, so negligible reduction in alcohol or calories.

Quick Guide

Alc ~ Alcohol (Grams)

Spirits/Liquors

Includes Bourbon, Brandy, Gin, Rum, Scotch, Tequila, Vodka, Whiskey.

Note: All spirits with same proof (alcohol) have similar calories and zero fat.

Average All Brands	C	Alc	Cb
80 Proof (40% Alcohol by Volume):			
1 fl.oz (1 shot)	**65**	9.5	0
2 fl.oz (Double shot)	**130**	19	0
½ Bottle, 350 ml	**810**	120	0
1 Bottle, 700 ml	**1620**	240	0
86 Proof (43% Alcohol):			
1 fl.oz (1 shot)	**70**	10	0
2 fl.oz (Double shot)	**140**	20	0
½ Bottle, 350 ml	**870**	125	0
1 Bottle, 700 ml	**1750**	250	0
100 Proof (50% Alcohol):			
1 fl.oz (1 shot)	**82**	12	0
½ Bottle, 350 ml	**1025**	150	0
1 Bottle, 700 ml	**2050**	300	0
Flavored Spirits ~ Average All Brands			
Includes Malibu Rum; Captain Morgan			
70 Proof (35% Alcohol)			
1 fl.oz (1 shot)	**70**	8.5	2
2 fl.oz (Double shot)	**140**	17	0.5

Hard Lemon(ade) & Sodas

	C	Alc	Cb
Doc's Hard Lemon (5%), 12 fl.oz	**170**	14	17
Henry's Hard L'ade (5%), 12 fl.oz	**285**	14	46
Hooch Hard (5.2%), 330ml	**215**	14	32
Hooch Ice (5.7%), 330ml	**230**	15	32
Mike's Hard Lem. (5.2%): 11.2 fl.oz	**240**	13	38
16 fl.oz bottle	**345**	19	54
24 fl.oz bottle	**515**	28	81
Mike's Light Lem. (4%), 11.2 fl.oz	**120**	10	12
Mike's Hard Iced Tea (5%), 11.2 fl.oz	**195**	13	27
Rick's Spiked (5.2%), 12 fl.oz	**250**	14	39
Two Dogs (4.2%), 355ml	**205**	12	30

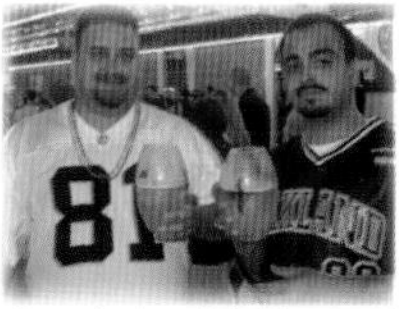

Enjoy a beer but watch the portion size. Those footballs hold 50 fl.oz!

Coolers & Premix Cocktails

Ready-To-Drink *Zero Fat Unless Indicated*	C	Alc	Cb
Arbor Mist: Blenders,			
all flavors (12.5%), 4 fl.oz	**100**	11	14
Bacardi: Silver (5%), 12 fl.oz	**230**	14	33
Silver O3 (5%), 12 fl.oz	**230**	14	33
Silver Raz (5%), 12 fl.oz	**230**	14	33
Silver Limon (5%)	**230**	14	33
Silver Low Carb Black Cherry (4%)	**100**	12	3
Ready to Pour (1.75 liter bottle)			
Bahama Mama (10%), 4 fl.oz	**130**	13	16
Hurricane (12.5%), 4 fl.oz	**144**	12	16
Rum Island Ice Tea (12.5%), 4 fl.oz	**150**	12	16
Bartles & Jaymes			
Malt Based Coolers (3.9% alc): *Per 12 fl.oz*			
Black Cherry; Classic Original	**200**	11	30
Exotic Berry, Juicy Peach	**210**	11	33
Fuzzy Navel; Hard Lemonade	**230**	11	38
Margarita, Pina Colada	**270**	11	48
Raspberry Daiquiri	**220**	11	38
Strawb. Cosmopolitan/Daiquiri	**230**	11	35
Raspb. Lemonade, Lusc. Blackb.	**230**	11	38
Cruzan Island Cocktails (5% alc): *Per 12 fl.oz*			
Jumbie Brew	**230**	14	32
Mojito	**300**	14	50
Wazi Koki	**285**	14	46
Jack Daniels Country Cocktails (5.9%)			
average all flavors, 6.8 fl.oz	**170**	10	25
Jack Daniels Hard Cola (5%) 12 oz	**234**	14	34
Jose Cuervo Authentic Margarita (5.9% alc)			
Margarita/ Lime.Strawb. 200ml	**180**	10	27
Sauza Diablo (5%), 12 fl.oz	**260**	14	40
Seagram's Coolers (5%)			
Smooth Red/Citrus 12 fl.oz	**240**	14	35
Skyy Blue (5%), 12 fl.oz	**280**	14	45
Stolichnaya Citr. (5%), 12 fl.oz	**240**	14	36
Smirnoff Ice (5%), 330ml	**220**	13	33
Black Ice (5.5%), 12 fl.oz	**240**	19	36
TGI Friday's: *Per 6 fl.oz*			
On The Rocks: Margarita (7.5%)	**180**	12	27
Long Island Ice Tea (15%)	**260**	22	27
Mudslide (10%)	**400**	15	36
White Russian (12.5%)	**410**	17	38
Blenders: Mudslide (12.5%)	**240**	17	31
Orange Dream (12.5%)	**240**	17	31
Strawberry Shortcake (12.5%)	**235**	17	24

Coolers & Premix Cocktails (Cont)

Ready-To-Drink	C	Alc	Cb
The Club *Premix Cocktails (8 oz Can): Per 4 oz Serving (½ can)*			
Long Island Ice Tea; Manhattan	**220**	16	30
Margar.; Screwdriver; Vodka Martini	**210**	7	40
Mudslide (9g fat)	**270**	12	41
Pina Colada; Or. Craze; Whisk. Sour	**260**	10	40
Zima (5.9%), 12 fl.oz	**235**	15	20

Shooters

Alc ~ Alcohol (Grams)

Alabama Slammer	**110**	14	2
Amaretto Sours	**120**	6	19
Cranium Meltdown	**75**	7	2
Duck Fart	**85**	7	5
Kamakazie	**150**	20	2
Kool-Aid	**160**	15	14
Liquid Cocaine	**130**	13	10
Mud Slide	**160**	13	17
Fuzzy Navel	**120**	13	7
Pineapple Bomber	**130**	11	13
Turbo	**110**	14	3

Cocktail Mixers

Non Alcoholic ~ No Alcohol Added

Bacardi: *Frozen Concentrate (Made Up from 2 fl.oz concentrate)*			
Margarita, 8 fl.oz	**90**	0	25
Pina Colada, 8 fl.oz	**170**	0	35
Strawberry, 8 fl.oz	**120**	0	35
Baja Bob's (Sugar Free), 4 fl.oz	**10**	0	2
Daily's Pina Colada, 3 fl.oz	**160**	0	37
J.Cuervo Margarita, 4 fl.oz	**100**	0	24
Mr & Mrs T: Mai Tai, 4.5 fl.oz	**140**	0	33
Bloody Mary, 8 fl.oz	**40**	0	9
Margarita, 4 fl.oz	**100**	0	26
Pina Colada, 4.5 fl.oz	**180**	0	43
Strawberry Daiquiri, 4 fl.oz	**200**	0	50
Sweet 'n' Sour, 4 fl.oz	**90**	0	23
Sauza Margarita, 3 fl.oz	**70**	0	18
Skyy Cosmo, 4 fl.oz	**140**	0	36
TGI Fridays: Hurricane, 2.3 fl.oz	**60**	0	15
Long Island Ice Tea, 3.3 fl.oz	**55**	0	14
Mudslide, 2.3 fl.oz	**120**	0	24

Cocktails

Alc ~ Alcohol (Grams)

Made to Standard Recipes

Main Reference: The New American Bartender's Guide

Zero Fat Unless Indicated	C	Alc	Cb
Bloody Mary	**95**	10	16
Blue Lady	**230**	15	16
Blushin' Russian (9g fat)	**365**	14	47
Bourbon & Soda	**130**	19	0
Brandy Alexander (10g fat)	**300**	20	17
Cerebral Hemorrhage (5g fat)	**290**	17	32
Chupa Naranjas (w. 1½ oz Tequila)	**150**	16	8
Collins (with 2 oz Gin)	**180**	20	11
Cosmopolitan	**215**	24	12
Daiquiri, average all types	**140**	19	4
Frozen Daiquiri: no fruit	**155**	19	6
with fruit (and less Rum)	**140**	14	10
Gin & Tonic	**220**	19	22
Grasshopper	**280**	13	30
Green Fantasy	**210**	23	11
Harvey Wallbanger (2 oz Vodka)	**200**	19	17
Highball (1½ oz Whiskey)	**110**	14	3
Irish Coffee (contains 5g fat)	**175**	14	6
Kahlua Mudslide: w.milk (3.5g fat)	**150**	11	10
w. cream (12.5g fat)	**230**	11	0
L.A. Sunrise	**280**	26	21
Lady Killer	**165**	13	20
Leprechaun's Libation	**285**	31	17
London Rock	**165**	18	10
Long Island Iced Tea (w. 8 oz Cola)	**290**	22	31
with Diet Cola	**190**	22	6
Mai Tai (with 2 oz Rum)	**220**	21	16
Manhattan	**130**	17	3
Margarita	**150**	18	4
Martini	**135**	20	0
Mind Eraser	**160**	17	10
Mint Julep	**210**	29	4
Mojito (with 2 oz Rum)	**160**	19	6
Pina Colada (contains 12g fat)	**325**	19	12
Rainbow Room	**265**	30	14
Screwdriver	**160**	14	14
Sex On The Beach	**240**	20	26
Singapore Sling	**210**	25	9
Spritzer (with 3 oz Wine)	**60**	8	2
Tequila Sunrise	**200**	14	25
Tom Collins	**210**	24	12
Tom & Jerry	**170**	9	8
Whiskey Sour	**150**	19	5
White Russian	**250**	20	16

Liqueurs (with Alcohol Counts)

Liqueurs/Cordials

Per 1 fl.oz	C	Alc	Cb
Advocaat (36 Proof; 2g fat)	**85**	4	9
Alizé: Cognac	**70**	11	2
Gold/Red Passion	**105**	4.5	11
Amaretto (56 Proof)	**110**	6	17
Baileys Irish Cream (34 Proof; 5g fat)	**95**	4	5
Lite (30 Proof; 2g fat)	**75**	4	7
Benedictine (80 Proof)	**90**	10	5
Chambord (33 Proof)	**105**	5	11
Chartreuse (80 Proof)	**100**	10	7
Cherry Brandy (48 Proof)	**80**	6	9
Coffee Liqueur (53 Proof)	**90**	6	11
Cointreau (80 Proof)	**100**	10	7
Creme de Cacao (54 Proof)	**100**	6	15
Creme de Menthe (60 Proof)	**120**	7	14
Curacao (70 Proof)	**95**	8	6
Drambuie (80 Proof)	**105**	10	9
Frangelico (48 Proof)	**80**	6	9
Galliano (80 Proof)	**100**	10	8
Grand Marnier (80 Proof)	**100**	10	7
Kahlua (53 Proof)	**90**	6	11
Kirsch (68 Proof)	**80**	8	6
Midori (42 Proof), average all types	**80**	5	11
Ouzo (80 Proof)	**90**	10	5
Pernod (80 Proof)	**75**	10	2
Sambuca (84 Proof)	**100**	10	7
Schnapps (80 Proof)	**100**	10	7
Southern Comfort (78 Proof)	**75**	9	3
Tia Maria (64 Proof)	**90**	8	9
Triple Sec (60 Proof)	**80**	7	4

Liqueur Coffee & Hot Drinks

Per Standard Drink	C	Alc	Cb
Liqueur Coffee, avg. all types	**200**	10	10
Egg Nog	**270**	10	25
Hot Toddy, w. 2 oz liquor	**200**	19	17
Irish Coffee, w. 2 Tbsp whip. crm	**80**	7	4
Mulled Wine (Glühwein), 5 oz	**175**	14	6

Flavorings/Syrups

Non-Alcoholic (Fat Free)	C	Alc	Cb
Angostura Bitters, ¼ tsp	**3**	0	0
Ginger Ale, 8 fl.oz	**80**	0	22
Grenadine/Cassis, 2 Tbsp, 1 oz	**70**	0	17
Lime/Lemon Juice, 2 Tbsp, 1 oz	**10**	0	2
Maraschino Cherry, 1 small	**8**	0	2
Pure Lemon Extract, 1 oz	**125**	0	17
Sugar Syrup, 2 Tbsp, 1 oz	**70**	0	17
Sour Mix, 2 Tbsp, 1 oz	**10**	0	2

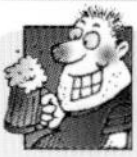

Ten Hints to Avoid Harmful Drinking

1. **Add up the alcohol** you typically drink each day and on social occasions. How does this compare with 'low risk' amounts?
2. **Compare the alcohol** content of different drinks and select the lowest. Request half ounces of alcohol in cocktails and mixed drinks. Dilute them and keep topping off with non-alcoholic drinks.
3. **Go easy on 'Light' beers.** At 4% alcohol, on average, they are still high in alcohol compared to regular beer (5% alcohol).
4. **Try low alcohol** or non-alcohol alternatives such as fruit juices and mineral water. Take your own to parties.
5. **Before drinking alcohol,** quench your thirst with water and non-alcoholic drinks - particularly after vigorous exercise or sport.
6. **Slow the rate of drinking.** Chugging or drinking fast is the major cause of illness and death from alcohol poisoning.
7. **Avoid drinking in 'rounds'.**
8. **Have a non-alcoholic 'spacer'** between drinks (e.g. mineral water, orange juice).
9. **Don't drink on an empty stomach.** Food slows the rate of alcohol absorption.
10. **Keep track of the number of drinks** and know when to stop. Stick to a set limit.

Note: • Alcohol can be very dangerous when taken with prescription or street drugs or when you are very tired.

Extra Info: www.CalorieKing.com

"The doctor told him to cut down to just one glass a day."

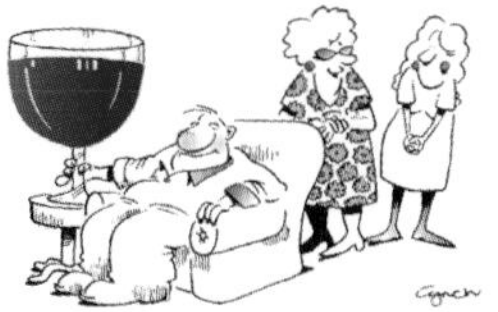

Cafeteria-Style Foods

	C	F	Cb
Apple & Cinnamon, 1.23 oz	**130**	1.5	26
Beef Stroganoff, 5 oz	**195**	13	7
Beef Stroganoff w. 4 oz noodles	**350**	14	36
Chicken Lasagna, 1 piece	**300**	11	32
Chicken Chop Suey w. 4 oz rice	**245**	4	37
Deep Dish Burrito, 7 oz	**265**	13	20
Grnd Beef Casserole, 2 scoop, 6 oz	**245**	13	17
Italian Meat Sce for Spagh., 5 oz	**150**	9	9
w. 5 oz Spaghetti	**350**	10	49
Lasagna, 1 piece	**275**	11	25
Meatloaf, 3 oz	**205**	13	4
Ranch Beans, 2 scoops, 6 oz	**350**	11	45
Red Beans & Rice, 7 oz	**280**	9	37
Scalloped Potato/Ham, 2 scp, 6 oz	**160**	6	20
Stuffed Shells in Sauce (1)	**105**	3	17
Swedish Meatballs (3)	**205**	12	9
Sweet & Sour Pork/Rice, 9 oz	**240**	3	40
Swiss Steak w/Mushr. Gravy, 6 oz	**280**	11	4
Tator Tot Casserole, 2 scoops, 6 oz	**260**	15	20
Tenderloin Tips/Mushr. Gravy, 5 oz	**210**	13	3
w. 5 oz noodles	**395**	15	38
Tuna Noodle Casserole, 2 scp, 6 oz	**180**	6	17
Turkey Tetrazini, 2 scoops, 6 oz	**195**	7	17
Vegetable Lasagna, 1 piece	**250**	13	21

Croissants

Unfilled: Medium 1½ oz	**180**	10	21
Filled: w. Ham (2 oz), Salad	**280**	14	24
w. Ham (2 oz), Cheese (2 oz)	**470**	30	20
w. Chick (2 oz) Cheese (2 oz)	**470**	30	20
w. Turkey/Ham/Chse (2 oz ea.)	**580**	36	20
Au Bon Pain: Ham & Cheese	**340**	10	46
Spinach & Cheese	**250**	9	32

7-Eleven: *Page 239*

Bagels

Plain: Large, 4 oz (no filling)	**320**	2	65
with 2 oz Cream Cheese	**500**	27	54
with 2 oz Lox (Smoked Salmon)	**400**	4	65

Also see Bagels Section: *Page 104*
Fast-Foods Restaurants: *Page 183*
Au Bon Pain: *Page 187*
Bruegger's: *Page 193*
Einstein Bros Bagels: *Page 207*

Sandwiches

No Spreads Unless Indicated
(Includes 2 Slices Bread ~ 3 oz)

	C	F	Cb
BLT (5 strips Bacon, 2 Tbsp Mayo)	**600**	40	46
Breaded Chicken & Salad	**540**	28	46
Chicken (5 oz) Salad w. Mayo.	**580**	30	49
Chopped Liver, Egg, Mayo.	**630**	25	44
Corned Beef (5 oz) w. Mustard	**560**	28	44
Cream Cheese w. Olives (5 large)	**340**	14	46
Egg Salad w. Mayonnaise	**570**	29	49
Egg Salad Club w. Bacon, Mayo.	**780**	53	49
Grilled Cheese (3 oz)	**540**	30	44
Ham (4 oz); Cheese (4 oz), Mayo.	**910**	56	44
Lobster Salad (4 oz) w. Mayo.	**530**	25	45
Overstuffed Tuna Salad (7 oz)	**870**	39	75
Philadelphia Cheese Steak S'wich	**550**	23	42
Reuben (6 oz Beef/Pastrami, 2 oz Cheese, 2 Tbsp Dressing)	**920**	60	28
Roast Beef (4 oz) w. Mustard	**460**	12	45
Roast Pork (4 oz) w. Apple Sauce	**500**	16	55
Shrimp Salad Club w. Bacon, Mayo.	**800**	57	48
Sloppy Joe w. Sauce (7 oz)	**600**	30	45
Steak Sandwich (5 oz cooked)	**680**	32	41
Triple Cheese (4 oz) Melt	**720**	45	46
Tuna (5 oz) Salad w. Mayo.	**610**	30	49
Turkey Breast (5 oz) w. Mayo.	**460**	18	44
Turkey Breast (5 oz) w. Mustard	**360**	7	44
Turkey Club w. Bacon, Mayo.	**830**	38	31
Vegetarian w. Avocado, Cheese	**820**	49	72

7-Eleven: *Page 246*
Schlotzsky's: *Page 247*
Subway: *Page 258*

Wraps & Roll-Ups

Average All Types
(Meat/Chicken/Fish/Veges)

	C	F	Cb
Small size, approx. 9 oz	**500**	25	48
Regular, approx. 15 oz	**830**	40	80
Large, approx. 22 oz	**1400**	70	134

Fast-Foods Restaurants: *Page 183*
Au Bon Pain: *Page 187*
Sonic Drive-In: *Page 252*
Subway: *Page 258*
The Wrap: *Page 263*
WAWA: *Page 266*

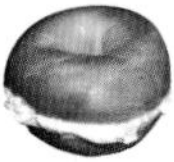

Fair & Carnival Foods

Fair & Carnival Foods

Mexican	C	F	Cb
Burritos w. Bean/Beef, 17 oz	**1100**	41	104
Carne Asada, 14.5 oz	**820**	44	58
Fish Tacos, 1 taco, 5 oz	**270**	13	31
Nachos w. Cheese, 9" plate	**860**	59	70
Taco Chicken, 3.3 oz	**210**	12	16
Tamale (1), 3.5 oz	**180**	8	21
Taquitos, 5 oz	**370**	17	43
Greek			
Baklava, 2" square	**245**	13	32
Falafel, 11.6 oz	**660**	27	85
Greek Salad, 14 oz	**520**	48	17
Gyros, 7.5", 12 oz	**680**	40	55
Spanakopita, 8 oz	**200**	7.5	23
Italian			
Garlic Bread, ½ loaf, 10 oz	**1135**	40	147
Pizza Bread Pepperoni, ½ loaf, 12 oz	**1115**	32	151
Pizza on a Stick, 1 piece	**535**	28	55
Personal Pizza, 7": Cheese (1)	**670**	24	80
Pepperoni (1)	**795**	35	80
Ham & Pineapple (1)	**800**	31	87
Low Carb			
Beef Patty, wrapped in lettuce, 4 oz	**480**	33	0
Sandwiches *(7½" Roll):*			
Ham, 11 oz	**645**	39	47
Hot Pastrami, 9 oz	**760**	17	62
Roast Beef, 11 oz	**620**	36	46
Philadelphia Cheese Steak, 13 oz	**680**	36	49
Tuna, 12 oz	**830**	60	46
Turkey, 11 oz	**665**	24	65
Veggie, 11 oz	**490**	23	49
Oriental			
Rice Bowl: *6" Bowl*			
Beef	**880**	13	136
Chicken	**870**	15	135
Egg Rolls (1), 1.7 oz	**80**	215	14
Hamburgers			
⅓ Pound Burger, 7.5 oz	**670**	41	26
Burger w. Cheese, 6 oz	**550**	36	25
Hot Dogs/Franks: *With Bun*			
Hot Dog: Regular, (1)	**215**	14	28
with Chili, 6 oz	**450**	32	32
with Chili & Cheese, 7.3 oz	**500**	36	31
⅓ Pound Hot Dog	**550**	41	31
Foot Long Hot Dog	**470**	26	41
Corn Dog: Regular, 4 oz	**250**	14	23
Jumbo, 6 oz	**375**	21	36
Jumbo Franks w. Bun:			
Bratwurst; Sausage; Kielbasa, avg.	**800**	60	28

Fair & Carnival Foods (Cont)

	C	F	Cb
Barbeque Items, *(Weights with Bone):*			
Beef Stew over Rice, 2 cups	**440**	14	61
Chicken, 15 oz	**740**	24	34
Chili, 1 cup	**280**	11	24
Corn on the Cob, 8" (1), 16 oz	**200**	1	42
Pork Ribs, 18 oz	**1360**	68	21
Smoked Turkey Legs (1), 19 oz	**1135**	54	0
Potatoes & Fries			
Australian Battered Potato, 12 oz	**1290**	66	155
Baked Potato, 14 oz	**435**	0.5	100
Fries: French, 7 oz	**560**	24	70
Cheese Fries, 10 oz	**645**	38	62
Chili Fries, 10 oz	**700**	36	83
Chili/Cheese Fries, 13 oz	**745**	45	57
Curly Fries, 7 oz	**620**	30	78
Tasti Chips, 40 chips, 6.5 oz	**780**	33	117
Sweet Potato, 14 oz	**405**	0.5	97
Ranch Dip, 3 oz	**165**	14	9
Finger Foods			
Artichoke: Steamed, 6 pieces	**65**	0	16
Fried, 9 pieces	**250**	14	24
Chicken Nuggets (6)	**340**	17	26
Chicken Strips (4), 4.5 oz	**445**	21	33
Finger Steaks (2), 4 oz	**400**	20	26
Mushrooms, Fried, 10-12 pieces	**395**	26	34
Onion Rings, 3 rings	**310**	13	40
Onion Flower	**1320**	72	140
Shrimp, Fried, 10-12 pieces, 5 oz	**555**	30	36
Sweet Potato Strips, Fried, 4 pces	**750**	30	106
Zucchini, Fried, 4 slices	**620**	40	42
Salads/Sides			
Baked Beans, 4 oz	**140**	2	38
Cole Slaw, 5 oz	**350**	21	37
Pickle, whole (6")	**30**	0	8
Potato Salad, 5 oz	**290**	15	35
Popcorn: Plain, small, 3 oz	**450**	24	48
Large, 6 oz	**900**	48	96
Kettle Corn: Small, 5 oz	**600**	15	110
Large, 10 oz	**1200**	30	220
Cakes, Donuts, Cookies			
Funnel Cake: Plain	**760**	44	80
Toppings: Cinn. & Sugar, 2 tsp	**30**	0	8.5
Apple Cinnamon, 2 oz	**85**	3	36
Strawberries & Cream, 2 oz	**70**	0	16
Cinnamon Roll, large	**730**	24	114
Churros, 1½ oz	**150**	8	18
Donuts, Jumbo Twist, 7.5 oz	**905**	49	109

Fair & Carnival Foods (Cont)

Cakes, Donuts, Cookies (Cont)	C	F	Cb
Fried Snickers, 5 oz	**445**	29	42
Fried Oreos, 3 cookies	**300**	10	33
Fried Twinkie, 1	**420**	34	45
Cotton Candy, 5½ oz bag	**625**	0	156
Red Rope Licorice, (24"), 2 oz	**200**	0	46
Cream Puff, 4.3 oz	**500**	43	22
Puff-on-a-Stick (4), 8.6 oz	**995**	86	44
Strawberry Crepe, 4.3 oz	**280**	14	36
Chocolate Dipped Straw, 1 pce	**125**	7	15
Fudge, 1.5 oz	**200**	11	25
Twinkie Dog (Sundae)	**500**	14	89
Key Lime Pie Bar, 6 oz	**635**	40	59
Cheesecake on a Stick, 6 oz	**655**	47	56
Cobbler, 5 oz	**350**	10	62
Soft Pretzel, 4.5 oz	**340**	2	70
Candied Apple, 7 oz	**330**	0.5	80
Ice Cream & Frozen Treats			
Dippin' Dots Ice Cream: Small, 4 oz	**150**	7	17
Medium, 8 oz	**305**	14	35
Large, 16 oz	**600**	28	70
Sno-Cone (includes 6 oz syrup)	**540**	0	132
Frozen Yogurt in sugar cone, 14 oz	**475**	2	94
Ice Cream: Small, sugar cone, 10 oz	**775**	42	83
Large, sugar cone, 14 oz	**935**	54	96
Sherbet, 8 oz	**270**	4	59
Frozen Banana, choc cover, 5 oz	**240**	4	53
Drinks			
Lemonade, 18 fl.oz	**210**	0	52
Orange Julius, 20 fl.oz	**490**	10	96
Strawberry Julius, 20 fl.oz	**430**	0	98
Icee, 16 fl.oz	**235**	0	59
Malt, 16 fl.oz	**690**	33	85
Slushies, 16 fl.oz	**260**	0	65
Soft Frozen Lemonade, 12 fl.oz	**300**	0	78
Smoothies: Berry Flavors, 16 fl.oz	**350**	1	80

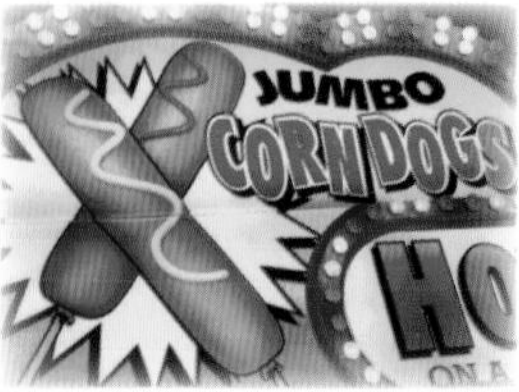

Chinese & Asian Dishes

Appetizers	C	F	Cb
Crab Cake, 63g	**105**	5	0.5
Curried Meat Triangles, 1 pce	**150**	5	12
Dumplings: Pork, steamed, 1	**40**	3	4
Pork, fried, 1 dumpling	**75**	7	4
Vegetable, steamed, 1	**25**	0.5	4
Egg Rolls, mini, 3 rolls	**100**	3	11
Rice Paper Roll, 1	**80**	2	10
Spring Roll: Small, 1½ oz	**100**	7	10
Medium, 3 oz	**200**	12	20
Large, 5 oz	**350**	15	33
Wonton, 1 only	**55**	3	4
Soup: Clear, 1 bowl	**30**	1	4
with Noodles	**100**	3	12
Chicken & Corn	**150**	8	8
Rice: Plain, 1 cup (½ Pint), 6½ oz	**240**	0.5	54
2 cups (1 Pint), 13 oz	**480**	1	108
Fried: 1 cup, 5 oz	**320**	13	42
Large dish, 16 oz	**1010**	40	134
Noodles: Chinese Egg, ckd, 1 cup	**200**	3	42
Entrees & Mains: *Per Whole Dish*			
Beef Satay, 17 oz	**760**	50	15
Beef in Black Bean Sce, 17 oz	**530**	33	17
Beef with Broccoli, 16 oz	**650**	30	31
Chicken & Almonds, 18 oz	**685**	50	18
Chicken (sliced) & Broccoli	**280**	12	13
Chop Suey: Chicken, 20 oz	**560**	37	7
Pork, 20 oz	**680**	50	12
Chow Mein, Beef/Chicken, 24 oz	**940**	60	50
Crab Puff/Rangoon, 1 dumpling	**80**	4.5	7.5
Crispy Fried Chicken, 8 oz	**485**	33	12
Egg Drop Soup: w. Noodles, 1 cup	**120**	3	15
w/out Noodles, 1 cup	**70**	3	3
Egg Foo Yung w. Sauce, 1 cup	**225**	12	11
Lemon Chicken, 10 oz	**580**	32	25
Lo Mein (stir-fried)	**620**	29	61
Moo Shu Chicken, 2 wrapped crepes	**430**	16	43
Omelet, Chicken/Shrimp, 16 oz	**990**	82	10
Steamed Whole Fish, ½ Red Snapper	**500**	11	1
Sweet & Sour: Fish, 20 oz	**1160**	58	106
Pork, 18 oz	**950**	50	92
Vegetable Combination, w. oil, 6 oz	**250**	17	19
Vegetables, Steamed (no oil), 6 oz	**120**	1	25
Bubble Tea, average, 12 fl oz	**240**	0	55
Fortune Cookie: each	**25**	0.5	5

Confucious say:
'Man who eat with one chopstick never have problem with obesity'

Cajun & Creole

	C	F	Cb
Alligator, 4 oz cooked	**160**	2	0
Baked Herb Chicken, 1 serving	**850**	53	2
Bouillabaisse	**400**	15	10
Cajun Fried Turkey, 1 serving	**630**	25	0
Cocktail Sauce, 1 Tbsp	**15**	0	3
Couche-couche, ½ cup	**80**	0	17
Crawfish Bisque, 1 serving	**500**	10	10
Crawfish, cooked, 2 oz	**45**	0.5	0
Creole Jambalaya, 1 serving	**550**	30	15
Dove, cooked, 1 oz	**60**	3.5	0
Frog's Legs, steamed (2)	**45**	0	0
Guinea Fowl, flesh, 1 oz, ckd	**40**	1	0
Hogshead Cheese, ¼ cup	**80**	5.5	0
Jambalaya, Shrimp & Crabmeat	**520**	14	12
Red Beans & Rice, 1 serving	**400**	17	52
Roasted Quail, w. Bacon on Toast	**550**	25	15
Remoulade Sauce, 1 Tbsp	**55**	5.5	1
Shrimp Creole, 1 serving	**450**	20	10
Stuffed Smothered Steak, w. 1 cup Rice	**890**	50	50
Squab, flesh, 1 oz cooked	**60**	3.5	0
Turtle, cooked, 1½ oz	**60**	1.5	0

Cuban

	C	F	Cb
Bl. Beans w. Rice (Moros con Cristianos)	**510**	22	76
Blk.-eyed Pea Fritters (Bollitos de Carita)	**80**	5	6
Casserole Corn Tamale (Tammal en Cazuela)	**445**	20	55
Chkn w. Yellow Rice (Arroz con Pollo)	**925**	49	87
Cuban Bread (Pan Cubano)	**80**	1.5	15
Donuts in Syrup (Bunuelos)	**170**	5	10
with Melado	**100**	5	10
Grilled Plantains	**145**	0	40
Gypsy's Arm Cake (Brazo Gitano)	**260**	18	42
Roast Pork S'wich (Pan con Lechon)	**640**	30	62
Seasoned Beef w. Olives & Raisins (Picadillo)	**435**	36	10
Shredded Beef (Ropa Vieja)	**550**	35	10
Taro Root Mash (Pure de Malanga)	**315**	3	69
Yuca with Citrus Garlic Dressing (Yuca con Mojo)	**190**	9	25

The cheapest slimming exercise is mind over platter.

French Foods

	C	F	Cb
Blanquette d'Agneau (Lamb Stew)	**800**	30	17
Brioche, 1 cake	**280**	14	34
Bouillabaisse (Fish Stew)	**400**	15	10
Coq au Vin (Chicken in Wine)	**800**	30	16
Coquilles St. Jacques, fried, 6 lge.	**300**	14	2
Crème Brulée, 1 serving	**460**	40	21
Creme Caramel (Caram. Custard)	**260**	10	38
Crepe Suzette, 1x6" crepe/sauce	**220**	10	13
Duck a l'Orange	**780**	35	47
Escargots (Snails), in garl. butter, (6)	**200**	10	4
French Stick Bread, 3 slices, 2.2 oz	**150**	1	35
Frogs Legs, fried, 4 med. pairs	**400**	20	10
Lamb Noisettes, fried, 2 chops	**500**	40	1
Mousse au Chocolat	**380**	15	33
Potage Creme Crecy (Carrot Soup)	**360**	18	14
Salade Nicoise (Tuna/Oliv./Veg.)	**450**	13	14
Veal Cordon Bleu (Veal/Ham/Ch)	**650**	25	18
Vichyssoise (Pot./Leek Soup), 1 c.	**200**	9	15

Baguette & French Stick: *Page 102, 103*
Croissants: *Pages 113, 173*

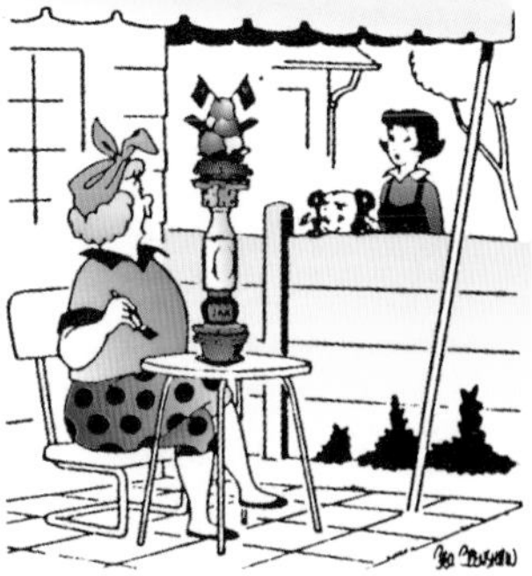

"My new diet allows me a small saucer of anything I want for lunch."

German

German	C	F	Cb
Bavarian Bread Dumpling, 3 small	**330**	10	28
Beef Goulash with Veges	**520**	20	46
Black Forest Cake, 1 slice	**380**	16	30
Bratwurst, grilled, 1 medium, 6 oz	**450**	37	2
Chicken: Fried, Viennese-style	**530**	20	28
Livers w. Apple/On., 6 oz	**460**	28	10
Herring, Pickled: Rollmops, 4 oz	**260**	16	3
with Sour Cream, 4 oz	**310**	20	3
Hot Sausage Curry	**300**	7	6
Kugelhupf Cake, 1 lge slice, 4 oz	**400**	23	40
Sauerbraten Pork (Pot Roast)	**650**	35	15
Torte: Linzer (Alm./Raspb. Jam)	**430**	18	58
Sacher (Choc./Apricot Jam)	**260**	12	23
Weiner Schnitzel, 1 medium	**750**	35	38

Greek

Greek	C	F	Cb
Baklava Pastry: Small	**240**	13	32
Large, 3¾ oz	**400**	21	45
Calamari, deep fried, 1 cup	**300**	13	17
Chicken Kebob Plate	**345**	13	8
Galactobureko, 1 only			
(Filo, Custard, Pastry in Syrup)	**360**	15	48
Greek Chicken Salad	**400**	18	9
Gyros, 4 oz	**380**	33	6
Hummus & Pita, 4 oz	**260**	12	30
Kataifi, (Filo, Nut, Pastry in Syrup)	**350**	11	56
Moussaka, 1 serve, 8 oz	**350**	22	22
Soup: Argolemono (Egg Lemon Soup			
with Chicken & Rice)	**85**	6	5
Souvlakia (Lamb), each, 2 oz	**120**	6	1
Stuffed Tomatoes, 2 only	**250**	12	17
Taramosalata, 1 Tbsp, ½ oz	**40**	3	2
Tyropita (Filo/Egg/Cheese Pastry)	**350**	26	31
Tzatziki (Cucumber/Yog. Dip), 1 T.	**20**	1	1
Vine Leaves, stuffed, 3 rolls, 6 oz	**200**	5	13

See Daphne's: *See Fast-Foods Section*

Hawaiian

Hawaiian	C	F	Cb
Ahi Tuna, grilled (6 oz fillet), no fat	**220**	2	0
Chicken Long Rice, 1 cup, 7 oz	**240**	14	12
Gyoza, 1 only	**55**	2	6
Haupia (Coconut Pudd.), 1 pce (4"x 2½")	**120**	6	17
Hawaiian Sweet Bread, ½" slice, 2 oz	**180**	4.5	29
Kalua Chicken, 4 oz	**280**	16	0
Pork, 4 oz	**350**	24	0
Kim Chee (pickled cabbage), ½ c., 4 oz	**20**	0	5
Kulolo (Taro Pudding), 1 slice	**125**	5	19
Lau Lau: Chicken (1) 7 oz	**280**	21	3
Pork (1) 7 oz	**320**	26	5
Loco Moco (rice/burger/egg/gravy)	**650**	27	63
Lomi Salmon, ¼ cup, 4 oz	**20**	1	2
Malasadas (Donut), 2 oz	**240**	13	26
Manapua (Char Siu Pork Bun), 2.3 oz	**180**	8	25
Poi (mashed ckd taro), 1 c., 8½ oz	**270**	0.5	65
Poke, avg all types, 3 oz	**90**	1	0
Portuguese Sausage, 2 oz	**180**	15	2
Potato Salad, ½ cup, 5 oz	**170**	10	17
Shave Ice *(Matsumoto)*, all flavors:			
w. Icecream, 1 large	**300**	4	64
w. Beans, 1 large	**290**	0	72
Spam Musubi: w. Regular Spam	**265**	11	34
(4 oz rice+1.3 oz Spam/7-Eleven Hawaii)			
Homemade: w. Lite Spam (50% less fat)	**220**	5	34
Taro Pancake Mix, ⅓ cup (makes 2)	**140**	2	26
Plate Lunches:			
Chicken Katsu (9 oz) w. 2 scp Rice	**1110**	48	108
+ Macaroni Salad, ¾ cup	**1360**	68	123
or Tossed Salad + Fr. Dress. (2 T.)	**1240**	61	111
Hamburger (5 oz) w. 2 scoops Rice	**710**	24	81
Gravy + Macaroni Salad	**1135**	49	112
MahiMahi (7 oz) w. 2 scoops Rice	**650**	12	90
+ Macaroni Salad + Tartar Sce	**1150**	58	109
or Macaroni Salad, no Tartar Sce	**935**	34	108
or Tossed Salad + Fr. Dress. (3 T.)	**815**	27	96
or Tossed Salad, no dressing	**670**	12	93
Teri Beef (5 oz) w. 2 scoops Rice	**790**	23	94
+ Macaroni Salad, ¾ cup	**1095**	47	113
or Tossed Salad, no dressing	**800**	23	95

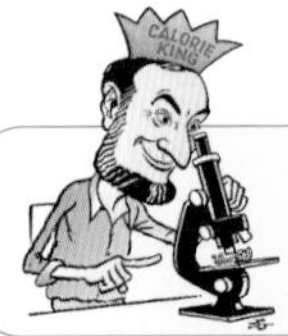

Indian & Pakistani

Per Serving
(Meat dishes allow 4 oz meat/serving)

	C	F	Cb
Aloo Samosa, each	**155**	12	12
Alu Gosht Kari (Meat/Pot. Curry)	**600**	40	23
Chicken Korma	**500**	35	6
Chicken Pilaf (Murgh Biriyani)	**700**	53	50
Chicken Tikka	**260**	16	2
Chicken Vindaloo	**400**	20	8
Chapati/Roti, 7" diam. piece	**60**	0.5	11
Dal (Lentil Puree): 1 cup, no oil	**230**	1	37
1 Tbsp Tadka (oil topping)	**120**	13	0
Dhakla (Lentil Dish), 1" sq., 1 oz	**105**	5	13
Dhansak, ½ cup	**105**	3.5	11
Gosht Kari (Meat Curry/Tom./Pot.)	**460**	25	17
Lamb Pilaf	**520**	35	40
Lassi (Sweet or Mango), 1 cup, 8 oz	**160**	4	24
Masala Gosht (Beef/Tom./Gravy)	**400**	25	18
Mulligatawney Soup, average	**300**	15	8
Murgh Tikka, 1 cup	**300**	4	7
Naan Bread, ¼ (8" x 2"), 1 oz	**75**	2	11
Pappadum, 1 large/2 small	**50**	3	5
Pesrattu (Lentil Crepe), 9", 2.6 oz	**130**	5	15
Pork Vindaloo Curry	**620**	47	3
Rajmah (Kidney Bean Curry), 1 cup	**225**	5	35
Rogan Josh (Lamb/Yogurt Sce)	**500**	30	3
Shahi Korma (Braised Lamb)	**430**	28	3
Tandoori Chicken: Breast	**260**	13	5
Leg/Thigh portion	**300**	17	6

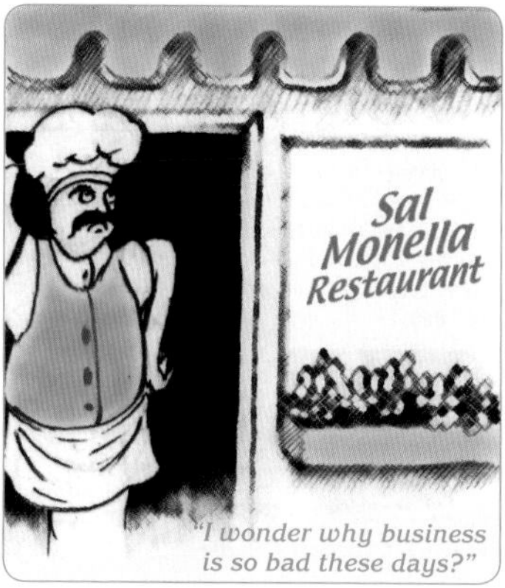

Sal Monella Restaurant
"I wonder why business is so bad these days?"

Italian Dishes

	C	F	Cb
Baked Ziti: Small	**370**	27	32
Regular	**575**	42	49
Breadstick (1), 2 oz	**120**	2.5	25
Broccoli Fettucine Alfredo, reg.	**815**	23	125
Bruschetta, 2 slices	**380**	17	53
Calzones, average, all types	**840**	34	101
Cannelloni, 1 tube, 6 oz	**280**	15	18
Cheese Breadstick (1), 2.4 oz	**180**	8	20
Cheese Ravioli w. Sauce	**495**	17	65
Chicken Alfredo	**775**	29	82
Chicken Parmigiana, 11 oz	**520**	22	16
Fettucine Alfredo: Small	**525**	15	80
Regular	**775**	22	119
Meat Lasagne, 16 oz	**700**	36	60
Meat Ravioli	**725**	22	102
Minestrone Soup, 1 bowl	**110**	2	18
Shrimp & Scallop Fettucine	**595**	16	81
Spaghetti w. Marinara: Small	**410**	6	74
Regular	**600**	8	111
Spaghetti w. Meatballs: Small	**710**	31	80
Regular	**1010**	42	119
Spaghetti w. Meat Sauce: Small	**425**	8	74
Regular	**625**	11	111
Vegetable Primavera	**610**	8	116
Pizza: *Per Slice (⅛ Medium)*			
Cheese: Thin Crust	**290**	8	21
Thick Crust	**275**	13	29
Pepperoni: Thin Crust	**215**	10	21
Thick Crust	**290**	15	29
Deep Dish Pizza: Pepperoni,			
Medium (11"), 1 slice, (⅙)	**445**	15	57
Personal (6"), whole	**380**	10	58
Desserts: Lemon Ice	**180**	0	45
Gelato: Vanilla (Milk Base), ½ cup	**200**	15	18
Choc. Hazelnut (Milk), ½ cup	**370**	29	26
Water Base, ½ cup	**100**	0	25
Tiramisu, 1 piece, 5 oz	**400**	29	30

For more listings see Fast-Foods Section.

Japanese

	C	F	Cb
Sushi Rice: cooked, 1 Tbsp	25	0	5
1 cup, 5¼ oz	380	3	82
Sushi (Maki) Rolls: *Per Piece*			
Average all types (California Rolls; Crm Cheese w. Crab; Eel; Salmon; Shrimp; Tuna; Yellowtail; Vegetable)			
Small (1⅛" diam. x 1⅛" high), 0.8 oz	22	0.5	0.5
Med. (1¾" diam. x 1¾" high), 1.6 oz	44	1	1
Large (2¼" diam. x ⅞" high), 2 oz	55	1.5	1.5
Sushi Packs: *Per Pack*			
Average all types: 6 large pces	335	7.5	7.5
9 medium pieces	405	9	9
12 small pieces	325	12	6
Futomaki (thick roll), 6 pieces	315	1.5	7
Hand Roll (Cone), 2, 6 oz	225	5	5
Inari (rice filled soybean pocket), 4 pce	260	5	46
Sushi-Nigiri (fish on rice):			
average all types, 1 piece	70	0.5	12
Sushi Plate: Assorted, 6 pieces	420	3	36
Combination (Sushi & Sushi Rolls)			
2 Sushi + 6 sm. & 3 med. rolls	400	7	72
Sashimi (Sliced Raw Seafood/Beef)			
Ika (Squid), 4 oz	105	2	0
Hamachi (Yellowtail), 4 oz	165	6	0
Naguro (Yellowfin Tuna), 4 oz	120	1	0
Niku (Beef), 5 oz	200	10	0
Saba (Mackerel), 4 oz	160	7	0
Suzuki (Sea Bass), 4 oz	110	0.5	0
Tako (Octopus), 4 oz	95	1	0
Dipping Sauces: Average, 2 Tbsp	30	0	7
Ginger Vinegar Dressing, 2 Tbsp	20	0	5
Edamame (young green soybeans):			
Steamed/Salad (in pods), 4 oz	60	3	5
Boiled beans (no pods), 4 oz	160	7	12
Katsu-don Pork w. Rice	1100	39	141
Miso Soup w. Tofu pces, 1 cup	85	3	11
Seaweed Salad, 1.5 oz	20	2	0
Sukiyaki (Beef/Tofu/Veg.), 8 oz	400	24	32
Tempura (Batter-fried Shrimp & Veges)			
3 large shrimp & veges	320	18	25
1 shrimp only	60	4	3
Teppan Yaki (Steak, Seafood & Veges)			
10 oz serving	470	30	15
Teriyaki: Beef, 4 oz serving	350	25	4
Chicken, 4 oz serving	260	9	7
Salmon, medium, 6 oz serving	270	8	3
Sake Wine (16% alc.), 3 fl.oz	115	0	7
Yakatori, 1 skewer, 2½ oz	140	5	1

Kosher/Deli Foods

	C	F	Cb
Bagel/Bialy, 1 small, 2 oz	160	2	32
Beiglach (Cheese Knish)	350	17	35
Blintzes: Average, 1 only	120	1	25
w. Sour Crm. & Preserves	370	10	30
Borscht: (no cream), 1 cup	85	3	14
Diet/Reduced Cal., 1 cup	30	1	7
Cabbage Roll (meat/rice), 5 oz	170	6	21
Chicken Broth: 1 cup	80	8	0
with vegetables	100	8	5
with noodles	150	9	16
Lowfat, plain, 1 cup	25	1	0
Cholent, 1 med serve, 1 cup	350	16	48
Chopped Liver: 1 serve, 3 oz	110	6	5
with Egg Salad, ¼ cup	100	7	3
Farfel, dry, ½ cup	90	0.5	21
Hallah (Yeast Bread), 1 sl., 1 oz	85	2	14
Gefilte Fish Balls: Reg., medium, 2 oz	55	2	4
with jelled broth	80	2	6
Cocktail size, 1 oz	30	1	2
Sweet, medium, 2 oz	65	2	4
with jelled broth	95	2	9
Herring: Smoked, 2 oz	120	8	0
in Sour Cream, 2 oz	150	10	0
Kasha, cooked, ½ cup	100	0.5	20
Kipfel (Vanilla/Almd. Cookie), 1 pce	60	2	7
Knaidlach, 1 ball	40	2	5
Knish: Kasha/Potato, 1 only	130	4	22
Cheese, 1 only	350	17	35
Knishette *(Gabila's)* Potato,			
4 piece, 4 oz	140	1	29
Spinach, 4 piece, 4 oz	110	1	20
Kreplach, beef, 1 piece	40	1	6
Kugel, potato/noodle, 1 serve	150	7	20
Latkes (Potato Pancake), 2 oz	200	11	22
3 Latkes w. Sour Cr./Apple Sce	750	25	95
Lochshen: Plain, 1 cup	130	2	26
Pudding, 1 cup	380	13	48
Lox (Smoked Salmon), 2 oz	65	2	0
Mandelbrot (Almond Bread),			
1 slice, ¼" thick	45	2	5
Matzo *(See Page 105)*, 1 oz board	110	0.5	21
Matzo Balls, 2 small, 1 large	90	3	12
Matzo Soup, with 1 large ball	180	7	24
New York Cheesecake, 4 oz	350	24	26
Pierogi, potato/cheese, 1 pce	90	4	11
Reuben Sandwich	920	60	28
Schmaltz (Rend'd chick. fat), 1 T.	90	10	0

Korean Food

	C	F	Cb
Bibimbab (Vege & Beef on Rice), 1 cup	**565**	15	89
Bulgogi (Barbeque Beef), 3.5 oz	**325**	12	15
Galbi (Short Ribs), 16 oz	**975**	61	16
Gujeolpan (Pancake w. Meat & Vegetables), cup w. 1 pancake	**340**	11	39
Japchae (Noodle w. Vege & Meat), 1¼ cup	**365**	19	34
Sides:			
Kimchee (Cabbage Relish), ½ cup	**30**	0	6
Namool (Assorted Veges) 1 cup	**125**	6.5	9
Soups: *Per Serving*			
Muguk (Radish & Chive Soup), 6 oz	**105**	7	6
Samgyetang (Ginseng Chicken Soup)			
no Chicken Skin, 1 cup	**520**	11	60
w. Chicken Skin, 1 cup	**725**	35	60
Yuk Gae Jang (Spicy Beef Soup), 1¼ cup	**180**	13	5

Lebanese/Middle East

	C	F	Cb
Baba Ghannouj, 2 Tbsp, 1 oz (Eggplant/Sesame Dip)	**70**	6	2
Baklava, 1 pastry, 1¾ oz (Pastry, Nuts, Syrup)	**245**	18	18
Cabbage Rolls, 1 roll, 3 oz (Cabbage Leaf, Meat, Rice)	**100**	3	12
Cous Cous, 1 serve (Semolina, Milk, Fruit, Nuts)	**400**	21	43
Felafel (Chick Pea Fritter):			
Fried, 1 medium, 1 oz	**60**	4	4
Hummus, ¼ cup, 2.2 oz	**105**	3	5
Fried Kibbi, 1 piece, 3 oz (Wheat, Meat, Pinenuts)	**180**	8	15
Kafta, 1 skewer, 1½ oz (Ground Lamb Saus. on Skewer)	**85**	5	2
Kibbeh Naye, 1 cup, 9 oz (Raw Lamb, Bulgur & Spices)	**450**	18	28
Lebanese Omelet, 1 serving, 4 oz (Egg, Spinach, Pinenuts, Onion)	**200**	12	13
Pilaf, 1 cup (Rice, Onion, Rais., Apr. Spice)	**400**	11	60
Shawourma, 1 serve, 4 oz (Spit Roast Beef)	**280**	15	2
Shish Kabob, 1 stick, 2½ oz	**130**	7	2
Spinach Pie, 1 piece, 3½ oz	**290**	21	20
Sweet Almond Sanbusak, 1 pce (Pastry, Almonds, Spices)	**200**	15	11
Tabouli, 1 serve, 4 oz	**170**	14	7
Tahini Sauce, avg., 1 Tbsp	**90**	8	2

Mexican

	C	F	Cb
Black Bean Soup, 1 bowl	**200**	3	34
Bueso Fresco, ¼ cup	**80**	4.5	8
Burritos *(Taco Bell):* Bean	**370**	10	55
Supreme® Beef	**440**	18	50
Chili, plain, ¼ cup	**90**	6	8
Chili con Carne: w. Beans, 1 cup	**310**	17	15
w/out Beans, 1 cup	**370**	28	10
Chimichangas, Beef, 5 oz	**400**	19	43
Chorizo Sausage, 2 oz	**265**	23	0
Churros, 1½ oz	**150**	8	18
Corn Chips, ½ cup, 1 oz	**160**	10	17
Costillas Ribs, 6 oz	**675**	52	0
Enchilada, average	**330**	10	49
Fajitas, Chicken (Soft)	**200**	7	20
Guacamole, 2 Tbsp, 1 oz	**120**	12	2
Horchata: *Don Jose*, 1 cup, 8 fl. oz	**140**	4	25
Cacique, 1 pint bottle, 16 fl. oz	**320**	7	62
Margarita (w. 1½ oz Tequila)	**160**	0	6
Menudo, ½ cup	**55**	1.5	10
Nachos: *Del Taco*, Regular	**395**	24	40
Macho Nachos	**1145**	63	113
Taco Bell: BellGrande®	**760**	43	80
Supreme®	**470**	26	42
Nachos: with cheese, peppers, 1 portion (6-8 nachos), 7 oz	**600**	33	60
with cheese, beans, ground beef, peppers, 1 portion (6-8 nachos), 9 oz	**570**	31	56
Nopal Cactus Salad, 1 serving	**130**	9	11
Papas Fritas (Fried Potatoes) (1), 6 oz	**325**	18	40
Piloncillo (Brown Sugar): 1 Tbsp, 13g	**50**	0	13
Cone, small, 3", 3 oz	**325**	0	81
Quesadilla, Cheese *(Taco Bell)*	**490**	28	39
Refried Beans, ¾ cup, 6 oz	**160**	3	26
Rice Pudding (Arroz Con Leche), 4 oz	**140**	3	24
Sopes (Gorditas), 2 oz	**120**	0	27
Taco *(Taco Bell)*: Regular, Crispy	**170**	10	13
Ranchero Chicken	**270**	15	21
Taco Supreme®	**220**	14	14
Double Decker® Taco	**340**	14	39
Taco Salad w. Salsa	**840**	52	85
Taco Sauce, average, ¼ cup	**15**	0	3
Taco Shell, regular	**50**	2	8
Tamales, Beef/Chicken, avg, 4.5 oz	**250**	11	27
Taquitos, Beef & Cheese, 4.5 oz	**330**	15	36
Tostada *(Taco Bell)*	**250**	10	29
Tortilla, Corn, 6" diam.	**70**	1	14
Tortilla Chips, 1 oz	**150**	8	18

Extra Listings of Mexican Dishes:

- **Fast-Foods Section** *(Taco Bell, Del Taco)*
- **Canned Bean/Chili Products:** *See Pages 77-83*

Mexican (Cont)

	C	F	Cb
Breads: Bolillos, 1 roll, 3½ oz	**240**	4	42
Telera, 2 oz	**150**	1.5	19
Mexican Cornbread, 4" square	**210**	11	19
French Baguette, 2 oz	**140**	1.5	26
Cakes, Cookies, Pastries			
Banderilla (Pastry Puff), 1 shell	**140**	10	8
Bigotes, 7"	**570**	22	44
Calvos, 2½ oz	**320**	18	38
Capirotada (Bread Pudding), 10 oz	**810**	38	107
Cinnamon Cookies, 2	**125**	8	13
Cocadas, 1 oz	**120**	6	15
Cortadillo, 1 cookie, 1.9 oz	**300**	11	48
Concha (All Colors):			
Small (3" diam), 2½ oz	**250**	8	38
Medium (4" diam), 3½ oz	**350**	11	53
Large (5" diam), 5½ oz	**550**	18	84
Cream Puff with Custard, 4¼ oz	**255**	14	25
Cuerno, 2 oz	**200**	4.5	34
Cuerno Fine, 2¾ oz	**330**	17	40
Donus (Donuts), 4", 3½ oz	**440**	21	58
Elotes, 3½ oz	**450**	24	51
Empanadas (Average all types):			
Small, 2 oz	**230**	10	28
Regular, 3 oz	**300**	14	42
Fiesta Cookie, 2¼ oz	**280**	8	47
Galletas Mixtas (1), 1 oz	**100**	2.5	16
Guayaba, 3¼ oz	**360**	14	53
Jelly Rolls, 3¼ oz	**240**	4	46
Mantecadites (Almond Shortbread), 4½ oz	**670**	42	64
Mini Pound Cake, 3 oz	**260**	12	33
Mini Cupcakes, 1¾ oz	**180**	8	25
Muffins/Nino Enbuelto, large, 6 oz	**465**	11	48
Novcias, 2¾ oz	**290**	9	46
Nuez, 3¼ oz	**380**	17	52
Ojo De Buey, 4 oz	**360**	15	55
Orejas Ears, 3 oz	**310**	15	38
Pan Dulce (Mexican Sweet Bread), 1 bun	**330**	10	45
Panquecitos, 2½ oz	**260**	11	36
Piedras, 4 oz	**470**	15	76
Polvorones, 3 oz	**370**	18	48
Puerquitos, 5 oz	**600**	24	88
Rebanadas, 3½ oz	**390**	18	51
Roles De Canela (Cin. Roll), 4½ oz	**490**	15	81
Roscas, 2¾ oz	**360**	18	44
Semitas, 3 oz	**300**	10	46
Sopapillas (flaky pastry puffs), 1 pce	**100**	7	10
w. Honey & Cream	**200**	14	18
Strawberry Crème Roll (1/6), 2½ oz	**240**	5	45

Extra Food Listings ~ See CalorieKing.com

Polish

	C	F	Cb
Cabbage Rolls w. Sour Cr., 2 sm.	**220**	10	30
Chicken Casserole w. Mush., 1 cup	**520**	27	5
Kielbasa (Sausages, Onions, fried), 2 large	**350**	28	2
Meatballs in Sour Cream, 3 x 1½" balls	**300**	16	11
Pierogi, Fruit/Veg, 3" ball	**80**	2	15
Pork Goulash (Pork/Veg. Stew)	**550**	21	38
Pot Roast with Vegetables	**630**	21	28

Soul Foods

	C	F	Cb
Breakfast Sausage, fried, 2 patties	**250**	17	0
Brunswick Stew, 1 cup, 8.5 oz	**320**	14	19
Cornbread, home-made, 3 oz	**200**	7.5	28
Fatback, raw, ¼ oz	**60**	6.5	0
Ham Hock	**90**	6.5	2
Hog Maw	**45**	2.5	0
Hominy, cooked, ¾ cup	**110**	0.5	25
Hush Puppies, 5 pieces	**260**	12	35
Kale, cooked, ½ cup	**20**	0.5	4
Opossum	**65**	3	0
Oxtail	**70**	3.5	0
Pig Ear, ¼ ear	**50**	3	0
Pig Foot, ½ foot	**70**	4.5	0
Pig Tail, 1/3 tail	**115**	10	0
Poke Salad, cooked, ½ cup	**16**	0.5	3
Pork Brains	**40**	2.5	0
Pork Chitterlings, simmered, 3 oz	**260**	25	0
Pork Cracklings, ½ oz	**80**	6	0
Pork Neck Bones	**65**	4	0
Pork Skin, 1 cup	**70**	4.5	0
Pork Tongue, 1/3 tongue	**75**	5.5	0
Sousemeat	**60**	4.5	0
Succotash, ½ cup	**80**	1	17
Sweet Potato Pie, 1/8 of 9" pie	**250**	12	34
Tripe, 2 oz	**55**	2	0
Vienna Sausage, 2 small	**90**	8	1
small	**45**	4	0.5

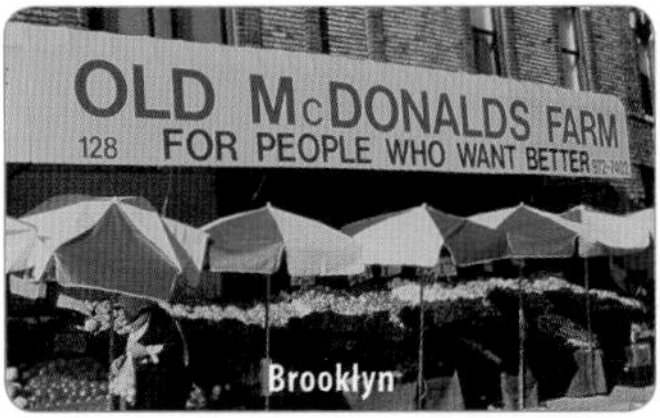
OLD McDONALDS FARM
128 FOR PEOPLE WHO WANT BETTER
Brooklyn

Spanish

	C	F	Cb
Arroz Abanda (Fish with Rice)	**340**	8	31
Arroz Con Pollo (Rice/Chick. Sal)	**500**	23	50
Clams Marinara, 8 clams	**330**	16	22
Cochifrito (Lamb w. Lemon/Garlic)	**650**	25	5
Cochinillo Asado, 2 sl. (Rst Suckling Pig)	**300**	15	3
Cocido Madrileno			
(Madrid-Style Boiled Dinner)	**450**	27	18
Flan de Leche (Caramel Custard)	**325**	9	52
Fritadera de Ternera (Sauteed Veal)	**450**	27	2
Gazpacho, 1 bowl	**60**	0	15
Paella a la Valenciana			
(Chicken & Shellfish Rice)	**900**	42	70
Pollo a la Espanola (Chicken)	**475**	30	4
Ternera al Jerez (Veal w. Sherry)	**660**	29	6
Zarzuela (Fish & Shellfish Medley)	**530**	27	40

Thai Foods

	C	F	Cb
Appetizers: Satay Pork, 1 oz	**100**	4	2
Spring Roll, 1¼ oz	**110**	6	13
Soups: Tom Yam (Hot & Sour):			
Spicy Shrimp/Seafood, 1 cup	**100**	4	6
1 bowl	**160**	7	10
Vegetarian, 1 cup	**50**	0	11
Curries: Chicken w. Ginger, 1 cup	**390**	34	4
Thick Red Curry w. Beef, 1 cup	**600**	50	7
Thai Chicken Curry, 1 cup	**340**	23	4
Massaman Curry, 1 cup	**680**	57	8
Green Curry w. Pork, 1 cup	**480**	44	5
Pad Thai, Large serving, 18 oz	**990**	38	125
Fish: Steamed w. Spicy Thai Sce	**450**	8	46
Crispy Fried, 5 oz	**290**	15	9
Spicy Chicken (w. veges), stir-fry	**450**	22	14
Spicy Garlic Tofu w. veges, stir-fry	**340**	18	18
Sticky Thai Rice: Plain 1 cup, 6 oz	**170**	0.5	36
w. Coconut & Sesame Seeds, 1 cup	**880**	28	120
Stir-fried Rice Noodles, 1 c., 5½ oz	**270**	9	40
Stir-fried Vegetables, 1 cup	**100**	3	18
Salads: Green Papaya Salad	**160**	0	40
Spicy Prawn, 9 shrimp	**170**	3	15
Thai Chicken, 1 serving	**330**	9	17
Thai Beef Salad, 1 serving	**260**	9	15
Thai Noodle, 1 serving	**410**	13	45
Satay Chicken & Peanut Sauce:			
1 satay stick	**390**	24	20
Sauces: Peanut Satay, ½ cup, 4 oz	**160**	10	13

Vietnamese

	C	F	Cb
Banh Cuon (Steam Rice w. Pork), 1 roll	**105**	7	8
Bo Nuong (Beef Satay), 2 sticks	**265**	9	4
Bo Xao Dau Phong			
(Ginger Beef w.Onion, Fish Sce.)	**750**	30	10
Ca Chien Gung (Whole Snapper/Ging.)	**600**	16	6
Canh Chay (Veg./Tofu Soup)	**80**	3	13
Cari (Curry) Chicken, 1 cup	**475**	29	16
Cari (Curry) Chicken, w. Rice Noodle,			
cup curry & cup cooked noodles	**660**	29	60
Cari (Curry) Chicken, w. Steam Rice,			
cup curry & cup rice	**650**	29	55
Cuu Xao Lan (Curried Lamb,			
Veges in Coconut)	**900**	40	80
Ga Chien (Crisp Chick + Plum Sce)	**900**	40	105
Ga Nuong (Chicken Satay + Sce)	**240**	10	4
Ga Xao Rau (Marinated Chicken			
Braised w. Veg.)	**800**	26	100
Gio Lua (Lean Pork Pie), ⅙ of pie	**245**	12	0
Goi Cuon (Cold Spring Rolls), each	**60**	1	7
Rau Cai Xao Chay (Stir Fried Vege.)	**400**	15	65
Thit Bo Vien (Beef Balls), 6 balls	**225**	14	2
Thit Heo Goi Baup Cai, each			
(Spicy Cabbage Rolls w. Pork)	**200**	7	11
Vietnamese (Cont)			
Soup: *Per Bowl (1½ Cup)*			
Bun Bo Hue (Hot & Spicy Soup			
no Pork Feet	**340**	9	35
w. Pork Feet	**830**	45	35
Chicken & Rice Noodle Soup	**400**	3	55
Pho Bo (Beef Noodle Soup)	**410**	7	59
Pho Ga (Chicken Noodle Soup)	**460**	6	58
Pho Tai (Rare Beef & Noodle Soup	**440**	7	73
Salad: *Per ½ Cup*			
Goi Du Du (Green Papaya Salad)	**155**	3	29
Sauce: Nuoc Cham (Hot Sauce)	**5**	0	1

Gourmet & Miscellaneous

	C	F	Cb
Ants Eggs/Larvae, 1 Tbsp	**20**	0	0
Ants, Choc. coated, 3 Tbsp	**140**	7	2
Bee Maggots, canned, 3 Tbsp	**65**	2	0
Caviar, black/red, 1 Tbsp	**40**	3	0
Caterpillars, canned, 2 oz	**60**	2	0
Frogs Legs, fried, 1 pair (large)	**125**	7	0
Haggis, boiled, 4 oz	**350**	24	22
Locusts, roasted, 1 oz	**35**	1	0
Silkworms, raw, 1 oz	**60**	2	0
Snails in garlic butter, 6 large	**200**	10	4
Snake, roasted, 4 oz	**160**	6	0

Fast-Food Chains & Restaurants

FOR MORE RESTAURANTS
See www.CaloriekKing.com

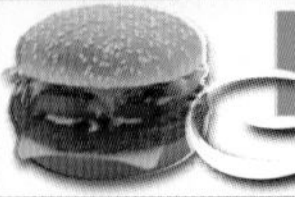

A&W®

Sandwiches	C	F	Cb
Cheeseburger	500	24	43
Cheeseburger Deluxe	540	28	43
Cheeseburger Deluxe Bacon	600	33	44
Cheeseburger Deluxe Bacon Double	835	49	49
Cheeseburger Deluxe Double	755	42	48
Cheeseburger Jr.	470	22	41
Crispy Chicken Sandwich	575	25	57
Grilled Chicken Sandwich	430	15	37
Hamburger	460	22	39
Hamburger Deluxe	500	26	40
Hamburger Jr	435	21	38
Chicken			
Chicken Grill	350	11	40
Chubby Chicken Burger	490	23	48
Chubby Chicken Pces: Breast	330	19	10
Drumstick	140	8	5
Thigh	410	31	9
Wing	205	14	6
Chicken Strips, 3 pces	500	29	32
Dipping Sauces: Barbeque, 1 oz	40	0	10
Honey Mustard	105	6	12
Sweet and Sour	50	0	12
Hot Dogs: Plain, 3.2 oz	285	17	22
Cheese Dog, 4.4 oz	325	20	25
Coney (Chili), 4.4 oz	310	18	24
Coney (Chili) Chse Dog, 5.4 oz	350	21	27
Fries & Sides: Per Serving			
Fries: Regular, 4 oz	310	13	45
Large, 5.5 oz	425	18	61
Cheese Fries, 6 oz	385	19	50
Chili Fries, 6 oz	370	16	49
Chili Cheese Fries, 7 oz	405	19	51
Poutine, small, 6 oz	420	24	38
Onion Rings, 4 oz	355	17	45
Salads: Coleslaw, Individual	90	6	7
Potato Salad, Individual	160	8	22
Macaroni Salad, Individual	175	9	22
Desserts			
Hot Caramel Sundae	340	9	57
Hot Fudge Sundae	350	11	54
Other Sundaes, avg.	310	8	52
Polar Swirl™: M&M; Oreo, small	720	25	107
Reese's, small	735	31	97
Soft Ice Cream Cone, regular, avg.	250	7	41

A&W® cont..

Milkshakes & Floats: Per 16 fl.oz	C	F	Cb
Chocolate Milkshake	705	29	100
Strawberry Milkshake	665	29	90
Vanilla Milkshake	715	31	97
A&W Root Beer Float	350	5	71
Drinks: Per 20 fl.oz			
A&W Root Beer	290	0	72
Diet A&W Root Beer; Diet Coke	5	0	0
Coca-Cola	300	0	75
Sprite	290	0	72

For Complete Nutritional Data ~ see CalorieKing.com

Applebee's®

Low Fat Menu: Per Serving	C	F	Cb
Asian Chicken Salad	715	9	121
Blackened Chicken Salad	425	8.5	39
Chicken Fajita Quesadilla	520	11	63
Chicken Quesadilla	740	14	89
Chicken Rancho Rollup	590	12	80
Chicken Roma Rollup	640	10	83
Chicken Pasta	530	10	76
Garlic/Lemon Chicken Pasta	530	11	78
Veggie Quesadilla	595	12	86
Whitefish w. Mango Salsa	435	10	54
Entree Meals			
Crispy Buttermilk Shrimp w. Garlic Toast	890	39	83
Crispy Orange Skillet	1710	69	209
Fiesta Lime Chicken	1285	47	136
Gr. Steak Caesar Salad w. Garlic Tst	1320	87	60
Madeira Steak Tips w. Garlic Toast	955	43	82
Oriental Chicken Salad Roll-Up	710	25	72
Southwest Philly Roll-Up	1880	121	122
without French Fries	1380	94	63
Riblets w. French Fries	2030	130	106
Sides			
French Fries	505	27	59
Garlic Toast, 1 slice	180	10	17
Desserts, Sundaes			
Low Fat Brownie Sundae	325	3	49
Bikini Banana Strawb. Shortcake	230	3	49
Marble Cheesecake	260	2	50
Sizzling Apple Pie	1085	56	146
Triple Chocolate Meltdown	730	31	107

Arby's®

Breakfast: Per Serving	C	F	Cb
Bacon 'n Egg Croissant	**410**	26	31
Bacon Biscuit	**295**	17	27
Biscuit: Plain	**230**	12	26
w. Butter	**330**	23	26
w. Scrambled Egg	**315**	18	28
w. Swiss Cheese	**270**	15	26
Ham 'n Cheese Croissant	**350**	19	30
Ham Biscuit	**275**	13	27
Sausage 'n Egg Croissant	**505**	36	31
Sausage Biscuit	**385**	27	26
Sourdough Bacon, Egg 'n Swiss	**495**	29	33
Sourdough Egg 'n Cheese	**330**	16	31
Sourdough Ham, Egg 'n Swiss	**445**	23	33
Roast Beef Sandwiches: *Per Sandwich*			
Arby-Q	**375**	11	51
Beef 'n Cheddar	**455**	21	44
Big Montana	**615**	29	41
French Dip 'n Swiss	**535**	21	51
Giant Roast Beef	**465**	19	41
Junior Roast Beef	**280**	9	34
Philly Beef Supreme	**715**	37	59
Regular Roast Beef	**335**	13	34
Super Roast Beef	**450**	19	48
Market Fresh Sandwiches: *Per Sandwich*			
Chicken Salad	**870**	44	92
Roast Beef & Swiss	**795**	39	74
Roast Ham & Swiss	**720**	31	74
Roast Turkey & Swiss	**720**	27	74
Roast Turkey Ranch & Bacon	**840**	38	75
Ultimate BLT	**805**	46	75
Market Fresh Low Carbys: *Per Wrap*			
Chicken Caesar	**560**	27	46
Roast Turkey Ranch & Bacon	**745**	39	48
Southwest Chicken	**590**	30	45
Ultimate BLT Wrap	**715**	47	48
Other Sandwiches: *Per Sandwich*			
Chicken Bacon 'n Swiss	**565**	27	49
Chicken Breast Fillet	**500**	24	46
Chicken Cordon Bleu	**580**	29	46
Grilled Chicken Deluxe	**385**	12	40
Hot Ham 'n Cheese	**315**	9	35
Hot Ham 'n Swiss Melt	**285**	8	35
Roast Chicken Club	**490**	25	39

Arby's® cont..

Market Fresh Salads: Per Serving	C	F	Cb
Asian Sesame:			
w. Almonds, Noodles & Dressing	**485**	25	40
no Almonds, Noodles or Dressing	**140**	1	15
Chicken Club Salad: No Dressing	**545**	33	32
w. Buttermilk Ranch Dressing	**870**	67	36
Garden Side Salad, no dressing	**40**	0	8
Martha's Vineyard Salad:			
w. Raspb. Vinaigrette & Almonds	**525**	27	41
no Vinaigrette or Almonds	**270**	8	23
Santa Fe: w. Dress. & Tortilla Strips	**865**	59	53
no Dressing or Tortilla Strips	**530**	29	40
Sauces & Condiments: *Per Serving*			
Mayonnaise, 0.5 oz	**100**	11	0
Dipping Sauce: BBQ, 1 oz	**40**	0	10
Buffalo, 2 oz	**20**	1	3
Honey Mustard, 1 oz	**130**	12	5
Dressing: Asian Sesame, 1.9 fl.oz	**190**	14	15
Buttermilk Ranch, 2 oz	**285**	30	3
Fat Free Italian, 2 oz	**30**	0	7
Light Balsamic Vinaigrette, 2 oz	**105**	6	13
Light Buttermilk Ranch, 2 oz	**105**	6	12
Raspberry Vinaigrette, 1.9 fl.oz	**170**	12	16
Santa Fe Ranch, 1.9 fl.oz	**270**	28	3
Sauce: Arby's, 0.5 oz	**15**	0	4
Bronco Berry, 2 oz	**120**	0	30
Cheddar Cheese, 1.5 oz	**60**	4.5	4
Horsey, 0.5 oz	**55**	5	3
Marinara, 1.5 oz	**15**	0	4
Red Ranch, 0.5 oz	**75**	6	5
Tangy Southwest, 2 oz	**340**	35	5
Sides: *Per Serving*			
Baked Potato: Plain	**200**	0	46
w. Broccoli 'n Cheddar	**475**	23	56
w. Butter & Sour Cream	**425**	23	48
Deluxe, 10.4 oz	**580**	34	50
Chicken Fingers: 4 Pack	**635**	38	42
Combo w. Curly Fries	**1045**	60	89
Snack w. Curly Fries	**595**	34	53
Fries: Curly, small, 3.7 oz	**335**	18	39
Homestyle, small, 4 oz	**305**	13	44
Potato Cakes (2)	**245**	15	26
Sidekickers: Jalapeno Bites (5)	**305**	19	29
Mozzarella Sticks (4)	**430**	23	38
Onion Petals, 4 oz	**325**	19	35
Shakes: Chocolate, reg., 13.2 fl.oz	**500**	13	83
Other flavors, regular, 13.2 fl.oz	**495**	13	81
Desserts: *Per Serving*			
Apple Turnover w. Icing	**375**	12	64

Arthur Treachers®

Meals: Per Serving	C	F	Cb
Cole Slaw, 5 oz	**220**	8.5	34
Fish N Chips	**1565**	101	132
Fish Sandwich	**390**	17	45
Hush Puppy (2), 2.3 oz	**275**	10	42
Seafood Sampler	**3560**	270	227
Shrimp N Chips	**2220**	124	225

Atlanta Bread Company®

Bagels: Per Bagel (4 oz)	C	F	Cb
Asiago; Banana	**350**	3	66
Blueberry; Plain; Cinnamon Raisin	**340**	1.5	68
Chocolate Chip	**330**	3	62
Everything; Poppy Seed; Sesame	**310**	1.5	61
Honey Wheat; Jalapeno	**330**	1.5	66
Onion; Pumpernickel	**300**	1.5	60
Bread: Per Thick Slice (2 oz)			
Asiago	**150**	2.5	26
Cinnamon Raisin	**170**	2.5	31
Cracked Wheat	**160**	2	30
French	**140**	0.5	29
Honey Wheat; Nine Grain; Pesto	**150**	1.5	29
Pumpernickel; Rye	**150**	1	28
Sourdough	**140**	0	29
Sundried Tomato	**150**	0	30
Bread Rolls: French, 2.6 oz	**180**	0.5	37
Sourdough, 2.6 oz	**190**	0	38
Muffins: Apple Cinnamon, 4 oz	**400**	19	52
Banana Walnut	**440**	22	53
Blueberry	**430**	20	55
Chocolate Chip/Mocha avg.	**470**	23	61
Cranberry Apple, 4 oz	**390**	18	51
Cranberry Orange Walnut	**440**	23	51
Honey Raisin Bran	**460**	21	65
Lemon Poppy Seed	**460**	23	57
Peaches/Creme	**530**	25	68
Pumpkin	**370**	13	58
Zucchini, 4 oz	**480**	24	60
Low Fat varieties, average, 4 oz	**320**	5	60
Muffin Tops: Blueberry, 3 oz	**320**	15	41
Banana Walnut, 3 oz	**330**	16	40
Chocolate Chip, 3 oz	**340**	16	45
Chocolate Mocha, 3 oz	**350**	17	45
Pumpkin, 3 oz	**280**	10	43

Atlanta Bread® cont...

Salads: Per Salad	C	F	Cb
Caesar	**220**	9	28
Chicken Salad	**310**	21	0.5
Chicken Caesar	**310**	11	28
Chicken Curry	**340**	24	10
Chicken House	**115**	2.5	8
Chopstix Chicken	**470**	24	38
Fruit Salad	**140**	1	32
Greek Chicken, no dressing	**210**	10	12
Greek Salad	**120**	8	12
House Salad	**35**	0	8
Tuna Salad	**240**	16	0
Sandwiches (Sourdough)			
ABC Special, no dressing	**510**	6	67
Avocado, no dressing	**630**	32	75
Bella Basil Chicken	**780**	37	76
Chicken Curry, no dressing	**630**	25	70
Chicken Salad, no dressing	**600**	23	61
Honey Maple Ham, no dressing	**420**	4.5	66
Pastrami, no dressing	**440**	7	62
Roast Beef, no dressing	**450**	5	62
Tuna, no dressing	**530**	18	61
Turkey Breast, no dressing	**420**	4.5	60
Veggie, no dressing	**290**	1	60
Panini: Cordon Bleu	**590**	15	76
Chargrilled Chicken Pesto	**740**	30	78
Cuban Pork Loin	**740**	30	82
Italian Vegetarian	**620**	21	81
Turkey Club	**780**	32	76
Soup: *Per Cup*			
Black Bean & Rice; Chkn Gumbo	**110**	3	14
Black Bean w/Ham	**200**	7	32
Chicken 'n Dumpling	**240**	13	21
Chicken Chili	**220**	6	27
Chicken Noodle	**110**	4	12
Chili w. Beans	**280**	11	24
Clam Chowder	**270**	16	22
French Onion	**60**	2	9
Garden Veg.; Mushr., Barley & Sage	**80**	1	15
Lentil & Roasted Garlic	**200**	2.5	33
Seven Bean w. Ham	**240**	12	27
Szechuan Hot & Sour	**80**	2	12
Tomato Florentine	**120**	3	17
Vegetable Chili	**180**	3.5	31
Wisconsin Cheese	**210**	11	20

For Complete Nutritional Data ~ see CalorieKing.com

Au Bon Pain®

Bagels: Per Bagel	C	F	Cb
Asiago Cheese	380	8	59
Cinnamon Raisin	340	1	71
Dutch Apple	485	4	99
French Toast	410	7	76
Plain	300	1	61
Spreads: Plain Cream Chse, 2 oz	130	11	4
Honey Walnut, 2 oz	140	9	12
Sundried Tomato; Veggie, 2 oz	140	12	3
Breakfast Sandwiches: *Per Sandwich*			
Egg on a Bagel	390	4	63
w. Bacon	480	12	63
w. Bacon & Cheese	555	18	63
w. Cheese	475	11	63
Sandwiches: *Per Sandwich*			
Arizona Chicken	585	19	58
Chicken & Mozzarella Foccacia	730	24	73
Chicken Tarragon w. Field Onions	800	42	71
Fresh Mozzarella, Tomato	465	24	40
Grilled Salmon Salad	265	7	40
Grilled Tarragon Chicken	320	13	35
Honey Dijon Cordon Bleu	575	12	71
Roasted Vegetable	280	8	42
Smoked Turkey Club	760	34	62
Turkey Tenderloin; Tuna	315	9	40
Wraps: Chicken Caesar	610	25	63
Fields & Feta	595	17	90
Mediterranean Wrap	605	23	80
Southwestern Tuna	680	26	68
Brownies: Blonde	575	36	57
Choc Chip	490	25	61
Soups: *Per Serving (8 oz)*			
Black Bean	155	0.5	27
Chicken Noodle	90	2	11
Corn Chowder	235	13	25
Garden Vegetable	45	1	7
Split Pea w. Ham	140	1	23
Vegetarian Chili	165	1	30
Breads: Average, 1.75 oz slice	130	1	27
Bread Bowl (1)	645	3	127
Foccacia (1)	735	9	137
Four Grain Bread, 1 slice	315	3	58
Rosemary Garlic Breadstick	200	5	33
Bread Rolls: Hearth (1)	240	2	44
Braided Pain Roll (1)	430	14	62

Au Bon Pain® cont...

Yogurt & Fruit Cups: Per Serving	C	F	Cb
Yogurt, average all types	220	3	43
Fruit Cup: Small, 1 cup	70	0	16
Large, 1 cup	145	1	32
Salads: *Per Serving (Container)*			
Caesar Salad	340	16	31
Charbr. Salmon Filet, Yellow Peppers	205	7	10
Chef's Salad	255	13	9
Chicken Caesar	400	18	32
Garden Salad, large	155	4.5	23
Gorgonzola & Walnut	345	28	10
Mediterranean Chicken	235	12	13
Thai Chicken	145	2.5	14
Tuna Garden	430	25	25
Turkey Medallion Cobb	440	24	27
Cookies: *Per Cookie*			
Chocolate Chip	265	10	41
English Toffee	195	6	33
Oatmeal Raisin	240	6	43
Shortbread	275	7	48
Cakes & Bars: Apple Strudel	410	18	56
Cinnamon Roll	410	12	67
Cherry Strudel	390	19	49
Pecan Roll	765	29	112
Croissants: Ham & Cheese	310	10	46
Spinach & Cheese	250	9	32
Filled: Plain	260	6	44
Almond	530	25	63
Apple	240	3	47
Chocolate	410	15	61
Raspberry	355	11	55
Sweet Cheese	370	14	52
Muffins: Blueberry	510	19	76
Cranberry Walnut	555	26	69
Chocolate Chip; Double Choc	550	20	83
Pumpkin	460	16	71
Raisin Bran	575	13	100
Lowfat: Chocolate Cake	330	2	74
Triple Berry	280	2	61
Drinks			
Mocha Blast, large, 20 fl.oz	460	14	68
Frozen Mocha Blast, 12 fl.oz	265	6	43
Iced Cappuccino, regular, 16 fl.oz	215	8	22
Iced Tea, 22 fl.oz	120	0	30

Auntie Anne's®

Pretzels: With Butter	C	F	Cb
Almond	400	8	72
Cinnamon Sugar	450	9	83
Garlic	350	4.5	68
Glazin' Raisin®	510	4	107
Jalapeno	310	4.5	59
Original	370	4	72
Parmesan Herb	440	13	72
Sesame	410	12	64
Sour Cream & Onion	340	5	66
Stix, 4 sticks	250	3	48
Whole Wheat	370	4.5	72
***Pretzels:* Without Butter**			
Almond Pretzel; Whole Wheat	340	1.5	72
Cinnamon Sugar	350	2	74
Garlic Pretzel; Sour Crm & Onion	320	1	66
Glazin' Raisin®	470	0.5	104
Jalapeno Pretzel	270	1	58
Original Pretzel	340	1	72
Parmesan Herb	390	5	74
Sesame Pretzel	350	6	63
Stix, 4 sticks	230	7	48
Dipping Sauces			
Caramel Dip, 1.5 oz	140	3	27
Cheese Sce; Hot Salsa Chse, avg.	100	8	4
Chocolate Flavored Dip, 1¼ oz	130	4	24
Light Cream Cheese, 1¼ oz	70	6	1
Marinara Sauce, 1¼ oz	15	0	4
Strawberry Cream Cheese, 1¼ oz	115	10	4
Sweet Mustard, 1¼ oz	50	1.5	8
***Beverages:* Per Serving**			
Auntie Anne's Lemonade, 22 fl.oz	170	0	43
Dutch Ice (14 fl.oz): Kiwi-Banana	175	0	44
Blue Raspberry	220	0	55
Lemonade	310	0	77
Mocha	400	10	73
Orange Crème	260	0	64
Pina Colada; Strawberry	350	0	87
Wild Cherry	195	0	48
Dutch Smoothie (14 fl.oz):			
Blue Raspberry	275	10	42
Kiwi-Banana	295	10	47
Lemonade	370	10	66
Mocha	410	10	63
Orange Crème	335	10	58
Pina Colada	325	10	55
Strawberry	305	10	50
Wild Cherry	310	10	52

Back Yard Burgers®

Burgers	C	F	Cb
Back Yard Burger ⅓ lb.	525	29	38
Cheeseburger ⅓ lb	580	34	38
Bacon Cheddar	675	42	38
Barbecue Bacon	680	39	47
Black Jack	620	39	36
Chili Cheese	620	36	41
Garden Veggie Sandwich	305	6	47
Jr Burger	375	17	38
Hawaiian	600	33	44
Miz Grazi's	585	34	39
Mushroom Swiss	605	36	37
Worcestershire	550	34	41
Chicken Sandwiches			
Bacon Swiss	455	20	37
Barbecue	345	8	44
Blackened	350	11	39
Buffalo Ranch	545	30	51
Hawaiian	350	8	45
Honey Mustard	385	11	46
Lemon Butter	325	9	37
Savory	295	6	36
Specialities			
BLT	335	16	36
Chicken Tenderloins, 3 piece	415	28	22
Chili Dog	340	20	29
Chili Cheese Dog	400	25	29
Hot Dog	310	18	27
Baked Potatoes			
Chili & Cheddar, 9 oz	340	11	48
Ranch, 7.7 oz	415	22	45
Salsa, 7.7 oz	260	5	47
Traditional/Plain, 6 oz	190	0	43
Fries			
Chili Cheese Fries, 6.7 oz	340	22	28
Seasoned Fries, regular, 3 oz	260	16	28
Waffle Fries, regular, 3 oz	245	22	28
Salads (No Dressing)			
Blackened Chicken	165	4	11
Charbroiled Chicken	155	3	11
Garden Fresh	25	0	5
Cobblers: Apple, 6 oz	430	20	60
Blackberry; Peach, 6 oz	435	20	60
Cherry, 6 oz	470	20	68
***Shakes:* Per 12 fl.oz**			
Chocolate/Vanilla	560	26	72
Strawberry	590	26	79

Baja Fresh®

Burritos: Includes Cheese	C	F	Cb
"Dos Manos": Steak, ½ meal	785	24	101
Chicken, ½ meal	735	20	101
Mexicano: Chicken	815	13	124
Steak	900	20	124
Ultimo Burrito: Steak, no sour crm	930	37	90
Chicken, no sour cream	850	30	90
Baja Burrito: Chicken	830	35	75
Steak	915	42	75
Bare Burrito	640	7	99
Bare Burrito Vegetarian	560	8	102
Bean & Cheese Burrito: Chicken	990	33	104
Steak	1080	41	104
Vegetarian	860	31	104
Enchiladas: Verano	580	9	87
Cheese Enchilada	855	35	91
Chicken Enchilada	765	23	91
Steak Enchilada	875	33	94
Ensalada: Mahi Mahi, no dressing	295	9	20
Shrimp, no dressing	190	4	17
Baja Ensalada: Chicken, no dress.	320	7	17
Fish, no dressing	385	15	27
Steak, no dressing	450	18	17
Fajitas: Chicken w. Corn Tortillas	1225	29	164
Steak w. Corn Tortillas	1380	42	164
Mini Tosta-Dita: Chicken	550	17	67
Steak	605	22	67
Mini-Quesa-Dita: Steak	685	23	81
Cheese; Chicken, average	630	21	81
Nachos: Cheese; Chicken, avg.	1900	104	166
Steak	2075	113	166
Picado: Chicken	670	31	31
Steak	835	45	31
Quesadilla: Chicken	1265	71	80
Steak	1355	79	80
Vegetarian; Cheese, avg.	1155	70	92
Tacos: Chilito Chicken	320	10	38
Chillito Steak	345	12	38
Baja Style Tacos: Chicken	200	5	26
Steak	225	7	26
Wild Gulf Shrimp	195	5	26
Fish Taco Baja	275	13	31
Mahi Mahi	270	10	32
Grilled Veggie Taco	440	10	72
Taquitos: Includes Sour Cream			
Chicken w. Beans/Rice, avg.	720	36	66
Steak w. Beans, Crema Salsa	815	42	69
Steak w. Rice, Crema Salsa	775	42	67
Tostada: Steak w. chse & sour crm	1210	60	102
Chicken w. chse & sour crm	1120	52	102
Vegetarian w. cheese & sour crm	990	50	102

Banana's®

Frosty: Per 8 oz Serving	C	F	Cb
Banana Berry Cream	180	0.5	40
Citrus Blend	110	0	26
Mango Magic	150	0	38
Melon Banana	140	0.5	36
Orange Swirl Creamy	170	0.5	37
P-nut Butter Cup Creamy	380	20	35
Raspberry Creamy	170	2	31
Strawberry	50	0.5	12
Strawberry Creamy	150	0	32
Smoothie: Per 8 oz Serving			
Banana Berry	130	1	32
Chococino	350	19	39
Cookies N Cream	300	4	57
Mocha ala Orange	160	1	37
Pina Colada	170	0	44
Raspberry Flavored Lemony Batch	290	0	73
Strawberry Flavored Lemony Batch	250	0	66

Ben & Jerry's®

Ice Cream & Frozen Yogurt ~ See Page 32
Novelty Bars ~ See Page 36

Big Apple Bagels®

	C	F	Cb
Bagels: All types, avg., 5 oz	380	2	72
½ bagel, 2.5 oz	190	1	36
My Favorite Muffin® Bagels: Per Bagel (4 oz)			
Honey Grain	310	3	61
Avg. other varieties	310	1	66
My Favorite Muffin® Muffins: Per Jumbo			
Blueberry	505	24	66
Blueberry, Fat Free	335	0	78
Chocolate Chip	655	33	81
Chocolate, Fat Free	360	0	84
Cream Cheese: Per 2 Tbsp (1 oz)			
Plain	105	10	2
Honey Cinnamon; Very Berry, avg.	130	12	3
Lite varieties, average	65	5	2
Soups: Per Cup (8 fl. oz)			
Boston Clam/Potato Chowder	210	13	20
Chicken Noodle; Beef Pot Roast	110	4	12
Garden Vegetable	110	1	18
Minestrone	150	3	26
Split Pea w. Ham; Hearty Vege	95	2	16

Baskin Robbins®

Hard Scooped Ice Cream	C	F	Cb
Classic: *Per Regular Scoop*			
Cherries Jubilee	240	13	29
Chocolate	280	14	33
Chocolate Chip	275	16	28
Chocolate Chip Cookie Dough	300	15	36
Chocolate Fudge	290	15	35
French Vanilla	280	18	26
German Choc Cake	310	16	36
Gold Medal Ribbon	275	13	34
Jamoca	240	13	26
Jamoca Almond Fudge	285	15	31
Mint Choc Chip	275	16	28
Old Fashion Butter Pecan	280	18	24
Oreo Cookies 'N Cream	285	15	32
Peanut Butter 'N Chocolate	330	20	31
Pink Bubblegum	270	14	34
Pistachio Almond	300	19	25
Pralines 'N Cream	280	14	34
Quarterback Crunch	290	17	32
Reeses Peanut Butter	310	18	31
Rocky Road	300	15	36
Vanilla	265	16	26
Very Berry Strawberry	225	11	28
World Class Chocolate	285	15	33
Chocolate Roll Cake: *Per Slice (4.1 oz)*			
Average all flavors	290	14	36
Lowfat Ice Cream: Espresso 'N Crm	185	4	32
No Sugar Added Ice Cream, avg.	160	4	27
Ices, Sherbets, Sorbets: *Regular Scoop*			
Ices, Daiquiri; Margarita	135	0	34
Sherbets, average all flavors	160	2	34
Sorbets, average all flavors	115	0	29
Lowfat Yogurt (Hard): *Regular Scoop*			
Average all flavors	215	4	38
Nonfat Yogurt (Soft Serve): *Per ½ Cup*			
Vanilla, 4 oz	150	0	32
Other flavors, 3 oz	115	0	25
Shakes, Smoothies, Blasts: *Regular (16 fl.oz)*			
Shakes: Chocolate Ice Cream	675	26	98
Vanilla Ice Cream	690	33	85
Smoothies: Average all flavors	365	1	82
Blasts: Cappuccino w/whip cream	325	14	44
Cones: Sugar Cone	60	3	7
Cake Cone	25	0.5	4
Waffle Cone: Large	120	1.5	14
Fresh Baked	145	2	30

Big Boy®

Sandwiches	C	F	Cb
Big Boy	600	26	35
Brawny Lad™	420	21	30
Buddie Boy	760	34	80
Fish Sandwich	690	48	41
Small Hamburger	445	30	30
Super Big Boy™	830	66	34
Swiss Miss	635	44	28
Tuna Salad Sandwich	545	40	30
Sides & Salad: French Fries	360	19	45
Chili	315	18	19
Onion Rings	580	41	45
Tartare Sauce, 2 oz	370	40	1
Trio Salad	620	46	18

Blimpie®

Cold Subs: *Per 6" Sub on White (w. Cheese)*	C	F	Cb
Blimpie Best	475	16	52
Club Sub	440	12	50
Ham & Cheese	435	12	52
Roast Beef	470	13	50
Seafood, no cheese	355	7.5	58
Tuna, no cheese	495	23	50
Turkey Sub	425	11	49
Hot Subs: *Per 6" Sub on White*			
BLT	590	32	49
Grilled Chicken	380	9	50
ChickMax w. cheese	510	13	71
Meatball w. cheese	575	27	56
MexiMax	425	9	66
Steak & Onion w. cheese	440	16	49
VegiMax	395	7	60
Grilled Subs: Reuben, 6"	630	33	55
Pastrami Special, 6"	460	14	52
Wraps: Zesty Italian, regular	640	33	74
Chicken Caesar, regular	645	35	56
Salads: Chef, regular	210	9	9
Coleslaw, 5 oz	180	13	13
Potato Salad, 5 oz	270	19	19
Turkey, regular	370	19	31
Dressings: Caesar, 1.5 oz	210	22	2
Buffalo Sauce, 1.5 oz	110	0.5	24
Soup: Chicken Noodle, 1 cup	120	2.5	18
Tomato Basil, 1 cup	115	1	22
Desserts: Oatmeal Raisin Cookie	190	8	27
Average other varieties	210	10	26

For Complete Nutritional Data ~ see CalorieKing.com

Bob Evans®

Beef & Pork: *Per Serving*	C	F	Cb
Country Fried Steak: w. Gravy	535	37	31
no Gravy	480	33	26
Meat Loaf	620	44	14
Steak Tips & Noodles	1050	39	98
Burgers: Bacon Cheeseburger	990	76	31
Cheeseburger	690	46	31
Hamburger	605	38	30
Chicken & Turkey			
Chicken Breast Dinner: Fried, 1 pce	290	15	9
Grilled, 1 piece	220	9	0
Chicken Pot Pie	755	49	46
Chicken-n-Noodles	405	22	32
Turkey, 1 slice, 1.5 oz	50	0	1
Sandwiches: Bob's BLT	800	57	48
Fried Chicken Club	890	59	40
Grilled Chicken	695	43	55
Grilled Chicken Club	820	54	32
Pot Roast	655	31	62
Pulled Pork Sandwich	465	18	54
Turkey Bacon Melt	825	47	56
Lunch Savors			
Salads: Country Spinach	545	38	11
Cobb w. Grilled Chicken	575	39	9
Frisco: w. Fried Chicken	495	26	26
w. Grilled Chicken	460	31	9
Wildfire Chicken: w. Fried Chkn	645	29	74
w. Grilled Chicken	610	29	57
Stir-Fry: Grilled Chicken	500	18	55
Grilled Shrimp (Combo)	230	7	4
Vegetable	280	4	55
Soups (Per Bowl): Bean	180	5	23
Cheddar Baked Potato	390	22	31
Pasta: Chicken Broccoli Alfredo	855	29	90
Spaghetti & Marinara Sauce	615	7	104
Spaghetti w. Meatballs	1085	45	116
Seafood: Fried Shrimp Dinner	330	20	8
Salmon Dinner	375	23	12
Side Items: Onion Rings, 6 oz	460	27	49
Baked Potato Seasoned: Loaded	475	18	57
Plain	250	0	54
Cheddar Broccoli Florets, 8 oz	175	9	14
Coleslaw, 4 oz	195	13	18
Corn, Buttered Sweet, 4 oz	155	9	18
Garden Side Salad	165	4	26
Grilled Garden Vegetables, 10 oz	260	20	16
Home Fries, 5 oz	190	7	28
Mashed Potatoes, 5 oz	120	6	15
Mushrooms, Grilled, 8 oz	165	12	10
Rice Pilaf, 5 oz	165	3	32

Bob Evans® cont...

Farm Fresh Salads	C	F	Cb
Chicken Salad Plate	820	46	77
Cobb w. Grilled Chicken	755	50	15
Breakfast Combinations			
Country Biscuit Breakfast	850	49	71
Fruit & Yogurt Plate	440	2	96
Home Fries, 5 oz	190	7	28
Lite Sausage Breakfast	405	20	48
Pot Roast Hash Breakfast	750	46	37
Sirloin Steak	415	29	3
Hotcake: Blueberry (1)	185	5	32
Buttermilk (1)	170	5	28
Eggs: Hardboiled (1)	65	4	1
Eggs Benedict, 9 oz	420	20	35
Over Easy (1)	90	7	1
Scrambled (1)	165	11	1
Scrambled Egg Beaters (1)	190	12	2
Omelettes: Cheese	480	40	3
Farmer's Market	615	50	11
Ham & Cheese	495	39	2
Western Chicken	515	39	6
Specialty Breads: Dinner Roll, 2.3 oz	200	5	34
Banana Nut Bread, 2.7 oz	195	7	30
Cinnamon Swirl, Frosted, 5.5 oz	560	24	76
English Muffin, 2 oz	140	1	28
Garlic Bread, 2 oz	220	16	16
Sourdough Bread, 1.8 oz	130	1	26
Texas Toast, 1.8 oz	120	1	12
Kids Items: Mac & Cheese	330	12	45
Hot Diggety Dog w. Bun	360	26	23
Mini Cheeseburgers (1)	240	14	20
Pizza Pizzazz; Spaghetti & Meatballs	525	21	57
Plenty-O-Pancakes	505	17	79
Quesadilla, Chicken	545	31	39
Sundae: Fudge Blast	250	10	37
Oreo Cookies 'n' Cream	385	13	64
Drinks: Iced Tea, 9.5 fl.oz	5	0	1
Raspberry Tea, 9.5 fl.oz	80	0	20
Strawberry Tea, 9.5 fl.oz	80	0	20
Desserts, Pies & Sundaes			
Apple Dumpling Pie, 1 slice	690	30	100
A La Mode, 1 slice	840	37	119
Banana Cream Pie, 1 slice	455	25	52
Cheesecake, Oreo, 1 slice	620	38	61
Coconut Cream Pie	465	23	57
Fudge Sundae	510	19	78
Hershey's Hot Fudge Cake, 1 slice	605	25	94
Lemon Meringue Pie, 1 slice	535	18	89
Pumpkin Pie, , 1 slice	545	27	69
Reese's Peanut Butter Cup Pie, 1 sl.	1130	60	129
Reese's Sundae	785	35	104

Boston Market®

Entrees: Per Serving	C	F	Cb
¼ Chicken:			
White meat w. skin & wing	280	12	2
No skin or wing	170	4	2
¼ Chicken: Dark meat w. skin	320	21	2
No skin	190	10	1
½ Chicken w. skin	590	33	4
Chicken Pot Pie, 1 pie	750	46	57
Crispy-Baked Country Chicken	425	22	31
Double-Sauced Angus Meatloaf	325	19	16
w. Beef Gravy	375	23	19
Double-Sauced Angus Meatloaf			
& Chunky Creole Sauce	365	19	25
Grilled Mango Chicken	400	12	26
Honey Glazed Ham (lean), 5 oz	210	8	10
Marinated Grilled Chkn, 1 breast	230	10	1
Rotisserie Turkey Breast: no skin	170	1	3
w. Stuffing & Gravy	600	18	67
Soup: Chicken Noodle, 1 cup	100	4.5	8
15 Vegetable Soup, 1 cup	130	2.5	24
Fire Roasted Tomato Bisque, 1 cup	385	29	25
Tortilla Soup w. toppings, 6 oz	170	8	18
Salads: Caesar Side Salad, 4 oz	300	26	13
Caesar Salad Entree, 9.5 oz	485	40	17
no Dressing, 8 oz	180	9	20
Grilled Chicken w. Chips	890	58	46
Oriental Gr. Ckn, no dress./noodles	320	10	20
Sandwiches			
Chicken Carver w. Cheese & Sauce	655	29	61
no Cheese or Sauce	420	6	60
Marinated Grilled Chicken	670	36	45
no mayo	465	13	45
Meatloaf w. Cheese	755	29	85
Open-Faced w. sides	730	36	74
Turkey Carver w. Cheese & Sauce	650	26	64
no Cheese or Sauce	420	4.5	61
Turkey on Honey Wheat			
no cheese or sauce	420	4.5	61
Side Dishes: Rice Pilaf, 1 cup	140	4	24
Whole Corn, ¾ cup	180	4	30
Hot Cinnamon Apples, ¾ cup	265	4.5	56
Macaroni & Cheese, ¾ cup	280	11	33
Mash Potatoes (¾ c.) & Gravy	230	9	32
Creamed Spinach, ¾ cup	260	20	11

Bojangles®

Cajun & Southern Style Chicken	C	F	Cb
Breast, average	280	17	12
Leg, average	265	16	11
Thigh, average	310	23	11
Wing, average	355	25	11
Sandwiches			
Cajun Filet: w/out Mayo	335	11	41
w. Mayonnaise	435	22	41
Grilled Filet: w/out mayo	235	5	25
w. Mayonnaise	335	16	25
Snacks: Buffalo Bites	180	5	5
Chicken Supremes	335	16	26
Biscuit Sandwiches: Bacon	290	17	26
Bacon, Egg & Cheese	550	42	27
Biscuit (plain)	245	12	29
Cajun Filet	455	21	46
Country Ham	270	15	26
Egg	400	30	26
Sausage	350	23	26
Smoked Sausage	380	26	27
Steak	650	49	37
Fixins': Botato Rounds	235	11	31
Cajun Pintos	110	0	18
Corn on the Cob	140	2	34
Dirty Rice	165	6	24
Green Beans	25	0	5
Macaroni & Cheese	200	14	12
Marinated Cole Slaw	135	3	26
Potatoes, no Gravy	80	1	16
Seasoned Fries	345	19	39
Sweet Biscuits: Bo Berry™	220	10	29
Cinnamon	320	18	37

Braum's®

	C	F	Cb
Cinnamon Rolls, with Icing	340	11	56
Frozen Custard, avg. all flavors	185	8	25
Frozen Yogurt: Per ½ Cup			
Banana Pecan	170	7	23
Bordeaux Cherry Amaretto	155	5	24
Capp. Chunky Choc.; Toffee Bark	170	6	26
Chocolate varieties, avg.	150	4.5	23
Coconut Chocolate Walnut	175	7	24
Peach; Strawberry/Banana	145	3.5	25
Pineapple Almond	155	5	24
Toffee Bark	170	6	25
Vanilla	115	0.5	24
Diet Yogurt: Avg. all flav., 2 ½ oz	140	5	20

Braum's® cont..

Frozen Yogurt (Cont)	C	F	Cb
Fat Free, No Sugar Added Yogurt:			
Brownie Fudge Sundae	100	0	21
Strawberry; Vanilla Bean	90	0	18
Yogurt Bars No Sugar Added:			
Chocolate Choc. w. Almonds	160	10	15
Chocolate Coated Vanilla	155	9	15
Choc. Covered Vanilla/Almonds	320	18	34
Fudge Bars	95	0.5	21
Ice Cream: *Per ½ Cup*			
Light: Average all varieties	165	5	26
Premium: Black Walnut	200	11	21
Dream Cooler	315	9	55
Peanut Butter Cups	235	14	23
Strawberry	165	7	22
Average other flavors	190	9	25
Low Carb: Butter/Choc. Pecan, avg.	195	13	17
Other flavors, average	180	12	17
Ice Cream Bars: Ice Cream Cups	160	7.5	20
Chocolate Covered Vanilla	215	14	19
Ice Cream Sandwiches: Brownie	370	17	49
Vanilla	295	11	44
Cones, avg. all varieties	325	19	34
Twin Pops, 2.5 oz	60	0	15
Sherbet: Avg. all varieties	170	3	36
Muffins: Banana Nut; Blueberry	415	21	50
Carrot Walnut	500	27	56
Cherry Pecan	435	21	56
Strawberry	470	21	64
Pies: Cappuccino; Chunky Choc	235	9	34
Ice Cream, Choc Pecan	235	13	27
Mint Choc. Chip; Pumpkin	220	10	30
Strawberry Cheesecake	210	8	31

Briazz®

	C	F	Cb
Paninis: Chicken Mozzarella	605	27	58
Chicken Pesto	680	12	104
Pepperjack Smoked Turkey	625	17	72
Philly Cheesesteak	700	32	75
Sunflower Chicken	790	44	52
Tuscan Turkey	590	29	50
Rustic Slice Sandwich: *Per Sandwich*			
Low Fat Turkey, 8.3 oz	295	3.5	38
Smoked Turkey & Havarti	455	25	36
Turkey Breast & Provolone	355	11	35
Subzz: *Per Sandwich w. Dressing*			
Beef & Cheddar	490	19	51
Briazz Tuna 'n Cheese	625	30	53
Demi Tuna 'n Cheese	390	24	26
Ham & Swiss	475	13	57
Italian Ham, Salami & Provolone	605	27	59
Turkey Provolone	500	17	54

Briazz® cont..

	C	F	Cb
Cafe Salads: Greek Orzo	260	10	33
Chicken Breast w. Dressing	200	12	11
Classic w. Dressing; Parisian	160	11	11
Greek Island w. Dressing	290	24	10
Orzo Almondine w. Dressing	430	21	50
Tuna w. Dressing	240	16	8
Togas: *Per Package*			
Chicken Club	680	42	46
Chop Chop Veggie	545	24	63
Classy Tuna	640	33	46
Italian w. Italian Dressing	760	47	49
Smokin' Turkey Club w. Ranch Dr.	740	43	55
Southwest Turkey	600	27	46
Cakes, Muffins, Desserts: *Per Serving*			
Banana Muffin	520	26	64
Chocolate Marble Pound Cake	410	21	49
Classic Brownie	375	16	55
Iced Lemon Pound Cake	505	23	69
Mixed Fruit Cup	110	0	25
Sour Cream Coffee Cake Muffin	710	40	78
Yogurt & Lowfat Granola Parfait	510	6	100

Bruegger's Bagels®

	C	F	Cb
Bagels: Plain/Salt/Sesame/Garlic	310	2	61
Blueberry/Cranb. Or./Cinn. Raisin	340	2	68
Chocolate Chip	360	5	69
Everything/Onion/Sundried Tom.	320	2	65
Cream Cheese: Average, 2 oz	180	15	8
Light varieties, average, 2 oz	115	8	6
Hummus, 2 oz	120	7	8
Breakfast Sandwiches: *Per Sandwich*			
Egg & Cheese	480	15	66
Egg & Cheese & Bacon	560	22	66
Egg & Cheese & Ham	530	17	66
Egg & Cheese & Sausage	695	33	66
Sandwiches			
Bagel: Chicken Fajita	515	12	74
Atlantic Smoked Salmon	475	12	66
Garden Veggie	405	2.5	80
Herby Turkey	530	14	73
Santa Fe Turkey	490	10	71
Deli: Chicken Breast	450	6	62
Chicken Salad	470	12	67
Ham	445	4.5	77
Turkey w. Mayonnaise	485	14	65

Burger King®

Breakfast	C	F	Cb
Croissan'wich: Egg & Cheese	**315**	19	24
Bacon, Egg & Cheese	**360**	22	25
Ham, Egg & Cheese	**350**	20	25
Sausage & Cheese	**425**	31	23
Sausage, Egg & Cheese	**525**	39	24
French Toast Sticks, 5 sticks	**390**	20	46
Breakfast Syrup	**85**	0	21
Hash Brown Rounds: Large	**400**	25	39
Small	**235**	15	23
Sourdough w. Bacon/Egg/Cheese	**380**	22	30
Biscuit, Plain	**300**	15	35
Biscuit & Gravy, 7 oz	**425**	23	45
Jam, Grape/Strawberry, 1 pkg	**30**	0	7
Cini-Minis with Vanilla Icing	**540**	26	71
Burgers & Sandwiches			
Baguettes (Chicken), all types	**390**	4	57
Burgers: Bacon Cheeseburger	**390**	20	31
Bacon Double Cheeseburger	**575**	34	32
BK Veggie Burger (with mayo)	**385**	16	46
without mayonnaise	**305**	7	46
Cheeseburger	**355**	17	31
Double Cheeseburger	**535**	31	32
Double Hamburger	**440**	23	30
Hamburger	**305**	13	30
The Angus Bacon & Cheese	**795**	44	64
Low carb (no bun)	**495**	40	7
The Angus Steak Burger	**645**	32	62
Low carb (no bun)	**350**	28	5
Original Whoppers®			
Original Whopper	**710**	42	52
without mayonnaise	**545**	24	52
Low carb (no bun)	**280**	20	3
Original Double Whopper	**965**	61	52
without mayonnaise	**810**	44	52
Low carb (no bun)	**545**	40	3
Original Whopper JR	**390**	22	31
without mayonnaise	**310**	13	31
Low carb (no bun)	**140**	10	1
Tacos (1)	**170**	8	16
Chicken & Fish			
BK Fish Filet sandwich, no sauce	**355**	13	42
w. tartar sauce	**520**	30	44
Chicken Whopper	**570**	25	48
without mayonnaise	**405**	7	48
Low carb (no bun)	**165**	3	3
Grilled Chicken Caesar Club	**480**	13	55
Original Chicken sandwich	**560**	28	52
without mayonnaise	**460**	17	52
Spicy TenderCrisp Chicken S'wich	**755**	39	73
TenderCrisp Chicken S'wich	**825**	47	72
without mayonnaise	**605**	23	71

Burger King® cont..

Chicken Tenders: *No Dipping Sauce*	C	F	Cb
5 pieces	**210**	12	13
8 pieces	**340**	19	20
Dipping Sauces (1 oz): Barbecue	**35**	0	9
Honey Flavored	**90**	0	23
Honey Mustard	**90**	6	9
Ranch; Zesty Onion Ring	**145**	15	1
Sweet & Sour	**40**	0	10
French Fries: Small, 2.6 oz	**225**	11	29
Medium, 4 oz	**360**	18	46
Large, 5.6 oz	**500**	25	63
King Size, 6.8 oz	**595**	30	76
Onion Rings: Small, 1.8 oz	**175**	9	22
Medium, 3.2 oz	**320**	16	40
Large, 4.8 oz	**475**	23	60
King Size, 5.6 oz	**555**	27	70
Sides: Chili, 7.6 oz	**190**	8	17
Crackers, 0.2 oz	**20**	0.5	4
Salads (Without Dressing)			
Fire-Grilled: Chkn Caesar, no toast	**200**	7	9
Chicken Garden, no toast	**215**	7	12
Shrimp Caesar, no toast	**205**	10	9
Shrimp Garden	**225**	10	13
Side Garden Salad	**20**	0	4
Garlic Parmesan Toast, ½ oz	**70**	2.5	9
Salad Dressings: Gdn Ranch, 2 oz	**120**	10	7
Creamy Garlic Caesar, 2 oz	**135**	11	7
Hidden Valley Fat Free Ranch, 1.5 oz	**30**	0	7
Vinaigrette (Sweet Onion/Tom.), 2 oz	**110**	8	9
Desserts: Dutch Apple Pie	**340**	14	52
Hershey's Sundae Pie	**300**	18	31
Nestle Toll House Cookies (2)	**435**	16	68
Drinks & Shakes: Coffee, Medium	**5**	0	1.5
Coca-Cola/Sprite/Dr Pepper (with ¼ Ice):			
Kids	**90**	0	22
Small	**120**	0	30
Medium	**170**	0	42
Large	**250**	0	62
King	**320**	0	80
Icee (Coke/Minute Maid): Small	**370**	0	92
Medium, 20 fl.oz	**450**	0	113
Lowfat Milk (1%), 10 fl.oz	**105**	2	12
Milk Shakes (Choc./Strawb.): Small	**420**	13	69
Medium	**590**	18	97
Large	**860**	26	142
Orange Juice, 10 fl.oz	**140**	0	33

For Complete Nutritional Data ~ see CalorieKing.com

Captain D's Seafood®

Platters: Per Platter	C	F	Cb
Broiled Chicken	1015	8	194
Broiled Fish	1010	8	194
Broiled Fish & Chicken	1005	7	194
Broiled Shrimp	1030	8	195
***Lunches:** Per Lunch Platter*			
Broiled Chicken	490	9	63
Broiled Fish	425	7	63
Broiled Fish & Chicken	460	8	63
Broiled Shrimp	420	7	63
Stuffed Crab	155	6	16
***Sandwiches:** Per Sandwich*			
Broiled Chicken	445	18	29
Broiled Fish	520	18	51
***Desserts:** Per Slice*			
Carrot Cake	430	22	49
Cheesecake	425	31	30
Chocolate Cake	300	10	49
Pecan Pie	455	20	64

For Complete Nutritional Data ~ see CalorieKing.com

Caribou Coffee®

Drinks: Per Serving	C	F	Cb
Caramel Hirise, 16 fl.oz	400	13	59
Lite White Berry, 16 fl.oz	310	5	57
Mint Condition, 16 fl.oz	510	19	75
Turtle Mocha, 16 fl.oz	540	19	82
Cappuccino: 2% Capp, 12 fl.oz	120	4	13
Skim Capp, 12 fl.oz	80	0.5	11
Latte: 2% Latte, 12 fl.oz	125	4.5	13
Skim Latte, 12 fl.oz	90	0.5	12
Chai Latte: 2% Chai Latte, 12 fl.oz	210	4	38
Skim Chai, 12 fl.oz	150	0	32
Mocha: 2% Mocha, 12 fl.oz	260	12	30
Skim Mocha, 12 fl.oz	225	9	26
Coolers: Caramel Cooler, 12 fl.oz	345	9	64
Chocolate Cooler, 12 fl.oz	190	2	40
Coffee Cooler, 12 fl.oz	175	2	36
Espresso Cooler, 12 fl.oz	140	2	28
Mint Oreo Cooler, 12 fl.oz	520	17	83
Vanilla Cooler, 12 fl.oz	195	3	39
Hot Apple Blast: Medium	235	8	41
Large	270	8	50
Smoothies: Raspberry, 12 fl.oz	220	0	53
Strawb. Banana; Green Tea, 12 fl.oz	190	0	46
Wild Berry, 12 fl.oz	175	0	42
Skinny Bon Latte: Small	80	0	12
Low Carb, small	780	84	7

Carl's Jr.®

Burgers/Sandwiches	C	F	Cb
Carl's Bacon Swiss Crispy Chicken	740	28	91
Carl's Catch Fish Sandwich™	550	27	58
Carl's Famous Star® Hamburger	585	32	50
Charbroiled: BBQ Chicken S'wich™	365	4	47
Chicken Club Sandwich™	545	23	43
Santa Fe Chicken Sandwich™	610	32	43
Dble Sourdough Bacon Chseburger	920	59	45
Dble Western Bacon Chseburger®	920	50	65
Guacamole Bacon Chicken S'wich	600	24	56
Hamburger	280	9	36
Ranch Crispy Chicken Sandwich	660	31	72
Sourdough Bacon Cheeseburger	550	29	41
Spicy Chicken Sandwich	480	26	48
Super Star® Hamburger	790	47	52
The Six Dollar Burger™	1000	62	72
Chili Burger	690	35	57
Low-Carb Burger	490	37	6
Western Bacon Burger	1045	61	79
Western Bacon Cheeseburger®	660	30	64
Western Bacon Crispy Chkn S'wich	755	38	72
Potatoes: Plain, no marg.	280	0	63
Bacon & Cheese	635	29	71
Broccoli & Cheese	520	21	71
Sour Cream & Chives	420	14	65
Breakfast: Breakfast Burrito	550	32	37
Loaded Breakfast Burrito	810	49	53
Breakfast Bowl, Low Carb	900	73	5
Breakfast Quesadilla	380	18	38
French Toast Dip (6), no Syrup	450	20	59
Sourdough Sandwich, no meat	410	20	39
Scrambled Eggs & Bacon	745	42	69
Sunrise Sandwich, no meat	360	21	28
Bakery/Desserts: Chocolate Cake	300	12	48
Blueberry Muffin	340	14	49
Bran Raisin Muffin	395	14	61
Chocolate Chip Cookie, 2.5 oz	350	18	46
Strawberry Swirl Cheesecake, 3.5 oz	295	17	30
Side Orders: Chicken Stars, 9 pces	410	26	23
Chicken Breast Stips (5)	630	34	45
CrissCut Fries®, 5 oz	410	24	43
French Fries, small, 3.2 oz	295	14	37
Hash Brown Nuggets, 4 oz	330	21	32
Onion Rings, 4.5 oz	440	22	53
***Salads:** No Dressing*			
Charbroiled Chicken Salad-to-Go	265	7	17
Garden Salad-to-Go	60	3	5
Buffalo Ranch Chicken Salad	390	16	42

Carvel Ice Cream®

Soft Serve Ice Cream: Per Serving (4 fl.oz)	C	F	Cb
Regular: Average all flavors	195	10	22
Fat Free: Average all flavors	120	0	28
No Sugar Added Vanilla	130	3	25
Sherbet, assorted flavors	140	1	31
Novelties: 98% Fat Free	190	1.5	40
Mini Sundae	210	2.5	42
Fountain Beverages: *Per small*			
Thick Shakes: Chocolate	735	31	96
Vanilla	655	30	79
Reduced Fat: Chocolate	540	8	100
Vanilla	465	7	84
Fizzlers®, regular	350	4.5	75
Carvelanche™ w. Topping (8 oz)	600	30	71
Creammaccino: Classic, 16 fl.oz	410	24	36
Caramel Cream, 16 fl.oz	585	26	74
Mocha Fudge, 16 fl.oz	615	35	61
Coladas *(16 fl.oz):* Pina Colada	400	17	61
Banana; Peach avereage	365	10	68
Uptown Smoothies: *Per 16 fl.oz*			
Berry Times Square	310	0.5	75
Broadway Banana	205	0.5	49
Thinny-Thin: *Per Small*			
Berry Times Square	300	0	73
Broadway Banana	270	0	66
Grand Central Cooler	260	0	63

For Complete Nutritional Data ~ see CalorieKing.com

Charley's Grilled Subs®

Grilled Sandwiches: *Regular w. Cheese & Dressing*	C	F	Cb
BBQ Cheddar	785	43	68
Bacon 3 Cheese Steak	940	63	53
Buffalo Chicken	590	23	57
Chicken Bacon Club	605	26	53
Chicken Cordon Bleu	585	21	57
Chicken Philadelphia	590	25	55
Chicken Teriyaki	500	14	56
Grilled Veggie Delight	435	17	59
New York Deli	690	36	55
Philly Ham & Swiss	625	30	55
Philly Steak Deluxe	820	53	55
Philly Steak	820	53	55
Steak Italiano	875	57	54
Turkey Breast	565	20	57
Ultimate Turkey Club	675	34	52
Gourmet Fries: *Per Regular Serving*			
Cheddar & Bacon	425	19	54
Cheddar Ranch & Bacon	780	56	57
Original	265	8	42
Ranch & Bacon	700	50	52
Fresh Salad: Garden, regular	300	22	13
Beverages: Natural Lemonade, reg.	170	0	40

Checkers®

~ Same Menu & Data as Rally's Hamburgers® See Page 240 ~

Cheesecake Factory®

Per Slice	C	F	Cb
Adam's P. B. Cup Fudge Ripple	940	59	95
Banana Cream Cheesecake	860	61	70
Brownie Sundae Cheesecake	960	62	96
Choc Chip Cookie Dough	1080	71	100
Dulce de Leche Caramel Ch/cake	1000	70	83
Kahlua Cocoa Coffee	840	55	80
Keylime Cheesecake	700	48	63
Original Cheesecake	640	45	55
Vanilla Bean Cheesecake	870	62	69
White Choc. Raspberry Truffle	900	60	80

Chevys Fresh Mex®

Burritos	C	F	Cb
Veggie w. Tortilla, Marinated Veges, San Antonio Veges, Pico de Gallo & Ranchero Sauce	430	19	49
Catch of the Day			
Fresh Fish, San Antonio Veges, Salsa & Tomalito	430	16	16
Fajitas			
Chicken w. San Antonio Veges & Tomalito	285	6	13
Shrimp w. San Antonio Veges & Tomalito	285	7	13
Veggie w. Marinated Veges, San Antonio Veges & Tomalito	345	28	16
Salad: *With Salsa Vinaigrette Dressing*			
Chicken, Grilled	535	18	53
Mixed Green	360	16	42
Sides			
Black Beans	60	0	11
Guacamole, 2 oz	105	10	3
Mexican Rice	210	3	39
Salsa for Chips, 5 oz	40	0	8
Sour Cream	120	12	2
Tortilla: Corn	80	1	17
El Machino	165	4	27

Chi-Chi's®

Low Fat Items	C	F	Cb
Acapulco Chicken	515	15	44
Chicken Enchilada	690	20	98
Santa Fe Grilled Chicken Salad	310	9	25
Chicken Soft Taco	605	15	88
Chicken Tortilla Soup	340	10	47

Chick-Fil-A®

Chick-Fil-A Sandwiches	C	F	Cb
Chicken Sandwich	**410**	16	38
Chargrilled Chicken Sandwich	**275**	3.5	33
Chargrilled Chicken, 1 fillet	**100**	1.5	1
Chicken Salad Sandwich	**350**	15	32
Cool Wraps®: Chicken Caesar	**440**	10	52
Chargrilled/Spicy Chicken, avg.	**395**	7	54
Breakfast: *Per Serving*			
Plain Biscuit	**265**	11	38
Hot Buttered Biscuit	**275**	12	38
Biscuit and Gravy	**315**	13	44
Biscuit: w. Bacon	**300**	14	38
w. Bacon, Egg & Cheese	**430**	24	38
w. Egg & Cheese	**395**	21	38
w. Sausage	**410**	23	42
w. Sausage & Egg	**495**	29	43
w. Sausage, Egg & Cheese	**540**	33	43
Danish (2), 4.6 oz	**430**	17	63
Hashbrowns, 3 oz	**170**	9	20
Salads: Chick-n-Strips® Salad	**385**	18	22
Chargrilled Chicken Garden	**180**	6	9
Southwest Chargrilled Chicken	**240**	8	17
Salad Dressing: *Per Packet (1.25 oz)*			
Caesar Dressing	**160**	17	1
Raspberry Vinaigrette	**80**	2	15
Bleu Cheese; Buttermilk Ranch	**150**	16	1
Fat Free Honey Mustard	**55**	0	14
Light Italian Dressing	**15**	0.5	2
Spicy Dressing	**135**	14	2
Thousand Island	**145**	14	5
Strips, Nuggets: Nuggets (8-pack)	**260**	12	12
Chick-n-Strips® (4-count)	**290**	13	14
Dipping Sauces: Polynesian, 1 oz	**105**	6	13
Barbecue; Honey Mustard, avg.,1 oz	**45**	0	10
Buffalo Sce, ¾ oz	**20**	1.5	1
Sides: Carrot & Raisin Salad, small	**170**	6	28
Fresh Fruit Cups, 4 oz	**60**	0	16
Coleslaw, small	**265**	21	17
Garlic and Butter Croutons, ½ oz	**50**	3	6
Side Salad	**55**	3	4
Tortilla Strips, 1 pkt, ½ oz	**70**	3.5	9
Waffle Potato Fries,small	**285**	14	37
Desserts: Cheesecake, 3.3 oz slice	**340**	21	30
Icedream® Cup, small	**230**	6	38
Icedream® Cone, small	**160**	4	28
Lemon Pie, 4 oz slice	**320**	10	51
Fudge Nut Brownie (1), 2.6 oz	**330**	15	45

Chili's®

Starters	C	F	Cb
Awesome Blossom w. Sauce	**2880**	222	191
¼ Whole w. Blossom Sauce	**720**	55	48
Boneless Buffalo Wings + Sauce	**1140**	74	64
Boneless Shanghai Wings	**1390**	84	90
Fajita Nachos: Chicken	**995**	36	94
Beef	**1130**	50	100
Buffalo Wings w. Dressing	**790**	66	5
Guiltless Grill®: Chicken Platter	**565**	9	83
Chicken Grill Pita	**545**	9	77
Chicken Sandwich	**535**	9	70
Tomato Basil Pasta	**670**	15	106
Burgers (No Fries): Ranch Burger	**1070**	66	64
Chipotle Bleu Chse Bacon Burger	**1120**	75	54
Grnd Peppercorn w. Strings, Dr.	**1200**	79	78
Bunless Burgers: Old Timer	**575**	38	11
Mushroom Swiss w. Mayo	**600**	38	14
Meals: Chili's Filet	**1215**	78	69
Bottomless Tostada Chips w. Salsa	**910**	46	109
Cajun Chicken Pasta	**1190**	56	103
Cajun Chicken Sandwich	**850**	41	77
Cheese Steak Sandwich (no Fries)	**740**	29	67
Chicken Caesar Pita (no Fries)	**520**	19	33
Citrus Fire Chicken & Shrimp	**660**	12	73
Country Fried Steak	**1335**	70	126
Flame Grilled Rib Eye	**1080**	66	70
Ginger Citrus Glazed Salmon	**710**	22	70
Grilled Baby Back Ribs	**1130**	54	109
Grilled Shrimp Alfredo	**1290**	53	142
Hawaiian Steak	**685**	13	88
Margarita Grilled Chicken	**725**	25	72
Margarita Grilled Tuna	**875**	25	97
South Western Egg Rolls	**830**	40	86
Veggie & Smoked Chse Quesadilla	**1160**	67	95
Fajitas: *Includes 3 Tortillas & Garnishes*			
Mushroom Jack	**1270**	60	103
Chicken	**1020**	41	97
Steak	**1070**	51	93
Knife & Fork Fajitas: *(w. veggies, sour cream, pico de gallo, guacamole)*			
Beef Chkn Fajita Combo, no tortilla	**600**	32	17
Chicken Fajitas, no tortilla	**555**	25	17
Salads: *Includes Dressing*			
Chicken Fajita Caesar Salad	**515**	24	11
Dinner Caesar Salad	**180**	15	5
Dinner House Salad w. Ranch	**320**	27	8
Desserts: Choc Chip Paradise Pie	**1250**	47	188
Molten Choc Cake	**1505**	67	207

For Complete Nutritional Data ~ see CalorieKing.com

Chipotle®

	C	F	Cb
Bol Salad: Per Bowl (no Rice or Tortilla)			
Burrito w. Beans: Meat & Chse	475	22	24
Meat & Corn Salsa	475	14	45
Meat & Sour Cream or Cheese	470	23	25
Meat & Tomato Salsa	395	13	29
Fajita w. Vege: Meat & Corn Salsa	435	21	28
Meat & Sour Cream or Cheese	435	30	8.5
Meat & Tomato Salsa	355	20	12
Vegetarian: w. Guacamole			
w. Beans/Corn Salsa	420	17	52
w. Beans, Tomato Salsa	340	16	36
Burrito Bol: with Rice & Beans			
Meat & Cheese	710	29	63.5
Meat & Corn Salsa	710	21	85
Meat & Sour Cream or Cheese	705	30	65
Meat & Tomato Salsa	630	20	69
Vegetarian w. Guacamole:			
Rice & Beans	545	23	70
Tomato Salsa	575	23	76
Corn Salsa	655	24	92
Fajita Burrito Bol: with Rice & Beans			
Meat & Corn Salsa	1040	30	139
Meat & Sour Cream	1040	39	119
Meat & Tomato Salsa	960	29	123
Vegetables: Meat & Cheese	675	36	46
Meat & Corn Salsa	670	28	68
Meat & Sour Cream or Cheese	670	37	48
Vegetables & Meat: & Tom. Salsa	590	27	52
& Cheese or Sour Cream	1005	45	100
& Corn Salsa	1005	37	122
& Tomato Salsa	925	36	106
Taco w. 4 Crispy Shells: Per Serving			
Meat, Corn Salsa: & Cheese	705	31	57
& Sour Cream	675	32	58
Meat, Tomato Salsa: & Cheese	600	30	41
& Sour Cream	595	31	42
Vegetarian Burrito: w. Rice, Beans & Guacamole			
Black Beans	880	32	124
Corn Salsa	990	33	146
Sour Cream	985	42	126
Tomato Salsa	910	32	130

CinnaMonster®

	C	F	Cb
Cinnamon Roll: Per Roll			
Caramel Pecan	840	32	120
Original	880	24	100

Chuck E. Cheese®

	C	F	Cb
Appetizers: Per Serving			
Blended Pizza Sauce, ¼ cup	35	0	7
Buffalo Wings, 4 pieces	220	15	1
Lamb Wesson French Fries, ckd, 4 oz	285	10	43
Sargento Mozzarella Sticks, 2	380	24	26
Sandwiches: Fries Not Included			
Grilled Chicken Sub	740	39	57
Ham & Cheese	770	41	60
Hot Dog	430	29	27
Italian Sub	770	47	52
Pizza (Medium): Beef, 2 slices	410	17	43
BBQ Chicken, 2 slices	410	13	51
Cheese, 2 slices	330	10	43
Pepperoni; Sausage, avg., 2 sl.	385	15	44
Breakfast: Per Serving			
Kellogg's Snack Um's: Cinn. Blast	140	5	24
Froot Loops; Rice Krispy, avg.	125	1	26
PCB Banana Loaf Cake (1)	350	11	50
PCB Cinn. Crumb Pound Cake (1)	385	17	55
Desserts: PCB Brownie (1)	380	18	46
PCB Choc Chunk Cookie (1)	410	19	56
PCB Original Krispy Treat (1)	340	9	50
Birthday Cake, Choc. or White, 1/12	210	11	25

Church's Chicken®

	C	F	Cb
Fried Chicken: Breast w. Skin, 1 pce	200	12	4
Leg w. Skin, 1 piece	140	9	2
Thigh w. Skin, 1 piece	230	16	5
Wing w. Skin, 1 piece	250	16	8
Krispy Tender Strips™, 1 piece	140	5	11
Tender Crunchers™, 6-8 pces	410	15	32
Side Items: Apple Pie, 3 oz	280	12	41
Honey Butter Biscuits (1)	250	16	26
Cajun Rice, regular, 3 oz	130	7	16
Chicken Fried Steak w. White Gravy	480	28	36
Cole Slaw, regular, 3 oz	100	6	8
Corn on the Cob, 1 ear	140	3	24
French Fries, regular	225	11	29
Mashed Potatoes & Gravy, reg.	90	3	14

Cinnabon®

	C	F	Cb
Classic	815	32	117
Caramel Pecanbon, 1 roll	1090	56	141
Minibon, 1 roll	335	13	49
MiniBon, Strawberry	250	5	45
CinnaPretzel	755	6	156
CinnaPoppers (3)	370	21	41
Cinnabon Stix (5)	350	11	54
Drinks: Frusia, 12 fl.oz	170	0	38
Mochalata Chill, 12 fl.oz	390	12	62

Coco's®

	C	F	Cb
3 Egg Omelette: California, 10 oz	**720**	60	5
Denver Cheese Omelette, 10 oz	**645**	51	6
Haystack Burger w. Chse & Sauce	**985**	54	82
Southern Style Chkn Strips, 11 oz	**940**	58	59
Cinn. Roll/French Toast, Combo	**1205**	76	96
Pot Roast Entree, 23 oz	**670**	28	65
Salads: Cobb Salad,14 oz	**510**	32	17
Oriental Chicken, 18 oz	**955**	57	86
Thai Chicken, 25 oz	**890**	53	65

Cosi®

	C	F	Cb
Pasta: Penne Marinara	**935**	4	190
Penne Pesto w. Chicken	**1510**	48	195
Penne a la Cosi	**1255**	34	194
Thai Chicken & Peanut Noodle	**1535**	45	208
Pizzas: Four Cheese	**950**	35	124
Meatlovers	**1280**	60	124
Spinach & Fresh Tomato	**905**	30	129
Sandwiches: Buffalo Blue	**700**	30	58
Cosi Club	**755**	38	62
Country Ham & Brie	**725**	35	71
Grilled Chicken TBM	**670**	29	58
Hummus & Fresh Vegetables	**435**	8	75
Sesame Ginger Chicken	**515**	7	71
Tandoori Chicken	**810**	34	78
Tuna & Cheddar	**940**	54	56
Turkey Light	**495**	8	75
Melts: Bacon Turkey Cheddar	**890**	39	79
Grilled Chicken Parmesan	**615**	19	60
Salads (No Dressing): Cobb	**460**	28	8
Bombay; Chicken Caesar, average	**310**	8	27
Caesar	**200**	6	25
Greek	**235**	17	10
Mixed Greens	**55**	1	9
Shanghai Chicken	**220**	5	16
Signature	**405**	21	39
Dressings (2 oz): Low-Fat	**85**	3	13
Balsamic Vinaigrette, Fat Free	**45**	0	11
Average other varieties	**330**	35	5
Desserts: Apple Pie, 14 oz	**990**	40	147
Caramel Coated Brd Pudding, 9 oz	**645**	31	84
Cheesecake, 8 oz	**740**	46	73
Dble Trouble Brownie Sundae	**1555**	77	198
Ice Cream, Double Scoop, 6 oz	**230**	14	22
Mud Pie, 9 oz	**915**	49	109
S'mmm...Oreos, for two, 7 oz	**850**	24	147
Sundae, medium, 8 oz	**410**	24	43

Cousins Subs®

	C	F	Cb
Cold 7 ½" Subs: *Per Sandwich*			
BLT	**615**	42	45
Club Sub	**745**	43	48
Club Sub, no mayo/cheese	**370**	6	48
Garden Veggie	**365**	11	49
Garden Veggie, no mayo/cheese	**245**	2	49
Genoa & Cheese	**730**	49	48
Ham, no mayo/cheese	**310**	5	47
Ham & Cheese	**645**	39	47
Provolone (Cheese) Sub	**690**	45	46
Regular	**685**	44	48
Roast Beef	**620**	36	46
Roast Beef, no mayo/cheese	**365**	8	46
Seafood with Crab	**560**	32	53
Tuna	**830**	60	46
Turkey Breast	**560**	32	48
Turkey Breast, no mayo/cheese	**305**	3	48
Hot 7 ½" Subs: *Per Sandwich*			
Cheese Steak	**540**	24	46
Double Cheese Steak	**850**	46	46
Chicken Breast	**620**	34	46
Chicken Breast, no mayo/cheese	**365**	6	46
Gyro	**680**	40	55
Hot Veggie; Italian Sausage, avg.	**490**	23	49
Meatball & Cheese	**585**	27	50
Pepperoni Melt	**785**	52	47
Philly Cheese Steak	**680**	36	50
Extras: Hot Dog	**300**	16	29
Italian/Wheat Bread, half loaf	**210**	3	42
French Fries, Medium	**400**	19	55
Soups: *Per Regular Serving*			
Cheese	**240**	16	18
Chicken w. Wild Rice	**230**	12	21
Chicken Dumpling; Clam	**170**	5	19
Chili	**250**	9	26
Cream of Broccoli w. Cheese	**190**	12	15
Cream of Potato	**190**	9	24
New England Clam Chowder	**150**	5	19
Salads: Chef Salad	**190**	10	7
Garden	**135**	8	7
Italian	**295**	25	15
Seafood	**175**	8	12
Side Salad	**70**	7	7
Tuna Salad	**310**	23	7

Cold Stone Creamery®

Sweet Cream Ice Cream	C	F	Cb
Like It, average	**390**	24	40
Love It, average	**660**	40	67
Gotta Have It, average	**920**	56	93
Cake Batter: Like It	**420**	23	48
Love It	**765**	39	80
Gotta Have It	**990**	54	112
Nonfat Frozen Yogurt: Like It, avg.	**220**	0	47
Love It, average	**390**	0.5	80
Gotta Have It, avg.	**545**	1	113
Italian Sorbet: Like It, avg.	**200**	0	50
Love It, average	**335**	0	84
Gotta Have It, average	**470**	0	118
Waffle Cone or Bowl	**160**	4	29

For Complete Nutritional Data ~ see CalorieKing.com

Culver's®

Butterburgers: Cheese, Single	**500**	31	32
Bacon Deluxe Double	**785**	51	35
Deluxe, Double	**700**	44	35
Double	**460**	23	32
Cheese, Double	**575**	32	32
Mushroom & Swiss Double	**590**	32	33
Sourdough Melt Double	**545**	26	37
Wisconsin Swiss Melt Double	**555**	27	36
Favorite Sandwiches: Chkn Filet	**515**	13	61
Beef Pot Roast	**340**	10	34
Chicken Salad	**665**	38	38
Grilled Chicken	**390**	11	46
Grilled Ham & Swiss	**405**	20	35
Norwegian Cod Filet	**625**	32	52
Philly Steak	**345**	21	43
Pork Tenderloin	**530**	27	72
Smoked Turkey	**315**	21	44
Turkey Sourdough BLT	**525**	24	38
Garden Fresh Salads: Club	**445**	21	24
Chicken Caesar	**410**	11	18
Chicken Cashew	**525**	29	21
Taco Salad	**700**	45	52
Side Salad, small	**35**	0.5	5
Fish & Chicken: Shrimp Basket	**1250**	63	119
Chicken Dinner, 2 pieces	**1660**	89	129
Chicken Tenders, 4 pieces	**390**	20	22
Norwegian Cod, 2 pce Basket	**1155**	58	120

Culver's® cont...

Sides	C	F	Cb
Cheese Curds	**600**	43	54
Chili Cheese Fries, regular	**620**	36	52
French Fries, regular	**355**	16	44
Mashed Potatoes & Gravy, small	**100**	5	32
Onion Rings	**395**	29	73
Desserts: Lemon Ice, 9 oz	**210**	0	46
Lemon Smoothie	**670**	28	94
Root Beer Float	**650**	18	116
Frozen Van. Custard: Dish, Single	**310**	18	32
Cake Cone, Single	**340**	18	38
Waffle Cone, Single	**410**	21	53
Sundaes: Turtle, 15.4 oz	**1245**	68	141
Caramel Cashew, small	**1185**	55	152
Hot Fudge Sundae, small	**1015**	65	91

D'Angelo's®

Sandwiches			
Number 9 Steak Sandwich: Pokket	**440**	18	36
Large	**940**	36	88
Chicken Stir Fry: D'Lite Pokket	**430**	10	45
Sub, small	**490**	11	57
Sub, large	**980**	22	114
Wrap	**510**	10	61
Classic Veggie: D'Lite Pokket	**380**	7	64
Wrap	**490**	14	69
Grilled Chkn Breast D'Lite Pokket	**395**	7	52
Italian: Sub, small	**645**	34	54
Sub, large	**1290**	68	108
Roast Beef: D'Lite Pokket	**360**	5	51
Sub, small	**355**	5	50
Sub, large	**710**	10	100
Steak: D'Lite Pokket, small	**480**	26	16
Wrap	**400**	13	41
Turkey: D'Lite Pokket	**515**	30	18
Sub, small	**495**	4	48
Sub, large	**990**	8	96
Salads: *No Dressing (Unless Indicated)*			
Asian Chicken Salad	**235**	4	23
Caesar Salad w. Dressing	**505**	39	23
Chef Salad	**275**	12	17
Chicken Stir Fry	**165**	3	10
Roast Beef	**155**	3	9
Lobster	**390**	27	11
Turkey	**160**	2	9

For Complete Nutritional Data ~ see CalorieKing.com

Dairy Queen®

Burgers/Sandwiches	C	F	Cb
BBQ Beef	**295**	9	37
BBQ Pork	**285**	8	36
Breaded Chicken Sandwich	**500**	27	47
Chili 'n' Cheese Dog	**330**	21	22
DQ® Homestyle: Hamburger	**290**	12	29
Bacon Double Cheeseburger	**610**	36	31
Cheeseburger	**350**	17	29
Double Cheeseburger	**540**	31	30
Ultimate Burger	**665**	43	29
Grilled Chicken Sandwich	**325**	16	25
Hot Dog, regular	**240**	14	19
Sides: Chkn Strip Basket w. Gravy	**1000**	50	102
Onion Rings	**475**	30	45
French Fries, medium	**375**	15	56
Salads: *With Dressing*			
Crispy Chicken w. Fat Free Italian	**460**	28	27
Grilled Chicken w. Fat Free Italian	**230**	9	13
Ice Cream Cones/Soft Serve			
DQ® Vanilla Soft Serve, ½ cup	**140**	4.5	22
DQ® Choc. Soft Serve, ½ cup	**150**	5	22
Chocolate Cone, medium	**345**	11	53
Dipped Cone, medium	**485**	24	59
Vanilla Cone, medium	**325**	9	53
Novelties: Buster Bar®	**455**	28	41
Chocolate Dilly® Bar	**215**	13	21
DQ® Fudge Bar, No Sugar Added	**70**	0	13
DQ® Sandwich	**195**	6	31
DQ® Vanilla Orange Bar, NAS	**75**	0	17
Lemon DQ Freez'r®; Starkiss®	**80**	0	20
Blizzards® & Sundaes			
Choc. Chip Cookie Dough, med.	**1030**	40	150
Oreo Cookie, medium	**700**	26	103
Chocolate Sundae, medium	**405**	10	71
DQ® Treatzza Cake® 1/8 cake	**370**	13	56
DQ® Treatzza Pizza™ 1/8 pizza	**180**	7	28
Royal Treats®: Banana Split	**525**	12	96
Peanut Buster® Parfait	**740**	31	99
Strawberry Shortcake	**435**	14	70
Drinks: Chocolate Shake, medium	**765**	20	129
Malts, medium	**890**	22	153
Misty Slushes, medium	**295**	0	74
MooLatte: Cappuccino	**460**	18	68
Mocha	**560**	23	80

For Complete Nutritional Data ~ see CalorieKing.com

Daphne's®

Meals	C	F	Cb
Chicken Kabob Lunch	**195**	9	2
Chicken Kabob Plate	**345**	13	8
Chicken White Meat	**365**	16	6
Humus & Pita, 4 oz	**260**	12	30
Humus Plate	**455**	21	51
Kids Chicken Kabob Plate	**145**	5	2
Salads: Greek Chicken Salad	**400**	18	9
Soup: Avgolemono	**85**	6	5
Extras: Feta Cheese, 2 Tbsp	**85**	7	1
Fire Feta, 2 Tbsp	**105**	9	2
Gyros, 4 oz	**380**	33	6
Pita Bread	**160**	1	32
Rice Pilaf	**265**	7	46
Salad Dressing, 1 Tbsp	**95**	9	2
Tzatziki Sauce	**75**	7	2

Davanni's®

Hoagies: *Per Half Hoagie (6"): Includes Mayonnaise*	C	F	Cb
Assorted	**405**	31	21
Chicken Breast	**495**	33	23
Chicken Parmigana	**385**	19	22
Club	**400**	27	22
Italian Sausage	**520**	37	28
Meatball	**465**	31	31
Mediterranean	**510**	38	22
Pastrami	**460**	27	22
Pizza	**315**	18	23
Cheese	**400**	29	21
Roast Beef	**385**	25	21
Salami	**485**	38	21
Tuna	**565**	44	24
Turkey	**370**	24	22
Vegie	**445**	29	29
Without Cheese ~ Deduct	**40**	3	0
Without Mayo ~ Deduct	**100**	11	1
Calzones: Average all varieties	**700**	35	66
Pizzas:			
Pepperoni & Vegie Works:			
Thin, 1 slice	**245**	12	18
Traditional, 1 slice	**295**	12	28
Solo	**775**	35	70
The Works: Thin, 1 slice	**250**	13	18
Traditional, 1 slice	**300**	14	28
Solo	**735**	32	70
Vegie Works: Thin, 1 slice	**210**	9	18
Traditional, 1 slice	**260**	9	28
Solo	**635**	22	70

Deep Dish ~ Similar to Traditional slice

Del Taco®

Breakfast	C	F	Cb
Breakfast Burrito	**235**	11	24
Bacon & Egg Quesadilla	**450**	23	40
Egg & Cheese Burrito	**465**	24	39
Macho Bacon & Egg Burrito™	**1030**	60	82
Steak & Egg Burrito	**600**	34	41
Hash Brown Sticks, 2.8 oz	**250**	19	20
Tacos: Big Fat Chicken Taco™	**340**	13	38
Big Fat Steak Taco™	**395**	19	38
Big Fat Taco™	**320**	11	39
Chicken Soft Taco	**210**	12	16
Steak Taco Del Carbon	**220**	11	19
Taco; Soft Taco, average	**160**	10	13
Ultimate Taco	**260**	17	13
Burritos: Combo Burrito™	**555**	22	61
Bean & Cheese Red/Green Burrito	**270**	8	38
Chicken Works Burrito	**540**	23	57
Del Beef Burrito™	**560**	30	42
Del Classic Chicken Burrito™	**585**	36	41
Deluxe Combo Burrito™	**600**	25	64
Deluxe Del Beef Burrito™	**605**	33	45
Half Pound Red/Green Burrito, average	**450**	12	65
Macho Beef Burrito™	**1155**	62	89
Macho Combo Burrito™	**1045**	44	113
Spicy Chicken/Veggie Works, avg.	**505**	17	68
Steak Works Burrito	**620**	31	58
Quesadillas: Cheddar	**490**	27	39
Chicken Cheddar	**575**	31	41
Spicy Jack Chicken	**560**	30	40
Spicy Jack	**480**	26	38
Salads: Deluxe Chicken Salad	**745**	34	77
Deluxe Taco Salad™	**795**	40	76
Taco Salad	**350**	30	10
Burgers: Cheeseburger	**330**	13	37
Double Del Cheeseburger™	**560**	35	35
Del Cheeseburger™	**430**	25	35
Nachos: Regular	**395**	24	40
Macho Nachos®	**1145**	63	113
Sides: Rice Cup, 4 oz	**140**	2	27
Beans 'n Cheese Cup, 7.7 oz	**265**	3	44
Fries: Chili Cheese, 10.5 oz	**685**	46	51
Deluxe Chili Cheese™, 12 oz	**720**	49	53
Large, 7 oz	**495**	32	47
Regular, 5 oz	**355**	23	34
Shakes: Chocolate, small, 11 fl.oz	**510**	12	89
Large, 15 fl.oz	**765**	16	117
Vanilla; Strawb., small 11 fl.oz	**410**	7	75
Large, 15 fl.oz	**550**	10	97

Denny's®

Breakfast	C	F	Cb
All American Slam®, no toast	**800**	67	3
Breakfast Dagwood, no toast	**1460**	90	81
Farmer's Slam, no syrup/marg.	**1250**	80	82
French Slam®, no syrup/marg.	**1160**	77	71
Grand Slam Slugger, no brd/pot.	**925**	55	74
Lumberjack Slam, no syrup/bread	**1020**	58	73
Moons Over My Hammy	**845**	51	42
Original Grand Slam®, no toast	**675**	49	33
w. Syrup & Margarine	**1030**	60	101
Scram Slam, no toast	**825**	68	8
Slim Slam (no topping/sides)	**400**	13	39
Extra Breakfast Items ~ See CalorieKing.com			
Soup: Chicken Noodle, 8 oz	**60**	2	8
Vegetable Beef, 8 oz	**80**	1	11
Sandwiches (No Fries/Sauces)			
Albacore Tuna Melt	**640**	39	42
BBQ Chicken	**1095**	62	86
BLT	**600**	38	50
Bacon Cheddar Burger	**910**	52	58
Boca Burger®	**630**	27	64
Buffalo Chicken Sandwich	**720**	28	80
Chicken Ranch Melt	**760**	45	44
Classic Burger	**700**	35	56
Club Sandwich	**645**	38	45
Grilled Chicken, no dressing	**495**	14	56
Ham & Swiss on Rye	**430**	16	39
Mushroom Swiss Burger	**900**	49	63
Patty Melt	**790**	50	37
The Super Bird® Sandwich	**485**	29	32
Turkey Breast on Multigrain	**290**	4	41
Appetizers/Entrees: *No Sides/Condiments*			
Buffalo Wings (9)	**860**	72	11
Buffalo Chicken Strips (5)	**740**	42	43
Chicken Strips (5)	**710**	33	56
Country Fried Steak	**645**	46	30
Fish & Chips	**955**	54	83
Fried Shrimp Dinner	**230**	10	18
Fried Shrimp & Shrimp Scampi	**350**	20	15
Buffalo Wings (9)	**860**	72	11
Grilled Chicken Dinner	**205**	5	15
Mozzarella Sticks (8)	**710**	41	49
Pot Roast Dinner w. Gravy	**290**	11	5
Roast Turkey & Stuffing w. Gravy	**505**	10	62
Sampler, no condiments	**1405**	80	124
Shrimp Scampi Skillet Dinner	**285**	19	3
Sirloin Steak Dinner	**330**	28	1
Steak & Shrimp Dinner	**645**	42	31
T-Bone Steak Dinner	**845**	65	0

Denny's® cont...

Sides	C	F	Cb
Bread Stuffing, plain, 3 oz	**100**	1	19
Carrots in Sauce, 3 oz	**40**	1	8
Corn in Butter Sauce, 3 oz	**100**	2	18
Onion Rings, 4 oz	**380**	23	38
Fries: Unsalted, 6 oz	**430**	20	57
Seasoned, 4 oz	**270**	12	35
Gravy, all types, average	**15**	0.5	2
Green Beans in Sauce, 3 oz	**35**	1	5
Potato: Baked, plain with skin, 5 oz	**225**	0	51
Mashed, 5 oz	**165**	7	23
Salads (No Dressing/Bread Unless Indicated)			
Albacore Tuna Salad	**570**	30	22
Fried Chicken Strips Salad	**470**	26	26
Grilled Chkn Caesar w. Dressing	**600**	41	20
Grilled Chicken Breast Salad	**270**	11	10
Side Caesar with Dressing	**360**	26	20
Side Garden Salad, no Dressing	**115**	4	16
Dressings & Sauces: BBQ Sce, 1.5 oz	**55**	1	11
Blue Cheese, 1 oz	**170**	18	1
Caesar; Ranch, 1 oz	**135**	14	1
French, regular, 1 oz	**105**	10	3
Honey Mustard, 1 oz	**215**	15	20
Italian Dressing, Low Calorie; Salsa	**15**	0.5	3
Marinara Sauce, 1.5 oz	**50**	2	7
Sour Cream, 1.5 oz	**95**	9	2
Tartar Sauce, 1.5 oz	**220**	23	3
Thousand Island, 1 oz	**120**	11	5
Desserts: Carrot Cake, 8 oz	**840**	45	99
Hot Fudge Brownie, 10 oz	**1015**	42	147
Pies (1/6 Whole): Apple, 7 oz	**485**	24	64
Cheesecake, no topping, 4 oz	**580**	38	51
Chocolate Peanut Butter, 6 oz	**665**	39	64
Sundaes: Banana Split	**930**	43	121
Single Scoop, no topping	**195**	14	14
Double Scoop, no topping	**385**	27	29
Dessert Toppings: Choc., 2 oz	**340**	25	27
Blueberry, 3 oz	**105**	0	26
Fudge, 2 oz	**210**	10	30
Strawberry, 3 oz	**115**	1	26
Drinks: Cappuccino, Orig., 8 fl.oz	**105**	3	17
Floats, Rootbeer/Cola, 12 fl.oz	**290**	10	47
Milkshake, Van/Choc., 12 fl.oz	**580**	26	76
Ruby Red Grapefruit Juice, 10 oz	**165**	0	41
Raspberry Iced Tea, 16 fl.oz	**85**	0	21

Dippin' Dots®

Ice Cream	C	F	Cb
Average all types, 5 oz	**190**	9	22
Red. Fat/No Sugar Vanilla, 5 oz	**120**	6	17
Fat-Free/No Sugar Fudge, 5 oz	**60**	0	14
Nonfat Yogurt, 5 oz	**110**	0	23
Flavored Ice, ½ cup, 2.6 oz	**90**	0	23
Flavored Sherbet, small, 5 oz	**100**	1	21
Vanilla; Strawb., large, 15 fl.oz	**550**	10	97

Donato's® Pizza

14" Traditional Pizza: *Per Slice (1/8 Large)*	C	F	Cb
Chicken Vegy Medley	**320**	9	42
Founders Fav.; The Works, avg.	**445**	20	45
Hawaiian; Serious Cheese, avg.	**400**	15	46
Mariachi Beef/Mariachi Chkn, avg.	**415**	15	46
Serious Meat	**475**	21	44
Vegy	**375**	13	47
Vegy (without Cheese)	**255**	3.5	45
Salads: Tuscan Chicken, no dress.	**210**	8	6.5
Tuscan Side Salad, no dressing	**95**	6	3
Tortilla Subs: Big Ham & Cheese	**400**	23	20
Big Don: Italian	**465**	30	19
Original	**400**	22	21
Sausage Italian	**740**	52	20
Sausage Original	**675**	44	22
Big Steak Hoagy, w. Sauce	**605**	41	19
Grilled Chicken Club	**615**	37	18
Low Fat Chicken Vegy	**280**	7	19
Roasted Vegy; Turkey	**415**	22	25
Steak & Cheese	**455**	22	20
Individual No Dough Pizza: *(Whole Pizza)*			
Chicken Vegy Medley	**495**	29	20
Classic Trio	**530**	37	18
Founder's Favorite	**565**	39	18
Hawaiian	**445**	27	28
Mariachi Beef	**555**	37	23
Mariachi Chicken	**495**	29	23
Pepperoni	**505**	35	16
Philly Cheese Steak	**525**	33	19
Serious Cheese	**460**	30	17
Serious Meat	**690**	49	18
Spinach	**530**	37	20
Vegy	**410**	25	22
White	**390**	26	15
Works	**560**	38	21

Domino's® Pizza

Classic Hand Tossed Pizza	C	F	Cb
Medium (12") Pizza: *Per 2 Slices (¼ Pizza)*			
Cheese Pizza (base only)	375	11	55
America's Favorite Feast	510	22	57
Bacon Cheeseburger Feast	550	26	55
Barbeque Feast	505	20	62
Deluxe Feast	465	18	57
Hawaiian Feast	450	15	58
MeatZZa Feast	560	26	57
Pepperoni Feast	535	25	56
Vegi Feast	440	16	57
Large (14") Pizza: *Per 2 Slices (¼ Pizza)*			
Cheese Pizza (base only)	520	15	75
America's Favorite Feast	710	30	78
Bacon Cheeseburger Feast	770	36	75
Barbeque Feast	700	27	85
Deluxe Feast	640	24	78
ExtravaganZZa Feast	780	36	80
Hawaiian Feast	630	22	80
MeatZZa Feast	760	34	78
Pepperoni Feast	740	34	76
Vegi Feast	620	22	78
Thin Crust Pizza			
Medium (12") Pizza: *Per 2 Slices (¼ Pizza)*			
Cheese Pizza (base only)	275	12	31
With Topping: Bacon	375	20	31
Beef	350	19	31
Cheddar Cheese	330	17	31
Pepperoni	350	19	31
X-tra Cheese & Pepperoni	400	23	32
Ham	300	13	31
Italian Sausage & Mushroom	360	18	34
Vegi (olive/mushr./onion/peppers)	340	17	34
Large (14") Pizza: *Per 2 Slices (¼ Pizza)*			
Cheese Pizza (base only)	380	17	43
With Topping: Bacon	530	30	43
Beef	490	27	44
Cheddar Cheese	450	23	44
Pepperoni	480	25	44
X-tra Cheese & Pepperoni	550	30	45
Ham	415	18	44
Italian Sausage & Mushroom	500	25	48
Vegi (olive/mushr./onion/peppers)	470	23	47
Personal Pizza (6"): *Per Pizza*			
Pepperoni	485	17	63
Pizza w. Cheese	420	11	63

Double Melt Cheese Pizza	C	F	Cb
12" Pizza: One Slice (⅛ Pizza)	320	16	32
½ Pizza (4 slices)	1280	64	128
Ultimate Deep Dish Pizza			
Medium (12') Pizza: *Per 2 Slices (¼ Pizza)*			
Cheese Pizza (base only)	480	22	56
With Topping: Bacon	580	30	56
Beef	560	29	56
Cheddar Cheese	540	27	56
Pepperoni	555	29	56
Ham	505	23	56
Italian Sausage & Mushroom	565	28	59
Vegi	550	27	58
Large (14") Pizza: *Per 2 Slices (¼ Pizza)*			
Cheese Pizza (base only)	675	30	80
With Topping: Bacon	830	43	80
Beef	785	40	80
Cheddar Cheese	745	36	80
Pepperoni	775	39	80
X-tra Cheese & Pepperoni	845	44	82
Ham	705	31	80
Italian Sausage & Mushroom	795	39	85
Vegi	765	36	83
Sides: Dots™, 1 oz	100	4	15
Breadstick, 1 stick	115	6.5	12
Cheesy Bread, 1 stick, 43g	125	6.5	13
Buffalo Chicken Kickers™:			
average 1 piece, 24g	47	2	3
10 pieces, 8.45 oz	470	21	32
Barbeque Wings, 1 piece	50	2.5	2
Hot Wings, 1 piece	45	2	0.5
Blue Cheese; Ranch Dress., 1.5 oz	220	23	2
Hot Sauce, 1.5 oz cup	15	0	4
Garlic Sauce	440	49	0
Marinara Dipping Sauce	25	0	5
CinnaStix®, 1 stick	125	6	15
Sweet Icing, 2½ oz cup	250	2.5	57

For Complete Nutritional Data ~ See CalorieKing.com

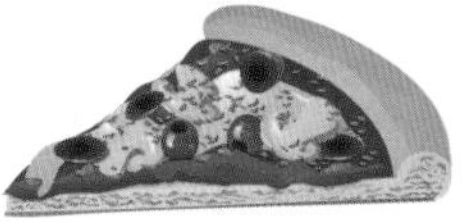

Don Pablos®

Appetizers: Per Serving	C	F	Cb
Beef Taquito (1), no garnish	65	6	5
Buffalo Chicken Wings (8)	1045	78	43
Chicken Flauta (1), no garnish	70	4	6
Nachos: Taco Beef	1625	113	85
Beef Fajita	1465	99	71
Chicken Fajita	1410	87	73
***Quesadillas:** Incl. Sour Cream & Guacamole (Whole)*			
Mesquite Grilled Chicken	1320	65	110
Mesquite Grilled Steak	1550	91	122
Portabello Mushroom & Veges	1525	83	136
Combo Grilled Chicken & Steak	1435	78	116
Combo Cheese & Vegetable	1440	81	120
***Dips:** Per Cup (No Chips)*			
Queso Blanco	345	27	13
Prairie Fire Bean w. Cheese	385	25	23
Spinach	320	28	8
Burritos (No Sides): Chicken	1090	42	114
Beef & Bean	1415	73	123
***Chimichangas:** Includes Rice & Refritos*			
Spicy Beef Chimi De Oro	1205	63	109
Chicken Chimi	1085	49	117
***Prime Combos:** Includes Everything on Plate*			
El Matador	1890	88	179
Conquistador (no rice)	1110	51	100
Primo Combo Chicken	1035	54	93
Primo Combo Steak & Chicken	1085	62	90
***Salads** (No Dress.):* Steak Fajita	630	35	27
Chicken Fajita	580	30	28
Traditional Taco Salad, average	1430	85	104
***Salad Dressing:** Per 3 oz*			
Blue Cheese	455	48	3
House Vinaigrette	345	31	10
Honey Mustard	300	27	17
Low Fat French	290	4	30
Ranch	330	34	3
Sides: Chips & Salsa, 1 order	345	17	43
Guacamole, 1.5 oz	60	5	2
Mexican Rice, 3 oz	100	1	21
Refritos, 5 oz	180	6	23
Salsa, 1 oz	5	0	1
Side Salad	110	7	8
Sour Cream, 1.25 oz	80	7	2
Sour Crema, 1 oz	60	5	1
Tortilla Shell	475	27	50

Dunkin Donuts®

Donuts	C	F	Cb
Apple/Blueberry Crumb Donut	240	10	36
Apple N' Spice Donut	200	8	29
Black Raspberry/Strawberry Donut	210	8	32
Blueberry Cake Donut	290	16	35
Boston Kreme Donut	240	9	36
Chocolate Coconut Cake Donut	300	19	31
Chocolate Frosted Cake Donut	360	20	40
Chocolate Frosted Donut	200	9	29
Chocolate Glazed Cake Donut	290	16	33
Cinnamon Cake Donut	330	20	34
Glazed Cake Donut	350	19	41
Jelly Filled Donut	210	8	32
Jelly Stick Donut	290	12	44
Kreme Filled (Choc./Vanilla)Donut	270	13	35
Lemon Cake Donut	240	14	28
Maple/Marble Frosted Donut	210	9	29
Old Fashioned Cake Donut	300	19	28
Powdered Cake Donut	330	19	36
Strawb./Van. Frosted; Bavarian	210	9	30
Sugar Raised Donut	178	8	22
Whole Wheat Glazed Cake Donut	310	19	32
Muffins: Banana Walnut	540	23	73
Blueberry: Regular	490	18	75
Reduced Fat	450	13	74
Chocolate Chip	585	23	85
Coffee Cake Muffin, 6.5 oz	710	29	102
Corn	515	17	81
Cranberry Orange	460	16	71
Honey Raisin Bran	490	14	81
Danishes: Apple	250	10	36
Cheese	270	14	32
Strawberry Cheese	250	12	33
Scones: Maple Walnut	470	22	62
Cinnamon Apple	460	19	67
Raspberry White Chocolate	460	22	59
Crullers: Plain Cruller	240	15	25
French Cruller	150	8	17
***Sandwiches:** Per Sandwich*			
Biscuit Sandwiches:			
Egg/Cheese Sandwich	360	20	31
Sausage/Egg/Cheese Sandwich	560	13	31
Croissant: Plain, each	330	18	37
Pizza; Spanish Cheese	520	35	33
Eng. Muffin S'wich:Ham/Egg/Chse	310	10	35

Continued Next Page . . .

Dunkin Donuts® cont...

Bagels: Per Bagel	C	F	Cb
Biscuit Bagel	**255**	13	29
Everything	**430**	7	75
Onion	**375**	4	71
Sesame	**455**	11	71
Salt; Plain	**360**	3	69
Cream Cheese (Per Packet): Lite	**130**	11	3
Average of other flavors	**180**	17	3
Cake Munchkins: Plain (4)	**270**	16	27
Cinnamon; Powdered, (4)	**250**	14	29
Coconut; Coconut Toasted (3)	**200**	12	23
Sugared (4)	**240**	14	28
Yeast Munchkins: *Per Serving*			
Glazed; Jelly Filled (5)	**210**	9	28
Lemon Filled (4)	**170**	8	23
Sugar Raised (7)	**220**	12	26
Cake Sticks: *Per Stick*			
Cinnamon	**455**	30	42
Glazed/Chocolate	**475**	29	50
Jelly	**260**	29	61
Plain	**420**	29	35
Powdered	**450**	29	42
Cookies: Chocolate varieties, avg. (1)	**220**	11	27
Oatmeal Raisin Pecan	**220**	10	29
Drinks: Dunkacinno, 10 fl.oz	**240**	10	35
Hot Chocolate, 10 fl.oz	**230**	8	38
Iced Coffee, 16 fl.oz	**5**	0	1
w. Cream, 16 fl.oz	**50**	6	1
w. Milk, 16 fl.oz	**15**	0	3
Vanilla Chai, 10 fl.oz	**235**	8	40
Coolatta®: Per 16 fl.oz			
Coffee Coolatta®: w. Cream	**370**	22	40
w. Milk	**220**	4	42
w. 2% Milk	**200**	2	41
Orange Mango Fruit Coolatta®	**270**	0	66
Strawberry Fruit Coolatta®	**290**	0	72
Vanilla Bean Coolatta®	**440**	17	70

Eat 'N Park®

Breakfast	C	F	Cb
Apple Waffles	**960**	45	126
Cornbeef Hash, 7.5 oz	**340**	23	17
Egg Beaters® Breakfast	**75**	0	5
Fruit Cup	**60**	0.5	15
Hash Browns, 6 oz	**235**	12	28
Homefries, 6 oz	**210**	12	24
Omelette: Cheese	**390**	30	2
Ham & Cheese	**465**	33	3
Supreme	**420**	30	9
Pancake, Plain (1)	**225**	3	43
Burgers: American Grill	**775**	50	31
Bacon & Cheese	**615**	36	33
Black Bean Burger	**780**	48	62
Cheeseburger	**540**	30	33
Classic Burger	**800**	50	40
Hamburger ⅓ lb	**495**	26	32
Mushroom & Onion	**875**	56	45
Southwest	**680**	37	57
Superburger	**705**	49	38
Swiss Burger	**570**	32	34
Swiss, Mushroom & Bacon	**870**	55	45
Turkey Burger	**500**	22	38
Sandwiches: Tuna Melt	**610**	41	35
Bacon Turkey Swiss	**525**	38	16
Chicken Bacon Deluxe	**565**	23	50
Chicken (Breaded)	**515**	20	50
Chicken Chargrill/Spicy, 4 oz	**320**	6	32
Chicken Fiesta, 4 oz	**325**	12	21
Dutch Ham & Swiss	**570**	31	36
Grilled Cheese	**505**	36	26
Hot Roast Beef	**290**	6.5	29
Hot Turkey	**255**	5	28
Reuben	**720**	49	31
Steak'n Cheese	**765**	51	43
Tuna Melt	**610**	41	35
Turkey Club	**775**	47	50
Turkey Pastrami	**715**	46	40
Croissants, Chicken Salad; Tuna	**595**	39	36
Pita: Chicken Fajita	**620**	19	69
Tuna	**640**	26	72
Turkey	**445**	5	68
Appetizers: Cheese Fries	**880**	50	93
Cheese Sticks	**410**	25	17
Onion Rings	**210**	13	20
Wings	**400**	28	0.5

Eat 'N Park® cont...

	C	F	Cb
Dinners: Chicken Breast, stuffed	**370**	17	28
Chicken Fillets (5)	**530**	26	28
Chicken Naturelle, small, 4 oz	**140**	3.5	0
Chicken Parmigiana, Meat	**900**	38	86
Chicken Stir-Fry	**555**	25	48
Country Fried Chicken Steak	**790**	41	43
Floridian Scrod, 4 oz	**120**	1.5	4
Rib Eye	**600**	42	1
Spaghetti Marinara	**620**	8	120
Veal Parmigiana w. Meat Sauce	**820**	27	108
Ziti w. Meat Balls & Meat Sauce	**960**	42	102
Salads & Dressings			
Buffalo Chicken Salad	**685**	42	42
Chicken Caesar Salad	**270**	9	16
Chicken Portabella Salad	**335**	13	22
Garden Salad	**100**	3	17
Steak Salad	**640**	39	35
Taco Salad	**820**	41	71
Dressings: Bleu Cheese, 2 Tbsp	**90**	7	7
French Fat Free	**70**	0	17
Italian Fat Free	**10**	0	3
House, 2 Tbsp	**115**	12	2.5
Thousand Island, 2 Tbsp	**95**	9	3
Desserts: Cheesecake	**505**	36	40
Banana Fudge Sensation	**975**	44	148
Grilled Sticky Loaf	**485**	28	53
Ice cream, 2 scoops	**285**	16	36
Pies: Apple (Reduced Fat)	**340**	11	62
Peach Lite	**300**	10	50
Pudding (Sugar Free)	**90**	2.5	13
Strawberry Shortcake	**685**	27	114

Edo Japan®

Meals: *Per Serving*	C	F	Cb
Beef Yakisoba	**585**	26	54
Chicken & Beef	**550**	17	68
Chicken Yakisoba	**425**	7	52
Curry Chicken Bowl	**490**	5	87
Ginger Pork	**510**	10	71
Grilled Vegetables	**330**	1	71
Hawaiian Chicken	**490**	7	71
Seafood Grill	**495**	8	73
Sukiyaki Beef	**625**	26	68
Teriyaki Chicken	**475**	7	68
Teriyaki Shrimp	**455**	6	72
Udon Soups: Beef or Chicken, avg.	**320**	11	36
Seafood	**280**	7	36
California Roll, 6 pieces	**250**	2	50

Einstein Bros®/Noahs®

	C	F	Cb
Bagels: Average, 4.2 oz	**350**	1	75
Chocolate Chip Bagel, 4 oz	**375**	3	76
Egg Bagel	**345**	3	69
Sesame Dip	**390**	5	75
Gourmet, average	**440**	6	78
Lower Carb 9 Grain	**245**	3.5	28
Cream Cheese: Plain, 2 Tbsp	**70**	7	1
Plain Reduced Fat, 2 Tbsp	**55**	5	2
Smoked Salmon, 2 Tbsp	**65**	6	2
Flavors, average, 2 Tbsp	**70**	5	5
Spreads: Fruit, 2 Tbsp	**75**	0	19
Honey Butter, 1 Tbsp	**90**	8	4
Peanut Butter, 2 Tbsp	**190**	15	8
Sandwiches: *Per Sandwich*			
Asiago Bagel Dog	**735**	34	78
Deli Roast Beef	**690**	26	76
Everything Bagel Dog	**730**	34	80
Challah: Club Mex	**750**	45	47
Cobbie	**625**	33	45
Deli: Chicken Salad	**490**	14	62
Egg Salad	**430**	20	45
Ham	**515**	25	43
Pastrami/Turkey	**495**	21	43
Tuna Salad	**380**	10	42
Lower Carb 9-Grain Bagel:			
Egg Salad Deli	**605**	41	41
Homestyle	**490**	20	31
Original Egg	**435**	17	31
Plain Bagel Dog	**595**	33	35
Tuna Salad	**390**	9	34
Turkey	**495**	17	40
Paninis: Cali Club	**765**	24	90
Italian Chicken	**775**	36	69
Taos Turkey	**775**	25	93
Salads: Mixed Greens, 3½ oz	**220**	18	13
Traditional Potato Salad, ½ cup	**285**	21	21
Soups: *Per Cup (6 oz)*			
Broccoli, Sharp Cheddar	**230**	15	13
Chicken Noodle	**215**	9	17
Chicken & Wild Rice	**190**	3.5	29
Clam Chowda	**165**	11	11
Lowfat Minestrone	**180**	4.5	27
Tomato Bisque	**200**	10	23
Turkey Chili	**135**	4.5	14
Cookies: Chocolate Chunk, 4 oz	**655**	31	87
Oatmeal Raisin, 4 oz	**600**	27	82
Coffee: Cafe Latte, 12 fl.oz	**135**	5	13
Cappuccino, 12 fl.oz	**90**	3.5	9

El Pollo Loco®

Flame-Grilled Chicken	C	F	Cb
Breast w. skin, 4 oz	**185**	7	0
Leg, 2 oz	**85**	3	0
Thigh, 2 oz	**120**	7	0
Wing, 2 oz	**80**	3	0
Tortillas: 6" Corn, 3 oz	**205**	3	42
6.5" Flour, 3 oz	**355**	12	48
Burritos: Bean, Rice & Cheese	**520**	18	70
Chicken Lover's	**515**	21	46
Classic	**610**	21	72
Spicy Chicken	**550**	22	56
Twiced Grilled	**1130**	56	93
Ultimate	**1030**	44	115
Bowls: Chicken Caesar Salad	**540**	29	45
Pollo Bowl	**550**	10	83
Veggie Bowl	**575**	15	90
Favorites: Cheese Quesadilla	**705**	43	43
Chicken Nachos	**1590**	102	88
Chicken Quesadilla	**760**	43	44
Chicken Soft Taco	**280**	15	17
Chicken Taquitos	**450**	21	48
Taco Al Carbon	**145**	4	18
Salads: Chicken Caesar, no dress.	**240**	10	16
w. dressing	**555**	43	18
Chicken Fiesta, no dressing	**585**	36	27
w. dressing	**890**	68	30
Chkn Tostada w. Shell/ Sour Crm	**775**	33	83
Monterrey, no dressing	**210**	7	15
w. dressing	**295**	14	20
Side Dishes: Cole Slaw, small	**200**	16	12
Corn Cobbette, small	**45**	0	10
French Fries, small	**440**	19	61
Garden Salad, small	**175**	12	8
Pinto Beans, small	**160**	4	24
Spanish Rice, small	**155**	1	33
Tortilla Chips, small	**415**	21	50
Condiments: Guacamole, 2 oz	**55**	4	5
House/Spicy Chipotle Salsa, 1 oz	**5**	0	1
Jalapeno Hot Sauce, 1 pkt	**5**	0	1
Sour Cream, 2 oz	**100**	10	2
Pico de Gallo Salsa, 1 oz	**20**	1	2
Desserts: Churros, 2 oz	**180**	11	18
Foster's Freeze without cone, 5 oz	**180**	5	30

For Complete Nutritional Data ~ see CalorieKing.com

Fatburger®

	C	F	Cb
Burgers: Baby Fat	**295**	13	25
Bacon & Egg Sandwich	**440**	27	31
Chicken Sandwich	**400**	15	32
Chili Dog	**510**	26	45
Fatburger	**600**	34	39
Fatburger w. Cheese	**625**	36	38
Kingburger	**825**	46	56
Kingburger w. Cheese	**1020**	58	65
Turkey Burger	**590**	33	41
Shakes: *Per 21 fl.oz*			
Chocolate Shake	**920**	43	115
Strawberry Shake	**850**	41	103
Vanilla Shake	**810**	44	85
Fries & Sides: Chili Cup, 7.2 oz	**345**	23	14
Fat Fries, 7.6 oz	**540**	26	70
Skinny Fries, 5 oz	**515**	26	65
Onion Rings, 6.1 oz	**235**	23	56

For Complete Nutritional Data ~ see CalorieKing.com

Fazoli's® Italian Food

Italian Specialities: *Per Serving*	C	F	Cb
Six Layer Lasagna w. meat sauce	**615**	26	63
Baked Chicken Alfredo	**775**	29	82
Baked Chicken Parmesan	**745**	20	99
Baked Spaghetti Parmesan	**680**	25	76
Broccoli Fettucine Alfredo, Reg.	**815**	23	125
Broccoli Lasagna 6 Layer	**695**	30	70
Cheese Ravioli w. Marinara	**480**	15	65
Cheese Ravioli w. Meat Sauce	**495**	17	65
Classic Meaty Ziti, Small	**370**	27	32
Regular	**575**	42	49
Classic Sampler w. 6 Layer Lasagna	**785**	25	108
Pizza Baked Spaghetti	**750**	31	78
Shrimp & Scallop Fettuccine	**595**	16	81
Twice Baked Lasagna	**810**	40	67
Twice Baked Ziti with Meat Sce	**660**	51	50
Ultimate Sampler Platter	**1000**	37	123
Pizza: *Per Double Slice*			
Cheese	**465**	15	58
Combination	**595**	25	63
Pepperoni	**550**	22	61
Soup & Breadstick: Breadstick (1)	**95**	1	17
Minestrone Soup	**105**	1	23

Fazoli's® cont...

Pasta: Per Serving	C	F	Cb
Fettucine Alfredo: Small	525	15	80
Regular	775	22	119
Fettucine Broccoli Alfredo	550	15	85
Garden Style Chicken Penne	790	28	100
Peppery Chicken Alfredo	590	16	80
Spaghetti w. Marinara: Small	410	6	74
Regular	600	8	111
Spaghetti w. Meat Sauce: Small	425	8	74
Regular	625	11	111
Spaghetti w. Meatballs: Small	710	31	80
Regular	1010	42	119
Spicy Marinara Penne w. Chicken	975	13	178
Salads & Dressings: Chicken Caesar	415	29	17
Chicken & Pasta Caesar	345	13	33
Chicken Finger	195	9	8
Chicken Finger w. Bacon & Honey Mustard Dressing	400	28	17
Garden, no dressing	30	0	6
Italian Chef, no dressing	300	21	13
Pasta, no dressing	575	25	70
Side Pasta	235	10	29
Dressings: Honey French	145	12	9
House Italian	100	9	5
Reduced Calorie Italian	55	5	3
Ranch	155	17	1
Thousand Island	135	13	4
Paninis: Chicken Caesar Club	675	35	51
Chicken Pesto	515	20	51
Four Cheese & Tomato	720	43	55
Ham & Swiss	605	30	53
Italian Club	670	37	54
Italian Deli	695	35	61
Smoked Turkey	700	38	57
Submarinos: Per ½ Sandwich			
Club	1085	44	121
Ham & Swiss	990	37	120
Meatball	1265	59	128
Original	1170	55	124
Pepperoni Pizza	1110	40	133
Turkey	960	34	121
Desserts: Lemon Ice	180	0	45
Milk Chocolate Chunk Cookie	375	15	54
Strawberry Topping, 28g	30	0	8
Cheesecake: Chocolate Chip	315	22	22
Plain	290	22	17
Turtle	435	34	24
Freezi: Strawberry	515	6	115
Strawberry Banana	525	6	118
Triple Berry	520	6	116

Firehouse Subs®

Subs: Per Medium	C	F	Cb
Chicken Salad	890	54	57
Engine Co	375	4.5	53
Engineer	370	3.5	56
Hero	445	7	55
Honey Ham	395	8	55
Hook & Ladder	370	5	54
Italian	625	33	55
La France	530	18	54
Roast Beef	670	32	55
Steak Sub	760	43	59
Tuna Sub	870	52	62
Turkey	350	3	53
Veggie Sub	730	44	61

Frisch's Big Boy®

Same Menu & Data as Big Boy

Freshens®

Yogurt Smoothies: Per 21 oz	C	F	Cb
Blueberry Sunset	385	0.5	84
Jamaican Jammer	475	1	110
Peachy Pineapple	405	1	91
Pina Collider	560	4	126
Raspberry Rapture	515	1	121
Raspberry Rocker	490	1	113
Strawberry Squeeze	390	0.5	88
Tropical Fruit Juice Smoothies: Per 21 oz			
Blueberry Wave; Caribbean Craze	330	0.5	84
Peach Sunset; Raspberry Rumba	365	0.5	93
Pineapple Passion	420	4	100
Raspberry Rhapsody	345	0.5	88
Strawberry Shooter	245	0	63
Orange Smoothies: Per 21 oz			
Aruba Orange; Orange Wave	420	3.5	97
Orange Shooter	370	3	81
Orange Sunrise	415	3	90
Coffee Smoothies: Per 21 oz			
Original Coffee	340	3.5	70
Caramel Coffee	425	4	89
Mocha Coffee	375	3.5	79
Oreo® Coffee	520	11	96
Decadent Smoothies: Per 21 oz			
Fudge Oreo® Supreme	640	11	126
Peanut Butter Cup	930	34	141
Pretzel Logic Pretzels (½), 3 oz	255	3	49
Freshen® Farms Ice cream, ½ cup	150	6	21
MET-Rx® Performance Supplements			
Protein Booster, 1 scoop, 10g	35	0	0
Soy Booster, 1 scoop, 16g	60	0.5	5
Average other varieties, 1 sachet	5	0	1

Gino's East®

	C	F	Cb
Deep Dish Pizza: *Medium 11" ~ Per Slice (⅙ Pizza)*			
Cheese	**410**	11	58
Crumbed Sausage	**420**	21	38
Pepperoni	**445**	15	57
Spinach	**405**	11	59
Deep Dish Pizza: *Small 6" ~ Per Whole Pizza*			
Cheese	**360**	8	58
Crumbed Sausage	**420**	21	38
Pepperoni	**380**	10	58

Gold Star Chili®

	C	F	Cb
Meals: *Per Serving*			
Cheese Coney	**345**	18	31
Cheese Fries	**525**	32	44
Chili	**215**	12	8.5
Chili Bean	**275**	10	22
Chili Cheese Fries	**595**	36	46
Chili Cheese Nacho	**420**	26	31
Chili Cheese Sandwich	**285**	13	30
Chili Salad	**675**	39	55
Chili Sandwich	**210**	5.5	32
Coney	**290**	14	31
Regular 2-Way	**415**	11	59
Bean	**280**	12	20
Onion	**260**	12	20
Onion Bean	**285**	12	20
Regular 3-Way	**645**	30	59
Regular 4-Way	**665**	30	63
Regular 5-Way	**735**	31	76
Super 5-Way	**1140**	51	109
Tex Mex	**220**	9	17
Veggie Chili Bowl	**165**	2	29
Sides: *Per Serving*			
Fries, 5.2 oz	**365**	19	44
Garlic Bread, 1.9 oz	**215**	13	20
Garlic Bread w. Cheese, 2.4 oz	**270**	18	20
Side Salad, 3 oz	**70**	5	2

Golden Corral®

	C	F	Cb
Meals: Bourbon Street Chkn, 3.5 oz	**210**	11	5
Fish Fillet w. Cajun style, 2 pces	**210**	9.5	18
Fresh Fried Chkn, Leg or Thigh (1)	**245**	19	2
Meatloaf, 3.5 oz	**195**	10	10
Sirloin Steak, Buffet, 3 oz	**215**	13	0
Steakburgers, Lunch, 6 oz	**715**	55	0
Turkey Breast w. Wing, 2 oz	**70**	3	1
Whitefish w. Cajun, 3 oz	**105**	7	0
Sides: Baked Potato, plain (1)	**110**	0	25
Carrot & Raisin Salad, ½ cup	**115**	5	17
Macaroni Salad, ½ cup	**190**	8	26

Godfather's™ Pizza

	C	F	Cb
Golden Pizza: *Per Slice*			
Cheese: Mini, ¼ pizza	**145**	4	20
Medium, ⅛ pizza	**215**	8	26
Large, 1/10 pizza	**165**	9	28
Combo: Mini, ¼ pizza	**195**	8	21
Medium, ⅛ pizza	**275**	13	27
Large, 1/10 pizza	**200**	15	30
Original Pizza: *Per Slice*			
Cheese: Medium, ⅛ pizza	**245**	7	34
Large, 1/10 pizza	**355**	15	37
Combo: Medium, ⅛ pizza	**340**	14	36
Large, 1/10 pizza	**280**	9	36
Thin Pizza: *Per Slice*			
Cheese: Medium, ⅛ pizza	**190**	9	19
Large, 1/10 pizza	**200**	10	19
Combo: Medium, ⅛ pizza	**260**	14	21
Large, 1/10 pizza	**285**	16	21

(The) Great American Bagel Co®

	C	F	Cb
Bagels: Plain	**390**	1.5	85
4-Grain Honey; Cinn. Raisin	**420**	1.5	88
Apple/Blueberry Crumb, average	**570**	8	106
Banana Nut; Cheddar Herb, avg.	**410**	5	82
Blueberry; Onion; Strawberry	**380**	1	83
Cheddar Salsa	**430**	11	63
Cheese Twist	**740**	20	107
Chocolate Chip	**390**	4	75
Cinnamon Sugar; Egg	**390**	2	83
Cranb. Nut; P'nut Butter Choc Chip	**400**	6	72
Hot Tomazzo; Tomazzo	**360**	7	57
Jalapeno Cheddar	**330**	4.5	58
Pumpernickel; Pumpkin, average	**330**	1.5	72
Pumpkin Chocolate Chip	**350**	3.5	67
Spinach Herb	**300**	1	60
Stuffed Pepperoni	**500**	12	74
Stuffed Spinach	**720**	22	98
Sun-Dried Tomato Basil	**390**	1.5	77
Veggie; Whole Wheat; Salt	**340**	1	70
Other varieties, average	**370**	2	75

(The) Great Steak & Potato Company®

Sandwiches	C	F	Cb
Cheeseburger, Kids	**340**	19	20
Chicken Philly	**715**	34	64
Chicken Teriyaki	**760**	34	74
Ham Delight	**675**	31	64
Ham Explosion	**530**	15	63
Phillyburger	**610**	41	23
Rueben Philly	**670**	32	64
Super Steak	**710**	34	60
Turkey Philly	**640**	28	60
Veggie Delight	**700**	38	62
Sides: Bacon Bits, 15g	**35**	1.5	2
Cheese: Average all types, 1 oz	**110**	9	0
Chicken Nuggets, Kids	**185**	10	11
Fries: Kids, 11.5 oz	**960**	44	128
Small	**1125**	55	142
Regular	**1265**	62	159
Large	**2230**	109	281
Potato Skins, 7 oz	**755**	57	54
Potato, Plain, 10.5 oz	**240**	0	52
Meat: *Per Serving (Sides Not Included)*			
Chicken, 4 oz	**165**	7	6
Corned Beef, 3 oz	**75**	2.5	0
Gyro, 4 oz	**345**	29	14
Ham, 3 oz	**115**	4	4
Salami, 2 oz	**135**	11	1
Steak, 4.5 oz	**65**	7	0
Turkey, 4 oz	**90**	1	2
Salad: Chef	**310**	12	12
Tossed	**40**	0	8
Sour Cream	**80**	7	3
Vegetables: Broccoli, 3 oz	**25**	0	4
Other Vegetables, avg., 1 serving	**10**	0	2
Salad Dressings: *Per Serving*			
1000 Island, 1½ Tbsp	**185**	18	6
Lo-Fat Mayo, 1 Tbsp	**40**	1.5	6
Mayonnaise, 1 Tbsp	**145**	16	0
Sauces: Cheese, 2 oz	**75**	5	6
Red Pepper, 1 oz	**90**	7	6
Teriyaki Glaze, 1.3 oz	**45**	0	10
Tzatziki, 1 oz	**90**	9	1
Bun: Regular, 3.5 oz	**290**	3	55
Wheat Bun, 4 oz	**310**	4	56
Pita, 3 oz	**185**	2	36
Wrap, Tortilla, 2 oz	**125**	3	17
Drinks: *Medium, 16 fl.oz*			
Lemonade	**225**	0	56
Cherry ; Root Beer	**250**	0	62
Mountain Dew	**265**	0	66
Pepsi; Sierra Mist	**220**	0	55

Haagen-Dazs®

Ice cream: *Per ½ Cup*	C	F	Cb
Baileys Irish Crm; Cookies & Crm	**270**	17	23
Bananas Foster	**265**	15	28
Belgian Chocolate; Pecan Pie	**335**	21	29
Butter Pecan	**310**	23	21
Cafe Mocha Frappe	**310**	19	30
Cherry Vanilla; Strawberry, avg.	**240**	15	23
Chocolate; Coffee, avg.	**270**	18	22
Chocolate Cheesecake; Rocky Road	**300**	18	29
Chocolate Chocolate Chip	**305**	20	26
Chocolate Peanut Butter	**355**	24	27
Chocolate Raspberry Torte	**265**	15	29
Coffee Almond Swirl	**315**	21	27
Cookie Dough Chip; Van. Cherry	**310**	20	29
Cookies & Cream	**265**	17	24
Dulce De Leche; German Choc.	**290**	17	28
Macadamia Brittle; Mint Chip	**295**	20	25
Mango	**255**	14	28
Mocha Almond Fudge	**340**	23	28
Peanut Butter Fudge Chunk	**355**	23	25
Pistachio	**290**	20	22
Rum Raisin; Vanilla, avg.	**260**	17	22
Strawberry Cheesecake	**270**	16	28
Tres Leche; Vanilla Fudge, avg.	**290**	19	26
Vanilla Caramel Brownie	**300**	18	30
Vanilla Chocolate Chip	**305**	20	26
Vanilla Fudge/Brownie; Pralines	**300**	18	28
Vanilla Swiss Almond	**295**	20	24
Sorbet, average other flavors	**120**	0	30
Gelato: Cappuccino; Raspberry	**240**	7	40
Chocolate	**240**	8	37
Hazelnut	**260**	12	33
Frozen Yogurt: *Per ½ Cup*			
Choc. Fudge Brownie	**200**	2.5	35
Coffee; Vanilla; avg.	**200**	4.5	31
Dulce De Leche	**185**	2.5	35
Strawberry Fat Free	**145**	0	31
Strawberry Banana	**170**	2	35
Vanilla Raspberry Swirl	**165**	2.5	31

Ice cream Bars ~ See Page 37

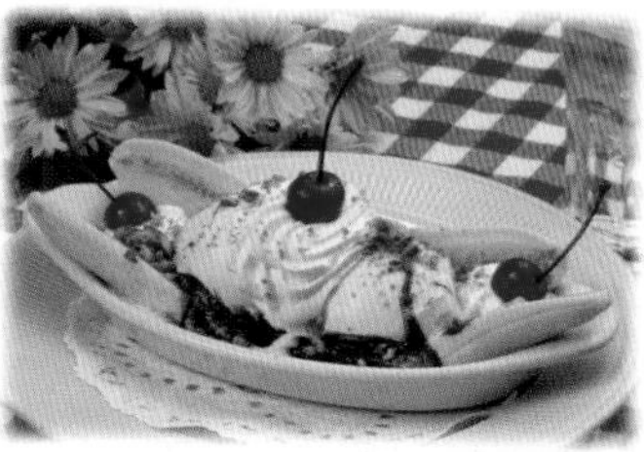

Hardee's®

Sandwiches	C	F	Cb
Bacon Cheese Thickburger ⅓ lb	900	63	50
Bacon Cheese Thickburger ⅔ lb	1330	96	60
Big Chicken Sandwich	770	36	73
Big Ham N Cheese	590	23	59
Big Roast Beef	475	23	38
Charbroiled Chicken	590	26	53
Cheeseburger ⅓ lb	675	39	51
Chili Cheese Thickburger ⅓ lb	870	54	55
Dble Bacon Chse Thickburger ⅔ lb	1290	96	51
Double Thickburger ⅔ lb	1230	90	53
Grilled Sourdough Thickburger ½ lb	1100	74	61
Hot Dog	420	30	22
Hot Ham N Cheese	440	18	39
Mushroom N Swiss Thickburger ⅓ lb	710	42	48
Regular Roast Beef	335	16	29
Six Dollar Burger ½ lb	1115	73	72
Slammer	235	12	19
w. Cheese	285	16	20
Spicy Chicken	440	22	46
Thickburger ⅓ lb	850	57	54
Low Carb: Thickburger ⅓ lb	420	31	5
Chicken Club Sandwich	425	24	11
Chicken: *Per Portion (edible portion, no bone)*			
Breast portion	365	15	29
Leg portion	175	7	15
Thigh portion	330	15	30
Wing portion	205	8	23
Sides: *Per Serving*			
American Cheese Slice, 25g	50	4	1
Chicken Strips (3)	385	21	27
Chicken Strips (5)	635	34	45
Chili Cheese Fries	705	39	67
Coleslaw, small, 4 oz	175	10	20
French Fries: Small, 4.4 oz	400	19	51
Medium, 5.2 oz	525	25	67
Large, 6 oz	610	29	78
Mashed Potato & Gravy, small	90	2	17
Breakfast Platters			
Bacon	975	56	90
Low Carb Breakfast Bowl	620	50	6
Breakfast Ham	965	52	90
Chicken	1145	61	105
Country Ham	970	53	90
Country Steak	1150	68	98
Dessert: *Per Serving*			
Apple Turnover	285	15	36
Chocolate Chip Cookie	290	11	44

Harvey's®

Main Menu	C	F	Cb
Big Harv	660	36	49
Big Harv w. Cheese	700	39	50
Big Harv Patty by Itself	405	29	7
Original Hamburger	355	18	32
Original Cheeseburger	405	21	32
Value Burger	300	13	30
w. Cheese	350	16	31
Hot Dog, 3.9 oz	315	12	39
Fish Sandwich	350	10	49
Harvey's Grilled Chicken	300	5	35
Harvey's Crispy Chicken	380	10	48
Chicken Nuggets, 2.3 oz	170	9	11
Veggie Burger, 3.2 oz	330	9	41
Crispy Fries: *Per Serving*			
Junior, 3.2 oz	290	15	34
Regular, 4.3 oz	380	20	45
Large, 5.3 oz	475	25	56
Onion Rings: Regular, 2.9 oz	285	20	23
Large, 4.3 oz	430	30	34
Side Orders: *Per Serving*			
Poutine, 10 oz	710	40	67
Gravy, 3 oz	45	0.5	9
Garden Salad	120	6	11
Caesar Salad	55	1.5	5
Chicken Caesar Salad	145	4.5	6
Chicken Garden Salad	210	8.5	12
Soup: Harvest Vegetable, 1 cup	120	1.5	25
Cream of Broccoli/Mushr., 1 cup	170	7	25
Chicken Noodle, 1 cup	100	1.5	17
Breakfast: Bagel, 4 oz	275	2	55
Breakfast Club Sandwich	310	15	26
Eggs (2): Fried	175	13	1
Scrambled Eggs	165	11	2.5
Hashbrowns	130	7	15
Home Fries, 4.6 oz	270	11	38
Muffins: Blueberry	375	19	62
Bran Muffin	435	17	57
Pancakes (2), 4 oz	225	3	42
Pancake Syrup, 1.4 fl.oz	165	0	42
Sausage	135	11	3
Toasted Western Sandwich	375	15	52
Dressings: Light Caesar/Italian	35	2.5	3
Average, other flavors	70	7	1
Desserts & Shakes			
Apple Turnover, 3 oz	245	15	25
Shakes: Choc.; Vanilla, 14.5 fl.oz	370	10	59
Strawberry, 14.5 fl.oz	355	9	56

Hogi Yogi®

Frozen Yogurt: Per ½ Cup	C	F	Cb
Chocolate Base, 2.5 oz	**80**	0	17
Vanilla (No Sugar Added): Base, 2.6 oz	**105**	0	22
Vanilla Base, 2.5 oz	**85**	0	18
Regular Sandwiches: Club	**335**	5	46
BBQ Chicken	**360**	4.5	59
Roast Beef	**310**	4.5	46
Smokey Turkey	**315**	3	46
Turkey	**325**	3	57
Vegetarian	**240**	2.5	45
Smoothies: *Per 24 oz*			
Berry Blast	**315**	0	70
Fruit Safari	**380**	3.5	84
Jungle Mist	**450**	4	101
Peach Treat	**450**	0	105
Pina Collision	**475**	4.5	105
Pure Passion	**450**	4	99
Ragin Rasberry	**385**	3.5	84
Strawberry Kist	**435**	0.5	98

Hot Dog on a Stick®

Menu Items	C	F	Cb
Hot Dog on a Bun	**470**	26	41
Hot Dog on a Stick	**250**	14	23
Veggie Dog	**175**	3	24
American Cheese on a Stick	**240**	13	22
Pepper Jack Cheese on a Stick	**240**	13	21
French Fries, 7 oz	**700**	37	83
Lemonade (12 fl.oz): Original	**140**	0	24
Cherry/Lime, average	**170**	0	42
Sugar Free Lemonade	**10**	0	2

Hot Stuff Pizza®

Pizza	C	F	Cb
Per Slice (⅛ Medium or 1/10 Large)			
Beef	**380**	15	39
Breakfast Pizza	**350**	21	36
Canadian Bacon	**340**	17	38
Cheese	**330**	11	38
Double Pepperoni	**420**	20	43
Garden Style	**360**	20	40
Italian Sausage	**400**	24	39
Masterpiece Supreme	**400**	19	40
Pepperoni	**370**	19	40
Pork Sausage	**410**	15	39
Western Omelet	**360**	21	37

Hungry Howie's Pizza®

Pizzas: Per Slice (Cheese Only)	C	F	Cb
Large, 1/12 of pizza	**175**	4	24
Medium, 1/10 of pizza	**160**	4.5	21
Small, ⅛ of pizza	**120**	2.5	17
Toppings: *Per Slice (For Medium or Large Pizza)*			
Bacon Only	**30**	0.5	0.5
Beef Only	**20**	1.5	0.5
Green Peppers Only	**5**	0	1
Ham Only	**5**	0.5	0
Mushroom Only	**5**	0	1
Olives Only	**5**	0.5	0.5
Onions Only	**10**	0.5	1
Pepperoni Only	**20**	1.5	0
Pineapple Only	**10**	0.5	1
Sausage Only	**20**	1.5	0.5
Sides: Howie Bread, Three Cheeser	**370**	13	47
Howie Wings, 6 wings	**180**	14	0

I Can't Believe It's Yogurt®

Original Frozen Yogurt: *Regular Serving (9 fl.oz)*	C	F	Cb
Awesome Amaretto	**280**	6	51
Cookies 'N Cream	**260**	3	54
French Vanilla	**260**	6	47
Peanut Butter Bliss	**310**	12	46
White Chocolate Mousse	**280**	7	49
Nonfat Frozen Yogurt: Regular	**220**	0.5	48
Small, 6.2 fl.oz	**160**	0.5	32
Nonfat *(with NutraSweet):* Regular	**190**	0.5	40
Small, 6.2 fl.oz	**140**	0.5	29

In-N-Out Burger®

	C	F	Cb
Burgers: Hamburger w. Onion	**390**	19	39
w. Mustard/Ketchup, no Spread	**310**	10	41
Protein Style, no Bun	**240**	17	11
Cheeseburger w. Onion	**480**	27	39
w. Mustard/Ketchup, no Spread	**400**	18	41
Protein Style, no Bun	**330**	25	11
Double Double® (2 patty/2 sl. chse)	**670**	41	39
w. Mustard/Ketchup, no Spread	**605**	32	41
Protein Style, no Bun	**520**	39	11
Grilled Cheese Sandwich	**470**	28	40
French Fries, 4.4 oz	**400**	18	54
Drinks: Milk, 10 fl.oz	**180**	6	18
Coca-Cola®; Dr. Pepper, 16 fl.oz	**200**	0	54
Lemonade, 16 fl.oz	**180**	0	40
Root Beer; Seven-Up® 16 fl.oz	**220**	0	54
Shakes, average all flavors, 15 fl.oz	**690**	36	83

For Complete Nutritional Data ~ see CalorieKing.com

IHOP®

Pancakes: (Syrup/Butter extra)	C	F	Cb
Buttermilk (1), 1.7 oz	**110**	3	17
Short Stack, 3	**330**	9	51
Full Stack, 5	**550**	15	85
Country Griddle Cakes (1), 2 oz	**120**	3.5	19
Harvest Grain 'N Nut (1) 2¼ oz	**180**	9	20
Crepe-Style, 2 oz	**120**	6	14
Syrup: 1 Tbsp	**50**	0	12
Whipped Butter, 1 Tbsp	**80**	9	0
Waffles (Plain): Regular (1), 3 oz	**310**	15	37
Belgian: Regular (1), 4 oz	**390**	19	48
Breakfast: *Per Serving*			
Classic Combos: Cntry Fried Steak/Eggs	**1530**	105	73
Fruity Country Griddle Cakes Combo	**960**	56	83
Harvest Grain 'N Nut Combo	**1035**	65	80
T-Bone Steak & Eggs	**1310**	86	63
Signature, Rooty Tooty Fresh & Fruity, average all flavors	**855**	45	84
Omlette Feast			
Colorado Omelette: No pancakes	**790**	68	5
with 3 buttermilk pancakes	**1205**	83	66
The Big Steak Omelette: No pancakes	**910**	72	14
with 3 buttermilk pancakes	**1325**	87	75
Burgers			
Sourdough Bacon Burger Melt:			
Burger Only	**690**	41	37
with French Fries	**1265**	74	104
with Onion Rings	**1230**	88	64
with Salad & 2 ½ T. Reg. Dress.	**870**	56	47
Entrees: Old Fashioned Pot Roast	**765**	48	30
with Mashed Potatoes	**965**	53	65
Signature Sampler	**1125**	67	14
Salad: Southwestern Chicken Fajita,			
with Tortilla Shell	**1090**	85	48
no Tortilla Shell	**870**	67	35

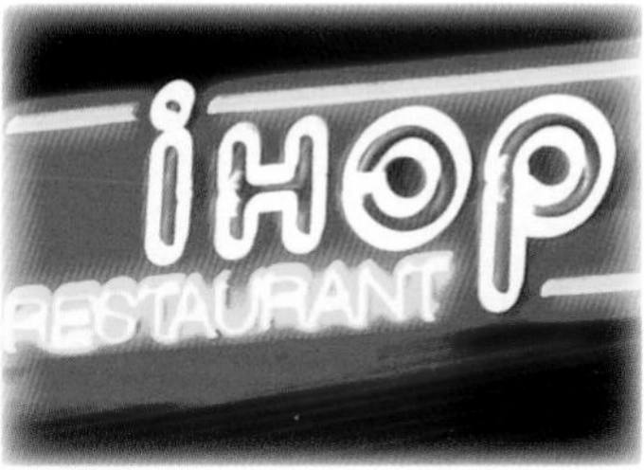

Jack's®

	C	F	Cb
Breakfast: Bacon Biscuit (1)	**290**	15	31
Biscuit (1)	**245**	11	31
Biscuit w. butter (1)	**350**	23	31
Bologna Biscuit (1)	**385**	24	32
Egg & Cheese Biscuit (1)	**550**	34	35
Eggs	**185**	13	3
Flapjacks	**365**	11	57
Gravy	**150**	11	11
Grits	**110**	8	8
Ham Biscuit (1)	**290**	13	31
Sausage, Egg & Cheese Biscuit (1)	**710**	48	35
Sausage Biscuit (1)	**400**	25	31
Steak Biscuit (1)	**430**	22	44
Chicken: Chicken Breast	**320**	19	9
Chicken Fingers (3)	**470**	24	33
Chicken Leg	**155**	10	5
Chicken Thigh	**260**	19	9
Chicken Wings	**170**	12	6
Pizzas			
Great Combinations (12"),			
Average all types, ¼ Pizza	**390**	18	40
Naturally Rising (12" Pizza),			
Canadian Bacon, ¼ pizza	**420**	14	51
Saus./Pepperoni/Bacon, avg., ¼	**510**	24	51
Naturally Rising (9" Pizza),			
Cheese, whole pizza	**900**	30	114
Saus./Pepperoni, avg., whole	**1200**	56	116
The Works Original (12" Pizza),			
Average all types, ¼ pizza	**300**	14	29
Original (9" Pizza), avg., whole	**760**	36	74
Pizza Bursts, avg. all types, 1 pce	**40**	2	4.5
Jack's French Fries: Regular	**250**	9	38
Medium	**355**	13	55
Mega	**455**	17	69
Sandwiches: Big Bacon	**700**	42	45
Big Jack	**505**	27	40
Cheeseburger	**380**	17	35
Chicken Fillet	**635**	31	69
Double Big Jack Cheese	**935**	60	43
Double Cheeseburger	**595**	33	37
Grilled Chicken	**410**	15	44
Hamburger	**270**	8	35
Side: Brown Gravy, 1 oz	**10**	0	2
Coleslaw, 4 oz	**215**	16	17
Green Beans, 4 oz	**20**	0	5
Mashed Potatoes, 4 oz	**65**	0.5	15
Desserts: Apple/Lemon Pie, avg.	**250**	10	37

Jack in the Box®

Breakfast	C	F	Cb
Biscuit	**190**	9	24
Breakfast Jack®	**310**	14	34
Extreme Sausage Sandwich	**720**	53	35
French Toast Sticks, 4 pces	**550**	18	89
Hash Brown	**150**	10	13
Sausage Biscuit	**540**	36	41
Sausage Croissant	**605**	41	42
Sausage, Egg & Cheese Biscuit	**915**	68	50
Sourdough Breakfast Sandwich	**450**	26	37
Supreme Croissant	**470**	27	41
Ultimate Breakfast Sandwich	**610**	31	58
Country Crock Spread	**25**	3	0
Grape Jelly, 1 packet	**35**	0	10
Syrup	**130**	0	32
Burgers: Hamburger	**315**	14	30
Hamburger w. Cheese	**360**	18	31
Bacon Bacon Cheeseburger	**780**	50	50
Bacon Ultimate Cheeseburger	**1030**	71	53
Big Cheeseburger	**700**	40	59
Big Texas Cheeseburger	**610**	32	55
Deluxe Hamburger, no Cheese	**385**	21	32
Ultimate Cheeseburger	**945**	65	52
Jumbo Jack®: Regular	**600**	35	52
w. Cheese	**690**	42	55
Philly Cheesesteak	**580**	22	55
Sourdough Jack®	**700**	51	36
Sandwiches: Chicken Chipotle	**380**	18	29
Chicken Fajita Pita	**300**	9	33
Chicken Sandwich	**410**	21	39
Chicken Supreme	**710**	39	62
Grilled Chicken Fillet	**430**	22	34
Jack's Spicy Chicken®	**620**	31	62
Roasted Turkey Sandwich	**580**	25	50
Sourdough Grilled Chicken Club	**500**	27	35
Ultimate Club Sandwich	**615**	29	52
Pannido: Deli Trio w. Sauce	**650**	35	53
Ham & Turkey w. Sauce	**620**	30	54
Zesty Turkey w. Sauce	**755**	44	51
Salads: *Includes Dressing*			
Asian Chicken Salad	**605**	33	58
Chicken Club	**825**	62	34
Greek Salad	**690**	50	32
Side Salad	**150**	7.5	16
Southwest Chicken	**685**	44	46
Salad Dressing: Ranch, 2.5 oz	**390**	41	4
Low Fat Balsamic Viniagrette, 2.5 oz	**40**	2	6
Mayo-Onion Sauce, 1/3 oz	**65**	7	1
Lite Ranch, 2.5 oz	**180**	18	3
Croutons, ½ oz	**60**	2	10

Snacks	C	F	Cb
Onion Rings, 4.2 oz	**500**	30	51
Bacon Cheddar Potato Wedges	**620**	41	45
Chicken Breast Strips, 8 oz	**640**	38	39
Curly Fries: Medium, 4.4 oz	**410**	23	45
Large, 6 oz	**550**	31	60
French Fries: Medium, 5 oz	**410**	20	55
Large, 7 oz	**570**	28	77
Egg Rolls, 1 piece, 2 oz	**180**	6	26
Fish & Chips	**845**	56	69
Monster Taco	**240**	14	20
Monster Chicken Taco	**180**	8	18
Stuffed Jalapenos, 3 pieces	**230**	13	22
Taco	**150**	8	15
Condiments			
American, Swiss Cheese, avg., 1 slice	**45**	3.5	1
Dipping Sauce: Buttermilk, 1 oz	**130**	13	3
Frank's Red Hot Buffalo®, 1 oz	**10**	0	2
Marinara, 1 oz	**15**	0	3
Barbeque; Sweet & Sour, 1 oz	**45**	0	11
Tartar	**210**	22	2
Packet Sauce: Ketchup; Salsa	**10**	0	2
Mayonnaise	**150**	17	0
Mustard; Soy Sauce	**5**	0	1
Taco	**0**	0	0
Sour Cream	**60**	6	1
Desserts			
Apple Turnover	**320**	16	41
Cheesecake	**310**	16	34
Double Fudge Cake	**310**	11	49
Ice Cream Shakes: *Per 16 fl.oz*			
Chocolate	**860**	38	117
Strawberry Banana	**700**	28	100
Oreo Cookie	**880**	44	107
Vanilla	**735**	38	85
Drinks: Barq's Root Beer®, 20 fl.oz	**180**	0	50
Coca-Cola Classic®, 20 fl.oz	**170**	0	46
Dr Pepper®; Minute Maid, 20 fl.oz	**190**	0	49
Orange Juice, 10 fl.oz	**140**	0	32

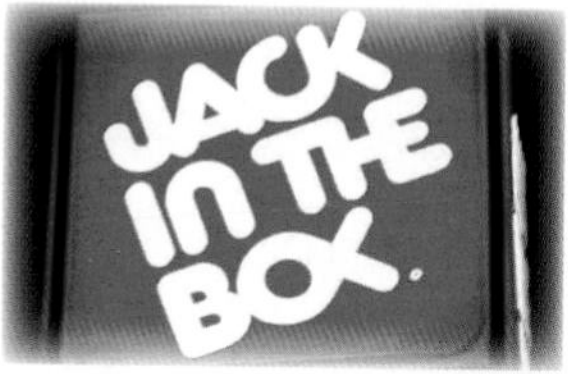

Jamba Juice®

Smoothies: Per 24 fl.oz	C	F	Cb
Aloha Pineapple™	515	1.5	117
Banana Berry™	480	1.5	112
Berry Fulfilling	300	1	64
Berry Lime Sublime®	455	2	106
Caribbean Passion™	440	2	102
Chocolate Moo'd™	730	8	148
Citrus Squeeze™	480	2	110
Coldbuster®	440	2.5	100
Cranberry Craze®	445	0.5	104
Endless Lime	610	2	140
Jamba Powerboost®	450	1.5	103
Kiwi Berry Burner™	470	0	112
Lime It UP	530	2	126
Mango-A-Go-Go™	440	1.5	104
Mango Mantra	335	1	71
Orange-A-Peel	440	2	102
Orange Berry Blitz™	420	2.5	94
Orange Divine	300	1	63
Orange Dream Machine®	540	2.5	111
Peach Pleasure®	465	2	108
Peanut Butter Moo'd™	885	22	149
Peenya Kowlada®	690	5	152
Protein Berry Pizzazz™	460	1.5	92
Razzmatazz®	480	2	112
Strawberries Wild®	450	0.5	105
Strawberry Nirvana	300	1	64
Strawberry Tsunami	545	2	128

16 fl.oz Size: Deduct 33% from figures of 24 fl.oz
32 fl.oz Size (Power): Add 50% of figures for 24 fl.oz size

Baked Items	C	F	Cb
Grin N' Carrot, 3½ oz	250	10	36
Honey Berry Bran, 4 oz	320	12	48
Lemon Poppyseed Bundt, 3½ oz	300	12	44
Pizza Protein Stick, 2.7 oz	230	6	33
Pretzels: Apple Cinnamon, 5 oz	410	5	78
Sourdough 'n Parmesan, 5 oz	460	11	75

For Complete Nutritional Data ~ see CalorieKing.com

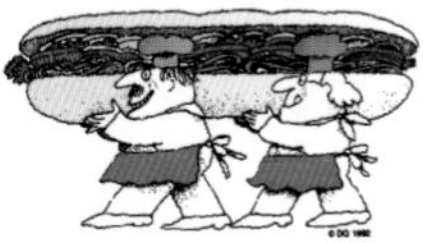

Jimmy John's®

Club Sandwiches	C	F	Cb
Figures based on 8" French Bread, Mayo, Chse, Sce			
Beach Club	900	47	79
Billy Club	845	42	75
Bootlegger's Club	695	29	71
Club Lulu Club	750	35	72
Country Club	780	39	74
Hunter's Club	780	39	74
Italian Night Club	950	54	75
Smoked Ham Club	830	42	73
Tuna Club	790	35	80
Veggie Club	1020	59	79
Low-Carb Club Unwich: *Deduct 345 calories, 68g Carb*			
Gargantuan™ Sandwich: Reg.	1070	57	75
Low-Carb Unwich	760	57	7
Plain Slim: *Figures based on 8" French Bread without Mayo/Sauce*			
Bacon	490	11	70
Double Provolone	545	16	71
Ham & Cheese	510	12	70
Roast Beef	400	2.5	69
Salami & Capicola	595	20	71
Tuna	570	20	74
Turkey Breast	385	0.5	69
Low-Carb Plain Slim Unwich: *Deduct 340 calories, 68g Carb*			
Subs: *Figures based on 8" French Bread, Mayo, Chse, Sce*			
Big John	550	28	52
JJBLT	630	37	53
Sorry Charlie	500	20	59
The Pepe	665	38	54
Turkey Tom	540	26	53
Vegetarian	720	43	58
Vito	555	24	56
Low-Carb Sub Unwich: *Deduct 245 calories, 50g Carb*			
Sides: Provolone Cheese, 1 oz	100	8	1
Real Guacamole, ½ oz	21	1	22
Grey Poupon Dijon Mustard, ½ oz	15	1	1
Hellman's Mayonnaise, 1.1 oz	230	25	0
Italian Vinaigrette, ⅓ oz	30	4	0

For Complete Nutritional Data ~ see CalorieKing.com

Johnny Rockets®

Original Hamburgers	C	F	Cb
#12	860	57	51
Chili Size	925	56	59
Original Burger	620	35	44
Patty Melt	945	60	51
Rocket Double	1250	84	57
Rocket Single	900	57	56
Route 66	900	61	45
Smoke House	1110	59	70
St Louis	1000	61	53
Streamliner	450	16	50
Sandwiches: Chicken Club	895	50	62
Bacon, Lettuce and Tomato	540	33	44
Egg Salad	705	49	40
Grilled Breast of Chicken	620	29	54
Grilled Cheese	535	31	42
Grilled Ham & Cheese	460	17	48
Tuna Melt	840	54	42
Tuna Salad	735	46	41
Other Favorites: Hot Dog	430	23	39
Chicken Club Salad			
with Chicken Tenders	685	40	37
with Grilled Chicken Breast	455	25	8
Chicken Tenders	525	22	47
Chili Dog	580	33	46
Garden Salad	275	20	5
Extras: Bacon, 0.7 oz	100	7	0
Extra Patty, 3 oz	270	20	1
Chili, 2½ oz	170	15	3
Grilled Onions or Mushrooms, 1 oz	25	2	2
Starters: American Fries	545	23	77
½ Fries & ½ Rings	730	36	92
Cheese Fries, 10 oz	774	42	77
Chilli Bowl	675	59	12
Chilli Fries, 12 oz	730	40	76
Onion Rings, 6.8 o z	500	34	22
Desserts: Apple Pie	920	59	88
Hot Fudge Sundae	805	47	93
a la mode	260	16	26
Drinks (Medium): Rootbeer	170	0	43
Coke; Sprite	170	0	43
Lemonade	190	0	49
Float	420	26	42
Shakes: Chocolate, 20 oz	1085	60	120
Strawberry, 20 oz	815	48	82
Vanilla, 20 oz	1125	60	130
Extra for Malt	65	2	10

Kenny Rogers Roasters®

Chicken	C	F	Cb
½ Chicken: No Skin or Wing	315	10	1
w. Skin	515	28	2
¼ Dark Meat: No Skin	170	7	1
w. Skin	270	17	1
¼ White Meat: No Skin or Wing	145	2	1
w. Skin	245	11	1
Pies: Chicken Pot Pie	710	33	78
Pitas: BBQ Chicken	400	7	51
Chicken Caesar	605	35	34
Roasted Chicken	685	35	42
Turkey: Sliced Breast	160	2	0
Sandwiches: Chicken Tender Pita	610	38	45
Chicken Tender Sandwich	725	47	55
Grilled Chicken	525	30	42
Turkey	385	12	30
Meals: Chicken Breast Platter	945	54	88
Chicken Tender Platter	1300	83	109
Salads (No Dressing): Per Serving			
Chicken Caesar	285	9	18
Pasta	230	12	28
Roasted Chicken	290	10	19
Side	25	0	5
Sour Cream & Dill Pasta	230	16	20
Tomato Cucumber	125	2	10
Side Dishes: Chicken Tenders (3)	510	37	24
Cinnamon Apples	200	5	41
Cole Slaw	225	16	18
Corn Muffin	160	6	25
Corn: on the Cob	70	0.5	14
Cornbread Stuffing	325	19	34
Muffin	175	8	24
Sweet Corn Niblets	115	0.5	28
Creamy Parmesan Spinach	120	6	10
Honey Baked Beans	150	1	32
Italian Green Beans	115	8	10
Macaroni & Cheese	200	6	24
Potatoes: Baked Sweet	265	0	62
Garlic Parsley	260	12	37
Potato Salad	390	27	34
Real Mashed	295	14	39
Rice Pilaf	175	5	43
Steamed Vegetables	50	0	8
Zucchini & Squash Santa Fe	70	5	8
Soup: Chicken Noodle, 1 bowl	90	2	12
Chicken Noodle, 1 cup	55	1	7

KFC®

	C	F	Cb
Extra Crispy™: Breast, 5.7 oz	**470**	28	19
Drumstick, 2.1 oz	**160**	10	5
Thigh, 4 oz	**370**	26	12
Whole Wing, 1.8 oz	**190**	12	10
Hot & Spicy: Breast, 6.3 oz	**450**	27	20
Drumstick, 2.1 oz	**140**	9	4
Thigh, 4.5 oz	**390**	28	14
Whole Wing, 1.9 oz	**180**	11	9
Original Recipe®: Breast, 5.7 oz	**370**	19	11
Breast, no skin or breading	**145**	3	0
Drumstick, 2 oz	**140**	8	4
Thigh, 4.4 oz	**360**	25	12
Whole Wing, 1.6 oz	**145**	9	5
Crispy Strips, 3 pieces	**400**	24	17
Sandwiches: Honey BBQ	**300**	6	41
Original Recipe Chicken: w. Sce	**445**	27	22
without Sauce	**360**	13	21
Tender Roast Chicken: w. Sauce	**390**	19	24
without Sauce	**270**	5	23
Triple Crunch Chkn: without Sce	**540**	26	41
Twister Wrap	**670**	38	55
Zinger: w. Sauce	**675**	41	42
without Sauce	**540**	26	41
Entrees: Chicken Pot Pie, 13 oz	**770**	40	70
Boneless Wings (7)	**600**	28	49
Honey BBQ Wings, 6 pces	**540**	33	36
Hot Wings, 6 pieces	**450**	29	23
Kentucky Nuggets, 6 pieces	**285**	18	15
Popcorn Chicken: Large, 6 oz	**660**	44	37
Individual, 4 oz	**445**	30	25
Chicken Caesar Salad w. Dressing	**570**	38	23
Chicken BLT Salad w. Dressing	**400**	25	16
Side Dishes: Per Serving			
BBQ Beans, 4.8 oz	**225**	1	46
Biscuit, 2 oz	**190**	10	23
Coleslaw, 4.6 oz	**190**	11	22
Corn on the Cob (3") 2.9 oz	**75**	1.5	13
Green Beans, 4 oz	**55**	1.5	5
Macaroni & Cheese, 10 oz	**135**	6	15
Mashed Potatoes: w. Gravy, 4.8 oz	**120**	4.5	18
without Gravy, 3.8 oz	**110**	4	16
Potato Salad, 4.5 oz	**175**	9	22
Potato Wedges, small,3.6 oz	**245**	12	30
Desserts: Per Serving			
Colonel's Pies: Apple Pie Slice, 4 oz	**275**	9	45
Pecan Pie Slice, 4 oz	**370**	15	55
Strawberry Creme Pie Slice	**270**	12	37
Double Choc. Chip Cake, 2.7 oz	**400**	29	31
Little Bucket™ Parfaits:			
Chocolate Cream, 4 oz	**275**	13	37
Fudge Brownie, 3.5 oz	**265**	9	44
Lemon Creme, 4.5 oz	**400**	14	65
Strawberry Shortcake, 3.5 oz	**200**	6	34

Kilwin's®

Ice cream: Per ½ Cup	C	F	Cb
Black Cherry; Caramel Revel	**90**	0	23
Butter Pecan	**190**	13	16
Butter Pecan Yogurt	**130**	6	17
Chocolate	**170**	10	17
Chocolate Chip Cookie Dough	**190**	10	22
Chocolate Ripple	**100**	0	23
French Silk; Mud	**190**	11	20
Lemon/Raspberry Sorbetto	**100**	0	25
Old Fashioned Vanilla	**180**	9	20
Toppings: Caramel, 40g	**160**	4.5	31
Fudge, 40g	**110**	6	28
Fudge: Per Piece (1.5oz)			
Chocolate	**150**	4.5	30
German Chocolate	**160**	7	27
Heavenly Hash	**200**	11	24
Other varieties, average	**160**	5	29

For Complete Nutritional Data ~ see CalorieKing.com

Kolache Factory®

Kolaches: BBQ Beef	**180**	6	18
Bacon & Cheese	**180**	7	23
Bacon, Egg & Cheese	**345**	16	35
Club	**260**	9	35
Cream Cheese	**185**	7	25
Fruit	**190**	3	38
Ham & Cheese	**185**	7	23
Italian Chicken	**190**	7	23
Jalapeno & Cheese	**185**	7	25
Pizza	**205**	9	24
Polish	**515**	29	47
Ranchero	**375**	18	35
Sausage	**125**	5	17
& Cheese	**245**	11	29
& Egg	**390**	20	35
Croissants: Per Croissant			
Fruit, 149g	**515**	24	67
Ham & Cheese, 191g	**625**	39	45
Ham & Egg, 194g	**615**	38	46
Italian Chicken, 213g	**550**	32	46
Sweet Rolls & Buns			
Cinnamon Roll: Reg. (1), 4.8 oz	**460**	14	74
Mini (1), 3.5 oz	**225**	7	37
Cinnamon Twist (1)	**465**	29	45
Raisin Nut Roll (1)	**610**	24	89
Sticky Bun (1)	**450**	20	61

Kolache is a pastry roll with savory or sweet fillings.

Koo•Koo•Roo®

Rotisserie Chicken	C	F	Cb
Leg & Thigh, 4.8 oz	**300**	18	1
Breast & Wing, 6.5 oz	**345**	16	1
Half Rotisserie Chicken, 11.3 oz	**635**	34	2
Original Skinless Flame Broiled Chicken™			
3 Piece Original Dark, 5 oz	**320**	16	5
Original Breast, 4.1 oz	**190**	5.5	0
Roasted Turkey: Breast, sliced, 4 oz	**180**	8	0
Hand-Carved Turkey Sandwich	**600**	32	31
Traditional Turkey Dinner	**690**	29	67
Turkey Pot Pie (1)	**870**	44	83
Salads: *Per Regular (no Dressing)*			
BBQ Chicken Salad	**365**	15	22
Chicken Caesar Salad	**285**	11	13
Chinese Chicken Salad	**570**	29	39
Koo Koo Roo House Salad	**125**	4	17
Chicken Bowls (No Sce): Chargrill	**560**	19	57
Southwest	**580**	19	67
Spicy Ginger Garlic	**475**	6	63
Tostade (no shell)	**540**	22	45
Soup: Ten Vegetable, 5 oz	**100**	2	17
Sandwiches: BBQ Chicken w. Sce	**560**	12	71
Original Chkn Breast w. Dressing	**670**	29	63
Chicken Caesar w. Dressing	**795**	36	63
Wraps: Caesar Chicken	**755**	39	60
Chipotle Chicken	**910**	44	89
Sides: Baked French Fries, 5 oz	**250**	7.5	42
Baked Yams, 6 oz	**200**	0	47
Black Beans, 6 oz	**145**	2.5	23
Buffalo Wings (no sauce), 6 wings	**590**	28	42
Creamed Spinach, 5 oz	**115**	6.5	10
Mashed Potatoes, 6.5 oz	**190**	5	33
Macaroni & Cheese, 6 oz	**340**	17	32
Roasted Garlic Potatoes, 5 oz	**135**	4.5	22
Extras/Dressings			
Lahvash (flatbread), each	**60**	0	12
BBQ Vinaigrette, 2oz	**90**	4	14
Caesar Dressing, 1½ oz	**235**	26	1.5
Chinese Salad Dressing, 3 oz	**340**	26	26
Chipotle Sauce, 1 oz	**130**	14	0.5
Cranberry Sauce, 1 oz	**45**	0	11

For Complete Nutritional Data ~ see CalorieKing.com

Kohr Bros®

Frozen Custard: *Per ½ Cup*	C	F	Cb
Chocolate	**140**	6	18
Orange Sherbet	**105**	2	21
Vanilla	**130**	6	16

Krispy Kreme®

Doughnuts	C	F	Cb
Caramel Kreme Crunch	**360**	19	43
Chocolate Brownie Deluxe	**300**	17	33
Chocolate Glazed Cruller	**290**	15	37
Chocolate Iced Cake	**280**	14	36
Chocolate Iced Custard Filled	**305**	17	35
Chocolate Iced Glazed	**250**	12	33
Chocolate Iced Kreme Filled	**345**	20	38
Chocolate Iced w. Sprinkles	**270**	12	38
Cinnamon Apple Filled	**285**	16	32
Cinnamon Bun	**270**	16	28
Cinnamon Twist	**225**	9	33
Dulce de Leche	**295**	18	30
Glazed Blueberry	**335**	17	43
Glazed Chocolate Cake	**310**	15	41
Glazed Cinnamon	**210**	12	24
Glazed Cruller	**240**	14	26
Glazed Kreme Filled	**345**	20	38
Glazed Lemon Filled	**295**	16	35
Glazed Raspberry Filled	**310**	16	39
Glazed Sour Cream	**340**	18	42
Key Lime Pie	**325**	17	40
Maple Iced Cake	**270**	13	35
Maple Iced Glazed	**245**	12	32
New York Cheesecake	**325**	19	35
Original Glazed	**205**	12	22
Powdered Blueberry Filled	**290**	16	33
Powdered Cake	**285**	14	37
Powdered Strawberry Filled	**290**	16	33
Pumpkin Spice Cake	**340**	18	42
Sugar Coated	**200**	12	21
Traditional Cake Doughnut	**230**	13	25
Doughnut Holes, 4 pieces	**210**	10	29
Beverages: *Per Container*			
Frozen Double Chocolate Blend/w. Coffee:			
large, 20 fl.oz	**740**	26	116
medium, 16 fl.oz	**595**	21	93
Frozen Latte Blend: large, 20 fl.oz	**740**	26	114
medium, 16 fl.oz	**595**	21	91
Frozen Original Kreme Blend:			
large, 20 fl.oz	**750**	27	119
medium, 16 fl.oz	**600**	21	95
Frozen Original Kreme w. Coffee Blend:			
large, 20 fl.oz	**725**	24	117
medium, 16 fl.oz	**580**	19	94
Frozen Raspberry Blend:			
large, 20 fl.oz	**720**	22	123
medium, 16 fl.oz	**580**	18	99

For Complete Nutritional Data ~ see CalorieKing.com

Krystal®

Burgers/Sandwiches	C	F	Cb
B.A. Burger	470	27	39
w. Cheese	530	32	40
Double B.A. Burger	800	53	41
Krystal	160	7	17
Krystal Chik	240	11	24
Bacon Cheese Krystal	195	10	16
Cheese Krystal	185	9	17
Double Krystal	265	13	24
Double Cheese Krystal	310	16	26
Chili Cheese Pup	210	12	17
Corn Pup	265	19	19
Plain Pup	165	9	15
Fries: Chili Cheese	540	28	59
Regular	410	20	53
Small			
Chik'n Bites & Salad			
Chik'n Bites, small	305	19	16
Chik'n Bites Salad	310	20	12
Sides: Krystal Chili	205	7	22
Breakfast Items			
Krystal Sunriser	230	14	14
Biscuit & Gravy	280	14	34
Biscuit: Bacon, Egg & Cheese	385	23	33
Chik Biscuit	345	15	40
Plain Biscuit	270	13	33
Sausage Biscuit	475	33	33
Country Breakfast	660	42	46
Kryspers	190	13	17
Scrambler	445	26	33
4-Carb Scrambler: Bacon	370	29	4
Sausage	600	51	3
Desserts			
Apple Turnover, fried	225	10	31
Lemon Icebox Pie	265	9	41
Drinks: *Per Serving (16 fl.oz)*			
Coca-Cola Classic	160	0	40
Coca-Cola Classic, frozen	145	0	36
Diet Coke	0	0	0
Sprite	155	0	39

For Complete Nutritional Data ~ see CalorieKing.com

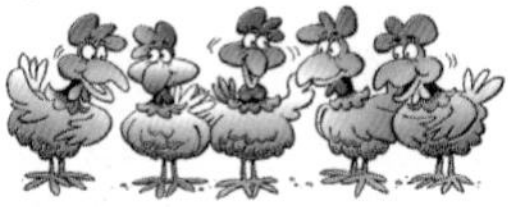

La Rosa's Pizzeria®

Pan Crust Medium Pizza: Per Slice	C	F	Cb
Blanca, 1/10 pizza	350	22	28
Cheese	300	16	30
Deluxe/Pepperoni Topper	370	21	31
Meat Topper	400	23	30
Veggie Topper	320	16	32
Traditional Crust Medium Pizza: *Per Slice*			
Blanca, 1/10 pizza	260	16	17
Cheese	200	10	19
Deluxe/Pepperoni Topper	280	16	20
Meat Topper	300	18	20
Veggie Topper	220	11	21
Calzones: *Per Calzone*			
3 Meat & 3 Cheese	1080	55	102
3 Veggie & 3 Cheese	860	34	105
Cheese	840	34	101
Cheese & Pepperoni	960	45	101
Philly Cheese Steak	865	39	90
Hoagy: *No Cheese/Dressing/Sauce*			
Baked Buddy, 8.7 oz	765	40	62
Baked Royal, 9 oz	595	22	62
Meatball, 11.7 oz	685	26	77
Original Steak, 11.3 oz	730	35	65
Philly Steak, 9.2 oz	615	25	64
Hoagy Dressing: Chse on Hoagy	220	18	0
Italian Dressing, 2 oz	320	34	3
Mayonnaise, 2 oz	400	11	0
Mushroom Sauce, 2 oz	20	0.5	3
Pizza Sauce, 2 oz	50	2	7
Tartar Sauce, 2 oz	260	24	11
Lite & Low Fat Menu			
Grilled Chicken Hoagy, low fat	520	9	56
Grilled Chicken Salad, low fat	380	10	40
Lite Deluxe Pizza, Medium, 1 slice	190	6	27
Minestrone Soup, 1 bowl	80	1	15
Pasta Dinner: *No Sides*			
Cheese Ravioli	675	26	80
Lasagna w. Meat Sauce	745	38	61
Meat Ravioli	725	22	102
Spaghetti: w. Meat Sauce	680	18	104
w. Meatballs	870	28	119
w. Traditional Sauce	640	12	113
Chicken Wings: BBQ Wings (12)	1295	77	48
Special Recipe Wings (12)	1270	87	21
Spicy Hot Wings (12)	1275	85	26

For Complete Nutritional Data ~ see CalorieKing.com

La Salsa Fresh Mexican Grill®

Appetizers	C	F	Cb
Nachos: Chicken	**1475**	83	129
Plain	**1375**	80	127
Burritos			
Bean & Cheese: Chicken	**735**	23	89
Plain	**605**	19	82
Steak	**755**	25	85
California: Chicken	**835**	36	97
Steak	**850**	38	93
Veggie	**795**	33	106
El Champion: Chicken	**1465**	55	180
Steak	**1490**	59	171
Grande: Chicken	**840**	37	99
Steak	**850**	39	95
Los Cabos Shrimp	**775**	36	78
Original Gourmet: Chicken	**655**	27	68
Steak	**675**	29	64
Sonora Mahi Mahi	**555**	22	57
Three Pepper Fajita: Chicken	**855**	37	86
Shrimp	**790**	36	80
Steak	**870**	39	82
Tacos: Baja Mahi Mahi	**415**	25	31
Baja Style Shrimp	**405**	21	44
Fajita: Chicken	**300**	13	26
Steak	**310**	14	23
La Salsa: Chicken	**295**	10	33
Steak	**305**	11	30
Mexico City: Chicken	**220**	5	31
Steak	**230**	6	28
Sonora Mahi Mahi	**225**	10	18
Meal Platters: *No Chips/Guacamole*			
Burrito Ranchero	**850**	31	295
Enchilada Platter	**870**	47	77
Steak Burrito Ranchero	**945**	36	109
Steak Enchilada	**695**	28	65
Taquitos: Chicken Quesadilla	**1740**	92	153
Plain Quesadilla	**1605**	88	146
Steak Quesadilla	**1750**	94	149
Three Pepper Fajita:			
w. Chicken & Corn Tortillas	**1150**	43	152
w. Steak & Corn Tortillas	**1170**	46	144
Two Soft Tacos: Chicken	**775**	25	111
Steak	**790**	27	105
Salads: Caesar w. Chicken	**660**	46	30

La Salsa Fresh Mexican Grill® cont...

Quesadillas	C	F	Cb
Classic: Chicken	**990**	59	64
Plain	**880**	55	57
Steak	**1030**	61	60
Grande: Chicken	**1165**	63	98
Steak	**1180**	65	94
Stuffed Fajita: w. Chicken	**920**	55	59
w. Steak	**1000**	61	58
Tacos: Baja Mahi Mahi	**375**	25	31
Baja Style Shrimp	**370**	25	45
Fajita Taco: w. Chicken	**260**	13	26
w. Steak	**270**	14	23
Mexico City Taco, average	**220**	6	30
Sonora Mahi Mahi	**200**	10	18
La Salsa, average	**275**	11	32
If Chips, Salsa added	**95**	4	11
Kids Plates: Nachos w. Beans	**700**	36	71
Burrito: Bean & Chse w. Beans	**875**	25	134
w. Rice	**655**	22	91
Quesadilla w. Beans	**700**	24	94
w. Rice	**450**	20	51
Taco: Chicken w. Beans	**450**	10	75
w. Rice	**335**	7	53
Steak w. Beans	**460**	11	75
w. Rice	**230**	6	28
Chips, Guacamole & Salsa	**970**	56	103
Sides: Nachos w. Beans	**1475**	81	143
½ Rice & ½ Beans	**440**	8	78
Black Beans	**500**	5	109
Rice	**155**	5	30
Corn Chips	**110**	7	10

LaMar's®

Bars: Caramel Iced, Unfilled	**430**	18	59
Chocolate Iced: Unfilled	**540**	22	81
Bavarian Cream Filled	**600**	22	96
Chocolate/White Fluff Filled	**800**	35	118
Bizmarks: Bavarian Cream	**620**	22	101
Blueberry/Lemon Filled	**530**	21	80
Cherry Filled	**550**	19	88
Donuts: Apple Spice Cake	**340**	17	44
Bluberry Cake	**350**	17	47
Chocolate Iced Cake	**330**	18	37
Old Fashioned Sour Cream	**420**	18	60
Ray's Chocolate Glazed	**290**	11	44
Ray's Original Glazed	**220**	10	31
White Iced Cake	**320**	17	38
Other Items: Apple Fritter	**650**	26	91
German Chocolate Knot	**480**	27	54
Cinnamon Roll	**690**	25	106
Cinnamon Twist	**770**	26	120
Raisin Nut Cinnamon Roll	**850**	27	137

Little Caesar®

Pizza: Per Slice	C	F	Cb
12" Round: Cheese, 1/8 pizza	185	6	23
Pepperoni, 1/8 pizza	205	7.5	23
12" Deep Dish: Cheese, 1/8 pizza	230	9	27
Pepperoni, 1/8 pizza	260	11	27
12" Thin: Cheese, 1/8 pizza	140	7	13
Pepperoni, 1/8 pizza	170	8.5	13
14" Round: Cheese, 1/10 pizza	200	6.5	25
Meatsa, 1/10 pizza	280	13	26
Pepperoni, 1/10 pizza	230	8	25
Supreme, 1/10 pizza	270	10	31
Veggie, 1/10 pizza	240	7.5	32
14" Deep Dish: Cheese, 1/10	320	12	37
Pepperoni, 1/10 pizza	350	14	38
14" Thin: Cheese, 1/10 pizza	160	7.5	14
Pepperoni, 1/10 pizza	180	9	14
16" Round: Cheese, 1/12 pizza	220	7	27
Pepperoni, 1/12 pizza	240	8.5	27
18" Round: Cheese, 1/14 pizza	230	7	30
Pepperoni, 1/14 pizza	260	9	30
Baby Pan! Pan!, 1 piece	360	16	34
Pizza By The Slice: Cheese (14"), 1/6	330	11	42
Pepperoni (14"), 1/6 pizza	390	14	42
Sandwiches			
Italian	800	45	66
Ham & Cheese	640	29	66
Veggie	600	28	67
Salads: Antipasto, 7 oz	140	7.5	6
Caesar, 4.5 oz	90	3	12
Tossed Salad, 6 oz	100	3	15
Greek, 9.5 oz	120	6.5	11
Dressings: Caesar, 1 oz	230	25	1
Greek, 1.5 oz	270	29	0
Italian, avg., 1.5 oz	220	23	2
Fat Free Italian, 1.5 oz	25	0	5
Ranch, 1.5 oz	230	24	2
Sides: Chicken Wings, 1 wing	70	5	0
Crazy Bread, 1 stick, 1.2 oz	90	2.5	15
Crazy Sauce, 4 oz	45	0	9
Italian Cheese Bread, 1 piece	130	6	13
Crazy Cinnamon Bread (2)	100	2	19

For Complete Nutritional Data ~ see CalorieKing.com

Lone Star Steakhouse®

	C	F	Cb
Chili: Lone Star, 6 fl.oz	225	15	8
Meals: Grilled Chicken, 6 oz	180	2.5	0
Grilled Pork Chops, 16 oz	1400	100	0
Ribs, 12 oz	960	80	0
Shrimp Dinner, 3½ oz	100	1.5	1
Sweet Bourbon Salmon, 6 oz	230	11	0
Mesquite Grilled Steaks: *Per Serving*			
Cajun Ribeye, 16 oz	1230	101	0
Chopped Steak, 12 oz	880	71	0
Delmonico, 11 oz	845	70	0
Five Star Filet, 9 oz	725	61	0
New York Strip, 14 oz	1015	80	0
San Antonio Sirloin, 12 oz	755	55	0
T-Bone, 20 oz	1515	124	0
Prime Rib: *Whole, ½" Fat*			
Smoked, 16 oz	1230	101	0
Sides: Baked Potato	670	18	114
Baked Sweet Potato	645	8	137
Sauteed Mushrooms	115	9	6
Sauteed Onions	100	7	8
Steamed Vegetables	85	1	14
Texas Rice	75	2	12
Soup: Black Bean, 6 fl.oz	200	4	31
Texas Teasers: Ribs, 6 oz	480	40	0
Dessert: Homemade Cobbler	250	8	43

Long John Silver's®

	C	F	Cb
Sandwiches: Ultimate Fish	480	22	51
Fish Sandwich	440	20	48
Chicken Sandwich	480	22	51
Sides: Fries: Regular	230	10	34
Large, 5 oz	390	17	56
Cheese Sticks (3)	140	8	12
Coleslaw, 4 oz	200	15	15
Corn Cobbette, no butter	90	3	14
Crumblies, 1 oz	170	12	14
Hushpuppies, 1 pup	60	2.5	9
Rice, 4 oz	180	3.5	34
Soup: Clam Chowder, 1 bowl	220	10	23
Chicken: Battered Plank, 1 piece	130	8	9
Seafood: Battered Fish, 1 piece	230	13	16
Battered Shrimp, 1 piece	45	2.5	3
Breaded Clams, 1 order	240	13	22
Desserts: *Per Pie*			
Chocolate Cream Pie	310	22	24
Pecan Pie	370	15	55
Pineapple Cream Pie	290	13	39

For Complete Nutritional Data ~ see CalorieKing.com

McDonald's®

Burgers/Sandwiches	C	F	Cb
BBQ Chicken Sandwich	340	8	48
Big Mac® Burger	595	33	50
Big N'Tasty Burger, no Cheese	535	32	38
with Cheese	590	36	39
Cheeseburger	330	14	36
Double Cheeseburger	485	26	38
Chicken McGrill	400	16	37
no mayo	300	5	37
Crispy Chicken	510	26	47
Deli Trio	415	7	61
Filet-O-Fish®	405	20	41
Grilled Chicken Flatbread, no dress.	355	6	50
Hamburger	280	10	36
McChicken	425	23	41
McChicken Hot & Spicy	455	26	40
McVeggie Burger	355	8	48
New York Corned Beef Reuben	565	23	58
New York Turkey Reuben	540	19	60
Quarter Pounder Burger	435	21	38
w. Cheese	535	29	39
Double Quarter Pounder w. Cheese	765	47	39
Turkey Club Flatbread	595	29	52
Turkey McDeli Wrap	775	50	54
Extra Value Meals			
Large Fries & Large Soda, add	825	25	141
French Fries			
Small, 2.6 oz	225	11	28
Medium, 4 oz	345	17	43
Large, 6 oz	515	25	64

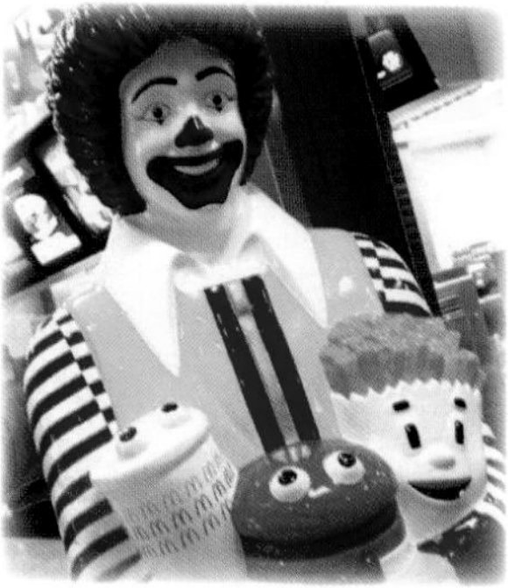

McDonald's® cont...

Chicken McNuggets®/Sauces	C	F	Cb
Chicken McNuggets®: 4 pieces	170	10	10
6 pieces	255	15	15
10 pieces	425	25	25
Sauce: Barbeque, 1 oz	40	0	10
Honey, ½ oz	50	0	12
Hot Mustard, 1 oz	65	3	7
Sweet 'N Sour, 1 oz	45	0	11
Chicken Selects® Breast Strips			
Strips: 3 pieces	380	19	28
5 pieces	630	32	47
10 pieces	1260	64	94
Sauces (1.5 oz pkg): Creamy Ranch	210	22	2
Spicy Buffalo	60	7	2
Tangy Honey Mustard	70	2.5	12
Breakfast Menu			
Bagel: Plain	260	1	54
Ham, Egg & Cheese	545	23	58
Spanish Omelete	705	40	59
Steak, Egg & Cheese	630	31	57
Big Breakfast Platter	700	47	45
Bacon, Egg & Cheese Biscuit	430	26	31
Cinnamon Roll: Regular	440	19	60
Deluxe	565	23	81
Deluxe Breakfast Platter	1190	61	130
English Muffin, 2 oz	145	2	27
Grape/Strawberry Jam	35	0	9
Hash Browns (1), 2 oz	130	8	14
Hotcakes: Plain (3)	340	8	58
w. Margarine (2 pats)	420	17	56
w. Margarine (2 pats) & Syrup (1)	605	17	104
Hotcakes with Sausage Platter	775	33	104
Low Fat Apple Bran Muffin	300	3	61
McGriddles®: Bacon, Egg & Chse	435	21	43
Sausage	420	23	42
Sausage, Egg & Cheese	550	33	43
McMuffin®: Egg	275	12	28
Sausage	375	23	28
Sausage w. Egg	450	28	29
Sausage, 1.5 oz patty	170	16	0
Sausage Biscuit	410	28	30
w. Egg	485	33	31
Sausage Breakfast Burrito	290	16	24
Scrambled Eggs (2)	155	11	1
***Breakfast Value Meal** (Extras)*			
If Hash Browns & Coffee (black/no sugar,) add	130	8	14
If Hash Browns & Orange Juice, add	270	8	47

Salads/Desserts/Drinks ~ Next Page ...

McDonald's® cont...

Salads: (No Dressing)	C	F	Cb
Bacon Ranch Salad, no chicken	140	8	7
Caesar Salad, no chicken	90	4	7
California Cobb Salad, no chicken	155	9	7
Chef Salad	150	8	5
Crispy Chicken Bacon Ranch	355	19	20
Crispy Chicken Caesar Salad	315	16	20
Crispy Chicken California Cobb	375	21	20
Fiesta Salad: with Salsa	395	22	26
Plain (no Salsa/Sour Cream)	360	22	19
with Salsa & Sour Cream	450	27	28
with Sour Cream	415	27	21
Fruit & Walnut Salad w. Yogurt	310	13	43
Grilled Chicken Bacon Ranch Salad	250	10	9
Grilled Chicken Caesar Salad	205	6	9
Grilled Chicken California Cobb	265	11	9
Side Salad, 3.1 oz	15	0	3
Butter Garlic Croutons,½ oz	50	1.5	8
***Salad Dressings:** Per Package*			
Newman's Own: Cobb Dressing	120	9	9
Low-Fat Balsamic Vinaigrette	45	3	4
Creamy Caesar Dressing	185	18	4
Ranch Dressing	175	15	9
Salsa	30	0	7
Desserts/Cookies/Shakes			
Apple Dippers w. Caramel Dip	100	1	22
Apple Dippers, 1 pkg	30	0	8
Caramel Dip	70	1	14
Baked Apple Pie	265	13	34
Cookies: Oatmeal Raisin (1)	160	6	24
Chocolate Chip Cookie (1)	170	8	22
Sprinkles Sugar Cookie (1)	170	8	23
Sugar Cookie	140	6	20
McDonaldland® Cookies, 2 oz	235	8	38
Chocolate Chip Cookies, 2 oz	285	14	37
Fruit 'n Yogurt Parfait: Regular	155	2	30
without Granola	135	2	25
Ice Cream: Kiddie Cone	45	1.5	7
Vanilla Reduced Fat Cone	150	4.5	23
McFlurry™: M&M®, 12 fl.oz cup	630	23	90
Oreo®, 12 fl.oz cup	570	20	82
Sundaes: Nuts (Topping)	50	3.5	2
Hot Caramel Sundae	360	10	61
Hot Fudge Sundae	350	12	52
Strawberry Sundae	290	7	50
Triple Thick Shakes, average all flavors:			
12 fl.oz cup	430	12	70
16 fl.oz cup	580	17	94
21 fl.oz cup	750	22	123
32 fl.oz cup	1150	33	187

McDonald's® cont...

	C	F	Cb
Drinks: 1% Low Fat Milk, 8 fl.oz	105	2.5	12
Coffee (black), 16 fl.oz	10	0	2
Half & Half Creamer, 1 pkg	15	1.5	0
Cappuccino: *Per 12 fl.oz*			
French Vanilla	215	6	38
Original; Swiss Mocha	205	4	39
White Choc. Raspberry	225	9	34
Coca-Cola or Sprite (with ⅓ Ice):			
Childs, 12 fl.oz cup	115	0	29
Small, 16 fl.oz cup	155	0	38
Medium, 21 fl.oz cup	205	0	51
Large, 32 fl.oz cup	310	0	77
Diet Coke	0	0	0
Hi-C Orange Drink (with ⅓ Ice):			
Childs, 12 fl.oz	130	0	32
Small, 16 fl.oz	170	0	42
Medium, 21fl.oz	225	0	56
Large, 32 fl.oz	340	0	85
Iced Tea	0	0	0
Orange Juice: 12 fl.oz cup	140	0	33
16 fl.oz cup	180	0	42
Powerade Mountain Blast (with ⅓ Ice):			
Childs, 12 fl.oz	70	0	18
Small, 16 fl.oz	95	0	24
Medium, 21 fl.oz	125	0	31
Large, 32 fl.oz	190	0	48
Whipped Hot Chocolate, 12 fl.oz	195	1	43

For Complete Nutritional Data ~ see CalorieKing.com

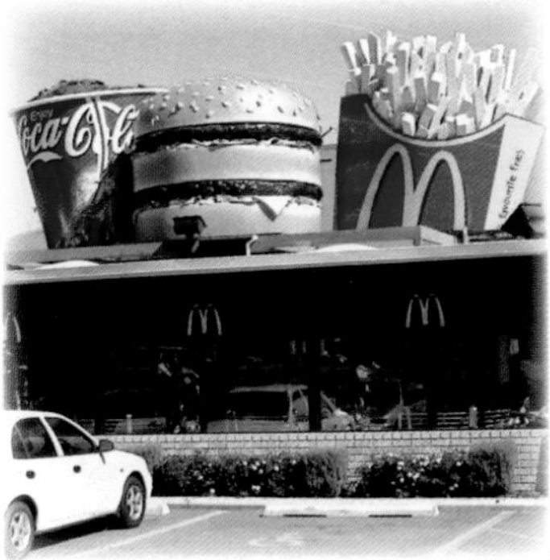

Manhattan Bagel®

Bagel: *Per Bagel (4 oz)*	C	F	Cb
Blueberry	**260**	1	54
Cheddar Cheese	**270**	4	48
Chocolate Chip	**285**	2.5	56
Cinnamon Raisin	**275**	1	57
Cranberry Orange	**270**	1	55
Egg, 4 oz	**265**	1.5	53
Jalapeno Cheddar	**265**	1.5	53
Marble Rye	**255**	1	52
Oat Bran	**260**	3	53
Plain, 4 oz	**255**	1	52
Pumpernickel; Rye	**255**	1	52
Sesame	**310**	5	55
Spinach	**265**	1	54
Sundried Tomato	**260**	1	53
Whole Wheat	**255**	1	52
Cream Cheese: Reduced Fat, 2 Tbsp	**70**	6	1
Fat Free, 2 Tbsp	**30**	0	3

For Complete Nutritional Data ~ see CalorieKing.com

Mazzio's® Pizza

Pizza: *Per Slice (1/8 Medium Pizza)*	C	F	Cb
Cheese: Thin Crust	**160**	9	18
Original Crust	**180**	6	29
Deep Pan Crust	**310**	16	37
Large Pizzeria Crust	**320**	15	42
Pepperoni: Thin Crust	**160**	10	18
Original Crust	**230**	11	29
Deep Pan Crust	**320**	16	37
Large Pizzeria Crust	**330**	15	42
Sausage: Thin Crust	**190**	12	18
Original Crust	**250**	12	30
Deep Pan Crust	**350**	19	38
Large Pizzeria Crust	**380**	20	43
Combo: Thin Crust	**200**	13	20
Original Crust	**250**	12	31
Deep Pan Crust	**350**	19	39
Large Pizzeria Crust	**370**	19	44
Supremebuster: Thin Crust	**190**	11	19
Original Crust	**240**	11	30
Deep Pan Crust	**340**	18	38
Large Pizzeria Crust	**360**	18	43

Mazzio's® cont...

	C	F	Cb
Meatbuster: Thin Crust	**220**	14	19
Original Crust	**270**	14	30
Deep Pan	**370**	21	38
Large, Pizzeria Crust	**410**	22	43
Chicken Club: Thin Crust	**180**	8	19
Original Crust	**250**	10	30
Deep Pan Crust	**350**	17	38
Large Pizzeria Crust	**360**	15	40
California Alfredo: Thin Crust	**210**	14	17
Original Crust	**260**	13	28
Deep Pan Crust	**370**	20	36
Large Pizzeria Crust	**390**	20	41
Mexican: Thin Crust	**280**	14	25
Original Crust	**330**	13	36
Deep Pan Crust	**440**	22	44
Large Pizzeria Crust	**490**	21	52
"Mazzio's Works": Thin Crust	**220**	14	20
Original Crust	**270**	14	31
Deep Pan Crust	**380**	21	39
Large Pizzeria Crust	**410**	22	44
Appetizers: *Per Serving*			
Cheese Nachos, ½ container	**440**	10	19
Cheese Dippers, ¼ container	**330**	16	38
Wings of Fire: Large	**370**	28	2
Small	**360**	26	3
Cinnamon Sticks, 3.2 oz	**350**	16	45
Breadsticks, 2.8 oz	**120**	2.5	25
Meat Nachos, 5 oz	**520**	18	20
Pasta: *Per Serving*			
Calzone: Pepperoni, 1/10 whole	**240**	8	33
Ham-Bacon-Cheddar, 1/10 whole	**280**	8	32
Fettuccine Alfredo, 14.7 oz	**1320**	42	195
Italian Sampler, 24 oz	**1640**	57	218
Lasagne w. Meat Sauce, 16 oz	**700**	36	60
Spaghetti: w. Meatballs, 21 oz	**1560**	53	206
w. Meat Sauce, 17 oz	**1210**	26	200
w. Marinara, 16 oz	**940**	10	208

Mimi's Cafe®

Menu Items: *Per Serving*	C	F	Cb
Broiled 10 oz Halibut Steak	**800**	16	94
Chicken and Fruit	**545**	9	59
EggBeater Fitness Omelette	**655**	8	110
Half-A-Turkey Sandwich	**410**	6	55
Roasted Turkey Breast	**540**	8	52
Spaghettini w. Tomatoes & Basil	**680**	8	130
Two "AA" Large Eggs	**395**	8	62

Miami Subs®

Burgers	C	F	Cb
Deluxe	765	59	32
Deluxe Cheeseburger	840	65	32
Deluxe Bacon Cheeseburger	890	70	32
Cheesesteaks: *Per 6" Sandwich*			
Original	405	11	46
Classic	420	12	48
Works	545	23	51
Chicken Philly Classic	550	27	47
Pitas: Gyros	665	39	47
Chicken	390	13	34
Subs: *Per 6" Sandwich*			
Ham & Cheese	450	18	49
Italian Deli	510	25	49
Meatball	505	22	49
Tuna	480	18	45
Turkey	485	19	52
Sides: *Per Serving*			
Mozzarella Sticks	745	57	34
Onion Rings	860	69	56
Spicy Fries, Regular, 6.4 oz	525	40	39
Platters: Gyros	1410	94	81
Chicken Breast	735	41	57
10 Wings w. Fries, Blue Cheese	995	67	50
Salads: Caesar w. Dressing	460	34	26
Chicken Caesar w. Dressing	605	39	28
Chicken Club, no Dressing	490	26	23
Garden, no Dressing	315	18	21
Greek, no Dressing	285	15	24
Side Greek w. Dressing	75	6	4

Mr. Goodcents®

Quartermeal: w. Chicken Noodle Soup			
Roast Beef	435	7	60
Turkey	460	9	62
Pasta: *w. Breadstick*			
Chicken Parmesan Mostiaccioli	680	10	110
Mostiaccioli w. Tomato Pasta Sce	505	8	95
Subs: *Per ½ Sub*			
Chkn Parmesan on Wheat, no dress.	480	10	63
Ham & Cheese on Wheat	510	12	71
Oven Roasted Chicken on White, standard dressing, no oil	445	4	74
Penny Club on Wheat	480	9	71
Roast Beef on Wheat	455	6	68
Turkey on Wheat	495	10	70
Veggie on Wheat	385	7	66

Mr. Hero®

Cheesesteaks: *Per 7" Serving*	C	F	Cb
Grilled Steak Philly	465	14	48
Hot Buttered Cheesesteak Deluxe	595	34	48
Pasta: *Per Serving*			
Breadsticks w. Sauce, 5 oz	295	9	47
Spaghetti Dinner, 16.8 oz	610	8	110
Spaghetti w. Meatballs, 19.8 oz	850	27	116
Salads			
Garden Salad	40	0.5	7
Grilled Chicken	220	10	7
Seafood Crab	455	37	18
Side Salad	30	0.5	6
Tuna Salad	740	69	8
Dressings: *Per Serving*			
Buttermilk, 2 oz	285	29	6
Creamy Italian, 2 oz	200	17	11
Croutons, ½ oz	60	2	8.5
Fat Free, French	75	0	18
Fat Free, Ranch	65	0	16
Sandwiches: *Per 7" Sandwich*			
Cold Subs: Classic Italian	610	36	50
Tuna & Cheese	685	47	47
Turkey & Cheese	470	21	46
Ultimate Italian	630	34	52
Hot Subs: Grilled Chicken Philly	455	14	48
Meatball	645	32	53
Romanburger	740	47	50
Round: Bacon Cheeseburger	355	23	23
Chicken	415	23	23
Fish Sandwich	415	23	31
Tuna	435	34	23
Side Orders: *Per Serving*			
Cheddar Cheese Sauce, 1.5 oz	65	4.5	5
Onion Rings, 6 oz	575	32	64
Potato Waffers, 3.7 oz	345	18	42
Desserts			
Cheesecake, plain, 3.5 oz	365	27	26
Cheesecake w. Cherries, 4.7 oz	405	27	35

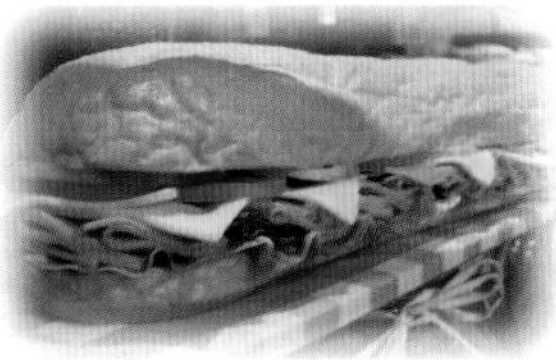

Mr Subb®

Subs (Regular Size)	C	F	Cb
Classic: Assorted	**665**	20	82
Ham	**500**	6	87
Meatball	**735**	26	78
Pizza	**590**	21	72
Salami	**570**	18	74
Vegetarian	**395**	3	73
Premium: Breaded Chicken	**755**	20	100
Canadian Club	**555**	11	78
Grilled Chicken	**570**	7.5	80
Louisiana Chicken	**585**	14	71
Seafood with Crab	**515**	5	89
Specialty Subs: BBQ Rib	**695**	26	73
BLT	**540**	14	75
Corned Beef	**505**	10	71
Roast Beef	**500**	9	70
Tuna	**565**	9	81
Turkey	**470**	5	75
Wraps: Louisiana Chicken	**360**	12	39
Roast Beef	**300**	8	38
Seafood with Crab	**325**	5.5	52
Tuna	**365**	9	46
Turkey	**285**	5.5	41
Sauces: *Per ½ oz (1 Tbsp)*			
Mayo Lite	**60**	5	2
MR SUB Secret Sauce	**80**	9	0
Other varieties, average	**20**	0	4
Soups and Chili			
Bean and Spring Vegetable	**125**	1	23
Caribbean and Black Bean	**110**	0.5	22
Chicken Noodle	**95**	2	14
Chili with Beef	**185**	1.5	31
Clam Chowder	**175**	8	21
Cream of Mushroom	**65**	1	10
Cream of Potato and Leek	**170**	8	20
French Canadian Pea	**145**	2.5	23
Garden Vegetable	**50**	0.5	11
Italian Wedding Style	**125**	3	21
Minestrone	**80**	0.5	15
Pasta Fagioli	**140**	1.5	25
Vegetable Beef and Barley	**85**	1	16
Salad: *No Cheese/Dressing*			
Garden Salad	**20**	0	4
Mediterranean Greek	**60**	4	6
Mighty Caesar Salad	**100**	4	8

For Complete Nutritional Data ~ see CalorieKing.com

Mrs Fields Cookies®

Per Cookie (2.3 oz)	C	F	Cb
Butter Toffee; Coconut	**290**	13	40
Chewy Fudge; Triple Choc	**220**	11	30
Cinnamon Sugar	**300**	12	41
Debra's Special	**280**	12	39
Milk Chocolate, no nuts	**280**	13	38
Milk Choc w. Walnuts/Macadamia	**320**	18	36
Milk/Oatmeal Chocolate Chip	**280**	13	39
Oatmeal Raisins & Walnuts	**280**	12	39
Peanut Butter	**310**	16	34
Peanut Butter Milk Chocolate	**300**	17	35
Pumpkin Harvest	**200**	10	24
Semi-Sweet Chocolate	**280**	14	40
w. Pecans/Walnuts	**310**	16	38
Snickerdoodle Jumbo	**640**	29	90
White Chunk Macadamia	**310**	17	37
Bite Size Nibbler™: *Per 2 Cookies (1 oz)*			
Chewy Chocolate Fudge; Butter	**110**	5	15
Cinnamon Sugar	**120**	4.5	17
Debra's Special Nibbler	**100**	4.5	13
Milk Choc w. Walnuts; Macadamia	**120**	6	14
Milk/Semi-Sweet Chocolate; M&M	**110**	5	15
Peanut Butter	**110**	6	13
Brownies: *Each (2.7 oz)*			
Double Fudge	**360**	19	49
Frosted Fudge	**440**	21	62
Pecan Fudge; Pie Brownie	**340**	21	40
Walnut Fudge	**380**	23	45
Bundt Cakes: *Per Piece (3 oz)*			
Banana Walnut	**350**	21	35
Banana Walnut w. Choc Chip	**370**	22	39
Blueberry; Raspberry	**270**	12	36
White Cake w. Choc Chips	**350**	17	45
Hand-Dipped Ice Cream: *Per ½ Cup*			
Butter Pecan	**260**	20	17
Chewy Chocolate Fudge	**270**	16	27
Chocolate; Pralines & Cream	**215**	13	21
Chocolate Chunk Cookie Dough	**210**	14	18
Lemon Meringue Pie	**235**	12	29
Oatmeal Raisin	**220**	12	25
Vanilla Bean	**195**	13	17
Very Berry Strawberry	**185**	11	19
White Chunk Macadamia	**250**	16	23

For Complete Nutritional Data ~ see CalorieKing.com

My Favorite Muffin®

~ Same Menu & Data as Big Apple Bagel (See Page 189) ~

Nathan's Famous®

	C	F	Cb
Burgers: ¼ lb Burger	**540**	30	43
¼ lb Burger w. Chse	**855**	62	46
Bacon Cheeseburger	**695**	44	44
Super Burger	**845**	62	42
Cheese Steaks: Original	**765**	43	51
Supreme	**810**	43	61
Chicken Cheesesteak	**575**	19	63
Sandwiches: Fish Sandwich	**405**	20	42
Sides: Nuggets (6)	**350**	27	20
French Fries: Regular, 9.6 oz	**550**	38	47
Large	**760**	52	65
Super, 21 oz	**1190**	82	100
Onion Rings: Small, 5.6 oz	**560**	44	36
Large, 7.5 oz	**735**	59	48
Hot Dogs: Nathan's Famous	**315**	20	23

For Complete Nutritional Data ~ see CalorieKing.com

O'Charley's®

	C	F	Cb
Appetizers: *Per Serving*			
Buffalo Wings, ½ order	**630**	46	24
Chicken Quesadilla, ½ order	**480**	30	26
Chicken Tenders, ½ order	**560**	15	74
Chips & Salsa, ½ order	**485**	23	62
Fried Cheese Wedges, ½ order	**270**	15	21
Loaded Potato Skins, ½ order	**570**	40	19
Spinach & Artichoke Dip, ½ order	**725**	44	69
Brunch: *Per Order (w. Fries & Bread)*			
Cajun Chicken Omelette	**1150**	80	48
Spanish Omelette	**975**	70	47
Ultimate Omelette	**980**	66	50
Waffles w. Strawberries, no fries	**975**	33	158
Chicken: *Per Order (No Sides or Salads)*			
Chicken Parmesan w. Vege	**835**	27	90
Chicken Tenders Dinner	**1325**	34	178
Chicken Teriyaki on Rice	**610**	17	69
Grilled Chicken Dinner	**525**	17	36
Salad: *Per Order*			
Black & Blue Caesar	**1000**	66	15
Caesar Salad	**445**	36	11
Cajun Chicken w. Ranch Dressing	**975**	78	21
Chicken Caesar	**610**	40	11
Island Salad w. dressing	**1465**	30	225
Southern Fried Chkn w. Dressing	**1770**	85	173
Sandwiches: *No Sides*			
Bacon & Cheese Chicken	**760**	45	36
Buffalo Chicken	**720**	32	65
Cajun Chicken	**480**	21	38

O'Charley's® cont...

Sandwiches (Cont): *No Sides*	C	F	Cb
Chicken Sandwich	**470**	21	35
French Dip	**925**	41	77
Half Pound Cheeseburger	**1135**	73	35
The O'Charley's Clu w. Dressing	**1160**	90	45
Three Cheese Bacon Burger	**1380**	88	36
Seafood: *Per Order (w. Sides & Salad)*			
Fisherman's Platter w. Fries	**1905**	95	180
Fried Shrimp Platter, 8 shrimp	**550**	28	26
Sides: Baked Potato, plain	**205**	0.5	46
Cole Slaw	**220**	14	21
French Fries	**410**	21	50
Loaded Baked Potato	**480**	25	53
Rica Pilaf	**220**	6	38
Smashed Potatoes	**305**	12	44
Vegetable Medley	**135**	8	13
Soup: Loaded Potato Soup, 1 cup	**205**	11	19
Steak & Ribs: *Per Serving (No Sides or Fries)*			
Steak Tips Monterey, 1 order	**1140**	82	46
Choice Sirloin, 10 oz	**480**	18	1
Filet Mignon	**745**	53	1
New York Strip Steak	**765**	56	0
Petite Sirloin, 7 oz	**305**	13	1
Prime Rib: 8 oz	**920**	80	0
10 oz	**1150**	100	0
16 oz	**1835**	159	0
Full Rack of Ribs w. Fries/Slaw	**2925**	193	164
½ Rack of Ribs w. Fries/Saw	**1820**	116	124
⅓ Rack of Ribs	**735**	51	28
Ribeye Steak	**885**	71	1
Shrimp, 4 oz	**335**	18	32
Chicken Breast, 5 oz	**240**	13	1

For Complete Nutritional Data ~ see CalorieKing.com

Olive Garden®

Garden Fare Selections (Lower Fat)	C	F	Cb
Lunch: Capellini Pomodora, 13 oz	**350**	11	52
Chicken Giardino, 15.5 oz	**350**	7	40
Linguine alla Marinara, 10.6 oz	**280**	6	48
Shrimp Primavera, 19 oz	**490**	15	65
Dinner: Chicken Giardino, 21.5 oz	**460**	8	59
Capellini Pomodora, 21 oz	**560**	18	84
Linguine alla Marinara, 17 oz	**450**	9	79
Shrimp Primavera, 26 oz	**730**	25	84
Extras: Minestrone Soup, 6 fl.oz	**100**	1	18
Breadstick, plain, 1 stick	**140**	1.5	26

(The) Old Spaghetti Factory®

	C	F	Cb
Garlic Cheese Bread, ½ srvg, 6 oz	**530**	25	60
Entrees: Fettuccine Alfredo	**1140**	87	61
Spaghetti Pot Pourri	**990**	40	110
Spaghetti: w. Clam Sauce	**720**	33	82
w. Meat Sauce	**520**	11	85
w. Meatballs/Tomato Sauce	**720**	18	95
w. Mizithra Cheese	**910**	57	76
w. Mizithra/Mushr./Tomato Sce	**680**	32	79
w. Mushroom/Tomato Sauce	**450**	6	83
w. Sausage/Meat Sauce	**730**	25	86
w. Tomato/Meat Sauce	**480**	8	84
Favorites: Baked Lasagna, 16 oz	**590**	32	35
Chicken Marsala, 19 oz	**1110**	69	61
Chicken Parmigiana, 19 oz	**630**	16	68
Spinach & Cheese Ravioli, 12 oz	**650**	19	87
Spinach Tortellini w. Alfredo, 12 oz	**1180**	68	104
Pies: Mud/Caramel Turtle, avg	**580**	31	68

Orange Julius®

	C	F	Cb
Original *(Orange, Strawberry):*			
Small, 16 fl.oz	**225**	0	55
Medium, 20 fl.oz	**280**	0.5	68
Large,32 fl.oz	**450**	1	109
Classic Smoothy® Drinks: *Per 16 fl.oz*			
Bananarilla; Tropical	**300**	7	56
Cool Cappucino	**415**	10	69
Pina Colada; Raspberry	**360**	7	70
Strawb. Banana; Tripleberry	**380**	7	75
20 fl.oz Size ~ Add 25% to above figures			
32 fl.oz Size ~ Double the above figures			
Julius Creations®: *Per 20 fl.oz*			
Berry Lively; Blackberry Toner	**450**	1	100
Blackberry Storm	**590**	8	130
Blueberrathon	**380**	1.5	90
Chai Tea Dragon	**515**	3	110
Cocoa Latte Swirl	**655**	9	122
Fruitasia	**395**	3	90
Muscle Peach	**290**	1	62
Orange Swirl	**490**	10	96
Pineapple Hardbody	**360**	0.5	80
Raspberry Crush	**360**	2	83
Strawb. Treasure; Raspb. Creme	**525**	8	103
Strawberry Xtreme	**385**	0.5	87
Tart 'N' Berry	**455**	1	102
Tropi-Colada	**550**	8	110
Add Banana, 1 medium	**110**	0.5	27
Nutrifiers: Avg. all types, ¼ oz	**16**	0	4

Outback Steakhouse®

Aussie-Tizers	C	F	Cb
Aussie Cheese Fries, 28 oz	**2900**	182	240
Bloomin Onion, w. dressing	**2210**	134	241
¼ serving	**550**	33	60
Gold Coast Coconut Shrimp	**690**	30	97
Grilled Shrimp on the Barbie	**660**	42	32
Kookaburra Wings w. Sauce (10)	**1160**	75	65
Lobster-Crab Cakes w. Sauce (2)	**840**	72	33
Steaks: *Meat Only ~ Add Extra for Sides*			
Michael J. "Crocodile" Dundee:			
New York Strip, 14 oz	**900**	60	0
Outback Special, 12 oz Sirloin	**810**	50	0
Prime Minister's Prime Ribs:			
8 oz cut	**450**	38	0
12 oz cut	**675**	57	0
16 oz cut	**905**	77	0
Rockhampton Rib-Eye, 14 oz	**730**	40	0
The Melbourne, P/house, 20 oz	**1230**	99	0
Lean meat only	**590**	32	0
Victoria's Filet, Tenderloin, 9 oz	**570**	44	0
Sides: Aussie Chips w Ketchup	**725**	32	100
Fresh Veggies	**80**	1	14
Grilled Onions, 7.5 oz	**180**	11	19
Jacket Potato, Plain	**270**	0	63
Jacket Potato, w. Butter/Cheese	**400**	14	63
Mushrooms, Sauteed	**150**	11	12
Desserts: Cheesecake Olivia	**700**	38	79
Choc. Thunder from Down Under	**1220**	78	134

Panda Express®

	C	F	Cb
Chicken: Black Pepper, 5.5 oz	**180**	10	10
Orange Chicken, 5.5 oz	**475**	21	50
w. Mushrooms, 5.5 oz	**135**	7	7
Spicy w. Peanuts, 5.5 oz	**205**	7	17
BBQ Pork, 4.5 oz	**350**	19	13
Beef & Broccoli, 5.5 oz	**150**	8	9
Sweet & Sour Pork, 4 oz	**415**	30	17
Mixed Veges, 5 oz	**70**	3	8
Fried Tofu w. Beans, 5.5 oz	**185**	11	11
Rice & Noodles: *Serving (8 oz)*			
Steamed Rice	**330**	0.5	74
Vegetable Chow Mein	**330**	11	48
Vegetable Fried Rice	**390**	12	61
Appetizers: Chkn Egg Roll (1)	**190**	8	21
Fried Shrimp, 6 pieces	**260**	12	26
Veggie Spring Roll (1)	**85**	2.5	14

Panera Bread®

	C	F	Cb
Bagels: Asiago Cheese	335	5	58
Blueberry	330	1.5	67
Chocolate Raspberry	375	7	67
Cinnamon Crunch	415	7	78
Dutch Apple & Raisin	345	2.5	70
Everything; Sesame Seed	300	1.5	60
Plain	280	1	57
Lower Carb: Plain	190	2	25
Asiago Cheese	235	9	20
Spreads: Per 2 oz			
Plain Cream Cheese	180	18	2
Reduced Fat, avg.	140	10	5
Roasted Garlic Hummus	100	5	11
Salad: Asian Sesame Chicken	415	17	34
Caesar Salad	375	26	22
Classic Cafe	400	37	14
Grilled Chicken Caesar	515	33	19
Greek	535	48	17
Sandwiches: Asiago Roast Beef	730	35	54
Bacon Turkey Bravo	775	28	84
Chicken Salad on Nine Grain	625	29	56
Frontega Chicken Panini	860	42	71
Garden Veggie	565	23	74
Italian Combo	1045	54	80
Peanut Butter & Jelly on French	445	15	63
Sierra Turkey	940	55	71
Smoked Ham & Swiss on Rye	660	34	47
Smoked Turkey Brst on Sourdough	425	15	44
Smokehouse Turkey on Artisan	665	23	68
Tuna Salad on Honey Wheat	700	43	50
Turkey Fresco	590	17	74
Tuscan Chicken	950	56	76
Soup: Per Serving (8 oz)			
Baked Potato	260	16	23
Boston Clam Chowder	200	11	19
Broccoli Cheddar	230	16	13
Chicken Noodle, Low Fat	100	2	15
Cream of Chicken & Wild Rice	205	12	19
French Onion	220	10	23
Vegetarian: Italian Vegetable	80	2	13
Black Bean	160	0.5	29
Garden Vegetable	90	0.5	17
Muffins: Banana Nut Muffie	265	12	34
Chocolate Chip Muffie	250	10	36
Pumpkin Muffie	240	6	43
Low Fat Tripleberry Muffin	305	3	63

Papa Gino's®

	C	F	Cb
Appetizers: Per Serving			
Buffalo Chicken Tenders, med., 4 oz	220	10	21
Cheese Breadsticks, medium, 2 oz	155	5	21
Cheese Garlic Bread, large	660	16	110
Chicken Tenders, medium	240	10	25
Cinnamon Sticks, 3.6 oz	315	9	52
French Fries, small, 6.5 oz	360	22	38
Mozzarella Sticks (1), large, 3.3 oz	300	15	27
Pasta: Entree Size			
Chicken Parmigiana Platter	1035	34	129
Penne or Spaghetti, plain	650	11	118
Papa Platter: Penne/Spaghetti	910	23	136
Spaghetti & Meatballs	805	19	123
Ravioli	445	20	49
Pizzas: Large (14") Thin Crust ~ Per Slice (⅛)			
Cheese	240	6	36
BBQ Chicken, 4.6 oz	280	6	41
Buffalo Chicken, 4.4 oz	255	6	35
Cheeseburger	335	13	37
Chicken Pepper; Garlic Chicken	300	9	37
Hawaiian	290	8	38
Meat Combo	340	14	36
PapaRoni	345	15	36
Pepperoni	285	10	36
Super Veggie	265	7	39
Works; Fenway	320	12	39
Salads: Buffalo Chicken Tender	330	15	31
Caesar Salad	190	8	19
Chicken Bacon Cheddar	475	21	24
Chicken Tender	325	15	29
Garden Salad	145	4	22
Italian Chopped Salad	580	50	10
Caesar Side Salad	70	3	6
Garden Side Salad	65	2	10
Dressings: Bleu Cheese, 1 oz	150	15	3
Caesar, 3 oz	400	43	0
Fat Free Ranch, 3 oz	85	0	23
Ranch, 3 oz	385	31	3
Subs (Small): BLT	685	30	75
Italian	785	36	74
Meatball	615	16	81
Seafood Salad	685	34	71
Steak	560	31	45
Tuna	740	38	70
Turkey	600	18	74

Papa John's®

Original Crust Large Pizza (14"): Per Slice (1/8 Whole)	C	F	Cb
All the Meats w. Beef	**410**	20	39
BBQ Chicken & Bacon	**370**	14	44
Cheese	**295**	10	39
Chicken/Spinach Alfredo	**315**	12	37
Fresh Garden, no Cheese	**210**	4	37
Garden Fresh	**290**	9	40
Hawaiian BBQ Chicken	**380**	14	46
Pepperoni	**345**	15	39
Sausage	**335**	14	38
The Works	**370**	16	40
Thin Crust Large Pizza (14"): *Per Slice (1/8 Whole)*			
All the Meats w. Beef	**380**	24	24
BBQ Chicken & Bacon	**340**	18	30
Cheese	**250**	13	23
Chicken Alfredo	**280**	15	22
Garden Fresh	**230**	11	24
Hawaiian BBQ Chicken	**330**	16	31
Pepperoni; Sausage	**310**	18	24
Spinach Alfredo	**265**	15	22
The Works	**320**	18	25
Side Orders: Bread Sticks, 1.9 oz	**140**	2	26
Cheese Sticks, 2.4 oz	**180**	8	20
Papa's Chickenstrips, 1.3 oz	**85**	4	5
Papa's Cinnapie, 6.6 oz	**115**	6	14
Sauce: Garlic, 1.2 oz	**235**	26	0
Honey Mustard, 1.2 oz	**190**	19	6
Pizza, 1.2 oz	**25**	2	3

Papa Murphy's®

Pizza: *Per Slice*	C	F	Cb
Deep Dish Traditional, 1/8 Pizza	**445**	24	34
Gourmet: *Per Slice (1/12 Family Pizza)*			
Chicken Garlic	**325**	15	30
Classic Italian	**365**	19	30
Gourmet Veggie	**310**	14	31
Calzones: *(1/8 Family):* Combo	**450**	20	45
Italian	**485**	23	46
Veggie	**415**	17	46
Papa's *(1/12 Family Pizza):* All Meat	**375**	19	31
Cheese	**260**	10	29
Cowboy	**365**	19	31
Hawaiian	**300**	11	34
Murphy's Combo; Papa's Fav.	**380**	20	32
Pepperoni	**315**	15	29
Perfect; Veggie Combo	**310**	13	32
Rancher	**330**	15	31
Specialty	**345**	17	31
Stuffed *(1/16 Family):* Big Murphy	**380**	17	39
Chicken & Bacon; Chicago	**370**	16	38

Papa Murphy's® cont...

Pizza (Cont): *Per Slice*	C	F	Cb
DeLites Thin Crust: *Per 1/10 Pizza*			
Cheese	**130**	6	11
Hawaiian	**155**	7	14
Meat	**195**	12	11
Pepperoni	**160**	9	11
Veggie	**150**	8	11
Salads: *Individual Size (No Dressing)*			
Club	**315**	21	11
Italian	**235**	17	7
Garden Salad	**180**	11	9
Cheesy Bread (2), 2 oz	**185**	7	23

Pepe's Mexican®

	C	F	Cb
Burritos: Beef & Bean	**510**	24	52
Beef & Bean Suizo	**645**	34	55
Chicken & Bean	**480**	21	51
Chicken & Bean Suizo	**615**	31	54
Pork & Bean	**470**	19	51
Pork & Bean Suizo	**605**	29	54
Flauta: Beef, plain	**155**	9	10
Beef, w. cheese & sauce	**190**	12	11
Chicken, plain	**185**	10	16
Chicken, w. cheese & sauce	**230**	13	17
Taco Salad			
Beef w. 4 oz salsa	**550**	26	52
Chicken w. 4 oz salsa	**520**	23	51
Pork w. 4 oz salsa	**505**	20	52
Without Taco Shell, deduct	**210**	7	32
Tacos: Beef Crisp	**210**	11	16
Beef Soft Corn	**255**	10	28
Beef Soft Flour	**245**	11	24
Chicken Crisp	**190**	9	15
Chicken Soft Corn	**230**	8	27
Chicken Soft Flour	**230**	9	23
Pork Crisp	**170**	6	16
Pork Soft Corn	**220**	6	27
Pork Soft Flour	**220**	7	24
Tostada			
Beef & Bean	**370**	23	26
Beef & Bean Suiza	**440**	29	26
Chicken & Bean	**335**	21	21
Chicken & Bean Suiza	**410**	26	25
Pork & Bean	**350**	20	26
Pork & Bean Suiza	**410**	25	26

Perkin's® Family Restaurant

Entrees	C	F	Cb
Chicken Dinner	**620**	13	60
Fish Dinner	**470**	7	60
Fruit Cup	**50**	0.5	12
'Lite & Healthy'	**105**	2	15
Omelettes: Country Club	**930**	79	6
Deli Ham & Cheese	**960**	79	8
'Everything' Omelette	**695**	54	9
Granny's Country Omelette	**940**	82	7
w. 9 oz Hash Browns	**1245**	90	57
Salads: Chef's, Mini	**215**	11	7
Muffins: Blueberry	**585**	26	78
Bran Muffin	**560**	16	94
Carrot	**495**	26	55
Chocolate Chips	**600**	26	81
Pumpkin	**585**	26	78
Raspberry & Cream	**600**	26	81
Reduced Fat: Banana	**520**	6.5	0
Blueberry; Honey Bran	**425**	6.5	0
Plain	**490**	8	0
Pancakes: Buttermilk, (3)	**440**	12	70
Harvest Grain: w. Low-Cal Syrup (5)	**475**	3.5	93
Short Stack (3)	**270**	2	56
Pies (Per Slice): Apple Pie, 1/6 pie	**375**	15	56
Brownie, Low Fat	**160**	0.5	0
Wildberry, 1/6 pie	**375**	15	56

Penn Station®

Subs (6")	C	F	Cb
Artichoke: w. mayo	**360**	18	37
No mayo	**260**	7	37
Cheese Bread	**255**	6	42
Chicken Salad	**360**	15	41
Chicken Teriyaki	**435**	13	48
Grilled Vegetarian	**255**	4	46
Ham Dagwood, no cheese	**430**	21	35
Philadelphia Cheesesteak	**500**	25	45
Philadelphia Cheesesteak, no mayo	**400**	14	45
Reuben	**500**	21	40
Reuben, no 1000 Island Dressing	**390**	12	37
Tuna Salad	**360**	16	41
Turkey Dagwood	**420**	18	36
Turkey Dagwood, no Cheese/Mayo	**250**	4	35

Petro's®

Petros	C	F	Cb
Pee Wee Petro, avg.	**290**	16	25
Small Petro: Original	**520**	30	43
Chicken	**470**	24	43
Medium Petro: Original	**740**	43	58
Chicken	**670**	36	59
Veggie	**750**	41	70
Large Petro: Original	**1080**	63	87
Chicken	**970**	52	88
Veggie	**1090**	60	105
Lite Petro: Small	**380**	12	48
Medium	**530**	16	66
Large	**790**	24	99
Pasta Petro: Small	**410**	17	46
Medium	**630**	27	68
Large	**850**	37	91
Lite Pasta Petro: Small	**335**	2.5	52
Medium	**495**	3.5	80
Large	**680**	4.5	108
Chili			
Chicken, medium	**275**	4	43
Original, medium	**370**	14	42
Veggie, medium	**385**	11	58
Baked Potatoes			
#1 Lite	**365**	0.5	74
#2 Butter Sour Cream	**480**	18	74
#3 Loaded	**680**	33	78
#4 Loaded w. Chili	**780**	37	90
#5 Broccoli 3 Cheese	**655**	30	77
Hot Dogs: Chili	**315**	17	28
Chili/Cheese; Loaded	**350**	19	30
Plain	**265**	14	22
Slaw	**350**	16	23
Tostitos™ Chips: Queso	**500**	27	60
Ransalsa	**560**	35	61
Salsa	**415**	18	62
Loaded Tostitos™: Ultimate Nachos	**880**	51	79
Petro Salads: Original	**570**	36	42
Grilled Chicken	**740**	41	42
Garden Salads: Small	**45**	0.5	8
Large	**85**	1	16

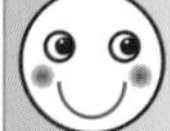

"Life is what happens to you when you're making other plans."
~ Betty Talmadge

Peter Piper® Pizza

Cheese Pizza: Per Slice	C	F	Cb
Personal Slice	**110**	3.5	13
Personal Pizza (7")	**430**	14	51
Small Pizza (10"), ½ pizza	**160**	5	19
Whole Pizza	**960**	31	114
Medium Pizza (12"), ⅛ pizza	**175**	5.5	20
Whole Pizza	**1385**	45	164
Large Pizza (14"), ⅛ pizza	**235**	8	28
Whole Pizza	**1885**	61	223
Extra Large Pizza (16"), 1/12 pizza	**205**	6.5	24
Whole Pizza	**2460**	79	291
Pepperoni Pizza			
Personal Slice	**150**	6.5	15
Personal Pizza (7")	**600**	25	60
Small Pizza (10"), ⅙ pizza	**185**	8	18
Whole Pizza	**425**	47	111
Medium Pizza (12"), ⅛ pizza	**270**	11	27
Whole Pizza	**1600**	68	160
Large Pizza (14"), ⅛ pizza	**270**	12	27
Whole Pizza	**2180**	92	218
Extra Large Pizza (16"), 1/12 pizza	**235**	10	24
Sides: Chicken Wings (4)	**210**	16	1
Breadsticks (1)	**120**	4.5	17

For Complete Nutritional Data ~ see CalorieKing.com

P F Chang's®

	C	F	Cb
Beef: Mongolian	**360**	20	17
Orange Peel	**450**	25	43
a la Szechwan, ⅓ dish	**265**	7	33
w. Broccoli	**230**	12	17
Buddha's Feast: Steamed, ⅓ dish	**60**	0.5	10
Stir Fried	**105**	3	13
Chicken & Duck: Crispy Honey	**375**	19	31
Almond Cashew, ⅓ dish	**215**	13	10
Cantonese Chicken	**255**	13	12
Cantonese Duck	**255**	12	18
Chang's Spicy Chicken	**330**	14	33
Chef Roy's Favorite	**185**	9	10
Chow Mein, ¼ dish	**207**	7	24
Kung Pao, ½ dish	**355**	18	16
Malaysian, ¼ dish	**180**	10	10
Moo Goo Gai Pan	**125**	5	6
Mu Shu	**235**	13	19
Orange Peel	**340**	16	28
Philip's Better Lemon Chkn, ¼ dish	**265**	11	24
Spicy Ground Chicken w. Eggplant	**220**	15	13
Szechwan Chkn Chow Fun, ¼ dish	**290**	21	16
w. Black Bean Sauce, ⅓ dish	**220**	10	12

P F Chang's® cont...

	C	F	Cb
Dumplings: Peking (1)	**165**	9	11
Shrimp (1)	**115**	4	11
Vegetable (1)	**105**	1.5	18
Pork: Mu Shu, ¼ dish	**245**	11	27
Cantonese Pork Medallions (1)	**195**	4.5	18
Sweet & Sour, ¼ dish	**315**	21	23
Rice & Noodles: Fried Rice, ⅙ dish	**285**	13	33
Combo Dble Pan Fried Ndles, ⅙ dish	**190**	7	22
Dan-Dan Noodles, ⅙ dish	**205**	7	25
Garlic Noodles, ⅓ dish	**250**	11	30
Singapore Ndles w. Curry, ⅓ dish	**210**	9	27
Salad: Ahi Tuna	**120**	6	5
Cantonese BBQ Chicken, ¼ dish	**250**	12	17
Cold Cucumber, ½ dish	**55**	3	3
Oriental Chicken	**220**	14	14
Peanut-Lime Chicken	**220**	14	6
Seafood: Crab Wonton (1)	**290**	16	26
Hot Fish	**200**	10	15
Lemon Scallops, ⅓ dish	**230**	8	24
Szechwan from the Sea, ⅓ dish	**230**	8	19
Paul's Catfish	**260**	15	6
Salt & Pepper Calamari	**320**	19	21
Seared Ahi Tuna, ½ dish	**125**	2.5	5
Shrimp: Crispy Honey, ½ dish	**395**	24	25
Lemon Pepper, ⅓ dish	**190**	10	13
Orange Peel, ⅓ dish	**265**	11	26
Treasures of the Sea:			
w. Shrimp, ⅓ dish	**140**	7	5
w. Lobster Sauce, ⅓ dish	**160**	11	5
Vegetables: Coconut Curry	**170**	11	12
Garlic Snap Peas	**260**	2	55
Poached Baby Bok Choy	**75**	1	13
Shanghai Snow Peas, ½ dish	**95**	2	15
Spinach w. Garlic, serving	**120**	10	3
Stir-Fried Spicy Eggplant, ⅓ dish	**225**	16	18
Szechwan Asparagus, ½ dish	**165**	11	12
Szechwan Long Beans	**190**	8	23
Temple Long Beans, ⅓ dish	**155**	7	12
Vegetable Chow Fun	**180**	5	30
Vegetarian: Ma Po Tofu, ¼ dish	**180**	10	12
Wraps: *Per Serving (⅓ Dish)*			
Chang's Vege in Lettuce Wraps	**175**	9	15
Minced Chkn & Cool Lettuce Wraps	**180**	9	15
Extras: Scallion Pancakes, ⅓ dish	**185**	9	21
Soup: Hot & Sour	**80**	6	3
Wonton	**70**	4	5
Harvest Spring Rolls, ½ roll	**170**	12	14

For Complete Nutritional Data ~ see CalorieKing.com

Philly Connection®

Cheesesteak: Regular Serving	C	F	Cb
The Original Cheesesteak	460	20	41
Cheesesteak Hoagie	485	23	42
Mushroom Cheesesteak	455	19	43
Pizza Steak	470	19	44
Steak Sandwich	355	11	40
The Works	485	19	52
***Chicken & Turkey:** Regular Serving*			
Cheese Chicken	325	12	43
Chicken Hoagie	365	19	42
Chicken Parmesan	360	14	45
Chicken Tenders	595	28	44
Chicken Works	395	14	54
Turkey Hoagie	430	20	41
***From the Sea:** Regular Serving*			
Tuna Hoagie	575	35	39
Italian Specialities: *Regular Serving*			
Italian Hoagie,	505	26	40
Meatball Parmesan	590	33	46
Large Size Hoagies have approximately 50% more calories, fat & carbs than regular size			
***Philly Lites:** Regular (No Cheese, Mayo or Oil)*			
Chicken Hoagie Lite	225	3.5	42
Chicken Parmesan Lite	255	6	44
Chicken Works Lite	290	5	54
Garden Salad	45	0.5	8
Grilled Chicken Lite	220	3.5	42
Grilled Chicken Salad	90	2	15
Turkey Hoagie Lite	290	4	42
Turkey Salad	145	2.5	11
Veggie Hoagie Lite	265	2.5	54
Specialty Salads			
Cheesesteak Salad	335	18	15
Chicken Tenders Salad	365	15	33
Grilled Chicken Caesar Salad	120	5	13
Grilled Chicken Salad	90	2	15
Tuna Salad	285	18	9
Turkey Salad	145	2.5	11
***Vegetarian:** Per Serving*			
Veggie Delite Hoagie	415	16	55
Veggie Delite Salad	240	10	27

Piccadilly Cafeteria®

Meals: No Sides Included	C	F	Cb
Beef: Chopped Steak Fried, 4.5 oz	220	12	2
Roast Leg, small, 4 oz	345	22	2
Steak New York Strip, 10 oz	865	71	1
Steak Ribeye, 10 oz	1025	91	2
Chicken: Breast, Mesquite Smoke	210	8	1
Baked Cajun Boneless Breast	420	27	9
Fish: Baked Tilapia,	205	11	10
Catfish Cajun Baked	390	28	5
Filet Stuffed	550	41	8
Trout Almondine Baked, large	440	18	10
Cajun Baked, large	505	27	6
Filets Baked, large	445	19	10
Pork Loin, Bone in Roast, 5 oz	355	13	10
Roast Beef, 5.5 oz	475	30	3
Shrimp, Fried,	480	22	45
Turkey Breast, Carved, 5.5 oz	285	11	2
Extras: Broccoli w. Cheese Sauce	110	7	9
Cabbage & Bacon, Seasoned	105	8	6
Cabbage Buttered, Steamed	75	5	6
Cauliflower Buttered	60	4	5
Spinach Buttered, Bacon Seasoned	80	6	3
***Soups:** Per Serving*			
Gumbo: Chicken & Sausage, no rice, 9.5 oz	225	15	10
Chicken, no rice, 9.5 oz	85	2	9
***Salads:** Per Serving*			
Caesar, 3 oz	145	11	7
Chef Salad, small, 6 oz	150	9	4
Italian Coleslaw, 3.75 oz	170	16	5
Louisianne Bowl	40	2	2
Mexican, 3.5 oz	65	3	8
Piccadilly Bowl	30	0	6
Shrimp Remoulade, 11.5 oz	515	29	33
***Dressings:** Per Serving*			
Au Jus, 3 fl.oz	5	0	1
Blue Cheese, 2 Tbsp	170	18	1
Cheese Sauce, 2 fl.oz	35	1	5
French, 2 Tbsp	135	13	5
Italian, 2 Tbsp	140	14	3
Ranch, 2 Tbsp	160	17	1
Ranch, Fat Free, 2 Tbsp	30	0	7
Thousand Island, 2 Tbsp	170	18	2
***Desserts:** Per Slice (Sugar Free)*			
Blueberry Pie	340	17	42
Cherry Pie	355	17	45
Chocolate Almond Pie	610	44	49

Pick-Up-Stix®

	C	F	Cb
California Rolls	**200**	8	27
Beef Dishes: Beef and Broccoli	**510**	27	37
House Special	**875**	27	48
Mongolian	**350**	20	20
Szechwan	**340**	20	20
Bowls			
Teriyaki Chicken	**1155**	22	148
Teriyaki Vegetable	**450**	1.5	96
Buddah's Feast: Dark	**105**	0.5	16
Light	**80**	0.5	16
Chicken Dishes *(Per Cup):* Cashew	**360**	16	33
Garlic	**285**	12	24
House	**755**	34	58
Kung Pao	**440**	22	33
Lemon Twisted	**260**	3	37
Orange Peel	**535**	15	76
Sweet n Sour	**475**	22	60
w. Vegetables	**195**	3	20
Chow Mein: *Per Cup*			
Beef	**350**	10	50
Chicken	**355**	9	52
House Special	**360**	9	52
Shrimp	**310**	5.5	51
Vegetable	**270**	3.5	49
Fried Rice *(Per Cup):* Beef	**505**	16	68
Chicken	**475**	13	70
Egg	**420**	8	74
House	**480**	14	69
Shrimp	**430**	10	68
Vegetable	**390**	8	67
Rice: White, 1 cup	**205**	0.5	45
Salad: *Per Serving*			
Chicken Salad w/out Dressing	**470**	20	35
Chinese Chicken Salad w. Lime Dressing	**675**	20	35
Chinese Chicken Salad w. Original Dressing	**650**	22	75
Shrimp: *Per Cup*			
Black Bean	**190**	5	23
Garlic	**185**	5	23
Orange Peel	**310**	5	54
Szechwan	**180**	5	21
w/Vegetables	**170**	5	19
Soup: *Per 2 Cup Bowl*			
Hot & Sour	**290**	5	38
Wonton	**290**	13	27
Vegetables: Szechwan, 1 cup	**105**	1	21

Pizza Hut®

	C	F	Cb
Lower Fat Pizzas: *Per Slice (1/8 Medium Pizza)*			
Diced Chkn, Red Onion, Peppers	**175**	4.5	23
Diced Chkn, Mushroom, Jalapeno	**175**	5	22
Ham, Red Onion, Mushroom	**160**	4.5	22
Ham, Pineapple, Diced Red Tomato	**165**	4	24
Peppers, Red Onion, Diced Tom.	**155**	4	24
Tomato, Mushroom, Jalapeno	**150**	4	22
Carb Tracker: *Per 6" Pizza*			
Pepperoni	**520**	29	37
Pepperoni & Mushroom	**490**	25	39
Meat Lovers	**740**	46	41
Pan Pizza: *Per Slice (1/8 Medium Pizza)*			
Buffalo Chicken	**280**	13	29
Cheese	**275**	13	29
Chicken Supreme	**280**	12	30
Ham	**260**	11	29
Sausage Lover's®	**330**	17	29
Meat Lover's®	**340**	19	29
Pepperoni	**290**	15	29
Pepperoni Lover's®	**340**	19	29
Super Supreme	**340**	18	30
Supreme	**320**	16	30
Veggie Lover's®	**270**	12	30
Personal Pan Pizza: *Per Pizza*			
Cheese	**640**	28	72
Ham	**600**	24	72
Pepperoni	**680**	32	72
Sausage Lover's®	**760**	40	72
Supreme	**760**	36	76
Veggie Lover's®	**600**	24	76
Thin 'n Crispy: *Per Slice (1/8 Medium Pizza)*			
Buffalo Chicken	**200**	7.5	21
Cheese	**195**	8	21
Chicken Supreme	**200**	7	22
Ham	**180**	6	21
Sausage Lover's®	**240**	13	21
Meat Lover's®	**260**	14	21
Pepperoni	**215**	10	21
Pepperoni Lover's®	**260**	14	21
Super Supreme	**260**	13	23
Supreme	**230**	11	22
Veggie Lover's®	**180**	7	23
P'zone Pizza: *Per ½ Pizza*			
Classic	**605**	21	71
Meat Lover's®	**685**	28	70
Pepperoni	**610**	22	69

Continued Next Page . . .

Pizza Hut® cont...

	C	F	Cb
Hand Tossed: *Per Slice (1/8 Medium Pizza)*			
Buffalo Chicken	**240**	7.5	29
Cheese	**240**	8	30
Chicken Supreme	**230**	6	30
Ham	**220**	6	29
Sausage Lover's®	**280**	12	30
Meat Lover's®	**300**	13	29
Pepperoni	**250**	9	29
Pepperoni Lover's®	**300**	13	30
Super Supreme	**300**	13	31
Supreme	**270**	11	30
Veggie Lover's®	**220**	6	31
Stuffed Crust: *Per Slice (1/12 Large Pizza)*			
Cheese	**360**	13	43
Chicken Supreme	**380**	13	44
Ham	**340**	11	42
Sausage Lover's®	**420**	19	43
Meat Lover's	**450**	21	43
Pepperoni	**370**	15	42
Pepperoni Lover's®	**420**	19	43
Super Supreme	**440**	20	45
Supreme	**400**	16	44
Veggie Lover's®	**370**	14	45
The Big New Yorker™: *Per Serving (1/8 Pizza)*			
Beef Topping	**520**	26	47
Cheese	**425**	18	46
Ham	**385**	14	46
Italian Sausage	**545**	29	47
Pepperoni	**410**	17	46
Pork Topping	**510**	25	47
Supreme	**490**	23	48
Veggie Lover's®	**500**	22	57
The Chicago Dish™: *Per Slice*			
Meat Lover's®	**465**	27	35
Pepperoni	**390**	20	34
Pepperoni, Italian Sausage & Mushroom	**415**	22	35
Supreme	**430**	23	36
Veggie Lover's®	**375**	18	36
The Insider: *Per Slice (1/8 Medium Pizza)*			
Cheese Pizza	**365**	17	35
Pepperoni Pizza	**360**	17	35
Supreme Pizza	**415**	21	36
Twisted Crust: Cheese	**455**	16	58
Pepperoni	**440**	15	58
Supreme	**480**	18	59

	C	F	Cb
Ultimate Lovers Big New Yorker: *Per Slice*			
Cheese/Pepperoni Lover's®	**470**	22	47
Meat Lover's®	**580**	33	47
Veggie Lover's®	**400**	16	50
Ultimate Lovers Hand Tossed: *Per Slice*			
Cheese Lover's®	**280**	13	28
Meat Lover's®	**330**	17	28
Pepperoni Lover's®	**290**	14	28
Veggie Lover's®	**230**	8	30
Ultimate Lovers Pan: *Per Slice*			
Meat Lover's®	**370**	22	29
Cheese Lover's®	**330**	17	29
Pepperoni Lover's®	**300**	16	29
Veggie Lover's®	**270**	12	30
Ultimate Lovers Personal Pan: *Per Slice*			
Cheese Lover's®	**740**	35	72
Meat Lover's®	**840**	45	72
Pepperoni Lover's®	**780**	39	72
Veggie Lover's®	**610**	24	75
Ultimate Lovers Stuffed Crust: *Per Slice*			
Cheese Lover's®	**400**	19	41
Meat Lover's®	**470**	26	41
Pepperoni Lover's®	**430**	22	40
Veggie Lover's®	**350**	15	42
Ultimate Lovers Thin 'n Crispy: *Per Slice*			
Veggie Lover's®	**200**	8	24
Cheese/Pepperoni Lover's®	**250**	12	22
Meat Lover's®	**330**	17	28
Sandwiches: Ham & Cheese	**550**	21	57
Supreme	**635**	28	62
Dessert Pizza: Apple Dessert	**260**	3.5	53
Cherry Dessert Pizza	**240**	3.5	47
Pasta: Cavatini Pasta	**475**	14	66
Cavatini Supreme Pasta	**560**	19	73
Spaghetti: w. Marinara	**490**	6	91
w. Meat Sauce	**600**	13	98
Meatballs	**845**	24	120
Sides: Breadsticks, 1.3 oz	**150**	6	20
Buffalo Wings, Hot (1)	**55**	3	1
Buffalo Wings, Mild (1)	**40**	2.5	0
Ranch Dipping Cup, 1½ oz	**210**	22	4
Garlic Bread, slice	**150**	8	16

Pizza Pizza® (Canada)

Pizza: Per Slice (1/8 Pizza)	C	F	Cb
Large: BBQ Chicken	240	5	37
Bacon Bonanza/Dble Chseburger	250	9	32
Canadian	260	9	33
Extreme Cheese	245	7	35
Four Seasons	265	9	37
Four Seasons, no Cheese	170	5	25
Hawaiian	260	7	38
Mediterranean Vegetable	235	7	35
Montreal Smoked Meat	220	5	33
Pepperoni & Mushroom	230	6	33
Sicilian	260	8	34
Super	230	6	33
Vegetarian	215	5	37

Medium Pizza: *Per Slice*
Deduct 10% fewer calories/fat/carbs from figures for large pizza

Extra Large Pizza: *Per Slice*
Add 10% more calories/fat/carbs from figures for large pizza

	C	F	Cb
Slices: Average all types, 1 slice	800	22	115
Vegetarian; Big Cheese, 1 slice	700	14	110
Stuffed S'wiches: Avg. all types	360	10	52
Oven Toasted Sandwiches			
BBQ Chicken	470	12	58
no Cheese	280	4.5	58
Deli Classic	560	24	55
Honey Mustard Club	490	15	62
Meatball	550	23	56
Mediterranean Vegetable	440	18	53
Roast Beef Supreme	440	14	53
Chicken Items			
Chicken Wings (6)	420	2.5	28
Dino/Chicken Nuggets (6)	320	29	22
Chicken Strips (4)	350	27	23
X-treme Chicken Sandwich	420	44	18
Fries: Regular, 5 oz	340	47	15
Large, 7 oz	470	66	20
Garlic Stix: Regular (3)	390	13	54
X-treme Cheese (3) w. 1 oz cheese	480	21	54
Garlic Bread: Regular bun	710	38	74
X-treme with Cheese	880	52	74
Drinks			
Crispy Crunch Milkshake, 11.5 fl.oz	350	11	50
Lipton's Brisk, 11.5 fl.oz	135	0	34
Gatorade Orange/Blue Raspb. 500ml	130	0	32
Mountain Dew Code Red, 20 fl.oz	320	0	70
Mug Root Beer, 11.5 fl.oz	160	0	39
Orange Crush, 11.5 fl.oz	180	0	45
7-UP, 11.5 fl.oz	140	0	35

Pizzeria Uno®

	C	F	Cb
Entrees: Veggie Burger Meal	610	15	104
Tomato Basil Chicken	570	8	83
Zesty Pasta Marinara	380	3.5	75
Thin Crust Pizza: *9" Individual*			
Vegetarian: w. Cheese	850	22	127
No Cheese	620	5	124
Soup: Light Lunch w. Soup	745	6	150
Tomato Garden Vegetable	125	1	25
Salads: Special House	90	1	17
Light Lunch w. Salad	710	6	141
Pasta Green Salad	410	9	69
Veggie Dip Platter	460	11	77

Planet Smoothie®

Cool Blended Smoothies *Per 22 fl.oz Unless Otherwise Stated*	C	F	Cb
Captain Kid, 12 fl oz	210	1.5	48
PBJ	600	17	97
Shag-a-delic	450	1	104
The Last Mango	375	3.5	83
Twig & Berries	325	0.5	74
Vinnie del Rocco	410	3.5	92
Energy Smoothies: *Per 22 fl.oz*			
Berry Bada-Bing	390	0.5	88
Chocolate Elvis	520	9	109
Frozen Goat	375	0.5	85
Grape Ape	320	0.5	78
Road Runner	300	0.5	72
Spazz	290	0.5	69
Low Carb Shakes, all flavors	150	2	8
Protein Smoothies: *Per 22 fl.oz*			
Big Bang	375	0.5	80
Chocolate Chimp	445	1	94
Merlin's Planet Living Pineapple	345	1	35
Strawberry	425	1.5	55

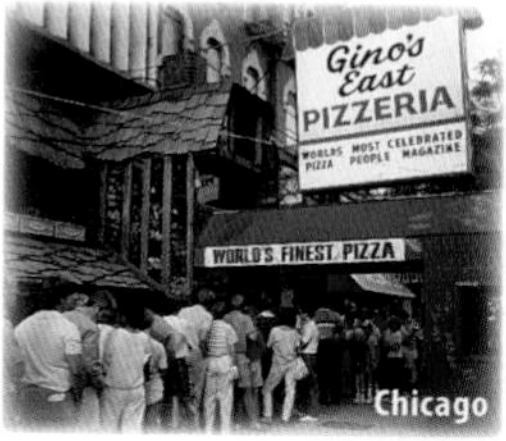

Chicago

Pollo Tropical®

	C	F	Cb
Grilled Chicken: ¼ Chicken White	295	14	1
¼ White no Skin, 4 oz	170	3	0
¼ Chicken Dark, 4.5 oz	300	18	0.5
¼ Dark no Skin, 3.5 oz	170	7	1
Bananas Tropical, 7 oz	500	13	90
Black Beans (combo portion), 5 oz	150	2	24
Black Beans, side, 8.5 oz	270	4	43
Boiled Yucs, 12 oz	330	0	81
Boneless Breast, 5 oz	140	4	1
Chicken Caesar S'wich, 6.5 oz	460	10	36
Chicken Sandwich, 8 oz	440	19	35
Chicken TropiChop	560	10	20
Congri, 7 oz	440	13	69
Corn, 3 oz	140	1.5	34
Grilled Chicken Salad (No Dressing)	210	4	na
Grilled Tropical Shrimp, 1 Skewer	90	1	0
Island Park, 5 oz	210	10	1
White Rice, 7 oz	340	6	65
Yucatan Fries, 5.3 oz	440	24	54

Popeye's®

	C	F	Cb
Chicken: Chkn Breast, Mild/Spicy	530	31	18
Chicken Leg, Mild/Spicy	200	12	7
Chicken Thigh, Mild/Spicy	390	29	12
Chicken Wing, Mild/Spicy	220	15	10
Sides: Biscuit, 2 oz	225	12	25
Cajun Rice	180	7	23
Cinnamon Apple Pie, 3 oz	250	10	37
Coleslaw	235	17	20
Corn on the Cob	255	4	48
French Fries, 4.5 oz	380	18	50
Mashed Potatoes: no Gravy	95	2	17
w. Gravy	120	4	18
Onion Rings, 4 oz	380	20	43
Red Beans & Rice	340	19	33

Port of Subs®

	C	F	Cb
BBQ Beef	560	6	87
Hot Pastrami	570	17	62
Meatball	645	25	76
Mesquite Chicken	545	11	68
Western Philly Cheese Steak	505	9	78
Breakfast Sandwiches: *Per 4" Sub*			
Egg & Smoked Ham w. Cheese	250	16	4
Soups *(Medium Bowl):* Minestrone	50	1	8
Boston Clam Chowder	105	4	13
Roasted Chicken Noodle	80	2	9

Port of Subs® cont...

	C	F	Cb
Original Submarines: *Per 5" White or Wheat Roll No Mayonnaise included in figures below.*			
If using mayo, add 1 Tbsp	110	12	0
BLT	400	19	43
Combination of Cheeses	495	25	44
Ham w. American Cheese	475	20	45
Ham & Salami/Turkey w. Provolone	425	15	47
Ham/Salami/Capicolla/Pepp./Prov.	525	26	45
Peppered Pastrami w. Swiss	415	17	44
Roast Beef Turkey w. Provolone	410	14	45
Rstd Chicken Breast w. Provolone	395	13	45
Salami w. Provolone	495	25	45
Salami & Pepperoni w. Provolone	525	27	45
Salami & Turkey w. Provolone	455	20	46
Smkd Ham & Turkey w. Smky Ched.	425	15	47
Smoked Ham w. Swiss	415	16	45
Tuna	420	18	45
Turkey w. Provolone	415	14	47
Vegetarian w. Avoc. & Olives, no chse	350	14	48
Hot Sandwiches: *Per 8" White or Wheat Roll*			
Salads: *Includes Vinegar & Oil Unless Indicated*			
Antipasto Salad, 12 oz	405	29	14
Chef Salad, 12 oz	395	26	14
Green Salad, 12 oz	125	7	13
Macaroni Salad, no oil, 8 oz	440	30	36
Mesquite Chicken Salad, 13 oz	315	13	16
Potato Salad, no oil, 8 oz	465	26	54
Tuna Salad, 11 oz	280	16	13

Pret A Manger®

	C	F	Cb
Bakery: *Per Serving*			
Almond Croissant	320	22	25
Carrot Cake	380	19	48
Elephant Poo	110	4	17
Ham, Cheese & Tomato	400	22	32
Muffin, Seville Orange	470	22	61
Pet Brownie	330	17	40
Pretzel	370	8	62
Slice, Orange & Fruit	340	16	45
Sandwiches			
Big BLT	540	25	52
Chicken Avocado w. Half Fat Mayo	480	25	38
Smoked Salmon	370	14	50
Super Club	540	25	47
Vegetarian	345	3.5	71
Sushi: Deluxe Sushi	490	8.5	89
Wraps: Avocado	540	37	40
Green Thai Chicken	325	12	34
Salads: Noodle & Chicken	295	5	43
Roast Vegetable	60	3.5	6.5

For Complete Menu ~ See CalorieKing.com

Pretzelmaker®

Pretzels	C	F	Cb
Caramel Crunch, 4.7oz	**390**	6	74
Cinnamon, 4.6 oz	**380**	5	74
Garlic, 4.6 oz	**375**	5	72
Original, 4.4 oz	**340**	2	70
Original, Butter Flavor & Salt, 4.6 oz	**370**	5	71
Parmesan, 4.7oz	**385**	6	72
Poppy Seed, 4.6 oz	**380**	6	71
Pretzel Dog, 5.6 oz	**1645**	159	38
Sesame, 4.6 oz	**380**	6	71
Stix, Butter Flavored & Salt, 4.9 oz	**385**	6	73
Stix, Plain, 4.6 oz	**355**	2.5	73
Sauces: *Per Serving (1.5 fl.oz)*			
Cheddar Cheese	**125**	10	6
Chili Spice	**375**	5	72
Cream Cheese	**205**	20	4
Nachos Cheese	**30**	0	4
Pizza Sauce	**35**	0.5	6
Drinks: *Per Serving*			
Mrs Fields: Lemonade, small, 20 fl oz	**170**	0	39
regular, 32 fl oz	**280**	0	65
large, 44 fl oz	**390**	0	91

Pretzel Time®

Pretzels	C	F	Cb
Caramel Crunch, 4.7 oz	**335**	4	66
Chili Spice, 4.2 oz	**300**	3	60
Cinnamon Sugar, 4.1 oz	**330**	4	65
Italian Parmesan, 4.2 oz	**305**	3.5	60
Plain, 3.8 oz	**275**	1	59
Poppyseed, 4.2 oz	**390**	4	80
Regular, Butter & Salt, 4 oz	**305**	4	59
Roasted Garlic, 4.2 oz	**300**	3	60
Sesame, 4.2 oz	**310**	4	59
Sour Cream & Onion, 4.2 oz	**305**	3.5	60
Deli Pocket: Ham & Swiss, 7.2 oz	**490**	16	61
Pepperoni, 6.3 oz	**505**	20	65
Turkey & Swiss, 7.2 oz	**515**	18	58
Pretzel Bites:			
Butter & Salt: Medium, 4.2 oz	**305**	4	59
Large, 4 oz	**270**	3.5	52
Plain: Small, 3 oz	**210**	0.5	45
Medium, 4 oz	**275**	1	59
Large, 3.5 oz	**245**	1	52
Pretzel Dog (1), 5.5 oz	**470**	28	38
Pretzel Stix, Butter & Salt, 4.7 oz	**370**	4.5	72
Stuffers: Cheese, 13 oz	**1215**	69	95
Jalapeno, Regular, 13 oz	**1225**	69	97
Small, 8 oz	**715**	38	64

Pretzel Time® cont...

Sauce: *Per Serving (2 oz)*	C	F	Cb
Caramel	**145**	0	35
Cheddar Cheese	**75**	5	4
Cream Cheese	**205**	20	2
Honey Mustard	**80**	0	20
Ketchup	**15**	0	4
Mustard	**5**	0	1
Nacho Cheese	**75**	5	4
Pizza Sauce	**35**	0.5	6
Vanilla Glaze	**180**	0	45
Drinks: Mrs Field's Lemonade,			
20 fl.oz	**170**	0	39
32 fl.oz	**270**	0	63
44 fl.oz	**370**	0	86

Quizno's Subs®

Signature Subs	C	F	Cb
Classic Italian Sub: (No Dressing)			
Small, 9 oz	**645**	30	60
Regular, 11½ oz	**728**	33	69
Large, 19½ oz	**1201**	58	102
Honey Mustard Chicken			
with bacon, large, 22½ oz	**1355**	40	137
Philly Cheese Steak, large, 10½ oz	**721**	16	92
Steakhouse Sub (6"), 6½ oz	**507**	21	52
Traditional (no dressing) (8"), 15 oz	**800**	24	94
Turkey Ranch Swiss (no dress.), 8"	**690**	18	89
Low-Fat Sandwiches (Small)			
Honey Bourbon Chicken	**330**	6	45
Sierra Smoked Turkey			
w. Raspberry Chipotle Sauce	**360**	6	53
Turkey Lite	**360**	6	52
Tuscan Chicken Salad	**325**	6.5	45
Veggie Lite	**300**	6	40
Dressings: Beef Au Jus, 4 oz	**20**	0.5	3
Honey Mustard, 2 oz	**140**	6	22
Italian Vinagarette, 1 oz	**130**	14	3
Ranch Dressing, 2 oz	**285**	30	3
Potato Chips			
Classic Potato Chips: Trad'l, 1.5 oz	**240**	14	25
Kettle Cooked, 1.375 oz	**200**	11	23
Jalapeno, 1.375 oz	**210**	12	22
Salt & Vinegar, 1.375 oz	**185**	9	23
Sour Cream & Onion, 1.5 oz	**250**	15	25
Cookies			
Peanut Butter, 3 oz	**380**	21	42
Average of other cookies	**360**	18	48

Quincy's®

Steak	C	F	Cb
Chopped, 8 oz	500	42	0
Country Style Steak w. Gravy	530	25	44
Cowboy Steak, 14 oz	580	33	9
Filet w. Bacon	340	17	2
N.Y.Strip Steak, 10 oz	450	26	1
Porterhouse Steak	680	46	0
Ribeye, 10 oz	450	29	0
Sirloin: Large	370	20	2
Regular	285	16	0
Sirloin Junior	195	10	0
Sirloin Tips	205	8	4
Smothered Strip Steak	620	41	12
T-Bone, 13 oz	520	35	0
Soups: Chili with Beans	235	11	21
Clam Chowder	180	9	21
Cream of Broccoli	170	10	18
Vegetable Beef	90	2	14
Entrees: Grilled Chicken	125	2	1
Homestyle Chicken Filet	220	9	21
Grilled Salmon	230	4	1
Sth Breaded Shrimp	545	31	47
Steak & Shrimp	680	39	33
Roasted Herb Chicken	875	65	4
Roasted BBQ Chicken	940	65	21
Grilled Trout	300	12	2
Sandwiches: No Mayo/Extras			
Bacon Cheeseburger	665	41	33
Grilled Chicken Sandwich	325	4	39
Philly Cheese Steak	590	30	38
Smothered Steak	430	15	36
Spicy BBQ Chicken	370	5	45
Breads: Banana Nut	165	7	22
Biscuit	270	15	29
Cornbread	140	5	17
Yeast Roll	160	4	29
Sides: Baked Potatoes	370	0	86
Corn on the Cob	140	1	33
Rice Pilaf	105	2	20
Desserts: Banana Pudding	240	12	30
Brownie Pudding Cake	310	5	66
Chocolate Chip Cookie	60	3	8
Apple Cobbler	255	8	49
Cherry Cobbler; Peach Cobbler	310	8	55
Frozen Yogurt	135	2	25
Sugar Cookie	60	3	8
Fudge Topping; Caramel	105	4	15

Rally's Hamburgers®

Burgers/Sandwiches	C	F	Cb
Rallyburger	435	22	35
with Cheese	490	27	35
Big Buford	745	48	35
Chicken Fillet Sandwich	400	15	43
Chili w. Cheese & Onion: 7 oz	360	22	20
13 oz size	670	41	37
Super Barbecue Bacon	595	31	49
Super Double Cheeseburger	760	48	37
French Fries: Regular	210	11	26
Large	320	16	39
X-Large	425	21	52
Shakes: Vanilla, small	320	11	49
Other flavors, small	410	12	73

Ranch 1®

Salads: Gourmet Greens, 12 ½ oz	220	7	31
Chicken on Gourmet Greens, 15 oz	350	11	31
Zesty Caesar Salad, 7 oz	180	3	31
Zesty Chicken Caesar Salad, 9 oz	290	6	31
Sandwiches: American Ranche	390	10	51
Club Sandwich	470	16	53
Grilled Chicken Philly	450	14	53
Ranch Classic	370	5	53
Spicy Grilled Chicken	420	11	58
Side Kicks: Fruit Cup, 8.3 oz	90	0.5	18
Ranch Fries, regular	350	14	51
Specialties: Chicken Tenders	370	15	7
Baked Potato: w. Broccoli	510	0.5	117
w. Cheese	790	25	118
w. Chicken	610	4	114
Grilled Chkn & Vegetable Platter	790	7	129
Grilled Chicken Fajita	330	16	25
Grilled Chicken Hot Pasta	590	10	86

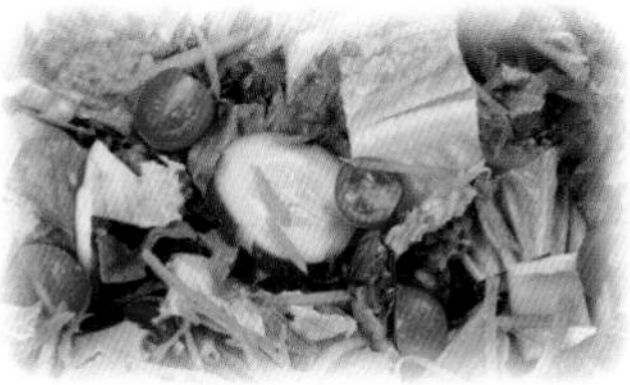

Rax®

Sandwiches	C	F	Cb
Regular Rax	**390**	22	32
Deluxe	**520**	35	35
BBC	**715**	51	37
Grilled Chicken: Philly Melt	**535**	32	35
Jr. Deluxe	**365**	25	25
BBQ Beef	**400**	20	43
Mushroom Melt	**600**	38	35
Turkey/Bacon Club	**680**	47	37
Turkey	**485**	32	33
Cheddar Melt	**345**	23	26
Potatoes: Plain	**205**	0	60
w. Butter	**305**	12	60
w. Sour Topping	**255**	4	62
Cheese/Broccoli	**285**	0	72
Soups: Cream of Broccoli	**95**	4	14
Chicken Noodle	**115**	1	21
Chili	**160**	9	12
Salads: Grilled Chicken	**160**	5	6
Side Salad	**40**	4	2
Garden	**220**	9	12
Salad Dressings: Fat Free Italian	**10**	0	2
Fat Free Catalina; Ranch	**30**	0	6
1000 Island	**130**	13	5
Buttermilk Ranch	**175**	20	1
Blue Cheese; Creamy Caesar	**145**	16	1
Honey French	**140**	5	9
Vinaigrette	**30**	2	4

Red Lobster®

Fresh Fish: *Per Plate*			
Atlantic Salmon (full portion)	**580**	31	0
(half portion)	**260**	12	0
Rainbow Trout (full portion)	**510**	25	6
(half portion)	**275**	14	2
Tilapia (full portion)	**345**	10	0
(half portion):	**185**	6	0
Specialties: *Per Serving*			
Broiled Flounder	**240**	5	0
Grilled Chicken			
w. Seasoned Fresh Broccoli	**380**	9	14
w. Wild Rice Pilaf	**530**	14	38
Signature Shellfish,			
Jumbo Shrimp Cocktail Dinner:			
plate	**250**	3	2
King Crab Legs, 1 plate	**490**	9	0
Live Maine Lobster, 1 plate	**145**	1	2
Rock Lobster Tail, 1 plate	**260**	3	2
Snow Crab Legs, 1 plate	**260**	4.5	0
Steamed Live Maine Lobster, 1 plate	**145**	1	2

Red Lobster® cont ...

	C	F	Cb
Lighthouse Menu: *Per Serving (Unless Otherwise Indicated)*			
Awesome Additions:			
100% Pure Melted Butter	**185**	21	0
Baked Potato w. topping	**185**	2	37
no topping	**180**	2	36
Cheddar Bay Biscuits	**160**	9	17
Cocktail Sauce, small	**35**	0	9
Fresh Buttered Vege (1)	**145**	12	9
Garden Salad (1)	**50**	2	9
Jumbo Shrimp Cocktail (1)	**145**	2	2
King Crab Legs (1)	**165**	3	0
Maine Lobster Tail (1)	**105**	5	2
Petite Shrimp Topping	**30**	1	1
Red Wine Vinaigrette Dressing	**50**	3	5
Seasoned Fresh Broccoli (1)	**60**	0	12
Snow Crab Legs (1)	**130**	2	0
Wild Rice Pilaf (1)	**210**	5	36
Beverages: *Per Serving*			
Coffee; Diet Coke	**0**	0	0
Michelob Ultra	**100**	0	2.5
Minute Maid Light Lemonade	**5**	0	1
Sutter Home Cabernet Sauvignon	**140**	0	4.5
Sutter Home Chardonnay	**150**	0	5

Rita's®

Cream Ice: *Per Serving*	C	F	Cb
Kids	**205**	3	45
Regular	**330**	4.5	72
Large	**520**	7	115
Quart	**880**	12	194
Gelati: Regular	**320**	10	56
Regular w. Cream Ice	**345**	12	59
Large	**545**	17	95
Large w. Cream Ice	**590**	21	101
Italian Ice: Kids	**170**	0	45
Regular	**275**	0	73
Large	**435**	0	115
Quart	**735**	0	195
Misto: Regular	**415**	7	90
Regular w. Cream Ice	**465**	11	88
Large	**620**	10	135
Large w. Cream Ice	**695**	17	132
Frozen Custard: Kids	**275**	14	31
Regular	**370**	20	42
Large	**535**	28	60

Rocky Rococo®

Pizza: Per Regular Slice	C	F	Cb
Cheese, 5.75 oz	**380**	9	54
Sausage, 7 oz	**495**	19	54
Pepperoni, 6.1 oz	**430**	13	54
Sausage & Mushroom, 7.6 oz	**500**	19	55
Garden of Eatin', 7.6 oz	**390**	10	56
Pizza: Per Super Slice			
Average all types	**700**	27	82
Pasta: Per Serving			
Spaghetti: w. Tomato Sauce, reg.	**470**	4	87
w. Meat Sce, regular	**500**	7	87
w. Meatballs, regular	**630**	16	89
Light Spaghetti: w. Tomato Sauce	**235**	2	44
w. Meat Sauce, regular	**315**	8	45
w. Meatballs, regular	**250**	3	44
Fettuccine: w. Alfredo, regular	**460**	14	66
Light w. Alfredo Sauce	**230**	4	33
Can't Decide, 14 oz	**465**	9	77
Bread: Muffin (1)	**200**	4	38
Breadsticks (6) w. Marinara Sce	**420**	7	72
Breadsticks (6) w. Jalapeno Chse	**530**	18	72

Roly Poly®

Sandwiches: Per ½ Sandwich	C	F	Cb
Baked Ham & Roast Pork:			
BarBQ Pork Melt	**290**	11	27
Italian Classic	**300**	13	30
Key West Cuban Mix	**305**	9.5	28
Peachtree Melt	**285**	12	29
Porky's Nightmare	**300**	12	28
Chicken: Basil Cashew Chicken	**270**	11	28
Catalina Chicken Salad	**290**	13	28
Chicken Caesar	**285**	12	30
Chicken Cordon Bleu	**305**	12	28
Chicken Fajita	**270**	8	28
Chicken Popper	**260**	7	31
Cobb Salad	**285**	14	30
Delhi Chicken	**315**	13	33
Hickory Chicken	**300**	11	29
Oriental Chicken	**255**	6	32
Popper w. Wheat bread	**255**	6.5	29
Santa Fe Chicken	**270**	8	29
Seafood: Salmon Club	**300**	14	30
Salmon Roll	**260**	11	27
Texas Tuna Melt	**300**	14	27
Thai Hot Tuna	**290**	13	29
Tuna Luau	**325**	15	30

Round Table® Pizza

Large Pizza (14") Per Slice (1/12 Whole)	C	F	Cb
Cheese: Thin	**210**	8	23
Pan	**290**	10	37
Chicken & Garlic Gourmet™:			
Thin	**230**	9	24
Pan	**320**	11	38
Chicken Rostadoro™: Thin	**250**	10	25
Pan	**330**	12	39
Gourmet Veggie™: Thin	**220**	9	25
Pan	**310**	11	39
Guinevere's Garden Delight®:			
Thin	**210**	7	25
Pan	**290**	9	38
Hawaiian: Thin	**210**	7	25
Pan	**290**	9	38
Hearty Bacon Supreme™: Thin	**270**	14	22
Pan	**360**	16	36
Italian Garlic Supreme™: Thin	**270**	14	23
Pan	**360**	16	37
King Arthur's Supreme®: Thin	**270**	14	24
Pan	**340**	14	38
Maui Zaui™ (Polynesian Sce):			
Thin	**240**	9	27
Large Pizza (14"): Per Slice (1/12 Whole)			
Pan	**330**	11	41
Maui Zaui™ (Red Sce): Thin	**240**	9	25
Pan	**320**	11	39
Montague's All Meat Marvel®:			
Thin	**290**	17	24
Pan	**350**	16	37
Pepperoni: Thin	**240**	11	23
Pan	**310**	12	37
Pepperoni Rostadoro™: Thin	**270**	12	26
Pan	**350**	14	40
Roastin' Toastin'™ Chicken Club:			
Thin	**260**	12	25
Pan	**350**	14	39
Ulti-Meat Premium: Thin	**290**	15	24
Pan	**370**	17	37
Western BBQ Chicken™: Thin	**240**	9	23
Pan	**320**	11	37
16" Pizzas: Per Slice (1/8 Whole)			
Aloha Vinnie Pepperoni™	**430**	14	55
Big Vinnie Pepperoni™	**460**	19	49
Maui Mama (Polynesian Sce)	**570**	22	63
Maui Mama (Red Sce)	**560**	22	61
Mama Zella Pizza	**550**	23	59

Round Table® cont...

Personal Pizzas: Per Pizza	C	F	Cb
Cheese: Thin	580	24	60
Pan	810	36	106
Chicken & Garlic Gourmet™: Thin	620	25	64
Pan	850	27	110
Chicken Rostadoro™: Thin	680	29	66
Pan	910	31	112
Hawaiian: Thin	560	19	66
Pan	780	21	109
Gourmet Veggie™: Thin	590	23	67
Pan	820	25	114
Guinevere's Garden Delight®: Thin	550	20	66
Pan	760	21	110
Hearty Bacon Supreme™: Thin	700	35	59
Pan	940	37	105
Italian Garlic Supreme™: Thin	760	41	63
Pan	990	43	109
King Arthur's Supreme®: Thin	750	39	64
Pan	900	34	109
Maui Zaui™ (Red Sce): Thin	590	22	66
Pan	820	24	111
Sides/Sandwiches			
Garlic Bread	470	21	59
w. Cheese	630	33	59
Garlic Parmesan Twists, 3 pce	510	14	76
Buffalo Wings, 3 pce	210	14	1
6 pce	420	28	2
Honey BBQ Wings, 3 pce	190	13	4
6 pce	390	25	8
Sandwiches: Chicken Club	820	39	75
Ham Club	810	37	76
RT Pizza	690	34	65
RT Veggie	680	29	79
Turkey Club	800	37	75

Roy Rogers®

	C	F	Cb
Breakfast Items			
Big Country Breakfast: w. Bacon	740	43	61
w. Sausage	920	60	61
w. Ham	710	39	67
Burgers			
Hamburger	260	9	33
Cheeseburger	300	13	34
¼ lb Hamburger	430	18	41
¼ lb Cheeseburger	470	22	42
Sourdough Grilled Chicken	500	21	46
Sandwiches: Roast Beef	260	4	30
Chicken Fillet	500	24	49
Grilled Chicken	340	11	32
Fries: Regular	350	15	49
Large	430	18	59
Desserts: Hot Fudge Sundae	320	10	50

Rubio's Fresh Mexican Grill®

	C	F	Cb
Burritos			
Especial: Cheesy Bean	840	37	92
Chicken	920	32	116
Carne Asada	970	37	117
Baja Grill: Chicken	640	26	61
Carnitas	660	30	64
Carne Asada	710	33	63
HealthMex: Chicken	520	11	75
Veggie	470	8	81
Baja Gourmet Seafood: Fish	780	41	76
Shrimp, grilled	650	25	77
Mahi Mahi, chargrilled	630	30	58
Lobster, grilled	660	26	82
Cabo Coconut Shrimp: Burrito	680	20	99
Burrito Sides: Chips, 1.5 oz	220	11	28
Rice, 3 oz	110	1.5	21
Tacos			
Chicken, whitemeat	300	16	23
Carne Asada	220	8	23
Mahi Mahi	310	16	24
HealthMex Chicken	170	2.5	23
Cabo Coconut Shrimp: Taco	300	8	43
Taco Meal Deal w. rice/beans	690	21	106
Fish Taco: Original	300	16	28
Especial	370	21	30
Street: Carnitas (1)	110	5	10
Carne Asada (1)	100	3.5	10
Rubio's Favorites			
3-Cheese Quesadilla	860	53	60
with Chicken	960	56	61
with Carne Asada	1010	61	62
Nachos Grande	1270	79	112
with Chicken	1380	82	112
with Carne Asada	1430	87	114
Chicken Taquitos (3)	310	11	37
Sides: Rice, 4 oz	150	2	28
Pinto Beans, 7 oz	190	3	44
Black Beans, 7 oz	220	2.5	37
Chips, 3 oz	430	22	56
Churro, 1.5 oz	170	8	22
Guacamole, small, 4 oz	170	16	8
Salads: Grilled Chkn Chopped Salad	540	33	33
HealthMex Chicken Salad	220	3.5	27
Low Carb Chicken Salad	480	34	11
Bowls: Chicken	710	31	69
Carne Asada	770	37	70

Ruby Tuesday®

Burgers: (No Sides or Sauces Incl.)	C	F	Cb
Bacon Cheeseburger	1010	67	52
Classic Burger	830	53	51
Colossal Burger	1680	114	78
Turkey Burger Club	780	41	52
Veggie Burger	805	41	69
Gourmet Sandwiches: *(No Sides or Sauces Included)*			
Ruby's Chicken Sandwich	640	25	58
Ultimate Roasted Turkey BLT	1120	66	71
Low-Carb: Roasted Turkey Wrap	275	7	25
Grilled Chicken/Caesar Wrap	395	18	21
Panini: Cuban/Ham, average	1170	82	56
Turkey & Bacon	1320	87	52
Steaks & More: *(No Sides or Sauces Included)*			
Top Sirloin	285	11	1
Petite Sirloin	220	8	1
Ruby's Ribeye	635	44	4
Smothered Sirloin Tips	990	52	53
Grilled BBQ Chicken: Single Breast	210	5	3
Platters: *(No Sides or Sauces Included)*			
Louisiana Fried Shrimp	1000	52	103
Chicken Tenders: Original	965	47	86
Spicy Buffalo	1190	70	92
Ribs, Half Rack: average all types	940	51	73
Full Rack	1430	84	87
Pasta: *(Garlic Toast Not Included)*			
Chicken Parmesan	1465	95	89
Pasta Marinara	660	10	115
Shrimp Alfredo; Roma Chkn, avg.	1180	50	107
Sonora Chicken	1170	41	121
Specialties: *(No Sides or Sauces Included)*			
Creole Catch	665	31	44
New Orleans Seafood	860	46	47
Oven Roasted Turkey Dinner	730	30	60
Low-Carb: New Orleans Seafood	800	50	28
Church Street Chicken	790	51	26
Creole Catch	610	35	23
Peppercorn Salmon	585	32	29
Oven Roasted Turkey Dinner	630	24	27
Appetizers: *Per ¼ Order (Sauces not Included)*			
Asian Pot Stickers	120	5	13
Chicken Quesadilla	190	11	12
Fried Cheese	170	11	13
Loaded Cheese Fries	290	18	21
Low-Carb Chicken Quesadilla	155	10	4
Low-Carb Spicy Buffalo Wings	230	16	1
Original Chicken Tenders	130	7	7
Queso Dip	320	22	23
Signature Sampler	280	17	19
Southwestern Spring Rolls	175	10	15
Spicy Buffalo Chicken Tenders	190	13	9
Spicy Honey BBQ Chicken Tenders	160	7	15
Spinach Dip	290	20	19
Tuesday Sampler	200	12	14

Salads (Entree)	C	F	Cb
Dressing Not Included Unless Indicated			
Carolina Chicken Salad	880	62	37
Low-Carb: Chicken Cobb	620	41	12
Chicken Caesar w. Dressing	500	35	16
Peppercorn Salmon w. Dress.	655	46	16
Spring Chicken Salad	400	24	10
Signature Sauces & Dressings: *Per 2 Tbsp (1 oz)*			
Barbecue Sauce	50	0	13
Cocktail Sauce	23	0	6
Marinara Sauce	15	1	2
Remoulade Sauce	160	17	1
Salsa	10	0	2
Sour Cream; Turkey Gravy	30	2	2
Steak Butter, 1 Tbsp, ½ oz	90	10	0
Thai Peanut Sauce	65	3	8
Dressings: Ranch	100	11	1
Light Balsamic Vinaigrette	35	2	4
Bleu Cheese Dressing	175	19	1
Honey Mustard Dressing	90	8	5
Caesar Dressing	100	10	2
Smoky Honey Dijon	100	8	7
Signature Soups: Onion Soup	200	13	20
Baked French Onion	550	39	30
Low-Carb Broccoli & Cheese	330	27	15
Side Items: Baked Beans	130	3	22
Baked Pot. w. Butter & Sour Crm	460	19	62
Broccoli, Fresh Steamed	130	8	8
Brown Rice & Black Beans	275	6	45
Brown Rice Pilaf	220	6	35
Cole Slaw	130	8	12
Creamed Spinach	205	17	11
Creamy Mashed Cauliflower	165	11	15
Fresh Sauteed Zucchini	55	3	5
Garlic Toast	220	12	24
Mashed Potatoes	330	15	46
Onion Straws	320	23	25
Ruby's Fries	185	9	24
Sugar Snap Peas	130	6	14
Desserts: Blueberry D'lite	215	5	37
Brownie	1000	46	129
Candy Bar Ice Cream Pie	830	42	102
Low-Carb: Cheesecake	400	32	6
Chocolate Lava Cake	630	40	24
Chocolate Sauce	75	2	9

For Complete Menu ~ See CalorieKing.com

Ryan's® Family Steakhouse

Mega Bar Buffet: Per Serving	C	F	Cb
Baked Fish, 3.5 oz	75	1.5	1
Black Eyed Peas, ½ cup	90	0	17
Breaded Okra, ¾ cup	90	0	19
Breaded Sweet Potato Nuggets (7)	125	3	22
Chicken Breast, 5.2 oz	230	5	0
Chicken Pot Pie, 3.5 oz	160	6	21
Chicken Salad, ⅓ cup	200	14	9
Chicken Tenders, 3 pieces	225	10	15
Clam Chowder, 8 oz	160	6	18
Corn, 3.5 oz	125	7	14
Crab Salad, 3.5 oz	160	10	10
Glazed Baby Carrots w. Salad, ½ cup	105	5	14
Lima Beans, ⅔ cup	120	2	21
Macaroni & Cheese, 8 oz	340	14	38
Marinated 7 Bean Salad, ⅓ cup	165	0	36
Mashed Potatoes, 3.5 oz	110	4.5	14
Meatloaf Patties, 3.5 oz	310	26	8
Mexican Style Beef Casserole, 8 oz	455	25	34
Nacho Cheese Sauce, ¼ cup	80	5	7
Petite Sirloin, 4.2 oz	230	9.5	0
Pinto Beans, 3.5 oz	85	2	13
Pork Chops, 3.5 oz	235	15	0
Pork Ribs (1 rib)	245	15	5
Salmon, 7 oz	225	7	0
Seafood Pasta Salad, 3.5 oz	145	6	16
Sirloin Tips, Plain, 3.8 oz	190	7.5	0
Sliced Pot Roast w. Gravy, 8 oz	175	8	10
Stewed Tomatoes w. Okra, 3.5 oz	50	0	11
Swt Potato w. M'mallows, 3.5 oz	130	0	32
Taco Meat, 3.5 oz	170	10	8
Turkey Breast, 1.3 oz	60	2	1
Vegetable Beef Soup, 8 oz	100	1.5	17
Vegetable Lasagna, 8 oz	390	20	32
Dressing: Ranch, 3.5 oz	355	36	6
Golden Italian; Blue Cheese 1 oz	125	13	2
Ranch, Fat Free, 2 Tbsp	45	0	11
Thousand Island, 3.5 oz	140	6	21
***Bakery Bar Buffet:** Per Serving*			
Pies, average, ⅒ pie	280	8	48
Choc. Pudding, Sugar Free, ½ cup	95	5	12
Chocolate Soft Serve, ½ cup	125	4.5	19
Cobbler, avg. all varieties	290	12	42
Cookies: Raisin Oatmeal (1)	105	3.5	18
Sugar Free (2)	95	6	10
Avg. other varieties	120	6	16
Frozen Yogurt ½ cup	100	0	21

Runza®

Sandwiches	C	F	Cb
Original Runza® Sandwich	545	20	66
Cheese Runza® Sandwich	605	25	68
BBQ Chicken Sandwich	370	11	36
Fish Sandwich	475	23	46
Polish Dog	405	26	25
Smothered Chicken Sandwich	280	9	25
Special Deluxe Chicken Sandwich	295	8.5	29
Kids-Size: Mini Corn Dogs	320	21	25
Chicken Nuggets	310	20	15
Runza® Sandwich	275	10	33
Hamburger	200	10	15
Hamburgers: Deluxe Hamburger	455	19	50
¼ lb Hamburger	345	14	28
¼ lb Cheeseburger	405	18	29
½ lb Double Hamburger	510	23	30
½ lb Double Cheeseburger	625	32	32
Bacon Cheeseburger Deluxe	515	28	30
Swiss Cheese Mushroom Burger	415	20	30
Onion Rings & Fries			
Fries: Regular, 3.3 oz	315	17	35
Large, 3.6 oz	345	19	39
Jumbo, 6.8 oz	640	35	72
Onion Rings: Regular, 4.3 oz	465	29	45
Large, 6.7 oz	715	44	69
Onion Ring Dip, 2 oz	90	6.5	4
Salads & Dressings			
Tossed Salad	90	4	4
Tossed Salad w. Chicken	210	8.5	5
Dressing: Ranch, 2.6 oz	290	30	4
Reduced Calorie Ranch, 2.6 oz	175	15	5
French, 2.6 oz	150	0	35
Lite Italian, 2.6 oz	40	1	5
Thousand Island, 2.6 oz	325	30	15
***Soups:** Per Serving (9.5 oz)*			
Boston Clam Chowder	305	17	30
Broccoli Cheese	280	16	27
Cauliflower Cheese	315	19	30
Chicken Noodle	110	1	16
Homemade Chili	250	8	21
Potato w. Bacon	205	9	27
Vegetable Cheese Medley	250	16	19
Wisconsin Cheese	365	25	27
Desserts & Drinks			
Brownie w. Nuts	465	16	74
Vanilla Shake, regular	520	15	84
Oreo® Shake, regular	655	24	97
Pepsi®, medium, 12 fl.oz	160	0	40

7-Eleven®

Breakfast Sandwiches	C	F	Cb
Big Bite: Breakfast Sandwich	330	19	23
⅓ lb Cheeseburger	410	33	71
Croissant: w. Bacon, Egg & Chse	420	26	34
w. Ham, Egg & Chse	390	22	34
Engl. Muffin w. Saus., Egg, Chse	450	24	37
Sausage, Egg & Cheese Biscuit	500	31	34
Hot Dogs (Big Bite)			
¼ Pound Hot Dog, no bun	360	34	6
⅓ Pound Hot Dog, no bun	480	45	11
Burritos: The Bomb (14 oz)	940	42	116
The Bomb w. Green Chillies	910	42	114
Reynoldos Jumbo Burritos (10 oz):			
Beef & Bean	680	22	93
Beef & Potato	590	20	82
Red Hot Burrito	640	20	88
Green Burrito	710	26	93
Sandwiches (7-Eleven)			
Big Eats Deli Sandwiches:			
Chicken Salad, 7.3 oz	630	35	47
Classic Chicken Caesar, 8.3 oz	590	27	45
Hearty Ham, 8.3 oz	570	30	48
Smoked Turkey w. Chse/Mayo	560	27	45
Stacked Turkey & Ham, 7.8 oz	630	34	46
Tuna Salad, 7.5 oz	550	22	56
Hot Pockets: Ham 'n' Cheese, 7 oz	480	19	55
Meatballs w. Mozzarella	490	18	59
Bakery Stix™ Treats: Per Stick (3.5 oz)			
BBQ Chicken	230	6	34
Pepperoni & Cheese	340	18	30
Other flavors, average	290	12	33
Sushi			
California Rolls, 8-Pack	560	8	80
Donuts & Muffins (World Ovens)			
Donuts: Boston Creme (1)	290	9	47
Blueberry Cake (1)	330	22	31
Chocolate Iced (1)	250	17	23
Glazed (1)	250	16	24
Jelly (1)	420	16	66
Muffins: Apple Spice, 7.5 oz	520	4	114
Banana Nut, 7 oz	660	26	97
Blueberry, 5.6 oz	450	14	73

7-Eleven® cont...

Go-Go Taquitos	C	F	Cb
Beef Taco & Cheese, 3 oz (1)	250	11	30
Fiesta Chicken, 3 oz (1)	220	12	22
Jalapeno & Cream cheese, 3 oz	240	13	27
Monterey Jack Chkn, 3 oz (1)	280	14	30
Fountain Drinks (Figures Assume ⅓ Ice)			
Coca-Cola/Pepsi/Dr.Pepper/7Up:			
Gulp, 20 oz	190	0	48
Big Gulp, 32 oz	300	0	75
Super Gulp, 44 oz	410	0	102
Double Gulp, 64 oz	600	0	150
Diet Coke/Diet Pepsi, 16 oz	1	0	0
Slurpees: Average All Flavors,			
12 oz size	165	0	41
22 oz size	300	0	75
28 oz size	385	0	96
40 oz size	545	0	136
Crystal Light, 12 fl.oz	60	0	12
Slurp & Gulp Combo,			
32 oz Big Gulp & 22 oz Slurpee	600	0	150
Café Coolers: Mocha, 12 oz	350	12	63
French Vanilla, 12 oz	380	16	58
Fruit Coolers			
Orange/Strawb. Creme, 12 fl.oz	280	1	68
16 fl.oz size	370	1	90
20 fl.oz size	470	2	113
Arizona Rasp. Green Tea, 12 fl.oz	230	0	56
Cafe Select Coffee: 12 fl.oz	7	0	2
16 fl.oz size	10	0	2
20 fl.oz size	12	0	3
24 fl.oz size	15	0	4
Hot Drinks: Hot Chocolate, 8 fl.oz	130	2	24
French Vanilla Cappuccino, 8 fl.oz	100	6	25

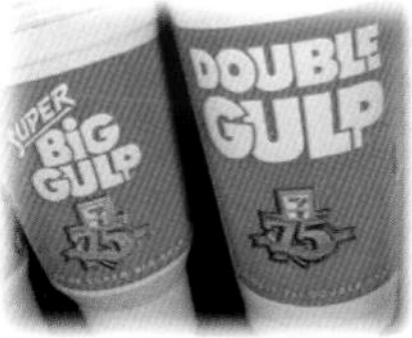

Sammy's® Woodfired Pizza

Healthy Dining Meals	C	F	Cb
Chinese Chicken Salad	480	13	49
Chopped Chicken Salad	385	11	20
Grilled Shrimp Wrap	560	19	57
Grilled Vegetable Penne	620	21	84
Tomato Angel Hair Pasta	670	18	105
Vegetarian Pizza, ½ Pizza	860	21	130

Samurai Sam's®

***Appetizers:** Per Serving*			
California Rolls	245	1	53
Grilled Egg Rolls	150	5	20
***Bowls:** Per Regular Bowl*			
Chicken	605	11	94
Chicken & Steak	610	10	94
Chicken & Steak, all white	565	7	91
Chicken, all white	525	3	89
Steak	615	9	93
Veggie	395	1	88
Salads: Oriental Chicken	495	8	89
***Specialties:** Per Serving*			
Chicken & Prawns	590	9	92
Chicken & Prawns, all white	555	4	92
Steak & Prawns	600	8	92
Teriyaki Prawns	480	2	88
YakiSoba	530	9	96

Sbarro's®

***Meals:** Per Serving*	C	F	Cb
Baked Ziti w. Sauce	700	41	43
Chicken Parmigiana, 11 oz	520	22	16
Meat Lasagne, 13 oz	640	37	36
Spaghetti w. Sauce, 20 oz	410	28	120
***Pizza:** Per Slice*			
Cheese, 7.7 oz	455	13	60
Pepperoni, 9.6 oz	720	37	61
Sausage, 9.7 oz	660	31	60
Supreme, 10.3 oz	620	27	63
***Stuffed Pizza:** Per Slice*			
Spinach & Broccoli	790	34	89
Pepperoni	940	42	89

Schlotzsky's®

Bread/Buns	C	F	Cb
Dark Rye, regular	330	2	68
Sourdough, regular	335	2	68
Wheat, regular	340	3	66
Jalapeno Cheese, regular	350	4	66
Pizza Crust	335	2	68
***Original Sandwiches:** Per Sandwich*			
The Original, regular	730	31	79
Large Original, family size	1390	58	152
Deluxe Original, regular	925	42	84
Ham & Cheese Original, regular	745	27	82
Turkey Original, regular	815	32	81
***Sandwiches:** Per Regular Sandwich*			
Albacore Tuna	520	10	77
Albacore Tuna Melt	770	29	83
BLT	580	24	70
Chicken Breast	500	4	80
Chicken Club	685	23	75
Corned Beef	595	12	78
Corned Beef Reuben	840	33	82
Dijon Chicken	500	6	74
Fiesta Chicken	840	36	79
Pastrami & Swiss	890	36	81
Pastrami Reuben	935	41	83
Pesto Chicken	520	9	73
Roast Beef	620	15	78
Roast Beef & Cheese	850	32	83
Santa Fe Chicken	620	14	81
Smoked Turkey Breast	500	7	75
Texas Schlotzsky's	765	32	76
The Philly	840	29	86
The Vegetarian	480	11	79
Turkey & Bacon Club	835	35	79
Turkey Guacamole	645	19	84
Turkey Reuben	825	34	80
Vegetable Club	540	18	76
Western Vegetarian	630	28	76
Wraps: Asian Almond Chicken	445	7	72
Chicken Caesar	505	27	40
Salsa Chicken w. Cheddar	435	17	44
Zesty Albacore Tuna	315	7	45
***Soups:** Per Cup (8 oz)*			
Boston Clam Chowder	235	15	24
Broccoli Cheese w. Florets	250	17	23
Chicken Gumbo	110	5	13
Chicken Tortilla	165	3	13
Chicken w. Wild Rice	380	19	36
Minestrone	90	1	17
Old-Fashioned Chicken Noodle	120	2	18

Continued Next Page . . .

Schlotzsky's® cont...

Deli Salads: Per 5 oz Container	C	F	Cb
Albacore Tuna, small, 4.4 oz	170	9	2
California Pasta	60	3	10
Elbow Macaroni	275	19	23
Homestyle Cole Slaw	190	10	24
Mustard Potato	250	13	31
Potato	290	15	35
Leaf Salads: w/out Dressing/Croutons/Noodles			
Caesar Salad	35	1	3
Chicken Caesar	105	3	4
Chinese Chicken	130	3	10
Garden Salad	50	1	7
Greek Salad	175	11	10
Ham & Turkey Chef's	225	11	13
Smoked Turkey Chef's	180	10	3
8" Pizzas: Bacon, Tom. & Mushr.	620	22	78
Barbeque Chicken	655	15	93
Chicken & Pesto; New Orleans	650	19	78
Double Cheese	580	19	76
Double Cheese & Pepperoni	730	32	77
Fresh Tomato & Pesto	540	16	76
Mediterranean	535	18	72
Smoked Turkey & Jalapeno	625	17	80
Thai Chicken	665	17	89
The Original Combination	625	23	79
Tuscan Herb	540	15	80
Vegetarian Special	555	17	76
Salad Extras: Chow Mein Noodles	75	4	9
Garlic Chinese Croutons, ½ oz, pkg	40	2	5
Greek Balsamic Vinaigrette, 1.5 oz	160	17	2
Light Italian Dressing, 1.5 oz	90	8	3
Olde World Caesar Dress., 1.5 oz	260	27	1
Ranch Dressing: Traditional, 1.5 oz	270	29	1
Spicy, 1.5 oz	230	25	2
Light Spicy, 1.5 oz	140	11	9
Schlotzsky's Deli Chips, 1.5 oz bag	210	11	26
Sesame Ginger Vinaigrette, 1.5 oz	170	15	8
Thousand Island Dressing, 1.5 oz	220	21	6
Kid's Deals: w/out Cookie/Drink			
Cheese Pizza	460	11	72
Cheese Sandwich	400	15	49
Ham & Cheese Sandwich	430	16	50
PBJ Sandwich	490	16	71
Pepperoni Pizza	510	16	72
Desserts/Cookies: Fudge Brownie	430	25	46
Cookies: Oatmeal Raisin	145	5	24
Cookies w. Real M&M's	135	5	20
Other varieties, average	165	7	23
Cheesecake: Cookies & Crème	330	18	36
New York; Strawberry Swirl	310	18	31

Shakey's®

Pizzas (12"): Per Slice (1/10 Pizza)	C	F	Cb
Cheese only:			
Thin Crust	135	5	13
Thick Crust	170	5	22
Homestyle Pan	305	14	31
Onion/Olives/Mushrooms:			
Thin Crust	125	5	14
Thick Crust	160	4	22
Homestyle Pan	320	15	32
Sausage Pepperoni:			
Thin Crust	165	8	13
Thick Crust	205	8	22
Homestyle Pan	375	20	31
Sausage Mushroom			
Thin Crust	140	6	13
Thick Crust	180	6	22
Homestyle Pan	340	17	31
Pepperoni:			
Thin Crust	150	7	13
Thick Crust	185	6	22
Homestyle Pan	345	15	31
Shakey's Special:			
Thin Crust	170	9	13
Thick Crust	210	8	22
Homestyle Pan	385	21	32
Other Items			
3-Piece Chicken & Potato	945	56	51
5-Piece Fried Chicken & Potato	1700	90	130
Hot Ham & Cheese Sandwich	550	21	56
Potato Wedges, 15 pieces	950	36	120
Shakey's Super Hot Hero	810	44	67
Spagh. w. Meat Sce/Garlic Bread	940	33	134

Sheetz®

Coffeez™: Per 16 fl.oz	C	F	Cb
Hot Chocolate, medium	195	3	39
Cupo'ccino®: Per Medium (16 fl.oz)			
Almond Amaretto; French Vanilla	215	8	34
Fat Free French Vanilla	220	0	47
M.T.O® Cold Subs:			
Per 6" Sub (No Cheese Unless Indicated)			
Cheese Sub w. American Cheese	410	11	75
Chicken, Salad	505	11	85
Club Combo Sub	445	5	76
Cold Cut Sub	520	17	77
Cooked Ham Sub; Roast Beef	410	5	76
Egg Sub	385	6	76
Italian Sub	455	9	77
Tuna Salad	520	12	84
Turkey Sub	405	3	76
Veggie Sub	330	2	75

Sheetz® cont...

M.T.O® Hot Subs: Per 6" Sub	C	F	Cb
Buffalo/Rstd Chicken, no Cheese	**475**	6	76
Meatball, no Cheese	**535**	17	80
Pepperoni Sub	**605**	28	75
Steak, no Cheese, 10 oz	**500**	9	77
M.T.O® Bagelz: *No Cheese Unless Indicated*			
Cheese Bagel w. American Cheese	**385**	11	60
Chicken Salad	**475**	11	71
Club Combo	**420**	5	62
Cheese Bagel w. American Cheese	**385**	11	60
Chicken Salad	**475**	11	71
Club Combo	**420**	5	62
Cold Cut	**495**	17	63
Cooked Ham; Roast Beef	**380**	5	62
Egg	**360**	6	62
Italian	**425**	9	63
Tuna Salad	**490**	12	70
Turkey	**375**	3	62
Veggie	**300**	2	61
M.T.O® Burgerz, no Cheese, 8 oz	**535**	28	41
M.T.O® Hot Dogs: *No Cheese*			
Big Deli Dog, 7 oz	**675**	33	77
Hot Dog, 2 oz	**265**	15	23
M.T.O® Nachos: *Per Serving*			
Nachos Bueno/Grande w. Cheese	**535**	32	42
Nachos Grande, no Cheese	**270**	12	36
M.T.O® Salads: *No Cheese*			
Caesar Salad	**20**	0	3
Chef Salad	**100**	3	5
Chicken Caesar; Roasted Chicken	**200**	4	3
Chicken Salad	**195**	9	14
Garden Salad	**20**	0	4
Oriental Chicken	**430**	12	37
Steak Salad	**190**	7	6
Taco Salad	**215**	9	27
Tuna Salad	**210**	10	13
M.T.O® Breakfast			
Bagels: Bacon Breakfast	**490**	19	62
Egg	**440**	15	62
Ham	**535**	18	64
Shmiscuits (Includes Cheese):			
Egg	**275**	15	26
Ham	**370**	18	28
Sausage	**415**	28	26
Shmuffins (Includes Chse): Egg	**285**	15	28
Bacon	**330**	19	28
Ham	**380**	18	30
Italian Meats	**320**	17	29

Shoney's®

Breakfast	C	F	Cb
All Star Breakfast, no extras	**185**	14	1
Deluxe Pancake Platter	**1600**	32	300
Half Stack Pancake Platter	**930**	14	187
Big Eater Steak Brkfast, no extras	**610**	41	1
Country Fried Steak Breakfast	**990**	66	49
Sunrise Breakfast	**975**	60	88
Sausage Biscuit (1)	**540**	34	42
Burgers			
All-American: Burger	**680**	32	44
Bacon Cheeseburger	**880**	49	44
Mushroom Swiss Burger	**970**	57	49
Famous Patty Melt	**935**	60	40
Half O-Pound Burger	**1350**	52	130
Sandwiches			
Blackened Chicken	**895**	21	122
Charbroiled Chicken Sandwich	**905**	22	122
Chicken Parmesan Sandwich	**750**	30	80
Corned Beef Reuben	**785**	53	37
Fish Sandwich	**830**	16	126
Fried Chicken Sandwich	**565**	14	76
Original Slim Jim Sandwich	**1010**	33	122
Potatoes & Gravy Sandwich	**770**	24	95
Raymond's French Dip	**510**	14	53
Turkey Club/Whole Wheat	**945**	52	46
Ultimate Grilled Cheese S'wich	**890**	46	77
Steaks			
BBQ Ribs	**1520**	78	124
Choice Sirloin, 6 oz	**1225**	51	127
Half-O-Pound w. Grilled Onions	**1335**	52	133
Half-O-Pound w. Grilled Mushr.	**1320**	52	127
Ribeye, 8 oz	**1475**	75	127
Southwest Half-O-Pound	**1290**	69	83
T-Bone, 12 oz	**1795**	100	127
Surf & Turf:			
Ribeye & 5 Fried Shrimp	**1640**	82	138
Ribeye & 6 Grilled Shrimp	**1590**	81	128
Sirloin & 5 Fried Shrimp	**1380**	58	138
Sirloin & 6 Grilled Shrimp	**1330**	57	128
T-Bone & 5 Fried Shrimp	**1965**	107	138
T-Bone & 6 Grilled Shrimp	**1900**	105	128
Rib Combos, w. Fries:			
¼ Rack & BBQ Chicken	**1230**	54	103
¼ Rack & Tenderloins	**1370**	70	120
¼ Rack & Fried Shrimp	**1145**	50	113
¼ Rack & Grilled Shrimp	**1125**	52	103

Continued Next Page . . .

Shoney's® cont...

Blue Plate Specials	C	F	Cb
Cajun Whitefish	475	10	56
Baked Whitefish	500	8.5	58
Grandma's Meatloaf w. Glaze	1080	46	92
Grandma's Meatloaf w. Gravy	1075	48	87
Original Country Fried Steak	1160	62	103
Grilled Liver & Onions	710	22	79
Ham Steak Dinner (no veges)	665	25	60
Roast Beef Platter (no veges)	885	30	96
***Pasta:** Per Serving*			
Chicken Alfredo	1725	78	170
Italian Feast	1480	45	204
Pasta Ya-Ya	1875	81	176
Shrimp Alfredo	1800	85	171
Spaghetti	495	16	63
Seafood: Fish 'n' Shrimp	1100	39	129
Fried Fish Platter	1035	38	122
Grilled Cod/Salmon Lite	200	4	0
Grilled Salmon	750	19	95
Grilled Shrimp	710	20	95
Grilled Shrimp Lite	305	8	30
Shrimper's Feast	1020	39	127
Shrimp Stir Fry	875	19	131
Sides: Baked Potato, Plain	350	6	67
French Fries, 4 oz	205	10	25
Onion Rings, 1 order (7 rings)	510	14	83
Chicken: Chicken Stir Fry	1200	35	172
Charbroiled Blackened Chicken	830	26	100
Charbroiled Chicken Breast	790	22	99
Fried Chicken Tenderloins	1150	60	121
Monterey Chicken	905	40	83
Smothered Chicken	890	34	90
Junior Meals: Fish 'N Chips	300	11	29
Chicken Dinner	190	10	12
Desserts, Ice cream, Sundaes			
Apple Pie: a la Mode	1220	53	173
w. NutraSweet	435	18	64
Cheesecake, 1 slice, 4 oz	340	25	23
Hot Fudge Sundae	600	30	75
Original Strawberry Pie, 1 slice	330	17	45
Ultimate Hot Fudge Sundae	605	30	75
Cherry/Peach Pie w. Nutrasweet	450	18	64
Caramel Sundae	615	27	83
Chocolate Milk Shake	1125	51	141
Strawberry Sundae	625	27	85
Walnut Brownie a la Mode	585	33	60

Sizzler®

Hot Entrees: (No Sides)	C	F	Cb
Hamburger	625	33	36
Dakota Ranch Steak: 6 oz	315	20	0
8 oz	420	27	0
9½ oz	500	32	0
Hibachi Chicken Breast, w. Pineapple	195	3	13
Lemon-Herb Chicken Breast	140	3	0
Malibu Chicken Patty, each	310	19	11
Salmon	250	12	0
Santa Fe Chicken Breast	150	3	0
Shrimp: Broiled	150	6	0
Fried, 4 only	225	2	35
Mini	150	1	24
Shrimp Scampi	145	3	0
Swordfish	315	14	0
Low Carb Grill Menu			
Grilled Salmon w. Broccoli	405	19	14
Hibachi Chicken w. Broccoli	295	6	15
Petite Sizzler Steak w. Broccoli	520	26	11
Hot Bar			
Broccoli Chse Soup, 4 oz	140	9	10
Chicken Noodle Soup, 4 oz	30	1	4
Chicken Wings, 1 oz	75	4	4
Clam Chowder, 4 oz	120	6	11
Focaccia Bread, 2 pces	110	7	9
Meatballs, 4 balls	155	11	5
Minestrone Soup, 4 oz	35	0	7
Pasta: Fettucine, 2 oz	80	1	15
Spaghetti, 2 oz	80	0	16
Potato Skins, 2 oz	160	8	22
Refried Beans, ¼ cup	60	1	11
Saltine Crackers, 2 crackers	25	1	4
Taco Filling, 2 oz	105	9	3
Taco Shells, each	50	2	7
Dessert Bar: Chocolate Syrup, 1 oz	90	0	21
Choc/Vanilla Soft Serve, 4 oz	135	4	24
Strawberry Topping, 1 oz	70	0	18
Whipped Topping, 1 Tbsp	10	1	1
Salads & Toppings			
Prepared Salads: *Per 2 oz*			
Carrot & Raisin	130	10	10
Chinese Chicken; Teriyaki Beef	55	2	6
Mediterranean Minted Fruit	30	0	7
Mexican Fiesta	55	1	10
Old Fashioned Potato	85	5	10
Red Herb Potato	120	9	9
Seafood	55	3	4
Seafood Louis Pasta	65	2	9
Spicy Jicama	15	0	4
Tuna Pasta	135	10	6

Sizzler® cont...

Sides	C	F	Cb
Baked Potato, plain	220	0	50
Cottage Cheese, 2 oz	50	1	2
Eggs, 1 oz	45	3	0
Garbanzo Beans, ¼ cup	65	1	11
Kidney Beans, ¼ cup	50	0	10
Olives, 1 oz	60	6	1
Peaches, ¼ cup	35	0	9
Peas, ¼ cup	30	0	6
Real Bacon Bits, 1 Tbsp	30	2	2
Turkey Ham, 1 oz	60	5	0
***Dressings:** Per 2 Tbsp (1 oz)*			
Blue Cheese	110	12	1
Honey Mustard	160	16	4
Italian, Lite	15	0	2
Japanese Rice Vinegar, Fat Free	10	0	2
Parmesan Italian	100	10	2
Ranch	120	12	2
Ranch, Reduced-Calorie	90	8	4
Thousand Island	145	15	3

Skyline Chili®

***Menu Items:** Per Serving*	C	F	Cb
Chili (Regular): Plain, ½ pint	250	15	4
w. Beans, ½ pint	260	12	17
Chili Spaghetti: Regular	400	14	44
Large	540	19	59
Chili Spaghetti: w. Onions: Reg.	415	14	47
Large	560	19	63
Chili Spaghetti w. Beans: Reg.	480	14	57
Large	650	19	79
Chili Spaghetti w. Beans/Onions:			
Regular	485	14	60
Large	665	19	82
Burritos: Regular	550	30	42
Deluxe Burrito	610	34	47
Coneys: Regular	270	14	23
Cheese Coney	390	24	23
Chili Sandwich	235	9	25
w. Cheese	340	18	24
Black Beans and Rice	330	12	44
3-Way (Spagh., Chili, Chse): Reg.	715	42	39
Large	1055	61	61
4-Way (3-Way w. Onions): Reg.	725	42	41
Large	1075	61	65
4-Way (3-Way w. Beans): Reg.	785	42	52
Large	1160	61	80

Skyline Chili® cont...

5-Way (3-Way + Onions + Beans)	C	F	Cb
Regular	795	42	54
Large	1185	61	84
Salads			
Garden Salads: Regular	80	5	4
Large	155	10	7
Greek Salads: Regular	385	36	9
Large	700	68	13
Nacho Salads: Regular	455	25	40
Large	760	42	66

Smoothie King®

***Weight Gain Smoothies:** Per 20 oz*			
Hulk™: Chocolate/Vanilla	870	29	128
Strawberry	980	29	156
Malts	915	41	118
Peanut Power®	535	21	72
Peanut Power Plus™: Grape	730	21	119
Strawberry	665	21	105
Shakes	900	41	117
***Lowfat Smoothies:** Per 20 oz*			
Angel Food™; Mangofest™, avg.	330	0.5	79
Blackberry Dream™	355	0.5	86
Blueberry Heaven™	265	1	58
Celestial Cherry High™	285	0.5	69
Cherry Picker™	420	0.5	98
Cranberry Cooler	535	0	132
Cranberry Supreme™	575	0.5	138
Grape Expectations™; Caribbean®	400	0.5	96
Grape Expectations II™	535	0.5	129
Hearthy Apple™	390	2	81
Immune Builder™; Island Treat®	350	1	80
Instant Vigor™	365	1	87
Lemon Twist® Banana	345	0.5	82
Lemon Twist® Strawberry	405	0.5	97
Light & Fluffy®	405	0.5	98
Muscle Punch®/Plus™	355	1.5	80
Orange Ka-Bam™	425	0	104
Peach Slice™	340	0	80
Peach Slice Plus®	475	0	113
Pep Upper®	340	1	80
Pineapple Pleasure®	315	0.5	76
Pineapple Surf™	455	1	104
Raspberry Sunrise™	360	0.5	85
Slim & Trim™: Chocolate	280	1.5	55
Strawberry	355	1	79
Orange-Vanilla	195	0.5	43
Vanilla	235	1	51

Continued Next Page . . .

Smoothie King® cont...

Lowfat Smoothies (Cont): Per 20 oz	C	F	Cb
Strawberry Kiwi Breeze™	**295**	0	70
Strawberry X-Treme™	**375**	0	91
Youth Fountain™	**275**	0.5	65
Specialty Smoothies: *Per 20 oz*			
Banana Boat	**540**	14	93
Coconut Surprise™	**480**	6	99
Mo'cuccino™	**430**	12	71
Pina Colada Island™	**570**	11	102
Yogurt D-Lite®	**335**	4	58
Workout Smoothies: *Per 20 oz*			
Activator®: Chocolate	**485**	1	90
Strawberry	**580**	1	123
Vanilla	**445**	1	90
Power Punch™	**445**	1.5	102
Power Punch Plus®	**510**	2	113
Super Punch™	**390**	0.5	95
Super Punch Plus®	**485**	0.5	118
High Protein Smoothies: *Per 20 oz*			
Almond Mocha; Chocolate	**420**	13	45
Banana	**440**	14	44
Lemon/Pineapple	**405**	13	41

Snappy Tomato®

Large Pizza: Per Slice (1/12 Pizza)			
Cheese Pizza	**160**	5	21
Sausage	**190**	8	22
Pepperoni	**200**	9	21
Snappy Supreme	**425**	28	24
Sides: Snappy Wings, 3 pces	**160**	11	0
Chicken Snappers, 2 pces	**150**	5	12

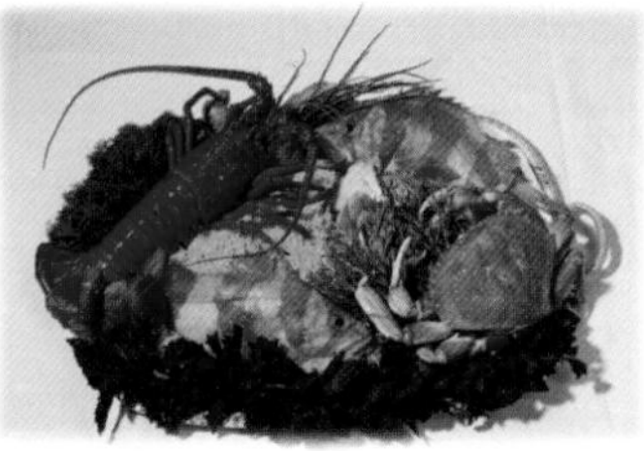

Sonic Drive-In®

Burgers	C	F	Cb
#1. Burger	**550**	36	43
#2. Burger	**455**	25	43
#1. Cheeseburger	**625**	42	44
#2. Cheeseburger	**525**	31	44
Bacon Cheeseburger	**710**	49	44
Super Sonic #1	**885**	66	45
Super Sonic #2	**790**	55	46
Junior Burger	**355**	21	27
The Little Cheese	**840**	66	28
Toaster Sandwiches: BLT	**615**	41	42
Bacon Cheddar Burger	**685**	38	60
Chicken Club	**715**	29	75
Country Fried Steak	**730**	45	55
Grilled Cheese	**310**	12	39
Sandwiches			
Country Fried Steak	**745**	47	56
Breaded Chicken	**585**	23	66
Grilled Chicken	**350**	13	31
Wraps			
Carb Friendly Chicken Club			
w. Carb Friendly Tortilla, 8.4 oz	**555**	30	34
Chicken Strip, w. Ranch Dressing	**560**	29	55
Fritos Chili Cheese	**740**	42	68
Grilled Chicken w. Ranch Dressing	**520**	27	40
Chicken			
Chicken Strip Dinner	**760**	32	86
Chicken Strip Snack	**280**	13	22
Salads: Grilled Chicken, no dressing	**365**	17	20
Jumbo Popcorn Chicken, no dress.	**495**	26	39
Santa FeGrilled Chkn, no dress.	**425**	18	33
Coneys			
Plain: Regular	**265**	16	22
Extra Long	**475**	27	44
Cheese: Regular	**365**	24	24
Extra-Long	**660**	42	47
Corn Dog	**270**	17	23
Breakfast			
Breakfast Burrito	**615**	37	45
Bacon Egg & Cheese Toaster®	**535**	29	40
Sausage Egg & Cheese Toaster®	**595**	36	44
Ham Egg & Cheese Toaster®	**470**	19	41
Sonic Sunrise® Breakfast: Regular	**240**	0	60
Large	**405**	0	100

Sonic Drive-In® cont...

Faves & Craves	C	F	Cb
French Fries: Regular, 3.7 oz	**185**	9	22
Large, 4.9 oz	**245**	12	30
Super Sonic™, 7.2 oz	**360**	18	44
Ched 'R' Peppers®	**255**	12	29
Cheese Fries: Regular, 4.3 oz	**270**	17	23
Large, 5.5 oz	**325**	22	29
Chili Cheese Fries: Regular, 5.1 oz	**300**	19	24
Fritos® Chili Pie, 6.7 oz	**610**	44	36
Mozzarella Sticks, 5.4 oz	**390**	19	35
Onion Rings: Regular	**340**	5	66
Large, 19 oz	**515**	7	100
Sonic™, 20.6 oz	**560**	8	108
Tater Tots: Regular, 4.2 oz	**235**	14	27
Large, 6.1 oz	**350**	21	40
Supersonic™, 8.1 oz	**465**	28	53
Cheese Tater Tots: Regular	**325**	22	28
Large, 6.8 oz	**425**	27	41
Chili Cheese Tater Tots: Regular	**360**	25	28
Large, 9 oz	**530**	36	43
Blasts: Regular, all types, avg.	**520**	27	58
Large, all types, average	**765**	39	89
Slushes: Small, average	**230**	0	58
Regular, average all flavors	**325**	0	81
Large, average all flavors	**510**	0	127
Wacky Pack®, average	**210**	0	50
Route 44®, average	**490**	0	123
Slush Floats/CreamSlush™			
Regular, average	**340**	12	52
Large	**485**	17	74
Desserts: Banana Split, 12½ oz	**425**	11	75
Chocolate Sundae, 8½ oz	**290**	11	41
Dish of Vanilla, 7 oz	**195**	11	19
Hot Fudge Sundae, 8½ oz	**320**	15	40
Ice cream Cone	**215**	11	23
Pineapple Sundae, 9 oz	**330**	11	53
Strawberry Sundae	**250**	11	32
Drinks: Barq's Root Beer, large	**360**	0	90
Coca-Cola, large	**325**	0	81
Coca-Cola Float, large	**425**	17	59

For Complete Nutritional Data ~ see CalorieKing.com

Souper Salad®

Soups: Per Serving (5 oz)	C	F	Cb
Beef Stroganoff	**105**	5	10
Chicken Creole	**95**	2	10
Chicken Tetrazini	**110**	4	10
Cream of Cauliflower	**60**	2.5	8
Cream of Spinach	**25**	1	4
German Potato; Potato Corn	**100**	5	11
Hungarian Mushroom	**115**	8	9
Mac and Cheese	**100**	4	13
New England Clam Chowder	**90**	3.5	11
Santa Fe Chicken	**100**	3.5	8
Other varieties, average	**80**	2	10
Potato Topping: *Per 5 oz*			
Vegetable Cheese	**105**	3	3
Bread: Blueberry, 4 oz	**260**	5	49
Corn, 4 oz	**265**	6	49
Focaccia Bread, 3.5 oz	**390**	7	69
Garlic Bread Stick (2)	**120**	2	23
Gingerbread, 3.5 oz	**290**	11	46
Focaccia, all varieties (1)	**70**	3	10

For Complete Nutritional Data ~ see CalorieKing.com

Souplantation®

Soups: Per Cup	C	F	Cb
Low Fat: Chicken Tortilla	**100**	3	5
Chicken Noodle	**160**	3	17
Vegetable Medley	**90**	1	14
Regular Soup: *Per Cup*			
Chesapeake Corn Chowder	**310**	13	43
Cream of Mushroom	**290**	21	15
Irish Potato Leek	**260**	16	23
Manhattan Clam Chowder	**130**	4	16
Minestrone w. Italian Sausage	**210**	11	14
Navy Bean w. Ham	**340**	10	30
Vegetarian Harvest	**190**	8	23
Chili: House Chili. 1 cup	**230**	3	26
Breads: Sourdough	**150**	0.5	27
Buttermilk Cornbread, 1 pce	**140**	2	27
Focaccia: Garlic Parmesan	**100**	3	15
Pizza /Tomatillo	**140**	6	16
Fresh Tossed Salads: *Per Cup*			
Antipasto Salad; BBQ, average	**140**	10	6
Caesar Salad Asiago	**190**	14	10
Won Ton Chicken Happiness	**150**	8	12

Continued Next Page . . .

Souplantation® cont...

Prepared Salads: Per ½ Cup	C	F	Cb
Aunt Doris' Red Pepper Slaw	70	0	18
Baja Bean & Cilantro	180	3	29
BBQ Potato	160	8	20
Broccoli Madness	180	14	11
Carrot Raisin	90	3	17
Dijon Potato w. Garlic Dill Vinegar	150	12	9
Greek Couscous w. Feta Cheese	170	9	19
Oriental Ginger Slaw w. Krab	70	3	8
Southern Dill Potato	120	3	20
Thai Noodle w. Peanut Sauce	170	8	17
Dressing & Croutons: *Per 2 Tbsp*			
Blue Cheese Dressing	140	14	3
Balsamic Vinaigrette	180	19	1
Italian Dressing	120	13	1
Fat Free	20	0	5
Honey Mustard Dressing	150	13	8
Fat Free	45	0	10
Ranch Dressing	130	13	1
Fat Free	10	0	2
Thousand Island Dressing	110	11	3
Croutons, Garlic Parmesan, 5 pces	40	3	2
Hot Tossed Pastas: *Per Cup*			
Bruschetta	260	4	41
Creamy Bruschetta	360	16	43
Garden Vegetable: w. Meatballs	270	7	42
w. Italian Sausage	300	10	42
Italian Vegetable Beef	270	6	43
Vegetarian Marinara w. Basil	260	4	44
Muffins: Chocolate Brownie	170	8	22
Georgia Peach Poppyseed	140	6	20
Lemon	140	4	19
Big Blue Blueberry, small	140	5	22
Fruit Medley Bran	80	0.5	17
Desserts: *Per ½ Cup*			
Apple Cobbler	350	10	64
Apple Medley (fat-free)	70	0	18
Banana Royale (fat-free)	80	0	20
Chocolate Chip Cookie, small	70	3	10
Chocolate Lava Cake	300	8	56
Jello, flavored	85	0	20
Rice Pudding	110	2	20
Vanilla Pudding	150	3	24
Chocolate Syrup, 2 Tbsp	70	0	18
Granola Topping, 2 Tbsp	110	4	16
Soft Serve: Chocolate, ½ cup	95	0	21
Vanilla Soft Serve (reduced fat)	140	4	22

For Complete Nutritional Data ~ see CalorieKing.com

Southern Tsunami®

Sushi: Per Serving	C	F	Cb
California Roll, 9 pieces	290	5	54
California Roll & Inari, 7 pieces	325	6	58
California Salad Roll, 6 pieces	570	20	83
Combos: Seaside, 12 pieces	300	3.5	49
Shoreline, 10 pieces	475	5.5	84
Stardust, 11 pieces	305	3	58
Vegetable, 9 pieces	230	4	45
Cream Cheese Roll:			
w. Imitation Crab, 9 pces	530	25	60
w. Salmon, 9 pces	570	29	53
w. Tuna, 9 pces	550	26	53
Crunchy Shrimp Roll, 9 pieces	650	19	83
Dragon Roll, 9 pieces	645	34	63
Eel Roll, 9 pieces	465	18	55
Fullmoon Combo, 6 pieces	305	7	50
Futomaki, 6 pieces	310	1.5	68
Futomaki & Inari, 6 pieces	355	4.5	68
Green River Roll, 9 pieces	490	20	55
Grilled Salmon Roll, 9 pieces	350	6.5	54
Inari, 4 pieces	260	5	46
Mix & Match (M & M) Roll:			
Eel & Carrot, 12 pieces	315	7	51
Imitation Crab & Carrot, 12 pces	245	0.5	53
Tuna & Cucumber, 12 pces	245	1	49
Shrimp & Avocado, 12 pces	280	4	50
Marina Plate, 6 pieces	425	5	73
Meteor Special, 11 pieces	370	3	67
Nigiri: *Per Piece*			
Eel	85	2	13
Octopus; Salmon; Yellowtail	65	0.5	12
Shrimp	90	1	12
Snapper; Squid; Tuna	60	0	12
Ocean Crab Roll, 9 pieces	345	8	54
Orange Roll, 9 pieces	395	8	65
Rainbow Roll, 9 pieces	480	10	92
Small Roll: *Per 12 Pieces*			
Avocado	295	7	52
Carrot	240	0.5	53
Cucumber	225	0.5	50
Eel	390	13	50
Imitation Crab	250	0.5	53
Salmon	330	6	47
Shrimp	265	1	49
Tuna	260	1.5	47
Yellowtail	290	3	49

Southern Tsunami® cont...

Snack Pack: *Per 12 Pieces*	C	F	Cb
Avocado	295	7	52
Carrot-Cucumber	230	0.5	51
Carrot	240	0.5	53
Cucumber	225	0.5	50
Imitation Crab & Cucumber	240	0.5	51
Spicy Roll: *Per 9 Pieces*			
Shrimp	335	5.5	52
Yellowtail	365	8	52
Salmon	360	9	52
Tuna	290	6	45
Sunshine Platter, 15 pieces	815	13	154
Tempura Roll, 9 pieces	605	13	92
Tofu Roll, 9 pieces	250	3	48
Tsunami Roll, 9 pieces	480	15	63
Salads: *Per Serving*			
Calamari Salad, 4 oz	185	2.5	20
Edamame (soybeans), 4 oz	170	7.5	12
Edamame Salad, 4 oz	60	3	4
Harusame Salad, 2 oz	60	0.5	13
Seabreeze Salad, 2 oz	55	1.5	11
Sauce: AFC Spicy Sauce, 2 oz	50	4.5	2

For Complete Nutritional Data ~ see CalorieKing.com

Spaghetti Warehouse®

Lunch	C	F	Cb
Minestrone Soup	80	1.5	12
Grilled Chicken Marinara	530	8	65
Seafood Marinara	385	5	65
Spaghetti: w. Tomato Sauce	425	5	82
w. Marinara Sauce #12	440	5	84
Spicy Marinara Sce Spaghetti	280	4	52
Vegetable Primavera	340	4	65
Dinner			
Minestrone, 1 bowl	110	2	18
Grilled Chicken Marinara	640	10	85
Grilled Halibut Dinner	880	14	106
Grilled Marinated Chicken Breast	910	17	116
Marinara Sauce #12	520	6	99
Seafood Marinara	520	8	86
Spaghetti w. Tomato Sauce	525	6	101
Spicy Marinara Sce Spaghetti	330	6	60
Vegetable Primavera	610	8	116

Starbuck's®

Figures Based on Grande (16 fl.oz)
Without Whip Unless Indicated

Drinks: *Per 16 fl.oz*	C	F	Cb
Apple Juice	230	0	57
Caramel Apple Cider	290	0	72
Chocolate Milk, Whole Milk	365	15	42
Hot Chocolate, Whole Milk	365	15	42
Steamed Apple Cider	230	10	57
Vanilla Creme	340	14	40
White Hot Chocolate, Whole Milk	480	18	63
Steamed Milk, Whole	280	15	21
w. Nonfat Milk	160	0	23
w. Soy Milk	210	6	28
Cafe Misto/Au Lait, Whole Milk	150	8	11
Caffe Americano	15	0	3
Caffe Latte, Whole Milk	265	14	21
w. Nonfat Milk	160	0	24
w. Soy Milk	210	6	28
Breve	555	47	20
Caffe Mocha, Whole Milk	325	12	41
w. Nonfat Milk	245	2	43
w. Soy Milk	280	6	46
Breve	540	37	40
Hot Drinks : *Per Grande (16 fl.oz)*			
Cappuccino: w. Whole Milk	150	8	13
w Nonfat Milk	90	0	14
w. Soy Milk	120	3	17
Breve	325	27	12
Caramel Macchiato: w. Whole Milk	320	14	37
w. Nonfat Milk	230	2	40
w. Soy Milk	300	8	49
Breve	565	42	36
Caramel Mocca w. Whole Milk	395	11	61
White Choc. Mocha: w. Whole Milk	410	15	56
w. Nonfat Milk	340	5	58
w. Soy Milk	420	14	62
Breve	630	40	55
Espresso (Hot): *Per Serving*			
Espresso: Doppio	10	0	2
Solo	5	0	1
Espresso con Panna: Doppio	40	3	2
Solo	35	3	1
Espresso Macchiato: Doppio	10	0	2
Solo	10	0	1

Continued Next Page . . .

Starbuck's® cont...

Cold Drinks: Per Grande (16 fl.oz)	C	F	Cb
Iced Caffe Americano	**15**	0	3
Iced Caffe Latte: w. Whole Milk	**155**	8	13
w. Nonfat Milk	**90**	0	14
w. Soy Milk	**125**	3.5	17
Iced Caffe Mocha: w. Whole Milk	**250**	8	35
w. Nonfat Milk	**200**	2	36
w. Soy Milk	**220**	4.5	38
Iced Caramel Macchiato, Whole Milk	**270**	10	34
Iced White Choc. Mocha, Whole Milk	**360**	11	56
Iced Shaken Drinks: *Per 16 fl.oz*			
Iced Shaken Coffee	**80**	0	20
Tazo® Iced Tea/Tea	**80**	0	20
Lemonade	**125**	0	31
Frappuccino® Blended Tea: *Per 16 fl.oz*			
Tazo® Chai Creme	**370**	4.5	69
Frappuccino® Blended Coffee: *Per 16 fl.oz*			
Caffe Vanilla	**345**	3.5	72
Caramel	**280**	3.5	57
Coffee	**260**	3.5	52
Espresso	**230**	3	46
Mocha varieties, avg.	**310**	4	58
Frappuccino® Light Blended Coffees: *Per 16 fl.oz*			
Caffe Vanilla	**235**	1	49
Caramel; Mocha	**185**	1.5	36
Coffee	**155**	1	30
Espresso	**140**	1	27
Java Chip	**280**	7	46
White Chocolate Mocha	**215**	2.5	40
Frappuccino® Blended Cremes: *Per 16 fl.oz*			
Double Chocolate Chip	**500**	12	82
Strawberries & Creme	**475**	5	93
Toffee Nut	**360**	4.5	65
Vanilla Bean	**395**	5	73
Tazo® Tea: *Per 16 fl.oz*			
Iced Tazo® Chai, Whole Milk	**285**	7	48
Tazo® Chai, Whole Milk	**285**	7	50
Drink Extras: *Per Serving*			
Flav. Sugar Free Syrup, 1 pump	**0**	0	0
Flavored Syrup, 1 pump	**20**	0	5
Mocha Syrup, 1 pump	**30**	0.5	6
Toppings: Chocolate, 4g	**5**	0	1
Caramel, 15g	**10**	0.5	2
Sprinkles	**0**	0	0
Whipped Cream Topping:			
Tall, 25g	**85**	8.5	1.5
Grande/Venti, 35g	**115**	12	2
Hot Beverage, 27g	**90**	9	2

	C	F	Cb
Bottled Frappuccino®: *Per 9.5 fl.oz Bottle*			
Caramel	**200**	3	37
Coffee	**190**	3.5	35
Hazelnut	**200**	3.5	37
Mocha	**200**	3.5	37
Bagels: Sesame	**460**	3	92
Other types, average	**440**	1	92
Bars: Caramel Apple	**310**	16	38
Lemon Bar	**310**	14	44
Peanut Butter Brownie	**460**	29	45
Raspberry Sammy	**300**	14	44
Carrot Cake; Enrobed Brownie	**430**	25	48
Cakes: Apple Walnut Coffee	**335**	17	41
Brownie, Sugar Free	**320**	19	34
Banana Pound; Coffee Cake	**360**	18	48
Choc. Big Baby Bundt	**330**	15	45
Iced Carrot Pound Cake	**540**	13	101
Pumpkin Pullman	**370**	17	51
Lowfat Cinnamon Coffee Cake	**360**	8	65
Reduced Fat Zucchini Lemon Cake	**310**	6	58
Cookies & Biscotti			
Biscotti, all types, 1 oz	**110**	5	15
Black & White	**440**	17	68
Crisp Cinnamon Twist	**60**	2	9
Madeline	**80**	3.5	11
Double Chocolate Chunk	**440**	21	58
Milk Chocolate Graham	**150**	8	17
Croissants: Chocolate Filled	**365**	19	43
Raspberry & Cream Cheese	**260**	12	34
Other varieties, average	**330**	18	39
Muffins: Blueberry	**380**	19	49
Chocolate Cream Cheese	**450**	24	53
Cranberry Orange	**410**	20	53
Morning Sunrise	**345**	12	54
Scones: Apricot Currant; Blueberry	**455**	17	67
Butterscotch Pecan	**520**	27	64
Cinnamon Chip w. Icing	**510**	23	71
Maple Oat w. Icing	**500**	22	69
Raspberry	**450**	18	65
Sweet Rolls			
Apple Danish	**370**	19	44
Caramel Pecan	**700**	40	75
Raspberry Danish	**370**	19	45

Ice cream & Ice cream Bars ~ See Page 35, 38

For Complete Nutritional Data ~ see CalorieKing.com

Steak Escape®

	C	F	Cb
Small Sandwiches (7"): No Cheese or Condiments			
Grand Gobbler	390	2	67
Grand Escape	430	6	64
Grandest Chicken	430	5	64
Great Escape	420	6	63
Hambrosia	395	2	69
Ragin' Cajun	420	5	63
Turkey Club	400	2	65
Vegetarian	305	1	64
Wild West BBQ	460	6	72
Large Sandwiches (12"): No Cheese or Condiments			
Grand Gobbler	680	2	116
Grandest Chicken	775	10	110
Great Escape; Grand Escape	760	12	108
Hambrosia	680	2	119
Ragin' Cajun	760	10	108
Turkey Club	690	4	111
Vegetarian	525	2	109
Wild West BBQ	830	12	126
Fresh Salads: No Cheese or Condiments			
Side Salad	50	0.5	8
Grilled Salad: w. Chicken	190	5	11
w. Ham	125	2	8
w. Steak	190	6	11
w. Turkey	125	2	8
Smashed Potatoes: Plain, 14 oz	255	0	53
w. Chicken	390	4	56
w. Ham	360	2	59
w. Steak	395	5	56
w. Turkey	360	2	59
Loaded: Bacon & Cheddar	650	26	91
Ranch & Bacon	710	34	87
Fresh Cut Fries: Per Serving			
Small, 12 oz	535	26	67
Medium, 16 oz	695	34	87
Large, 25 oz	980	48	123
Loaded: Bacon & Cheddar	820	44	88
Ranch & Bacon	1045	71	84
Condiments			
Mayonnaise, 1 oz	100	11	0
BBQ Sauce, 1 oz	35	0	9
Cheddar Cheese, 1 oz	70	9	1

For Complete Nutritional Data ~ see CalorieKing.com

Steak 'n Shake®

Meals	C	F	Cb
All-American Melt Sandwich	1310	103	53
Chicken Fingers, no fries	610	46	22
Chili 3-Way	655	36	63
Chili 5-Way	1025	67	66
Chili Deluxe, 6 oz cup	505	38	17
Fish Fillet Sandwich w. Cheese	820	58	54
Frisco Melt Sandwich	1170	93	43
Grilled Cheese Sandwich	690	51	40
Grilled Chicken Breast Sandwich	475	26	33
Original Double w. Cheese	585	38	29
Original Single w. Cheese	405	23	29
Philadelphia Sandwich	870	52	63
Triple Steakburger	700	47	29
Tuna Melt Sandwich	925	77	27
Fries: French, reg., 5 oz	470	23	62
French, large, 7.25 oz	695	34	90
Cheddar Cheese, reg., 5 oz	635	35	70
Salads: Beef Taco Salad	940	59	75
Chicken Chef Salad	470	32	10
Fried Chicken Salad	1060	81	47
Soups: Chicken Gumbo, 6 fl.oz cup	95	2.5	10
Chicken Noodle, 6 fl.oz cup	70	1	9.5
Cream of Broccoli, 6 fl.oz cup	125	8	11
Vegetable Beef, 6 fl.oz cup	125	6.5	10
Breakfast: Bacon 'n Egg (1), Works	890	70	38
Biscuits, Gravy 'n Hash Browns	1615	99	154
Classic Stack 'O Cakes (2)	255	4	47
Country Scrambler (1)	1040	78	51
Cinnamon Swirl French Tst, 3 sl.	285	7	44
One Egg, cooked w. Margarine	140	12	1
Hash Browns	385	25	35
Steak 'n Eggs Breakfast	1030	80	36
Sandwich on Bagel: Egg & Chse	360	20	30
Egg, Cheese & Bacon	475	30	31
Healthy Morning Cholesterol-Free Egg Product, w. Melted Margarine	190	15	2
Desserts: Apple Cobbler	515	22	76
Hot Fudge Brownie	505	23	69
Hot Fudge Sundae	515	26	64
Outrageous Parfait, no cream	775	40	95
Pumpkin Pie, ⅛ w. topping	395	14	61
Beverages: Root Beer Float	570	22	87
Hot Chocolate, 7 fl.oz, no topping	180	6.5	29
Orange Freeze, regular	630	19	101
Shake: Chocolate, no Cream reg.	710	22	110
Banana; Vanilla, regular	670	21	106

Subway®

'7 Under 6' Sandwiches (6")	C	F	Cb
Figures based on Italian bread and toppings: lettuce, tomato, onion, green peppers, olives and pickles.			
Ham; Roast Beef	**290**	5	45
Honey Mustard Ham	**310**	5	54
Oven Roasted Chicken Breast	**330**	5	47
Savory Turkey Breast	**280**	4.5	46
Savory Turkey Breast & Ham	**290**	5	46
Sweet Onion Chicken Teriyaki	**370**	5	59
Turkey Breast, Ham & Roast Beef	**320**	6	47
Veggie Delite	**230**	3	44
6" Hot Sandwiches: *Figures based on Italian bread and following toppings: lettuce, tomato, onion, green peppers, olives, pickles, cheese, oil, vinegar, salt and pepper.*			
Cheese Steak	**360**	10	47
Chipotle Southwest Cheese Steak	**440**	19	49
Dijon Turkey, Ham & Bacon Melt	**470**	21	48
Meatball Marinara	**500**	22	52
Turkey Breast, Ham & Bacon Melt	**380**	12	47
6" Cold Sandwiches: *Figures based on Italian bread and following toppings: lettuce, tomato, onion, green peppers, olives, pickles, cheese, oil, vinegar, salt and pepper.*			
Classic Tuna	**430**	19	46
Cold Cut Combo	**410**	17	46
Italian BMT	**450**	21	47
Subway Seafood Sensation	**380**	13	52
Deli Style Sandwiches: Ham	**210**	4	35
Classic Tuna	**300**	13	36
Roast Beef	**220**	4.5	35
Savory Turkey Breast	**210**	3.5	36
Double Meat Subs (6"): *Per Sub*			
Cheese Steak	**450**	14	50
Chicken; Subway Club	**430**	8	50
Classic Tuna	**580**	32	48
Cold Cut Combo	**550**	28	48
Ham; Roast Beef	**360**	7	49
Italian BMT	**630**	35	49
Meatball Marinara	**740**	38	61
Seafood Sensation	**490**	20	60
Sweet Onion Chicken Teriyaki	**450**	7	59
Turkey Breast/& Ham, avg	**360**	7	48
Turkey Breast, Ham & Roast Beef	**410**	8	49
Turkey Breast, Ham & Bacon Melt	**490**	17	51

Footlong ~ *Double figures for 6"*

Atkins Friendly Wraps	C	F	Cb
Chicken Bacon Ranch	**440**	26	17
Mediterranean Chicken	**350**	18	17
Turkey Bacon Melt	**430**	27	20
Turkey Breast & Ham	**390**	23	19
Breakfasts: French Toast w. Syrup	**235**	17	2
Omelets, average all types	**235**	16	3
Breakfast Sandwiches *(6"):*			
Deli Style (Round), average	**320**	13	35
Subs: Italian or Wheat Bread, average	**440**	18	43
Salads: *Dressing Not Included*			
Classic Club	**390**	21	13
Garden Fresh	**60**	1	11
Grilled Chicken & Spinach	**420**	26	10
Mediterranean Chicken	**170**	4.5	11
Salad Dressings & Toppings: *Per Package*			
Bacon Bits, 0.5 oz	**60**	4.5	0
Croutons	**70**	3	8
Diced Eggs	**45**	3	0
Garlic Almonds	**80**	7	3
Dressings: Atkins Honey Mustard	**200**	22	1
Greek Vinaigrette	**200**	21	3
Kraft Fat Free Italian Dressing	**35**	0	7
Kraft Ranch Dressing	**200**	22	1
Red Wine Vinaigrette	**80**	1	17
Select Sauces: *Per 1½ Tablespoons*			
Chipotle Southwest; Dijon Horseradish	**90**	10	1
Fat Free, average all types	**30**	0	7
Breads: 6" Honey Oat	**250**	3.5	48
6" Italian Herbs & Cheese	**240**	6	40
6" Italian (White)	**200**	2.5	38
6" Parmesan Oregano	**210**	3.5	40
6" Wheat	**200**	2.5	40
Atkins Friendly Wrap	**120**	4.5	13
Deli Style Roll	**170**	2.5	32
Value Meal Extras			
If 21 oz Drink + Chips, add	**335**	2	77
If 21 oz Drink + 2 Cookies, add	**640**	20	111
Kids Pak: *(Deli Sandwich + Juice + Fruit Roll-Up)*			
If Ham or Beef or Turkey Deli S'wich	**370**	5	71
If Classic Tuna Deli Sandwich	**450**	14	72

Subway® cont...

	C	F	Cb
Extras: *Spreads, Cheese, Vegetables*			
Cheese (slices for 6"), avg., ½ oz	**50**	4	0
Shredded Swiss/Monterey, 1 oz	**110**	9	1
Feta, ½ oz	**30**	2	0
Bacon, 2 strips	**45**	3.5	0
Cucumber, Lettuce, Pickles, Peppers	**0**	0	0
Tomatoes (3 slices), Olives, Onion	**5**	0	1
Mayonnaise, 1 Tbsp, ½ oz	**110**	12	0
Light Mayonnaise, 1 Tbsp, ½ oz	**45**	5	1
Mustard (Yellow or Brown), 2 tsp	**5**	0	1
Olive Oil Blend, 1 tsp	**45**	5	0
Vinegar, 1 tsp	**0**	0	0
Cookies: Average all types, 1½ oz	**220**	10	30
Atkins-Friendly Double Choc, 1 oz	**100**	6	17
Fruit Roll-Up (1), ½ oz	**50**	0.5	12
Chips, *Lay's* Baked Potato, 1.1 oz bag	**130**	2	26
Soft Drinks: *Average all types with ⅓ Ice*			
Small, 16 fl.oz	**155**	0	38
Medium, 21 fl.oz	**205**	0	51
Large, 32 fl.oz	**310**	0	77
Fruizle Express: Small Cup			
Berry Lishus	**110**	0	28
Berry Lishus with Banana	**140**	0	35
Sunrise Refresher	**120**	0	29

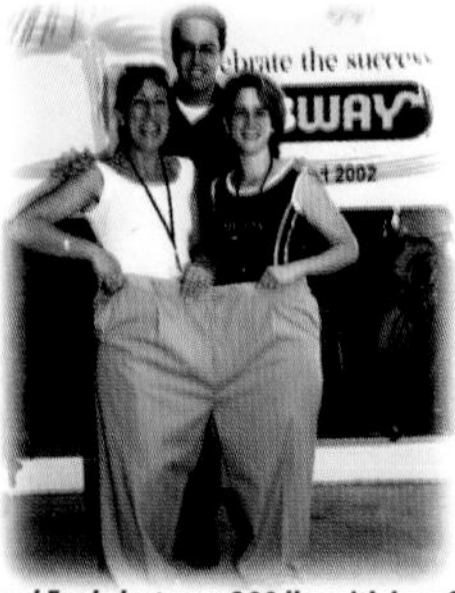

Jared Fogle lost over 200 lbs with low-fat Subway® Sandwiches and lots of walking.

Sub Station®

	C	F	Cb
Sandwiches			
Per ½ Sub (Incl. Oil, Vinegar, Salad)			
Ham & Cheese	**505**	30	40
Ham, Turkey & Cheese	**510**	30	40
Turkey & Cheese	**525**	31	40
Roast Beef & Cheese	**525**	31	39
Ham, Salami, Pepperoni, Cappicola, Bologna, Turkey & Cheese	**635**	42	40

Sweet Tomatoes®

~ Same Menu & Data as Souplantation (See Page 253) ~

Swiss Chalet®

	C	F	Cb
Burgers: *Includes Garnishes*			
Bacon Cheese Burger	**835**	43	52
Big Beef Burger	**635**	30	48
Veggie Burger	**405**	11	51
Rotisserie Chicken: *Meat Only*			
Double Leg	**625**	34	0
Half Chicken, no Skin	**455**	18	0
w. Skin	**695**	39	0
Quarter Chicken: Dark, no Skin	**230**	10	0
Dark meat w. Skin	**315**	17	0
White meat, no Skin	**225**	8	0
White meat w. Skin	**380**	22	0
Starters: *Per Serving*			
Baked Garlic Cheese Loaf, 8 oz	**695**	29	85
Hot Wings, 11.6 oz	**955**	50	63
Mild Wings, 11.6 oz	**915**	53	50
Perogies w. Cajun Sauce, 6.5 oz	**395**	11	62
Ranchero Corn & Chkn Quesadilla	**930**	42	90
Soup: Chalet Chicken, 1 cup	**100**	2	11
Creamy Chicken, 1 cup	**180**	6	17
Entree Garden Salads: *Includes Flatbread*			
Golden Grilled Chicken Caesar	**830**	53	41
Santa Fe Grilled Chicken	**275**	9	17
Warm Chicken Salad Amandine	**870**	60	42
Side Salads: Garden	**35**	0	7
Hall Caesar Salad	**345**	19	12
Fire Grilled: *Meat Only Unless Indicated*			
Chkn Breast on Rice w. Flatbread	**625**	9	91
Chicken & Rib Combo	**1065**	72	5
BBQ Ribs: Feature Cut	**500**	37	3
Regular	**755**	55	5
Large	**1505**	110	10

Continued Next Page . . .

Swiss Chalet®cont...

Stir Fry/Pot Pie: Per Serving	C	F	Cb
Chicken on Rice w. Flatbread	370	7	40
Veggie on Rice w. Flatbread	220	3	42
Chicken Pot Pie	495	24	53
Sides: Baked Potato	270	0	62
Bread Roll	145	0.5	29
Butter, ½ oz	100	11	0
Coleslaw, 2.2 oz	90	6.5	7.5
Corn, 3.5 oz	95	2	16
French Fries, 5.6 oz	470	25	53
Gravy, 3.5 oz	40	1	6
Mashed Potatoes, 6.4 oz	215	8.5	31
Rice Pilaf, 6.2 oz	230	1.5	49
Sour Cream & Chives, 1 oz	50	4	2
Vegetables, 5.5 oz	60	2	7
Sandwiches: Chicken on Kaiser	435	9	37
Chicken on Kaiser and Soup	530	11	48
Club Wrap	620	24	58
Grilled Santa Fe Chicken Breast	525	15	59
Messy Chicken	1010	41	102
Salad Dressings: Per Serving			
Creamy 1000 Isle Dressing, 15 ml	60	6	2
Garlic Peppercorn, 15 ml	65	7	1
Famous Chalet Sauce, 100g	25	0.5	4.5
French Dressing, 15 ml	60	5.5	2
House Dressing, 15 ml	65	6	3.5
Light Italian, 15 ml	30	2	2.5
Mayonnaise, 15 ml	100	11	0
Raspberry Vinaigrette, 15 ml	10	0	3
Dipping Sauce: BBQ, 33 ml	55	0	13
Honey Mustard, 33 ml	75	1	19
Plum, 33 ml	65	0	17
Sweet & Sour, 33 ml	50	0	13
Desserts: Apple Blossom	565	30	67
Apple Pie	425	17	66
Carrot Cake	660	38	73
Chocolate Eruption Cheesecake	785	45	84
Coconut Cream Pie	410	27	41
Colossal Caramel Fudge Chsecake	655	38	68
Cranberry, Raspberry Yogurt	215	4	39
Ice cream: Butter Pecan	340	20	38
Chocolate	275	16	26
Vanilla	335	21	32
Sauce: Butterscotch	315	0	78
Chocolate	240	0.5	57
Strawberry	215	0	53
Lemon Meringue	410	16	66
Pecan Pie	410	24	53
Sugar Pie	395	21	52
Tuzedo Truffle Mousse	680	42	66

Taco Bell®

Burritos	C	F	Cb
7-Layer Burrito	530	22	67
Bean Burrito	370	10	55
Burrito Supreme® Beef	440	18	50
Burrito Supreme® Chicken/Steak	420	16	50
Chili Cheese Burrito	390	18	40
Fiesta Burrito Beef	390	15	50
Fiesta Burrito Chicken; Steak	370	13	48
Grilled Stuft Beef	730	33	79
Grilled Stuft Chicken; Steak	680	27	76
Tacos: Taco, regular/Crispy	170	10	13
Taco Supreme®	220	14	14
Soft Taco Chicken	190	6	19
Soft Taco Ranchero Chicken	270	15	21
Soft Taco Steak	280	17	21
Soft Taco Supreme Beef	260	14	22
Soft Taco Supreme Chicken	230	10	21
Double Decker® Taco	340	14	39
Double Decker® Taco Supreme	380	18	40
Gorditas: Gordita Baja™ Beef	360	19	31
Gordita Baja™ Chicken; Steak	340	16	29
Gordita Supreme® Beef	320	16	30
Gordita Supreme® Chicken; Steak	300	12	28
Gordita Nacho Cheese Beef	295	13	32
Gordita Nacho Cheese Chkn; Steak	290	10	30
Chalupas: Chalupa Baja® Beef	410	27	32
Chalupa Baja® Chicken; Steak	390	25	30
Chalupa Supreme® Beef	370	24	31
Chalupa Supreme® Chicken	350	20	30
Chalupa Supreme® Steak	350	22	29
Chalupa Nacho Cheese Beef	360	22	33
Chalupa Nacho Cheese Chkn; Steak	340	19	31
Fresco Style (Less Than 15g Fat)			
Burritos: Bean	350	8	56
Fiesta Chicken	340	9	49
Supreme Chicken/Steak	350	9	50
Enchiritos: Beef	275	9	35
Chicken	245	5	34
Steak	255	7	34
Gordita Baja: Beef	250	9	30
Chicken; Steak	230	7	29
Tacos: Regular, crunchy	145	7	14
Soft Taco Beef	195	8	22
Soft Beef Chicken/Steak	170	5	21
Tostada	205	6	30
Nachos and Sides: Nachos, 3.5 oz	350	19	33
Nachos Supreme®	470	26	42
Nachos BellGrande®	760	43	80
Pintos 'n Cheese, 4.5 oz	180	7	20
Mexican Rice, 4.6 oz	210	10	23
Cinnamon Twists, 1.25 oz	165	5	28

Taco Bell® cont...

Big Bell Value Menu: Per Serving	C	F	Cb
½ lb Bean Burrito Especial	600	21	82
½ lb Beef & Potato Burrito	535	24	65
½ lb Beef Combo Burrito	465	19	52
Caramel Apple Empanada	295	15	37
Cheesy Fiesta Potato	285	18	27
Taco, Grande Soft	445	21	44
Specialities: Tostada	250	10	29
Cheese Quesadilla	490	28	39
Chicken Quesadilla	540	30	40
Enchirito® Beef	370	18	35
Enchirito® Chicken; Steak, avg.	350	16	33
Express Taco Salad w. Chips	610	31	60
Fiesta Taco Salad	870	46	82
Meximelt®	290	16	23
Mexican Pizza, 7½ oz	550	31	46
Taco Salad w. Salsa & Shell	830	42	73
Taco Salad w. Salsa, w/out Shell	410	21	33
Southwest Steak Bowl	660	32	73
Zesty Chicken Border Bowl	720	42	65
w/out Dressing	460	19	60

Taco Cabana®

Grilled Chicken: Per Serving	C	F	Cb
¼ Chicken White, 5 oz	300	14	1
No Skin, 4 oz	170	3	0
¼ Chicken Dark, 4.5 oz	300	18	0.5
No Skin, 3.5 oz	170	7	1
Fajitas: Beef, 4 oz	245	12	4
Chicken White, 4 oz	190	6	3
Chicken Dark, 4 oz	235	11	2
Sides: Black Beans, 4 oz	110	0.5	21
Borracho Beans, 4 oz	110	2.5	17
Calabacita, 4 oz	70	5	6
Chips, 2 oz	290	14	36
Elotes (1)	220	11	27
Guacamole, 1 oz; Sour Cream, 1 oz	50	4	2
Queso, 3 oz	170	12	7
Refried Beans, 4 oz	170	6	21
Salsa, all types, 1 oz	10	0	2
Spanish Rice, 4 oz	180	5	30
Tortillas: 6" Flour	130	3.5	22
6" Table Corn	60	1	11
Tortilla Soup: Small, 8.5 oz	250	8.5	26
Large, 19 oz	375	13	32
Tacos: Bean & Cheese	295	12	35
Black Bean	225	5	37
Carne Guisada	210	8	20
Crispy Beef	150	7	13
Soft Chicken	220	9	21

Taco Cabana® cont...

Burritos	C	F	Cb
Bean & Cheese	695	27	85
Beef/Chicken, average	640	24	76
Black Bean	545	11	95
Breakfast Tacos: Barbacoa	230	15	2
Chorizo & Egg	250	12	22

Taco John's®

Tacos	C	F	Cb
Taco Bravo®	340	14	39
Taco Burger	280	12	28
Beef Taco In A Bag	180	12	6
Chicken Taco In A Bag	140	7	4
Crispy Taco	180	10	13
Softshell Taco	220	10	21
Softshell Chicken	190	6	19
Low Carb: Chicken Soft Shell	160	6	15
Beef Soft Shell	190	10	16
Burritos: Bean Burrito	380	12	53
Beef/Chicken Grilled, avg.	590	32	49
Beefy Burrito; Super Burrito, avg.	445	20	44
Combination Burrito	400	16	47
Meat and Potato Burrito	490	23	55
Favorites: Bean Tostada	160	6	19
Cheese Crisp	210	14	11
Chilito	430	22	38
Double Enchilada	720	40	54
Mexi Rolls®	480	30	33
Tostada	180	10	14
Specialities			
Chicken Festiva Salad, no dressing	580	24	60
Crunchy Chken Festiva, no dressing	750	37	71
Chicken Super Nachos	780	45	62
Chicken Taco, no dressing	530	27	45
Potato Oles Bravo	580	36	55
Cheese Quesadilla	480	26	39
Super Nachos	830	51	73
Super Potato Oles®	980	62	82
Taco Salad, no dressing	580	32	46
Platters: Beef and Bean Chimi	760	34	88
Beef Enchilada	780	37	80
Chicken Enchilada	700	32	73
Smothered Burrito	830	33	102
Sides: Mexican Rice	240	8	35
Nachos	380	23	38
Potato Oles, Medium, 7 oz	620	36	67
Refried Beans	400	14	50
Crunchy Chicken Side, 5 oz	450	27	24
Desserts: Apple Grande, 3 oz	240	9	36
Choco Taco, 4 oz	300	15	38
Churros, 2 oz	230	11	13

Taco Mayo®

Beans	C	F	Cb
Refried w. Cheese	315	9	43
No cheese	285	6.5	42
Burritos: Bean w. Cheese	505	15	71
No cheese	445	11	70
Chicken Supreme Burrito	405	18	39
No cheese & sour cream	335	12	38
Fajita Steak Grilled Burrito	480	24	41
No cheese	420	19	41
Taco: Crispy, with cheese	160	9.5	10
No cheese	135	7	10
Soft Taco: with cheese	225	11	17
No cheese	195	9	16
Chicken Soft Taco: with cheese	180	8	16
No cheese	155	5.5	16
Extreme Fajita Chicken Soft Taco	260	13	19
No cheese & sour cream	190	7	18
Rice: Mexicalli	165	1	35
Salads			
Fiesta Acapulco	725	53	33
No cheese, guacamole & corn stix	410	32	7.5
Fiesta Monterey	510	31	32
No corn stix	295	19	9
Fiesta Santa Fe	590	36	38
No cheese & corn stix	320	19	14

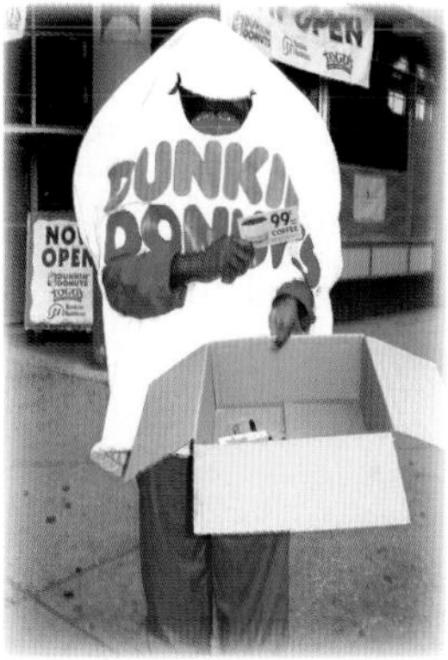

Taco Time®

Burritos	C	F	Cb
Beef, Bean & Cheese	630	23	66
Big Juan Beef Burrito	645	25	71
Big Juan Chicken Burrito	630	24	69
Casita Burrito, Beef	650	31	54
Chicken & Black Bean	420	18	45
Chicken BLT	595	39	38
Crisp Burrito: Bean	435	18	53
Meat	560	30	39
Chicken	420	25	32
Soft Bean Burrito	385	10	58
Soft Meat Burrito	505	21	48
Veggie Burrito	510	16	70
Tacos: Cheeseburger Taco	640	36	48
Crisp Taco	305	17	16
½ lb Chicken Soft Taco	390	16	41
½ lb Soft Taco	525	23	46
Soft Taco	325	15	23
Super Soft Taco	525	23	50
Specialties: Crustos®, 3.5 oz	375	15	47
Cheddar Fries, Medium, 7 oz	525	36	40
Cheddar Melt	210	11	17
Mexi Fries®, Medium, 6 oz	410	26	40
Mexi-Rice, 4 oz	150	2	30
Nachos: Regular, 10.5 oz	690	38	61
Deluxe, 15.25 oz	1060	57	91
Stuffed Fries, Medium, 6.2 oz	740	55	50
Refritos, 7 oz	340	10	44
Salads: *Per Serving*			
Chicken Fiesta, 12 oz	390	19	35
Chicken Taco	375	21	27
Taco Salad, regular	490	28	30
Tostada Salad	635	33	48
Sauces & Dressings: *Per 1 oz*			
Green Sauce	10	0	2
Original Hot Sauce	10	0	2
Salsa Fresca	65	0	16
1000 Island Dressing	120	12	3
Desserts: Cinnamon Crustos	360	15	47
Fruit Filled Empanadas	250	9	37

For Complete Nutritional Data ~ see CalorieKing.com

Tacone®

Gourmet Wrapped Sandwiches	C	F	Cb
Campfire	740	21	92
Pilgrim	770	39	52
Samurai	805	12	124
Thai Cone	800	20	106

TCBY®

Frozen Yogurt (Soft Serve)	C	F	Cb
96% Fat-Free: Small, 7 oz	260	6	47
Regular, 9 oz	340	8	61
Large, 11 oz	420	10	74
Non-Fat: Small, 7 oz	220	0	47
Regular, 9 oz	280	0	60
Large, 11 oz	340	0	73
Non-Fat/No Sugar Added, Regular	210	0	45
Low Carb Lovers™ (No Toppings)			
Choc/Vanilla: Small Cup, 7 oz	240	15	9
Regular Cup, 9 oz	300	19	11
Large Cup, 11 oz	370	24	14
(Note: Carb figures do not include fiber or sugar alcohols)			
Sorbet (Non-Fat): Small, 7 oz	195	0	49
Regular, 9 oz	250	0	63
Large, 11 oz	305	0	77
Ice Cream			
Mrs Fields: *(Regular Size, 9 oz)*			
Butter Pecan	700	54	46
Chocolate Chunk Cookie Dough	540	38	49
Vanilla Bean	570	35	46
Very Berry Strawberry	490	30	51
Arthurs, avg., 1 scoop (approx. ½ cup)	150	9	16
Chillers & Shivers			
Made with Frozen Yogurt *(96% Fat-Free)*			
Cappuccino Chiller, regular, 20 fl.oz	510	21	65
Shivers: Fruit, regular, 20 fl.oz	600	14	106
Hot Fudge, regular, 20 fl.oz	725	21	120
Cones: Sugar or Jnr Waffle	70	1	15
Waffle Cone	110	2	22
Smoothies: with Yogurt (20 oz)			
A Lotta Colada	575	17	99
Berry Slim; Healthy Balance	425	3	95
Holy-Cal; Peachy Lean; Workout	500	3	114
Raspberry DeLITE; Revitalizer	385	3	85
Tropical Replenisher	390	3	87
Without Yogurt (20 oz): Deduct	120	3	30
32 oz Size *(with Yogurt):* Add 50% of 20 oz size			

Teriyaki Stix®

	C	F	Cb
Bowls: Beef Bowl	620	7	102
Chicken Bowl; Hot & Spicy	730	15	101
Chicken Curry	680	17	92
Teriyaki Chicken Salad	360	13	26
Teriyaki Special	740	13	111
Veggie Bowl	440	1	99
Yakisoba	360	4.5	56

The Taco Maker®

Burritos	C	F	Cb
Bean	295	9	44
Beef	440	17	44
Chicken	370	12	44
Crisp Bean; Crisp Beef, avg.	420	27	30
Enchiladas: Beef	375	20	23
Cheese	585	39	26
Chicken	315	13	21
Nachos: Cheese	605	36	49
Chips 'n Beans	295	16	32
Macho Nacho w. Beef	815	50	57
Macho Nacho w. Guacamole	845	55	62
Salad: Chicken Fiesta	620	35	39
Taco	680	43	40
Tacos: Crisp	180	9	16
Crisp Super	300	16	25
Soft	180	6.5	21
Soft Super	390	15	43
Tater Gem Fries, Regular	490	31	49

The Wrap®

Breakfast Wraps: Per 10" Wrap	C	F	Cb
Bacon & Eggs	395	16	41
Harvest Fruit	405	11	68
Huevos Rancheros	485	17	56
Truck Stop	635	34	56
Special Wraps: Jason's Lite, 12"	695	13	119
Buffalo Chicken, 12"	730	23	94
Greek Salad, 12" wrap	655	37	65
Burritos: Per 12" Burrito			
Bean & Cheese	635	13	107
Grilled Chicken	795	20	107
Roasted Veggie	685	14	115
Tofu	820	23	111
Bowls: Per Large Bowl			
Bean & Cheese	390	11	57
Grilled Chicken/Steak, avg.	550	18	57
Just Veggies	335	7	59
Papas	545	16	81
Pepp's Paella	325	4	60
Roasted Veggie	440	12	65
Shrimp	480	13	58
The Caesar w. Chicken Salad	495	33	12
Tofu	575	21	61
The Teriyaki w. Chicken	475	7	71
The Tuna Salad	330	5	12
Veggie Patch Salad	180	6	23

Tim Horton's®

	C	F	Cb
Sandwiches: *Incl. Dressing Unless Indicated*			
Albacore Tuna Salad	370	10	50
Blk Forest Ham & Swiss, w. dress.	475	18	51
Chunky Chicken Salad	375	9	50
Fireside Roast Beef, w. dressing	385	11	50
Garden Vegetable, w. dressing	450	23	51
Harvest Turkey Brst, w. dressing	380	10	52
Soup: *Per Bowl (10 fl.oz)*			
Beef Noodle	140	1.5	23
Clam Chowder	240	9	31
Cream of Broccoli	240	11	26
Cream of Mushroom	220	10	27
Hearty Vegetable; Vege Beef	115	3	19
Italian Florentine	170	5	27
Minestrone	150	2	28
Tim's Own, Chicken Noodle	110	3	16
Turkey & Wild Rice	135	2	25
Cakes: *Per Slice (1/8 Cake)*			
Black Forest	480	27	54
Double Chocolate Delight	465	20	65
Tim's Own Coffee Cake	455	22	59
Cookies: *Per Cookie*			
Apple Cinnamon	135	5	20
Chocolate Chunk	150	7	20
Oatcakes	195	9	25
Peanut Butter	165	8	20
Peanut Butter Chocolate Chunk	175	9	21
Plain Macaroon	150	8	18
Donuts: *Per Donut*			
Cake: Chocolate Glazed	375	22	40
Old Fashion Plain	215	12	23
Sour Cream Plain	285	19	26
Filled: Apple Dumpling	280	9	44
Blueberry; Strawberry	275	8	47
Boston Cream; Canadian	255	8	42
Honey Stick	355	15	51
Sugar Twist	220	10	29
Walnut Crunch	350	18	42
Yeast: Apple Fritter	345	15	47
Chocolate/Honey Maple	230	10	31
Dutchie	305	13	42
Baked Goods			
Southern Country Biscuits (1)	490	20	71
Croissant: Butter (1)	220	11	25
Cheese (1)	240	12	27
Cherry Cheese Danish (1)	365	23	33
Tea Biscuit: Plain, 3 oz	235	7	38
Raisin, 3 oz	275	7	48
Pies: Apple, ¼ pie	485	22	66
Lemon Meringue, ¼ pie	440	15	71

Tim Horton's® cont...

	C	F	Cb
Muffins: *Per Muffin*			
Blueberry Bran	320	11	49
Carrot Whole Wheat	410	20	51
Chocolate Chip Plain	425	16	65
Fruit Explosion	355	10	62
Low Fat Carrot/Cranberry	315	2	67
Low Fat Honey	285	2	61
Oatbran 'n Apple	335	11	53
Oatbran Carrot 'n Raisin	335	11	53
Oatmeal Raisin	405	11	72
Raisin Bran	365	11	60
Timbits (Lowfat):			
Chocolate Glazed	55	3	6
Old Fashion Plain	45	2	6
Sour Cream Glazed	55	3	6
Filled, average	35	1	6
Yeast: Dutchie; Honey Dip	45	2	6
Bagels			
Average all types	305	3	59
Cream Cheese: *Per 1 ½ oz*			
Plain	140	14	1
Plain Light	90	7	3
Garden Vegetable; Strawberry	140	13	3
Beverages: *Per Serving*			
Cafe Mocha, 10 fl.oz	120	5	18
Cappuccino: Eng. Toffee, 10 fl.oz	140	5	21
French Vanilla, 10 fl.oz	140	5	21
Iced w. 2% Milk, 10 fl.oz	155	1.5	32
Coffee w. sugar/cream, 10 fl.oz	80	4	10
Fruit Punch, 10 fl.oz	150	0	38
Hot Chocolate, 10 fl.oz	190	5	34
Iced Tea, 15 fl.oz	130	0	33

T.J. Cinnamons®

	C	F	Cb
Cinnachips, 10 oz bag	1135	50	157
Cinnamon Twist, 2.5 oz roll	260	13	33
Coffee, 12 fl.oz	5	0	1
Mocha Chill (with cream): 12.5 oz	290	6	49
Large, 18.5 oz	440	8	73
Original Roll: with Icing, 6.5 oz	775	37	103
w/out Cream Cheese Icing	510	17	81
Pecan Sticky, 6.5 oz roll	695	28	97

Togo's Eatery®

Sandwiches: Regular 6" Roll	C	F	Cb
Albacore Tuna	455	10	69
Avocado & Cucumber	615	26	79
Avocado & Turkey	690	27	78
BBQ Beef	525	13	64
California Chicken	620	15	68
Cheese	670	30	70
Chunky Chicken Salad	1087	63	93
Hot Pastrami	810	42	72
Hummus	807	31	104
Meatball,	690	23	80
Philly Cheesesteak	720	21	102
Reuben	660	25	69
Roast Beef	670	22	68
The Italian	745	37	68
Turkey & Cheese	600	18	71
Turkey, Ham & Cheese	600	19	70
Turkey, Roast Beef & Cheese	670	23	70
Large Size: Add 50% to Regular Size			
***Salads:** Per Serving*			
Chicken Caesar, 9 oz	315	13	13
Farmers Market, 9 oz	120	3	18
Oriental Salad, 21.3 oz	390	7	53
Taco, 24.5 oz	1050	66	79
Dressings: Caesar Dressing	125	9	9
Ranch Dressing	100	9	3
Low Fat Balsamic Vinaigrette	55	2	9
Oriental Sesame Salad Dressing	140	9	15
Sesame Orange Ginger	330	28	19
Soup: Black Bean	200	7	27
Chicken Noodle; Chili, avg.	150	3.5	20
New England Clam Chowder	105	6	6

Topz®

	C	F	Cb
Burger: Ahi Fillet Burger	365	8	42
Cheeseburger	495	23	38
Chicken Breast	315	5	37
Double Cheeseburger	730	36	45
Garden Cheeseburger	485	17	62
Jr. Kids Burger	200	6	21
Spicy Chicken Breast	355	6	43
Topz Burger	425	15	44
Topz Jr Burger	230	9	21
Turkey Burger	390	11	38
Chili: Half Order	110	5	4
Fries: Aero, 5.6 oz	380	14	58
Chili Cheese, 9 oz	665	35	68
French Fries, 6 oz	500	22	68

Tropical Smoothie Cafe®

	C	F	Cb
Tortizzas: BBQ Chicken	595	13	88
Cheese	530	19	66
Hawaiiwan	590	19	81
Pepperoni	760	40	68
***Sandwiches:** Per Sandwich (no Cheese)*			
BBQ Chicken	395	2	63
Blazin Buffalo	395	3	57
Golden Roasted Chicken	395	2	63
Half Hoagie: BLT	285	16	21
Pastrami	245	6	21
Turkey	250	2	26
Wraps: Blazin BBQ	590	13	87
Buffalo Chicken	625	28	59
Totally Turkey	655	27	57
Veggie Veggie	615	26	72
***Salads:** Per Salad*			
Specialty: Chef, no chse or dress.	245	8	12
Garden Salad w. chse, no dress.	140	8.5	6
Chicken Caesar w. cheese, no dr.	160	4.5	8
Sesame Chicken, no chse/dress.	535	11	77
Tuna, no cheese/dressing	215	7	15
Dressings: Blue Cheese, 1 Tbsp	80	8.5	0.5
Caesar, 1 Tbsp	80	8.5	0.5
Sesame, 1 Tbsp	45	2.5	5.5
Vinaigrette, 1 Tbsp	45	3	1.5
Dessert Smoothies *(with Turbinado):*			
Beach Bum (Chocolate)	565	5	125
Beach Bum (Vanilla)	570	5.5	126
Chocolate Chiller	555	7	117
Coffee Cooler	450	7.5	90
Mocha Madness	645	12	126
Strawberry Cheesecake	405	4	90
Tropi-colada	300	5.5	61
With Splenda, deduct 200 calories & 50g carbs			
Kids Smoothies *(with Turbinado):*			
Chocolate Chimp,	260	2.5	57
Groovy Grape	290	0	71
Jetty Jr	85	0.5	19
With Splenda, deduct 100 calories & 25g carbs			
Low-Fat Smoothies *(with Turbinado):*			
Berry Blast	345	0.5	84
Blimey Limey	410	0	102
Blue Lagoon	330	1	79
Cool Breeze	410	0	99
Cranberry Cove	445	0.5	109
Grape Gumbo, w. Turbinado	470	0.5	115

Tubby's®

Subs: Per 6" Sandwich	C	F	Cb
Burger Subs: Big Tub	665	45	41
Cheeseburger	615	41	37
Pizza Burger	630	41	39
Taco Burger	575	31	48
Deli Style Subs: Ham & Cheese	455	24	39
Turkey & Cheese	425	23	37
Turkey Club Sub	480	27	38
Specialty Subs: BLT	530	36	35
Tuna Salad	385	20	35
Veggie Stir Fry	410	20	46
Tubby's Subs: Tubby's Famous	500	29	40
Grilled Chicken Subs: *Per 6" Sub*			
Chicken & Broccoli	460	20	40
Chicken & Cheddar	390	16	38
Chicken Club Sub	445	21	36
Chicken Fajita Sub	350	9	40
Grilled Chicken	240	2	35
Grilled Steak Subs: *Per 6" Sub*			
Mushroom Steak & Cheese	630	42	39
Pepper Steak & Cheese	625	42	38
Pizza Steak & Cheese	620	41	39
Steak & Cheese	610	41	37
Salads: Side, no dressing	50	1	8
Antipasto Salad, no dressing	455	30	18
Chicken Salad	410	23	16
Taco Salad	655	46	25
Tuna Salad	340	26	11

Una Mas®

Burritos	C	F	Cb
El Cheapo	555	9	98
Fajita Burrito: Chicken	715	21	89
Steak	735	26	89
Gallito	590	30	62
Thai Chicken Burrito	500	16	62
Vegetariano Burrito	540	20	69
Una Mas Burrito: Chicken	585	15	76
Steak	605	20	76
Tacos: Crispy Chicken Taco	240	17	12
Fish Taco Cabo Style	265	6	36
Una Mas Taco: Chicken	340	9	48
Steak	345	11	48
Veggie	275	7	45
Favoritos: 5-Layer Dip	345	22	25
Chicken Enchiladas (2)	480	20	37
Nachos	1220	81	91
Verde Salad	210	5	19

Wahoo's Fish Taco®

Lower Fat Menu Items	C	F	Cb
Bowls: Carne Asada, Steak	760	22	90
Chicken, Skinless Breast	750	18	90
Fish of the Day	705	16	90
Burrito: Bonzai Chicken	650	18	87
Carne Asada, Steak	690	18	60
Carnitas, Pork	780	27	60
Chicken	510	15	43
Fish of the Day	430	12	44
Veggie	580	13	94
Tacos: Carne Asada, Steak	330	7.5	30
Carnitas, Pork	380	12	30
Chicken, Skinless Breast	260	6	27
Fish of the Day	225	5	27
Veggie	230	4.5	42
Sides: 1/2 Rice, 1/2 Beans	320	6	49
Beans	315	1	46
Rice	335	10	52
Salads: Carne Asada, Steak	605	35	12
Chicken, Skinless Breast	575	30	12
Fish of the Day	575	29	12

WAWA®

Breakfast & Baked Goods	C	F	Cb
Bagel: Plain	295	1	61
w. Butter	505	23	64
w. Cream Cheese	390	8	66
Avg. other varieties	320	2	66
Bagel Melts: Ham & Cheese	500	13	67
Pepperoni & Cheese	705	31	67
Turkey Club w. Mayo	720	32	70
Breakfast Bowls: *Per Bowl*			
Crmd Chipped Beef on a Biscuit	425	21	45
Sausage Gravy on a Biscuit	455	25	43
Croissant: Regular, 2 oz	300	15	35
Hash Brown: (1), 1.7 oz	90	5	10
Muffins: Banana Walnut, 4 oz	435	24	48
Blueberry, 4.2 oz	420	19	55
Chocolate Chip, 4 oz	425	21	52
Corn, 4 oz	395	17	55
Sizzli Bagels: Bacon Egg & Chse	470	19	53
Sausage Egg & Cheese	500	22	54
Sizzli Biscuits: Bacon Egg & Chse	500	31	37
Sausage Egg & Cheese	525	34	37
Sizzli Muffins: Bacon Egg & Chse	385	21	31
Sausage & Egg	410	24	31

WAWA® cont...

	C	F	Cb
***Hot Sandwiches:** No Cheese Unless Indicated*			
BBQ Pork Kaiser	560	20	61
Chicken Breaded Club	715	36	56
Classics: BBQ Pork w. Cheese	1090	48	112
Chicken Grilled, no Dressing	470	16	40
Meatball w. Cheese	660	37	49
Roast Beef Homestyle w. Cheese	665	21	67
***Cold Sandwiches:** No Cheese Unless Indicated*			
Italian w. Pesto & Rstd Peppers	900	64	40
Pepper Turkey w. Rstd Tomato	705	44	41
Roast Beef & Horseradish	460	18	26
Healthy Choice: Chkn on White	220	3	27
Ham on White	255	5	28
Smoked Turkey on White	270	4	31
Roast Beef on White	255	4	31
Turkey Carolina on White, avg.	250	2	30
Turkey on White	440	6	67
Roast Beef	375	7	37
Seafood Salad	450	21	46
Tuna Salad	465	22	43
Veggie	200	2	37
Veggie Supreme	325	11	43
Cold Shortis: American	425	18	40
BLT; Cheese, average	500	28	37
Chicken Salad	480	22	41
Egg Salad w. Cheese	630	40	43
Healthy Choice: Ham; Roast Beef	320	6	40
Honey Smoked Turkey	335	5	42
Hot Shortis: Chicken Grilled	325	3	42
Meatball w. Cheese	660	37	49
Roast Beef Homestyle w. Cheese	425	14	40
Wraps: Buffalo Blue Chicken	340	16	33
Roast Beef & Pepper Jack	430	17	42
Roasted Chicken Caesar	390	20	33
Smoked Turkey Supreme	325	7	44
Turkey Bacon & Colby Jack	455	22	37
Hot Dogs: ¼ lb Beef Frank	390	28	20
All Beef Hot Dog	270	17	20
Big Bacon Cheese Dog	730	50	37
Hot Sausage	300	17	21
Kielbasa	215	17	21
***Bowls:** Per 12 oz Bowl*			
Chicken Teriyaki	535	9	94
Chili	550	13	86
Steak & Vegetable	480	6	46
Southwest Chicken Bowl	455	5	82

WAWA® cont...

	C	F	Cb
***Sides:** Per Medium (11 oz)*			
Beef Stew	265	13	24
Chili, 11 oz	275	9	31
Homestyle Chicken & Noodles	325	16	26
Macaroni & Cheese	430	20	45
Mashed Potatoes	520	33	49
Meatballs in a Cup	375	27	14
Shepherd's Pie	400	24	37
***Soups:** Per Medium (11 oz)*			
Boston Clam Chowder	290	15	26
Chicken Corn Chowder	370	24	29
Potato Au Gratin	465	28	40
Potato w. Bacon	260	15	25
Drinks: Cappuccino, 12 fl.oz	170	7	27
French Vanilla, 12 fl.oz	195	7	30
Fat Free Cappuccino, 12 fl.oz	160	0	37
Frozen Cappuccino, 12 fl.oz	250	7	47

Weinerschnitzel®

	C	F	Cb
***Breakfast:** Per Serving*			
Biscuit: w. Egg	285	18	20
Egg, Sausage & Bacon	410	29	22
Egg, Sausage, Bacon & Cheese	465	34	22
Sausage & Bacon, 3.7 oz	325	23	21
Burrito: Breakfast, 9 oz	575	33	41
Chili Cheese, 9.2 oz	500	24	44
Country Breakfast, 10.1 oz	630	45	31
Croissant, 6.5 oz	580	36	41
French Toast, 5.2 oz	495	30	50
Hash Browns, 2.8 oz	285	25	14
Platter, 9.8 oz	700	48	42
Sandwich, 5.5 oz	370	22	28
Burgers: Chili Cheeseburger	345	13	32
Deluxe Cheeseburger	430	23	33
Deluxe Hamburger	385	19	33
Double Chili Cheeseburger	535	24	35
Tamale: Chili Cheese	445	27	33
***Fries:** Per Serving*			
Regular, 4.6 oz	350	25	28
Large, 6.4 oz	480	34	39
Chili Cheese, 8.1 oz	545	38	39
Hot Dogs			
BBQ Bacon Dog	370	20	33
Chili Dog	285	13	31
Chili Cheese Dog	335	17	31
Deluxe; Kraut; Mustard; Relish	270	12	30
All Beef: BBQ Bacon Dog	470	28	35
Chili Dog	385	21	33
Chilli Cheese Dog	435	25	33
Deluxe; Kraut; Mustard; Relish	360	20	32

Continued Next Page . . .

Weinerschnitzel® cont...

Hot Dogs (cont)	C	F	Cb
Healthy Choice: BBQ Bacon Dog	320	12	38
Chili Cheese Dog	295	10	36
Chili Dog	235	5	36
Deluxe; Kraut; Mustard; Relish	220	4	35
For Pretzel Bun add extra	140	3	26
Sandwiches: Bacon Ranch Chkn	540	31	41
Bratwurst	335	17	30
Cheddar Sausage Melt	670	38	58
Fish	390	17	48
Italian Sausage	345	17	31
Polish Sausage	495	28	39
Southwest Smoky Sausage	460	27	35
Sides: Jalapeno Poppers	485	32	37
Onion Rings	475	25	56
Ranch Dressing	120	12	2
Dessert: Apple Turnover, 3.2 oz	300	19	31

Wendy's®

Sandwiches	C	F	Cb
Bacon Mushroom Melt	550	28	41
Big Bacon Classic®	575	29	45
Classic Single with Everything	420	19	37
Grilled Chicken Sandwich	295	6	36
Chicken Temptations: Ultimate	365	7	44
Spicy Fillet	515	19	57
Homestyle Fillet	540	22	57
Kids' Meal: Jr. Hamburger	275	9	34
Jr. Cheeseburger	310	12	34
Jr. Cheeseburger Deluxe	350	15	36
Jr. Bacon Cheeseburger	385	19	34
French Fries: Medium, 5 oz	395	17	56
Biggie®	445	19	63
Great Biggie®	530	23	75
Kid's Meal	255	11	36
Chicken: Crispy Nuggets, 5 pce	220	14	13
Homestyle Strips (3), no sauce	405	18	33
Sauce: Heartland Ranch, 1 pkt	195	21	1
Other varieties, avg., 1 pkt	175	17	5
Garden Sensations Salads			
Chicken BLT Salad: no Dressing	345	19	10
w. Croutons/Dressing	690	48	30
Mandarin Chicken™: no Dressing	185	3	17
w. Dressing/Nuts/Noodles	630	35	50
Side Salad, no Dressing	35	0	7
Spinach Chkn, no Dressing/Croutons	300	14	10
w. Bacon Dressing and Croutons	485	19	43
Spring Mix Salad: no Dress./Pecans	190	11	12
w. Dressing/Pecans	530	42	25
Taco Supremo: no Dressing	370	16	29
w. Chips/Sour Cream/Salsa	670	32	64

Wendy's® cont...

Hot Stuffed Baked Potatoes™	C	F	Cb
Plain	270	0	61
Bacon & Cheese	555	25	67
Broccoli & Cheese	455	15	70
Sour Cream & Chives	335	6	62
Whipped Margarine	65	7	0
Chili: Small, 8 oz	200	5	21
Large, 12 oz	295	7.5	32
Hot Chili Seasoning	10	0	2
Cheddar Cheese, shredded, 2 Tbsp	75	6	1
Saltine Crackers, 2	30	0.5	5
Frosty™ Dairy Dessert: Per Cup			
Junior, 6 oz	165	4	28
Small, 12 oz	330	8	56
Medium, 16 oz	435	11	73

For Complete Nutritional Data ~ see CalorieKing.com

WesterN SizzliN®

Steaks (Meat Only, Raw Wts)	C	F	Cb
New York Strip, 14 oz	900	60	0
Ribeye, 10 oz	520	28	0
Sirloin: 8 oz Steak	540	33	0
16 oz Steak	1080	66	0
T-Bone, 20 oz	1230	99	0
Baked Potato, plain, 8 oz	245	0	58

Whataburger®

Burgers/Sandwiches	C	F	Cb
Whataburger®	605	30	53
No Bun	270	18	4
Double Meat Whataburger®	850	48	53
No Bun	345	36	4
Whataburger® w. Bacon/Cheese	790	45	53
Triple Meat Whataburger®	1090	66	53
Justaburger®	315	15	28
Whatacatch®	495	26	45
Whatachick'n®	550	21	63
Whataburger Jr.®	315	15	29
Grilled Chicken S'wich: w. Dressing	495	20	49
No Bun	190	7	10
Grilled Chicken Fajita Taco	350	13	35
Whatameals: Includes Drink & Fries			
Whataburger® Meal	1275	50	169
Whataburger® w. Bacon & Chse	1420	62	170
Chicken Strips w. Toast & Gravy	1055	49	127
Chicken Strips Kids Meal	740	38	92
Double Meat Whataburger®	1515	67	169
Grilled Chicken S'wich Meal	1115	39	165
Justaburger® Kids Meal	655	26	97
WhataChick'N® S'wich Meal	1240	51	172
Whataburger Jr.® Meal	705	29	110

Whataburger® cont...

Sides	C	F	Cb
French Fries: Small	265	13	33
Medium	400	20	50
Large	535	26	66
Onion Rings: Medium	195	10	23
Large	305	16	35
Chicken & Salads			
Chicken Strips (2)	380	24	22
Chicken Strips Salad	425	25	29
w. Cheddar Cheese, no Bacon	610	39	32
Garden Salad	55	0	10
w. Cheddar Cheese	225	15	10
Grilled Chicken Salad	240	7	18
w. Cheddar Cheese	400	21	18
Dressings: Ranch, 2 oz	315	33	3
Low Fat Ranch, 2 oz	80	4	10
Low Fat Vinaigrette, 2 oz	25	1.5	6
Thousand Island, 2 oz	160	13	11
Shakes			
Chocolate; Strawberry:			
Small, 20 fl oz	615	16	100
Medium, 32 fl oz	905	25	146
Vanilla: Small, 20 fl oz	535	17	81
Medium, 32 fl oz	800	26	122
Breakfast			
Bacon, 2 slices	75	5.5	0
Cinnamon Roll	860	34	126
Hashbrown Sticks (4)	135	8	16
Texas Toast	325	14	42
Biscuit: Buttermilk	300	16	34
w. Bacon	375	22	34
w. Bacon, Egg, Cheese	470	29	35
w. Egg & Cheese	440	27	35
w. Sausage	515	35	34
w. Sausage Gravy	520	33	47
w. Sausage, Egg, Cheese	655	46	35
Breakfast-On-A-Bun®: w. Bacon	400	23	28
w. Sausage	540	36	28
Ranchero: w. Bacon	410	23	29
w. Sausage	545	36	29
Breakfast Platters (Biscuit/Eggs/Hash Brown):			
w. Bacon, 2 slices	685	42	52
w. Sausage, 1 patty	830	56	51
Pancakes: Plain (3)	610	7.5	117
w. Bacon, 2 slices	680	13	118
w. Sausage, 1 patty	835	27	118
Taquito: Bacon & Egg	385	22	25
Potato & Egg	370	20	33
Sausage & Egg	375	23	26
Desserts: Hot Apple Pie	240	12	31
Chocolate Chunk Cookie, 2 oz	215	8	33
White Choc Macadamia Cookie	230	11	30

Winchell's®

Baked Products	C	F	Cb
Bagel	130	1	22
Banana Nut Muffin	560	28	63
Blueberry Muffin	480	25	54
Blueberry Muffin, Low Fat	220	3	42
Bran Muffin	405	20	48
Bran Muffin, Low Fat	230	3	44
Cheese Muffin	485	25	51
Chocolate Chip Muffin	450	22	54
Croissant	285	17	28
Cake Donuts: *Per Donut Unless Indicated*			
Buttermilk Bar Glazed	275	16	29
Cinnamon Crumb Cake	290	18	30
Glazed Old Fashion	290	18	28
Iced Cake	255	15	28
Iced French	230	13	24
Iced Old Fashion	300	19	28
Iced Donut Holes (4)	255	15	28
Plain Donut Holes (4)	235	14	26
Raised Donuts: Apple Fritter	615	41	55
Bear Claw	480	30	47
Chocolate Bavarian	330	18	36
Chocolate Rounds/Twist/Bar	275	16	29
Glazed Cinnamon Roll	290	24	12
Glazed Jelly; Sugar Jelly	320	17	36
Glazed Rounds/Twist	250	15	27
Iced Bar	240	16	29
Sugar Rounds/Twist	250	15	27
Drinks: Frozen Orange Chilla	340	8	66
Frozen Mocha Cappuccino	490	19	74

White Castle®

Hamburgers	C	F	Cb
Hamburger	140	7	11
Cheeseburger	160	9	11
Bacon Cheeseburger	200	13	12
Double Hamburger	240	14	16
Double Cheeseburger	290	18	16
Sandwiches: Chicken	190	8	21
Fish Sandwich	200	7	27
Breakfast Sandwich	340	25	17
Sides: Cheese Sticks, 3 piece	255	14	22
Chicken Rings, 6 piece	210	14	11
French Fries, small	115	6	15
Onion Rings, 6 piece	260	13	31
Drinks: Coca-Cola, 16 fl.oz	215	0	54
Chocolate/Vanilla Shake, 16 fl.oz	270	8	40
Iced Tea, 16 fl.oz	95	0	24

Yoshinoya®

Bowls	C	F	Cb
Beef Bowl: Regular, 15 oz	840	30	109
Large, 21 oz	1160	41	153
Kids, 9 oz	340	11	48
Chicken Bowl: Regular, 19 oz	760	15	125
Large, 30 oz	1110	22	180
Kids, 10 oz	370	9	53
Combo Bowl: Regular, 17 oz	750	19	117
Large, 27 oz	1220	36	171
Vegetable Beef Bowl: Reg.,18 oz	770	23	114
Large, 28 oz	1090	32	163
Vegetable Bowl: Regular 19 oz	530	3.5	116
Large, 32 oz	780	5	169
Tempura: Fish Tempura, 22 oz	990	24	168
Fish & Beef Tempura, 30 oz	1450	45	214
Fish & Chicken Tempura, 31 oz	1450	37	225
Shrimp Tempura, 20 oz	890	19	160
Shrimp & Beef Tempura, 28 oz	1350	40	206
Shrimp & Chicken Tempura, 29 oz	1340	32	217
Extras			
Beef, 5½ oz	370	28	6
Chicken & Vegetables, 9½ oz	300	12	21
Rice, 10 oz	460	2.5	104
Vegetable, 9 oz	60	0.5	12

Note: Yoshinoya Beef Bowl Restaurants are based in California.

Zoup!®

Soups: Per Cup (8 fl.oz)	C	F	Cb
Chicken & Dumplings	110	1.5	14
Corn & Crab Chowder	280	18	21
Gazpacho (chilled)	100	1.5	16
Ginger Butternut Squash	150	6	16
Jamaican Bay Gumbo	115	1.5	15
New England Clam Chowder	185	7	21
Old Fashion Chicken Noodle	80	1.5	7
Potato Cheddar	265	14	26
Spicy Black Bean Chili	110	1	21
Turkey Chili	115	1	21
Vegetarian Split Pea	160	1	28
Paninis: *Per ½ Sandwich*			
Italian Chicken	370	21	23
Smoked Ham and Swiss	185	8	17
Turkey Club	455	28	22
Bread: *Per Piece (2 oz)*			
Extra Low-Carb French, 2 oz	105	2	7
Extra Multigrain, 2 oz	190	4	30
Extra Sourdough, 2 oz	170	1.5	31

Zero's Subs®

Oven Baked Subs (6") (Includes cheese, lettuce, tomato, onions, oil & vinegar)	C	F	Cb
BLT	410	19	48
BLT, no Mayo	330	12	43
Cosmo Vegetarian	470	23	46
Cosmo Deluxe	500	25	48
Grinder	565	31	48
Grinder, Multigrain	570	32	50
Ham & Cheese	445	19	44
Meatball & Cheese	560	30	50
without Cheese	460	22	50
Pepperoni & Cheese	550	31	42
without Cheese	345	15	41
Roast Beef & Cheese	465	19	45
The Club	505	23	44
Tuna & Cheese	525	26	47
Turkey & Cheese	450	17	44
6" Subs: *Per Sub (No Cheese, Oil or Vinegar)*			
Cosmo Deluxe	245	3	47
Cosmo Vegetarian	220	2	45
Grilled Veggie	265	3	51
Grinder	400	17	47
Grinder, Multigrain	405	18	49
Ham & Cheese	285	5	43
Roast Beef & Cheese	310	5	45
The Club	360	10	43
Tuna & Cheese	370	12	46
Turkey & Cheese	285	3	43
12" Size Subs: *Double the figures for 6" size*			
6" Subs From The Grill			
Grilled Veggie	410	14	52
Hot Italian Sausage & Cheese	655	37	45
Philly Chicken & Cheese	410	10	48
w. Mushrooms/Green Peppers	415	10	49
without Cheese	325	4	45
Philly Steak & Cheese	495	21	49
w. Mushrooms/Green Peppers	500	21	50
without Cheese	410	15	46
Drinks			
Pepsi (with ⅓ Ice):			
Small, 12 fl.oz	110	0	29
Medium, 16 fl.oz	150	0	37
Large, 22 fl.oz	210	0	55
Potato Chips, 1 oz pkg.	150	10	15

Notes on Cholesterol

- **Cholesterol** is a white waxy substance produced mainly by our liver. It is also found in animal food products. Plant foods have no cholesterol.

- **Cholesterol is essential to life.** It is a structural part of every body cell wall and is the building block for vitamin D, sex hormones, and bile acids which help in the digestion of dietary fats.

- **The body makes sufficient cholesterol** for its needs and does not rely on cholesterol in the diet. Dietary fats have a major influence on blood cholesterol levels - more so than dietary cholesterol.

- **A high blood cholesterol increases** the risk of atherosclerosis - the thickening of arteries that can reduce or block blood flow to the heart muscle, brain, eyes, kidneys, sex organs and other body parts.

 This in turn increases the risk of heart attack, stroke, blindness, kidney failure, impotence and other blood circulatory problems.

 Other risk factors which increase the risk of atherosclerosis include high blood pressure, tobacco smoking, obesity and diabetes (uncontrolled).

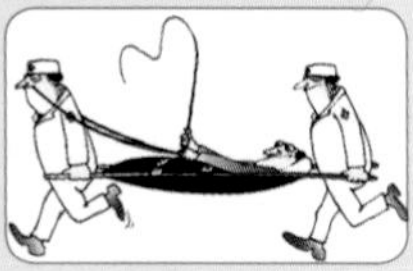

BLOOD CHOLESTEROL

Check Your Risk!

Cholesterol Level (mg/dL) ▼	Risk of Heart Attack ▼
240 and above ~	High Risk
200 - 239 ~	Borderline/High
Below 200 ~	Desirable

- ❤ Know your cholesterol level, particularly if there is a family history of heart disease or stroke. If high, see your doctor.

- ❤ All adults should have their cholesterol, HDL and triglycerides tested at least every 5 years.

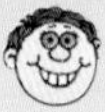

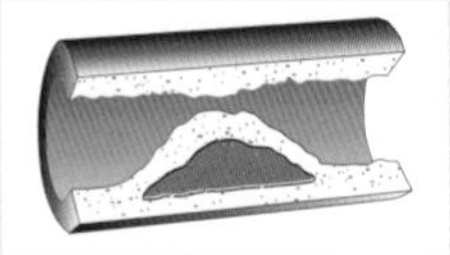

▲ Atherosclerosis can clog arteries and impede blood flow to the heart muscle or other body organs.

▼ A thrombus (blood clot) can form on unstable, festering atherosclerotic plaque and rapidly block blood flow. A heart attack or stroke can result.

HEART ATTACK WARNING SIGNALS

Many victims die before reaching hospital by ignoring warning signals and delaying medical help.

Symptoms vary and commonly include:

- **Chest pain**, vice-like squeezing or burning sensation in centre of chest or between shoulder blades, or feeling of severe indigestion.

- **Pain** may spread to shoulders, neck, jaw or arms.

- **Sweating**, nausea, dizziness, shortness of breath, irregular pulse.

If you experience any of the above symptoms seek IMMEDIATE medical attention!

Every minute counts.

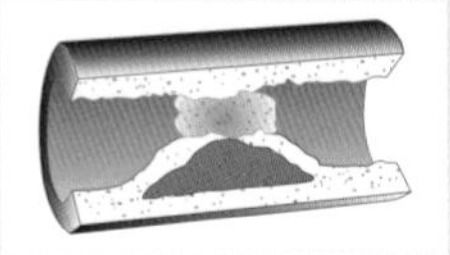

Fats & Cholesterol Guide

The amount and type of dietary fat has the greatest influence on blood cholesterol levels.

Fats in food are a mixture of 3 basic types: saturated, monounsaturated, and polyunsaturated. Animal fats are mainly saturated while plant oils and fish oils are mainly mono- and polyunsaturated.

Saturated fats have subgroups known as long chain, medium chain, and short chain fats. Most of the long chain fats raise blood cholesterol; and increase the risk of blood clots and thrombosis leading to artery blockage.

Long chain saturated fats are found mainly in full cream milk, cheese, butter, cream, fatty meats and sausages, and processed foods.

Monounsaturated fats tend to more selectively lower 'bad' LDL-cholesterol and maintain the protective 'good' HDL-cholesterol in the bloodstream - but only if they replace saturated fats in the diet.

Foods rich in monounsaturates include canola and olive oils, canola margarine, peanuts, and avocados.

Polyunsaturated fats consist of two main classes. **Omega-6** polyunsaturates tend to lower blood cholesterol. Rich sources include safflower, sunflower and corn oils.

Omega-3 polyunsaturated fats can lower blood cholesterol, and also confer extra benefits by lowering blood triglycerides, and reducing the risk of thrombosis, heart arrhythmias, and artery spasm.

Best practical omega-3 sources include canola oil and margarine, soybean oil and fish.
(See adjoining chart)

A balanced intake of the two omega classes is important for optimal health. Increasing slightly omega-3 intake by Americans would help to attain a more ideal balance. Adequate vitamin E intake is also important.

All fats are high in calories and need to be limited for weight control.

DIETARY FATS COMPARISON

■ Saturated Fat ■ Monounsaturated Fat
Polyunsaturated Fats:
■ Linoleic (Omega-6) ■ Alpha-Linolenic (Omega-3)

OILS	Saturated	Monounsaturated	Linoleic (Omega-6)	Alpha-Linolenic (Omega-3)
CANOLA OIL	7	63	20	10
LINSEED/FLAX OIL	9	19	17	55
SAFFLOWER OIL	9	14	77	
GRAPESEED OIL	10	22	68	
SUNFLOWER OIL	11	23	66	
CORN OIL	14	32	52	2
OLIVE OIL	14	76	10	
SOYBEAN OIL	15	23	54	8
PEANUT OIL	19	45	34	2
COTTONSEED OIL	26	16	58	
PALM OIL	51	39	10	

PERCENTAGE CONTENT

SPREADS & FATS
Saturated Fat includes 'Trans Fats' ☐ WATER CONTENT

SPREADS & FATS	Saturated	Monounsaturated	Linoleic (Omega-6)	Alpha-Linolenic (Omega-3)	Water
LIGHT MARGARINE	14	14	21		51
CANOLA MARGARINE	18	45	12	6	19
POLYUNSATURATED MARG	24	20	36		20
BUTTER	57	18	2		24
LARD	41	47	12		
BEEF FAT	44	37	4		15

GOOD SOURCES OF OMEGA-3 FATS

Plant Sources	Omega-3 Fats (Grams)
Canola Oil, 1 Tbsp, ½ fl.oz	1.5g
Flaxseed Oil, 1 Tbsp	8g
Soybean Oil, 1 Tbsp	1.2g
Canola Margarine, 1 Tbsp, ½ oz	1g
Soybeans, cooked, ½ cup, 4 oz	0.5g
Walnuts, ½ oz	0.5g

FISH - *Per 4 oz Serving*

High Content: Salmon (Chinook), Tuna, — 3g
Trout (Lake), Sardines, Herring, Mackerel — 3g

Medium Content:
Salmon, (Pink/Red/Coho), 4 oz — 2g

Fair Content: *Per 4 oz Serving*
Bass, Catfish, Cod, Grouper, Hake, Halibut, Kingfish, Perch, Pollock, Shark, Trout (Rainbow), Tuna (Skipjack), Crab, Oysters, Blue Mussel, Shrimp, Squid — 0.5-1g

How Much Is Needed?

As little as 1-2 grams daily of omega-3 fats may benefit general health. High doses of fish oil supplements should only be taken as directed by your doctor.

Dietary Cholesterol

Cholesterol in food varies in its effect on blood cholesterol level (BCL) from person to person. Much depends on the amount and type of fat, and fiber eaten at the same meal.

Any elevating effect of dietary cholesterol on BCL is more likely to occur when the diet is high in saturated fat. Little elevation, if any, generally occurs when dietary fats are balanced in favor of mono- and polyunsaturated fats (including omega-3 fats).

For example, while fish does contain cholesterol, the omega-3 fats can prevent any increase in BCL. Conversely, a meal containing no cholesterol but rich in saturated fat, may result in a significant increase in BCL.

Consequently, the need to be overly concerned about dietary cholesterol is being de-emphasized in favor of a stricter approach to limiting total fats, as well as saturated fat and trans fats in particular.

The liver usually cuts back its own cholesterol production in response to cholesterol in the diet. Many people can consume normal amounts of high cholesterol foods without concern.

However, it is difficult to identify just who is at risk - the so-called 'hyper-responders' - and because over 50% of Americans have a BCL above ideal levels, the **American Heart Association** advises all Americans to be prudent and limit their cholesterol intake to less than 300mg daily – as well as adopting a heart-healthy diet.

This limitation still allows the inclusion of most foods regularly eaten - even the overly maligned egg.

Note: Eggs contain a modest 5 grams of fat per large egg of which barely 2 grams are saturated, the rest being mono- and polyunsaturated.

By comparison, a cup of whole milk has almost 10g fat of which 6g are saturated.

Cholesterol Counter

Cholesterol is found only in foods of animal origin. Plant foods contain no cholesterol.
AHA recommends limiting dietary cholesterol to less than 300mg/day.

	Chol mg
Meat - Average all types:	
Lean Meat, cooked, 4 oz	70
Fatty Meat, cooked, 4 oz	105
Fat, thick strip, 2 oz	35
(Note: While lean meat and fat have similar amounts of cholesterol, choose lean meat to limit fat intake.)	
Chicken/Turkey, average, 4 oz	90
Organ Meats: Liver, fried, 4 oz	500
Brains, beef, pan fried, 3 oz	1700
Sausages: Frankfurter, 1.5 oz	25
Salami, 2 slices, 2 oz	40
Bacon: 3 slices, cooked, 1 oz	20
Fish: Fish fillets, average, ckd, 4 oz	70
Tuna/Salmon, canned, 3 oz	30
Scallops, 9 medium, 3 oz	30
Shrimp, 12 large, raw, 3 oz	130
Oysters, raw, 6 medium, 3 oz	45
Lobster, Crab, raw, 3 oz	80
Eggs (Chicken), 1 large	210
1 medium	180
Egg White, *Egg Beaters*	0
Milk/Yogurt: Whole, 1 cup, 8 fl.oz	35
1% Milk, 1 cup	10
Skim/Non-fat, 1 cup	5
Soy Milk, Tofu, Tempeh	0
Cheese: Natural/Hard/Cream, 1 oz	30
Cottage, lowfat, 4 oz	5
Ricotta, part skim, 4 oz	25
Fats: Butter, 2 Tbsp, 1 oz	60
Margarine, Oils (vegetable)	0
Mayonnaise, 1 Tbsp	10
Cream: Heavy, whipping, 2 T, 1 oz	40
Half & Half/Sour, 2 Tbsp, 1 oz	10
Icecream: Regular, ½ cup, 4 fl.oz	30
Fruit, Vegetables, Avocados	0
Nuts, Seeds, Grains	0
Coffee, Tea, Soda, Beer, Wine	0

For Comprehensive Food Listings ~ see CalorieKing.com

DIETARY HINTS TO LOWER BLOOD CHOLESTEROL

1. **Maintain a healthy weight.**
   If overweight, lose weight with lowfat eating and daily exercise.

2. **Reduce saturated fat intake by:**
   (a) eating less dairy fat. Choose lowfat or fat-reduced varieties of milk, yogurt, cheese, and icecream. Enjoy soy drinks.

   (b) replacing saturated fats with fats and oils rich in mono- and polyunsaturated fats; and carbohydrate-rich foods. Choose vegetable oils such as canola, olive, sunflower and soybean. Avoid solid frying fats.
   Take Control and *Benecol* (spreads) contain plant stanol esters which can lower total and LDL cholesterol.

   (c) eating less fat from meat and poultry. Choose lean cuts of meat and skinless chicken. Go easy on luncheon meats, salamis and fatty sausages. Enjoy fish.

   (d) eating less saturated and trans fats from baked and fried fast-foods. Avoid deep-fried foods. Avoid donuts, cakes, pastries and cookies unless made with healthier fats and oils.

3. **Increase your 'soluble' fiber intake.**
   Foods rich in 'soluble' fiber include dried beans, baked beans, lentils, chick peas, hummus, nuts, seeds, psyllium seed husks and psyllium fiber supplements. Oat bran, rice bran and barley are also useful, as are fruit, veggies and avocados.

4. **Eat more soya bean products** such as: soy drinks, tofu, tempeh (cultured soya beans), soy flour and soy vegetarian foods.
   Soy protein in place of animal protein can significantly decrease high blood cholesterol levels - as well as 'bad' LDL-cholesterol and blood triglycerides. Good' HDL-cholesterol is maintained. For best results, eat at least 25g of soy protein per day (from 3-4 servings).

5. **Eat more fruit and vegetables in place of high-fat foods.**
   Aim for 2 fruits and 5 servings of vegetables per day. They also contain valuable antioxidants. The fat of avocados (and most nuts and seeds) is mainly unsaturated and lowers blood cholesterol levels.

6. **Limit cholesterol to 300mg per day.**
   (Extra Notes ~ See Previous Page)

7. **Avoid brewed unfiltered coffee** (espresso; plunger-style). It contains oil compounds (diterpenes) which can raise blood cholesterol. American style filtered coffee is fine.

8. **Spread your food intake over the day.**
   Have 5-6 small meals per day rather than just 2-3 large meals. Nibbling, versus gorging, favors lower blood cholesterol.

ALCOHOL - WINE

Alcohol is a mixed bag. Moderate amounts of 1-2 drinks daily appear to reduce the risk of heart attack and ischaemic stroke in older persons.

However, larger amounts increase the risk of high blood pressure, obesity, heart failure and hemorrhagic stroke; and can aggravate hypertriglyceridemia - in addition to many other health hazards.
(See Alcohol Guide - page 166)

The over-riding harmful effects of excess alcohol do not allow its recommendation for any aspects of health promotion.

Notes On Wine:
Red wine (more so than white) contains antioxidants which may help protect cholesterol in the blood from becoming oxidized.

Many fruits, vegetables and tea also contain protective antioxidants.

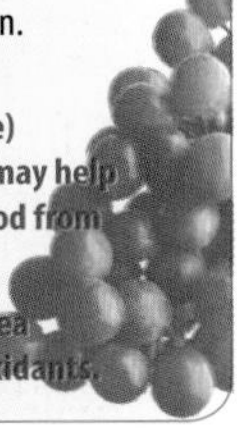

How Fats Affect Blood Flow

Fats in the diet not only affect blood cholesterol levels. They can also strongly influence blood clot formation and thrombosis, as well as blood flow and ultimate oxygen delivery to body parts and organs.

While advanced atherosclerosis can impede blood flow to the heart and other organs, it is thrombosis (complete blockage by blood clots) or arterial spasm which commonly result in a heart attack or stroke.

Plant and fish oils rich in omega-3 fats lessen the risk of blood clots, thrombus formation and artery spasm by reducing platelet stickiness and adhesion to artery walls. This reduces the risk of atherosclerotic plaque becoming unstable and reactive.

Omega-3 fats also improve blood flow by reducing blood viscosity; and increasing the flexibility of red blood cells (RBC) that need to flex and twist on themselves in order to squeeze through tiny narrow capillaries often half their diameter.

A diet high in saturated fats has the opposite effect by stiffening RBC membranes and increasing blood viscosity thereby hindering blood flow. The stiffening of the RBC membrane also reduces its ability to release vital oxygen to body cells and take up carbon dioxide.

Stiff red blood cells may also form aggregates like coin stacks. In narrow blood vessels, this further impedes blood flow and impairs oxygen release through the much lessened surface area of red blood cell membranes exposed to blood. (Smoking, lack of exercise, and stress can have similar adverse effects on thrombosis, red blood cell flexibility and blood flow.)

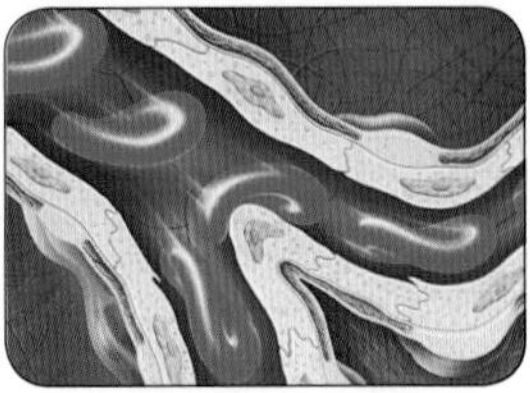

▲ **Picture of Healthy Blood Flow**

Flexible red blood cells twist and slide through tiny capillaries - often half the diameter of red blood cells.

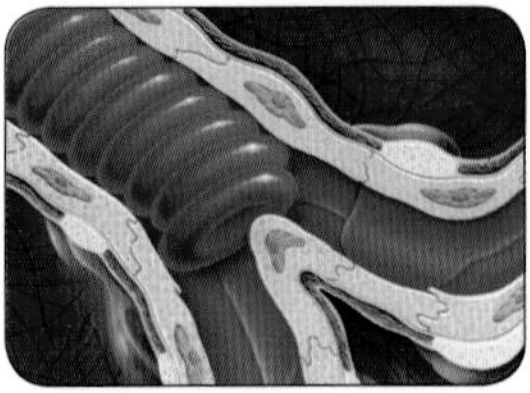

▲ **A Not-So-Healthy Picture!**

Red blood cells have lost their flexibility and ability to twist and slip through capillaries. They are stacked up thereby impeding blood flow.

A diet high in saturated fats can contribute to this picture - as can smoking, lack of exercise and stress.

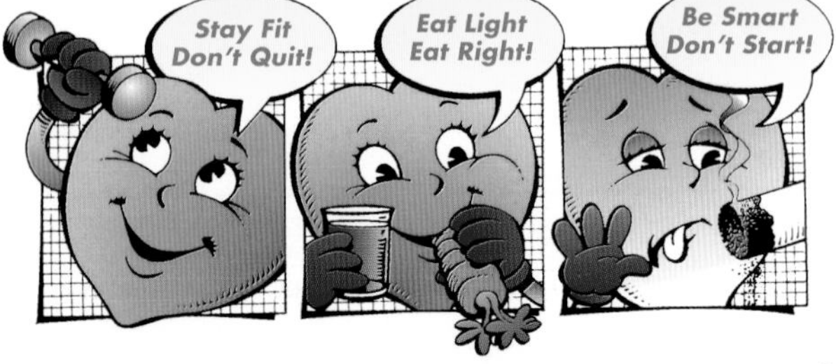

Introduction

Fiber is the general term for those parts of **plant** food that we cannot digest (although bacteria in the large bowel partly digests fiber through fermentation). It is not found in foods of animal origin (meats, dairy products).

Fiber promotes intestinal health, bowel regularity, can benefit diabetes and blood cholesterol levels, and may help prevent colon cancer. High fiber foods also assist weight control.

Most Americans don't eat enough fiber - less than 20 grams/day - instead of a healthier **25 to 35 grams/day.**

Fiber promotes good health, and better control of diabetes and cholesterol.

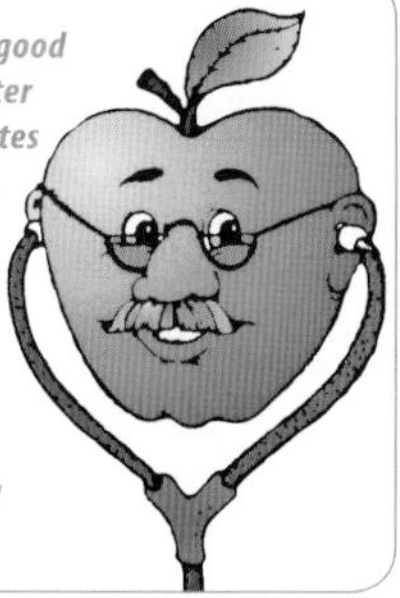

'An apple a day keeps the doctor away.' ... it just might!

Types of Fiber

Plant foods contain a mixture of different fibers in varying proportions. Insoluble and soluble fiber categories are based on their solubility in water. All types of fiber are beneficial to the body.

- **Insoluble fibers** (cellulose, hemi-celluloses, lignin) make up the structural parts of plant cell walls. The **best sources** are wheat bran, corn bran, rice bran, wholegrain cereals and breads, dried beans and peas, nuts, seeds and the skins of fruits and vegetables.

These fibers absorb many times their own weight in water. They create a soft bulk and hasten the passage of waste products through the intestines.

They promote bowel regularity, and aid in the prevention and treatment of uncomplicated forms of **constipation, diverticulosis and haemorrhoids.**

The risk of colon cancer may also be reduced by fiber's diluting effect of potentially harmful substances.

- **Soluble fibers** (pectin, gums, mucilages) are found mainly within plant cells, soy milk (whole bean) and products.

Types of Fiber (Cont)

Best Sources of Soluble Fiber:
Fruits and vegetables, oat bran, barley, dried beans and peas, psyllium and flax seed.

These fibers form a gel which slows both stomach emptying and the absorption of sugars from the intestines. This helps to control **blood sugar** levels.

Weight control is also aided by the slower emptying of the stomach and the feeling of **fullness provided by soluble fiber.**

Some soluble fibers can lower **blood cholesterol** by binding bile acids and excreting them. More body cholesterol must then be broken down to supply bile acids for emulsification of dietary fats. **Rice bran, while not high in soluble fiber can also lower blood cholesterol.**

- **Resistant starch** is that part of starchy foods (approx. 10%) which is tightly bound by fiber and resists normal digestion. Friendly bacteria in the large bowel ferment and change the resistant starch into short-chain fatty acids which are important to bowel health and may protect against colon cancer.

Starchy foods include bread, cereals, rice, pasta, potatoes and legumes.

Fiber & Weight Control

Fiber can assist weight control in several ways. Fiber-rich foods such as fresh fruit and vegetables, potatoes and whole-grain bread contain few calories for their large volume (due to their lowfat, high water content).

Their bulk fills the stomach and satisfies appetite much earlier than fiber-depleted foods. The extra chewing time also contributes to satiety, and gives the stomach time to register a feeling of fullness. Excessive calories are less likely to be consumed.

Fiber-depleted foods and drinks are more concentrated in calories; e.g. fats, sugar, candy, soft drinks, fruit juices, alcohol. They require little or no chewing. Large amounts with excessive calories can be consumed before appetite is satisfied.

Example: Whereas one fresh apple might satisfy our appetite, an apple juice drink with the equivalent sugars and calories of 2-3 apples does little to satisfy appetite. (See illustration below.)

High Fiber Foods fill the stomach. Fewer calories are consumed.

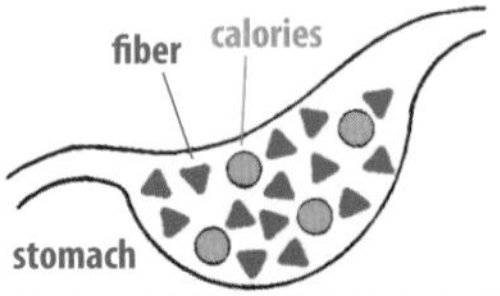

Low Fiber Foods are more concentrated in calories. More food must be eaten to fill the stomach.

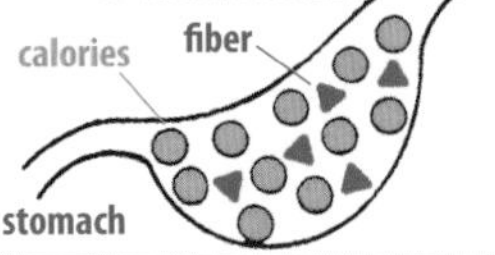

EFFECTS OF REMOVING FIBER FROM FOOD

2-3 pieces of fresh fruit produces 1 glass of fruit juice. The removal of fiber concentrates the sugar and calories.

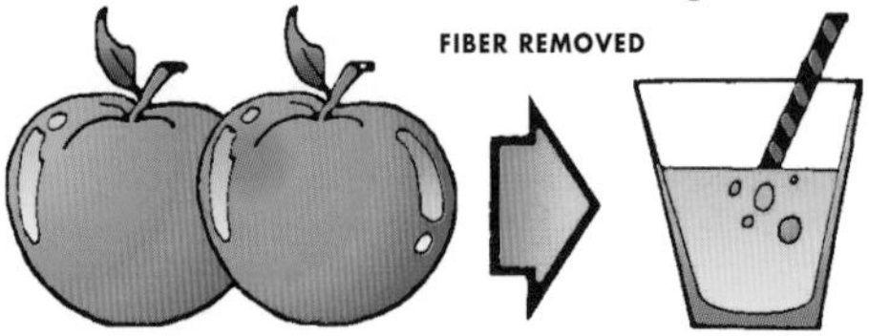

Fresh Fruit		Fruit Juice
High Fiber	✦	Negligible Fiber
Low Calorie Density	✦	High Calorie Density
Long Eating Time	✦	No Eating Time (Drink)
Satisfies Hunger	✦	Does Not Satisfy Hunger
Sugar Slowly Absorbed	✦	Sugar More Quickly Absorbed
Less Insulin Required	✦	More Insulin Required

Constipation

Constipation can reasonably be defined as a failure to have a bowel movement at least every second day - and just as importantly, without straining or pain.

Typically, stools are too hard, too narrow, and too small . . . *sinkers* rather than *floaters*.

The **main cause** is simply a lack of dietary fiber. Other contributing factors include insufficient fluids, too little exercise, emotional stress, gastro-intestinal disease, lack of proper dentition to chew high-fiber foods, and some medications (e.g. some antacids, antidepressants, tranquilizers).

Note: Check with your doctor to rule out any underlying medical problem – especially if you have a change in bowel habits in middle-age or later years.

DESIRABLE FIBER INTAKE

Adults: 25-35gm per day
Children (under 18): Age + 5gm
Example: 6-year old (6 + 5)= 11gm

SAMPLE FOOD QUANTITIES

For 35 Grams of Fiber/Day		Fiber
	Breakfast Cereal (higher-fiber)	5g
plus	4 slices wholegrain Bread	6g
plus	3 servings fresh Fruit	9g
plus	1 medium Potato (w. skin)	4g
or	1 cup Brown Rice	
or	½ cup wholegrain Pasta	
plus	3-4 servings Veges/Salad	6g
plus	1 cup Bean Soup	5g
or	¼ cup Baked/Soy Beans	
or	½ cup Corn/Peas/Lentils	
or	1¼ oz Almonds (natural)	
or	3 medium Figs	

HINTS TO INCREASE FIBER AND AVOID CONSTIPATION

1. **Breakfast is an important** contributor to daily fiber intake. Eat high-fiber breakfast cereals (bran-based cereals, oatmeal etc.). Add 1-2 tablespoons of unprocessed bran (wheat/ barley/ rice) and wheat germ if required.

Dried fruits, chopped nuts, soy grits, and seeds are also excellent additions to cereals.

Note: A gradual increase in fiber will prevent bloating, gas or pain. People intolerant to bran may benefit from psyllium-based fiber supplements and cereals.

2. **Drink 6-8 glasses of water daily.** Fiber works by absorbing many times its own weight of water.
3. **Eat whole-grain breads,** or fiber-enriched breads. One slice of wholegrain bread has over double the fiber of regular white bread.
4. **Enjoy fruit as fresh fruit** with skins rather than as fruit juice. Enjoy wholegrain pasta, barley, brown rice, nuts and seeds.
5. **Eat more vegetables,** salads and legumes - especially dried beans, baked beans, lentils, potatoes with skins, avocado, broccoli, brussel sprouts, cabbage, carrots, celery, and peas.
6. **Add bran** (barley/rice/wheat) or soy grits to soups, casseroles, yogurt, desserts, biscuits, cakes. Also use wholemeal flour or soy flour in place of white flour. Use nuts and seeds.
7. **Snack** on fresh or dried fruits, carrot or celery sticks, popcorn, nuts or seeds, wholegrain crackers, high-fiber bars (low-fat). Limit amounts if overweight.
8. **Exercise regularly** to strengthen abdominal muscles and stimulate the gut. Keep up fluids, especially in warm weather.
9. **Avoid** indiscriminate and regular use of harsh laxatives. They can overstimulate the intestinal muscles and may make normal bowel activity impossible. It may take several weeks to restore normal bowel function.

FOODS WITH ZERO FIBER

- **Dairy Products (Milk, Cheese, etc)**
- **Meats, Poultry, Fish, Eggs**
- **Fats/Oils, Sugar/Syrups**
  (Only foods of plant origin contain fiber.)

Breakfast Cereals

	Fiber
General Mills:	
Basic 4, 1 cup, 2 oz	3
Cheerios (Honey Nut; Multigrain), 1 c., 1 oz	3
Multi-Bran Chex, 1 cup, 2 oz	8
Oatmeal Crisp Almond, 1 cup, 2 oz	4
Raisin Nut Bran, ¾ cup, 2 oz	5
Total, average all types, 1 oz	3
Wheat Chex; Wheaties, 1 cup	5
Wheaties Energy Crunch, 1 cup	4
Health Valley:	
Amaranth Flakes, ¾ cup	4
Corn Bran Flakes, ¾ cup	4
Fiber 7 Flakes, ¾ cup	4
Golden Flax, ¼ cup	6
Granola (Fat Free), ⅔ cup	6
Healthy Crunches & Flakes, ¾ cup	4
Healthy Fiber Flakes, ¾ cup	4
Oat Bran Flakes, all types, ¾ cup	4
Oat Bran O's, ¾ cup, 1.95 oz	4
Real Oat Bran, ½ cup	5
Kellogg's: All-Bran, ½ cup, 1 oz	10
All-Bran w. Extra Fiber, ½ cup, 1 oz	13
Bran Buds, ¾ cup, 2 oz	12
Corn Flakes, Fruit Loops, Smacks, ¾ cup	1
Cocoa/Rice Krispies Treats, ¾ cup, 1 oz	0
Complete: Wheatbran Flakes, ¾ c., 1 oz	5
Oatbran Flakes, ¾ cup	4
Corn Pops, 1 cup, 1 oz	0
Cracklin' Oat Bran, ¾ cup, 2 oz	6
Frosted Mini Wheats, 1 cup, 2 oz	6
Healthy Choice, all types, 1 cup	5
Nutri-Grain, 1¼ cup, 2 oz	4
Cereal Bars, 1 bar, 1.3 oz	4
Mueslix (Almond. Raisin Date), ⅔ cup	4
Raisin Bran, 1 cup, 2 oz	8
Smart Start Original, 1 cup	2
Soy Protein, 1 oz	2
Special K; Product 19, 1 cup	1
Special K Red Berries, 1 cup	4
Wheat Chex, 1 cup	3

Fiber ~ **Fiber (grams)**

Breakfast Cereals (Cont)

	Fiber
Kashi: GoLEAN Cereal, ¾ cup, 1.4 oz	10
GoLEAN Crunch!, 1 cup, 1.8 oz	8
GoLEAN Bars, each	6
Breakfast Pilaf, ½ cup, cooked, 5 oz	6
Good Friends, ¾ cup, 1 oz	8
Cinna-raisin Crunch, 1 cup, 1¾ oz	10
Heart to Heart, ¾ cup, 1.2 oz	5
Puffed Kashi, 1 cup, 0.9 oz	2
Quaker: Captain Crunch, ¾ cup	1
100% Natural Granola, average, ½ cup	3
Crunchy Corn Bran, 1 cup, 1 oz	5
Fruity Oh's, 1 cup	2
Honey Nut, 1 cup	3
Life Cereal (¾ cup), Oat Squares (½ c.)	2
Oat Bran, ⅓ cup	6
Oatmeal, average, 1 packet	3
Puffed Rice, 1 cup	1
Puffed Wheat, 1 cup	2
Shredded Wheat, 3 biscuits	3
Post: 100% Bran, ½ cup	8
Blueberry Morning, 1 cup, 2 oz	2
Cocoa/Fruity Pebbles, 1 cup	0
Cranberry Almond Crunch, 1 cup, 2 oz	3
Frosted Alpha Bits, 1 cup	1
Fruit & Bran, 1 cup, 2 oz	5
Grape-Nuts, ½ cup, 2 oz	5
Great Grains, ⅔ cup, 1.8 oz	4
Honey Bunches of Oats, ¾ cup, 1 oz	1
Shredded Wheat 'n Bran, ½ cup	3

Brans & Supplements

Oat Bran: 1 Tbsp (level)	1
⅓ cup, (5⅓ Tbsp), 1 oz	4.2
Rice Bran: ¼ cup, 1 oz	6
Wheat Bran: unprocessed: 1 Tbsp	1.5
2 Tbsp (level), ¼ oz	3
¼ cup, (4 Tbsp), ½ oz	6.5
½ cup, 1 oz	13
Corn Germ: ¼ cup, 1 oz	5
Wheat Germ: ¼ cup, 1 oz	3
Psyllium Seed Husks, 2 Tbsp	8
Metamucil, 1 dose	3.4

Hot Cereals, Oatmeal

Bulgur (cracked Wheat), ckd, 1 cup	8
Cream of Wheat, ckd, ⅔ cup	1
Hominy Grits, dry, 3 Tbsp, 1 oz	1.2
Oatmeal (uncooked ⅓ cup), ckd, ⅔ cup	2.7

Fiber Guide

Breads & Crackers

	Fiber
Bread: White, 1 slice, 1 oz	0.7
Whole-wheat, 1 slice, 1 oz	1.5
Whole-grain, 1 slice, 1 oz	2
Rye, Pumpernickel, 1 oz	1.5
Bagel/Roll/Bun, 1 medium, 2 oz	1.5
Pita, whole wheat, 5" pocket	4.5
Crackers: Graham, average, 2	1.4
Saltine, 4 crackers	0.3
Crispbreads (Rye), average, 2	4
Matzo 1 board, 1 oz	1
Rice Cakes: Average, 1 cake	0.3
Tortilla: Regular, 6"	0.5
Whole-wheat, 6"	1.3

Barley, Pasta, Rice & Flours

Barley, pearled, raw, ¼ cup, 1.7 oz	5
Rice: White, cooked, 1 cup, 7 oz	1.6
Brown, cooked, 1 cup	3.2
Rice-A-Roni, average, 1 cup	1.5
Spaghetti/Noodles: cooked, 1 cup	2
Whole-grain, cooked, 1 cup	7
Amaranth *(Health Valley)*, 1 cup	9
Flour: Wheat, All-purpose, 1 cup, 4½ oz	3.5
Whole-grain, 1 cup, 4½ oz	15
Cornmeal, stone ground, 1 cup, 4½ oz	13
Carob Flour, 1 cup, 3½ oz	13
Rye Flour, 1 cup, 3½ oz	15
Soy Flour: Defatted, 1 cup, 3½ oz	17
Full-fat, raw, 1 cup, 3 oz	8
Soy Meal, defatted, 1 cup, 4½ oz	14

Frozen Entrees & Dinners

***Average All Brands:** Per Serving*	
Beans/Chili base, average	6-10
Potato/Pasta base, average	4-6
Vegetable base, average	3
Meat/Chicken base, average	2-3
Pizzas, ¼ large, average	3
Vegetarian Soy Burgers, 1 pattie	5

Soups

Chicken Noodle, 1 cup	0
Tomato Soup, average, 1 cup	0.5
Vegetable Soup, average, 1 cup	3
***Health Valley:** Per 1 Cup Serving*	
Black Bean; Minestrone	10
Tomato	4
5-Bean Vegetable; Lentil & Carrots	13
Mushroom & Barley; Split Pea; Vegetable	7
Rotini & Vegetables	4

Fast Foods & Restaurants

	Fiber
Hamburgers: Small, average	1.5
Large/Whopper, average	2.5
Hot Dog, Regular	1.5
French Fries: Small serving, 2½ oz	2.5
Regular/Medium, 3½ oz	3.5
Chicken Nuggets, 6 pack	0.5
Chicken Sandwich, average	2
Taco, average	4
Sundaes, Shakes, Soft Drinks	0
Arby's: Baked Potato w. Broc. & Cheddar	6
Roast Beef Sandwich, regular	2
Denny's: Grilled Chicken Caesar Salad, no bread	4
Classic Burger w. fries	4
Club Sandwich, no fries	2
Grilled Chicken Sandwich, no fries	4
***Domino's* (Classic):** Vegi Feast, 2 sl. (12")	2
Hawaiian Feast, 2 slices, (12")	2
Pepperoni Feast, 2 slices (12")	2
McDonald's: Big Mac; McChicken	4
Ham/Cheeseburger; Quarter Pounder	2
Egg McMuffin	2
Grilled Chicken Caesar Salad	3
McVeggie Burger	8
***Pizza Hut:** Per 2 Slices, Medium*	
Pan Pizza: Cheese, Pepperoni	2
Supreme	4
Thin 'n Crispy, Supreme	4
Hand-Tossed, average	4
Personal Pan Pizza, 1 whole	5
Subway: Sandwich, white roll, avg.	4
w. Honey Wheat Roll, average	3.2
Footlong w. Wheat Roll, average	8
Salads, average	3

Cakes, Cookies, Snack Bars

Apple/Fruit Pie, 1 serving	2
Cake: w. plain flour, 1 serving	1
w. whole-wheat flour, 1 serving	3
Carrot Cake, 1 serving	2
Cookies, oatmeal, (3 small/1 large)	3
Donuts	0
Fruit Cake, 1 serving	3
Fig Bars, 2	1.3
Muffins, Oat Bran (2 small, 1 large), 4 oz	5
Granola Bars, average, 1 bar	2
Atkins Advantage Bars, average	9
Cliff Bars, 1.7 oz	5
Fi-Bar Nectar, 1 bar	4
Health Valley: Fruit/Granola Bars	4
Cereal Bars	7
Luna Bars, 1.7 oz	3

Chocolate, Chips, Popcorn	Fiber
Cheese Balls/Curls/Twists	0
Chocolate, Hard Candy, Cheese Balls	0
Chocolate with nuts/fruit, 2 oz bar	1
Mars Bar	1
Potato Chips, corn chips, 1 oz	1
Popcorn, 3 cups	2
Pretzels, Twists, 6	1
Nuts, Seeds	
Almonds: Natural, 25 kernels, 1 oz	4
Blanched (skins removed), 1 oz	3
Cashews, Filberts, Pecans, 1 oz	1.7
Peanuts, Mixed Nuts, Coconut, 1 oz	2.5
Peanut Butter, 2 Tbsp, 1 oz	1.8
Pistachio Nuts, dried, shelled, 1 oz	3
Walnuts, Black/English, dried, 1 oz	1.5
Seeds: Amaranth, 2½ Tbsp, 1 oz	3.5
Flax Seeds, 3 Tbsp, 1 oz	7
Psyllium Seed Husks, 5 Tbsp, 1 oz	20
Quinoa Seeds, 3 Tbsp, 1 oz	2.7
Sesame Seeds, whole, 1 oz	3
Sesame Butter/Tahini, 2 Tbsp, 1.1 oz	3
Sunflower kernels, ¼ cup, 1 oz	4.4
Teff Seeds, 1 oz	3.8
Fruit – Fresh	
Apples: 1 medium, 6 oz (whole)	
with skin + core	5.5
with skin, no core	4.5
without skin, no core	3.7
Apricots, 2 medium, 4 oz	2
Avocado, average, ½ medium	3
Banana, 1 medium, 6 oz (w. skin)	2
Blueberries, raw, ½ cup, 5 oz	4.4
Cherries, sweet, raw, 10 fruits, 2½ oz	1.5
Grapefruit, average, ½ fruit, 8½ oz	1
Grapes, 1 medium bunch, seedless, 7 oz	3
Kiwifruit, 1 medium, 3 oz	3
Mango, 1 medium, 11 oz (whole)	1.6
Melons, cantaloup, 4 oz (edible)	1
Nectarine, 1 medium, 4 oz	1.8
Olives, average all types, 7 jumbo, 2 oz	1.5
Oranges, 1 medium (7-8 oz w. skin)	
5½ oz (peeled)	3.8
Passionfruit, 2 medium, 2½ oz	5
Peaches, 1 large, 6 oz	2
Pears, raw, 1 medium, 6 oz	4.5
Pineapple, 1 slice, 3 oz	1.8
Plums, 2 medium, 6 oz	2.8
Strawberries, 6 medium/3 large, 2 oz	1.5
Watermelon, 4 oz (edible)	0.5

Fruit – Dried, Juice	Fiber
Dried Fruit: Apricots, 8 halves, 1 oz	2.2
Dates (3 med); Raisins (2 Tbsp), 1 oz	1.5
Figs, 3 medium, 1½ oz	5
Prunes, 4 medium, 1 oz	2
Fruit Juice: Orange/Apple etc, 1 glass	<0.5
Prune Juice, 5 oz	1.4
Carrot Juice, 8 oz	1.8
Vegetables	
Asparagus, 4 spears	2
Bean Sprouts, ½ cup, 2¼ oz	1.5
Beans: Snap/Green, ½ cup, 2½ oz	2
Baked Beans in Tom Sce, ½ c, 4½ oz	10
Dried Beans, ckd, average, ½ cup	7
Beets, ckd, slices, ½ cup, 3 oz	1.5
Broccoli, cooked, ½ cup, 3 oz	2.2
Brussels Sprouts, ckd, ½ cup, 3 oz	3.5
Cabbage: White, ckd, ½ cup, 2½ oz	1
Red, ckd, ½ cup, 2½ oz	2
Carrots, 1 medium (7½"), ½ cup, 3 oz	2.7
Cauliflower, cooked, ½ cup, 3 oz	2.8
Celery, raw, diced, ½ cup, 2½ oz	1
Chick Peas (Garbanzos), ckd, ½ c., 3½ oz	6
Corn, kernels, ckd, ½ cup, 2½ oz	2.5
Cream-style, ½ cup, 4½ oz	1.5
Cucumber/Lettuce/Mushrooms, 2 oz	0.5
Eggplant, raw, sliced, ½ cup	2.5
Lentils, cooked, ½ cup, 3½ oz	4
Onions, 1 medium, 4 oz	2
Spring Onions, chop., ¼ cup, 1 oz	1.5
Peas: Green, ½ cup, 3 oz	3
Cowpeas (Black-eyed), ckd, ½ cup	10
Split Peas, ckd, ½ cup, 4½ oz	6.5
Peppers, sweet, raw, 1 large, 3½ oz	1.5
Potatoes: 1 medium, with skin, 5 oz	4
without skin	2
½ cup mashed, 3½ oz	1.5
French Fries, 3 oz serving	3
Spinach, cooked, ½ cup, 3 oz	2
Squash: Summer, cookd, 3 oz	1.2
Winter, cooked, 3 oz	2.4
Tomatoes: 1 medium, 5 oz	2
Tomato Sauce, 1 cup	0.3
Frozen: Mixed Vegetables, ckd, ½ cup	3
Soybean Products: Miso, ½ c., 5 oz	7.7
Tempeh, 1 piece, 3 oz	2
Tofu, 4 oz	1.4
Salads: Side Salad, average	1
Bean Salad, ½ cup	5
Coleslaw, ½ cup	1
Potato Salad, ½ cup	2

Protein Guide

General Notes

- **Protein has many important body functions.** It builds and repairs muscle, and is the basis of our body's organs, hormones, enzymes, and antibodies to fight infection.
- **Protein is also an emergency fuel** in the absence of sufficient carbohydrate and fats. For this reason, weight loss should be gradual so as to preserve protein levels in muscle, the heart and other body organs.
- **It is easy to obtain sufficient protein,** even if vegetarian. **Plant proteins are not inferior to animal proteins.** In fact, eating more soy and other plant proteins, and less animal protein, may help to build stronger bones and prevent osteoporosis; and may help to control blood cholesterol levels.
- **When changing to a vegetarian diet,** include soybeans, and other dried beans, soy milk drinks (calcium-enriched), lentils, tofu, tempeh, nuts, and wholegrain breads and cereals. Milk, yogurt, cheese and eggs may enhance nutrient intake.

Protein & Muscle

- Although muscles are built of protein, protein is not a special fuel for working muscle cells - carbohydrates and fats are.
- In fact, a diet high in protein (and fat) and low in carbohydrate, can significantly reduce the performance of endurance sports athletes. **Carbohydrate** is the best fuel for muscles exercised for long periods.
- Any **extra protein** required by athletes and body-builders, can easily be obtained from the extra food eaten to satisfy hunger and energy needs - even allowing an excessive 120g protein daily for a 170 lb athlete (0.7g/lb body wt; twice the RDI).
- Remember, **excess protein** in food will not build bigger muscles. Any excess is converted and stored as fat. Excess protein can also strain the kidneys which excrete the waste products of protein metabolism.

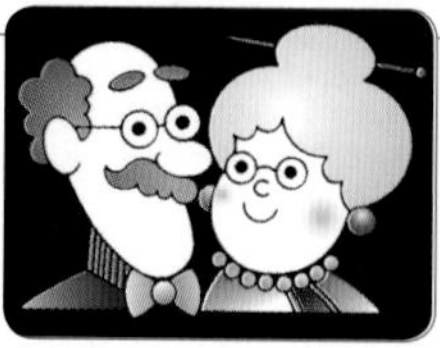

Elderly people (and dieters) must eat sufficient food to ensure adequate protein intake.

Inadequate protein leads to a drop in immune response with greater susceptibility to illness and infections. Muscle strength and muscle mass also drop.

Protein needs are easily met with sensible eating. Athletes who eat enough food for their energy needs, can obtain sufficient protein.

PROTEIN

RECOMMENDED DAILY INTAKE (Grams)

(Figure in brackets - Recommended amount of protein per lb of ideal body weight.)

		Pro	
Infants:	0-6 mths	**9-13g**	(1g/lb)
	6-12 mths	**14g**	(0.7g/lb)
Children:	1-3 yrs	**13g**	(0.6g/lb)
	4-8 yrs	**19g**	(0.5g/lb)
	9-13	**34g**	(0.5g/lb)
Males:	14-18	**52g**	(0.4g/lb)
	19+	**56g**	(0.36g/lb)
Females:	14+	**46g**	(0.36g/lb)
Pregnancy:		**71g**	
Breastfeeding:		**71g**	

Note: Above figures allow for a large safety margin for most persons.

Iron & Anemia Guide

- **Iron deficiency** is one of the most common nutritional deficiencies in women. The risk is increased in dieters who do not eat well-balanced meals. Chronic shortage of iron leads to anemia.
- **Women** between 11 and 50 years of age are at greater risk because of the monthly loss of menstrual blood. Pregnancy, growth, and endurance sports also demand extra iron.
- **In red blood cells,** iron combines with protein to form **hemoglobin** - the red pigment which carries oxygen in the blood. A lack of iron limits the production of hemoglobin and hence the amount of vital oxygen delivered to body cells.

Note: A blood test will tell you if your Hb and Iron stores (ferritin) are adequate. (Iron stores can be low even when Hb is normal.)

- **Vitamin C** (in fruits/veges/salads) enhances absorption of 'non-heme' iron in bread, cereals, milk, vegetables, nuts, eggs and iron supplements. Small amounts of meat, fish or poultry also help. (They contain 'heme' iron).
- **Iron absorption is lessened** by up to 60% when high calcium foods are consumed with iron-rich main meals. Tea, coffee, phytates (in bran) and oxalates lessen absorption of non-heme iron.
- **For infants to 1 year,** use iron-fortified milk/ soy formula if not breast-feeding. Introduce iron-fortified baby cereals at 4-6 mths.

Note: Iron deficiency in children (even without anemia), can result in lethargy, irritability, repeated infections, and developmental problems.

Iron Supplements

- **Most people** can obtain adequate iron from their diet. **A wide variety** of animal and plant foods contain iron. (See Iron Counter)
- **Iron supplements** are only recommended for women with heavy menstrual blood losses, during pregnancy (if tests show a low-iron status), endurance athletes with low blood ferritin (iron stores) and for persons with diagnosed anemia. Check with your doctor.
- While the 5 mg of iron in multi-vitamin/mineral supplements is safe for most people, large amounts can be toxic, (especially in persons with hemochromatosis iron-overload condition).

ANEMIA SYMPTOMS

Anemia reduces the amount of oxygen carried in the blood.
The body tissues become starved of oxygen. Symptoms include:

- **Pale skin; brittle finger nails (may turn up into spoon shape).**
- **Excessive tiredness or fatigue**
- **Breathlessness**
- **Feeling of malaise and irritability.**
- **Always feel cold.**
- **Decrease in attention span.**

Note: Other medical conditions may also cause similar symptoms. Check with your doctor.

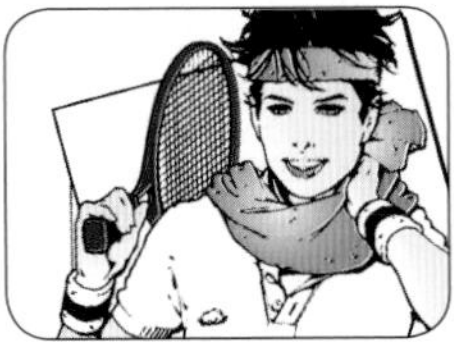

A nutritious diet with adequate iron is important - particularly for women and athletes.

RECOMMENDED DAILY IRON INTAKE (mg)

			Iron
Infants (0-6 mths):			
	Breastfed	~	**0.5mg**
	Bottlefed	~	**3mg**
	6-12 mths	~	**9mg**
Children:	1-11 yrs	~	**6-8mg**
Males:	12-18 yrs	~	**10-13mg**
	19+ yrs	~	**7mg**
Females:	12-50yrs	~	**12-16mg**
	51+ yrs	~	**5-7mg**
	Pregnancy	~	**22-36mg**
	Breastfeeding	~	**12-16mg**

Protein & Iron Counter

Pro ~ Protein (grams) **Iron** ~ Iron (mg)

Meat

	Pro	Iron
Steak: Average all cuts, lean (no fat)		
Small (4 oz raw/3 oz ckd)	23	2.3
Medium (6 oz raw/4¼ oz ckd)	34	3.4
Large (10 oz raw/7¼ oz ckd)	57	5.7
Roast Beef: lean, 2 slices, 3 oz	24	2.5
Ground Beef patty, lean, ckd, 3 oz	21	2
Lamb chop, broiled, 3 oz	22	1.5
Liver, cooked, 3 oz	23	5.5
Veal cutlet, 1 medium	23	1
Pork, cooked, lean, 3 oz	24	1
Bacon, 3 medium slices	6	0.3
Ham, roasted, 2 pieces, 3 oz	18	1
Ham, luncheon, 2 slices, 1½ oz	7	0.3
Pastrami (Oscar Mayer), 3 sl., 1¾ oz	10	1.3
Sausages: Bologna, 2 sl., 2 oz	7	1
Braunschweiger, 2 sl., 2 oz	8	5.3
Pork link, thick, 2 oz	6	0.4
Frankfurter, 1⅓ oz	5	0.5
Salami, hard, 3 slices, 1 oz	7	0.5
Vegetarian (BocaBurger), 1 pattie	13	2

Chicken/Turkey

	Pro	Iron
Chicken, ckd; Breast portion, 3 oz	27	1
Leg/Thigh, lean, 3 oz	24	1
½ Whole Chicken	60	2.5
Drumstick, 1 medium, 3 oz	12	0.6
Turkey, cooked, Light meat, 3 oz	24	2
Dark meat, lean, 3 oz	24	2

Fish

	Pro	Iron
Finfish: Per 4 oz, cooked		
Cod, Flounder/Sole, Pollock	28	0.5
Catfish, Haddock, Halibut, M/Mahi	28	1.3
Ocean Perch, Swordf., Orange Roughy	28	1.3
Canned Fish: Tuna, Light, 3 oz	25	1.5
White, 3 oz	23	0.5
Salmon, pink, 3 oz	17	0.7
Salmon, red, 3 oz	17	1
Sardines, 3 whole (3"), 1¼ oz	9	1
Anchovies, 1 can, 1½ oz	13	2
Shellfish: Crabmeat, 3 oz	17.5	0.7
Clams, raw, 4 large/9 sml, 3 oz	11	12
Crayfish, cooked, 3 oz	20	2.7
Lobster, cooked, 3 oz	17	0.5
Oysters, raw, 6 medium, 3 oz	7	5
Scallops, 2 lge/5 small, 1 oz	5	0.1
Shrimp, raw 6 large, 1½ oz	8.5	1
Fish Products: Fish Sticks, 4 sticks	10	0.5
Fish Portions, in batter, 4 oz	13	0.6
Gefilte Fish, 1 medium ball, 2 oz	8	1

Eggs

	Pro	Iron
1 Large Egg, whole	6	0.7
Egg Yolk	3	0.7
Egg White	3	0
Omelet: Plain, 2 eggs	13	1.7
Ham & cheese	17	3
Egg Substitutes (liquid):		
Eggbeaters, 1 egg equiv.	4.5	1
Scramblers, ¼ cup, 2 oz	6	0.7

Milk, Yogurt, Icecream

	Pro	Iron
Milk: Whole/Lowfat/Skim, 8 fl.oz cup	8	0.1
Protein Enriched, 1 cup	10	0.1
Carb Countdown (2% or Fat Free)	12	0
Chocolate Milk, 1 cup	8	0.6
Thick Shake, Chocolate, 10 oz	9	1
Vanilla, 10 oz	11	0.3
Soymilk (fortified), average, 1 cup	7	1
Yogurt: Plain, 6 oz	10	0.1
Fruit flavors: 6 oz	8	0.3
8 oz	11	0.5
Ice-Cream: Rich, ½ cup	2	0
Regular, Vanilla, ½ cup	2.5	0
Sherbet, ½ cup	1	0
Custard, baked, ½ cup	7	0.5

Cheese

	Pro	Iron
Hard Cheeses, average, 1 oz	7	0.2
4 oz piece	28	0.8
Cottage Cheese, ½ cup	13	0.3
Ricotta, part skim, ½ cup	14	1

Bread, Bagels, Biscuits

	Pro	Iron
Bread (w. enriched flour): 1 slice, 1 oz	2	1
4 slices, 4 oz	8	4
4 thick slices, 6 oz	1.2	6
Bagel, plain 2 oz	6	1.5
Biscuits, 1 oz	2	0.7
Pita Bread, 1 pita, 1½ oz	4	1
Pumpernickel, 1 slice, 1 oz	3	1

Infant/Baby Foods

	Pro	Iron
Infant Formula Milk:		
Enfamil/Gerber/Similac, 5 fl.oz		
Regular/Low Iron	2.2	0.2
With Iron	2.2	1.8
Isomil/Nursoy/ProSobee	3	1.8
Baby Cereals: Average All Brands		
Dry, 4 Tbsp, ½ oz	1	7
Jars (w. fruit), 4½ oz	1	7

Breakfast Cereals

	Pro	Iron
Hot Type, cooked:		
Bulgur, cooked, 1 cup, 5 oz	9	2
Oatmeal: Reg., non-fortified, 1 cup	6	1.5
Instant, fortified, average, 1 pkt	4	8
Quaker, all flavors, ½ cup	5	18
Total, all types, 1 pkt	4	18
Corn/Hominy Grits: Reg., 1 cup	3	1.5
Quaker: Reg., 3 Tbsp, 1 oz	2	0.8
Instant White, 1 packet	2	8
Cream of Wheat, 1 cup	4	10
Ready-To-Eat: *Per 1 oz Serving Unless Shown*		
Arrowhead: Average, all varieties	3	1
General Mills: Basic 4, 1 cup, 2 oz	4	3.8
Cheerios, regular, 1 cup, 1 oz	3	6.8
Cocoa Puffs, 1 cup, 1 oz	1	3.8
Kix, 1⅓ cups, 1 oz	2	6.8
Multi-Bran Chex, 1 cup, 2 oz	4	16
Total Corn Flakes, 1⅓ cups, 1 oz	2	6.8
Total Raisin Bran, 1 cup, 2 oz	4	18
Wheaties Energy Crunch, 1 cup, 1.95 oz	6	18
Health Valley: Oat Bran O's, ¾ cup	3	0.9
Amaranth Flakes, ¾ cup	3	0.6
Bran Cereal w. Raisins, ¾ cup	5	1.5
98% Fat Free Granola, ⅔ cup	5	1.2
Real Oat Bran, ½ cup	6	0.6
Golden Flax, ¼ cup	6	1.2
Kashi GoLean: ¾ cup, 1.5 oz	8	1.5
Crunch!, 1 cup, 1.9 oz	9	1.8
Seven in the Morning, ½ cup	7	1.5
Kellogg's: All Bran, ½ cup	4	4.5
Complete Oatbran Flakes, ¾ cup	3	8.5
Cocoa Krispies, ¾ cup	2	1.8
Corn Flakes, 1 cup	2	8.4
Just Right, 1 cup	4	16
Nutrigrain, 1¼ cup	4	1.4
Product 19, 1 cup, 1 oz	2	18
Raisin Bran, 1 cup, 2 oz	6	4.5
Rice Krispies, 1¼ cup	2	1.8
Special K: Regular, 1 cup, 1.1 oz	6	8
Low Carb, ¾ cup, 1 oz	10	8
Post: Raisin Bran, ½ cup, 1 oz	3	4.5
Grape Nuts, ½ cup, 1 oz	3	1
Quaker: Crunchy Corn Bran, 1 cup, 1 oz	2	8
100% Natural Granola, ½ cup	3	1
Life, ¼ cup, 1 oz	3	4.5
Puffed Rice/Wheat, 1 cup, ½ oz	1	0.5
Shreaded Wheat, 3 biscuits	4	1

Brans & Wheatgerm

	Pro	Iron
Oat Bran, raw, 1 Tbsp	2	0.5
Rice Bran, raw, 2 Tbsp	1	1
Wheat Bran, unprocessed, 2 Tbsp	1	1
Wheat Germ, 2 Tbsp, ½ oz	4	1.3

Grains & Flours

	Pro	Iron
Amaranth, 1 cup, ½ oz	10	3
Barley, ½ cup, 3½ oz	8	2
Buckwheat Flour: Dark, 1 cup	11.5	2.7
Light, 1 cup	6	1
Carob Flour, 1 cup	5	3
Corn Flour, 1 cup, 4 oz	9	2
Corn Meal, enriched, 1 cup	11	3.5
Flour: White, enriched, 1 cup, 4½ oz	13	6
Wholegrain, 1 cup, 4¼ oz	16	5
Millet, wholegrain, 1 cup, 3½ oz	10	7
Rye Flour: Dark, 1 cup, 4½ oz	21	6
Light, 1 cup, 3½ oz	10	1
Soy Flour, full fat, 1 cup, 3 oz	32	5.5
Yeast: Brewer's, dry, 1 Tbsp	3	1.5

Rice, Spaghetti

	Pro	Iron
Rice: Brown/White, average		
1 cup cooked, 6½ oz	5	1
Spaghetti/Macaroni/Noodles (enriched):		
Cooked, 1 cup, 4½ oz	7	2
Canned: in Tomato Sauce, ½ cup	2	0.5
w. Meatballs, 1 cup, 8 oz	9	2

Soups

	Pro	Iron
With Noodles/Vegetables, 1 cup	3	0.5
With Meat/Beans/Peas, 1 cup	8	1.5

Fruit

	Pro	Iron
Fresh/Canned: Average, all types, 1 serving		
1 medium/2 small fruit	1	0.5
Avocado, ½ medium	2	1
Dried Fruit: Apricots, 8 halves, 1 oz	1	1.3
Dates, 6 dates, 2 oz	1.5	0.7
Figs, 4 medium figs, 2 oz	2	1.7
Prunes, 5 medium, 1½ oz	1	1
Raisins, 1 oz	1	0.7
Fruit Juice: Average, 1 cup	0.5	0.5
Prune Juice, 6 fl.oz	1	2.5
Tomato Juice, 6 fl.oz	0.5	1

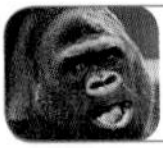

King Kong was a vegetarian!

Protein & Iron Counter

Vegetables	Pro	Iron
Beans: Snap/green, ½ cup	1	0.8
Dried: Average all types, cooked, ½ cup	7	2.5
Baked Beans, ½ cup 4½ oz	5	2
Bean Sprouts, mung, 1 cup	3	1
Broccoli, ¾ cup pieces, 4 oz	4	1.4
Cabbage; Cauliflower, 1 cup	1	0.6
Corn, ½ cup kernels, 3 oz	2.5	0.3
1 ear trimmed to 3½"	2	0.4
Lentils, cooked, ½ cup, 3½ oz	9	3.3
Mushrooms, raw, ½ cup, sliced	0.5	0.5
Peas: Green, ½ cup, 3 oz	4	1.2
Split Peas, cooked, 1 cup	16	2.5
Potatoes, cooked:		
1 medium, with skin, 5 oz	3.3	2
without skin, 4 oz	2.3	1
French Fries, 3 oz	3	1
Potato Salad, ½ cup	3.5	2.5
Pumpkin, ½ cup mashed	1	2.5
Seaweed, kelp, 1 oz	<1	2.5
Spinach, cooked, ½ cup, 3 oz	2.7	2.5
Squash, ckd, all types, ½ cup	1	0.3
Tomatoes, 1 medium, 4½ oz	1	0.6
Vegetables, mixed, ckd, 1 cup	2.5	0.7
Soybeans, cooked, ½ cup, 3 oz	14	4.4
Tofu, Tempeh, Miso		
Tofu, raw, firm, ½ cup, 4½ oz	10	1.5
Tempeh, ½ cup, 3 oz	16	2
Miso, ½ cup, 5 oz	16	4
Miso Soup, 1 cup	3	0.4
Soybean Protein (TVP), 1 oz	18	3
Cakes, Pastries, Pies		
(Made with enriched flour)		
Carrot w. cream cheese frosting, 4 oz	4	1.3
Cheesecake, 1 piece, 3½ oz	5	0.5
Chocolate, 1 piece, 2 oz	2	2
Fruitcake, 1 piece, 1½ oz	2	1.2
Plain, 1 piece, 3 oz	4	1.2
Croissant, plain, 2 oz	5	2
Danish Pastry, 1 pastry, 2¼ oz	4	1.3
Donuts, average, 2 oz	4	1.2
Muffins, average, 1 medium, 1½ oz	3	1
Pancakes, 4" diam., two, 2 oz	4	1
Pies: Fruit, 1 piece, 5½ oz	4	1.5
Pecan, 1 piece, 5 oz	7	4.5
Puddings, average, ½ cup, 4½ oz	4	0.3
Waffles, 1 large, 2½ oz	7	1.5

Sugar, Honey, Jam	Pro	Iron
Sugar: White	0	0
Brown, 1 Tbsp	0	0.3
Molasses: Light/Medium, 1 Tbsp	0	1
Blackstrap, 1 Tbsp, ¾ oz	0	3
Corn Syrup, 1 Tbsp, ¾ oz	0	1
Honey, Jams, Jelly	0	0.2
Candy, Chocolate, Carob		
Candy, sugar-based	0	0
Chocolate: Plain, 2 oz bar	4	0.8
with nuts, 2 oz bar	6	0.8
Carob, plain, 2 oz	6	0.7
Cookies, Crackers, Chips		
Cookies, average, 4 cookies	2	1
Crackers, Graham, 2½" sq., (2)	1	0
Rice Cakes, average, one	1	0
Corn/Potato Chips, 1 oz	2	0.3
Nuts: Almonds, shelled, 20-25 nuts	6	1
Brazil Nuts, 7-8 medium nuts, 1 oz	4	1
Cashews, 12-16 nuts, 1 oz	5	1.5
Macadamias, 1 oz	2	0.5
Peanuts, dry roasted, 40 nuts, 1 oz	6	0.5
Pecans, 24 halves, 1 oz	2	0.5
Walnuts, 15 halves, 1 oz	4	0.7
Peanut Butter, 1 Tbsp	1	0.5
Seeds: Sesame Seeds, dry, 1 Tbsp	2	0.6
Pumpkin Kernels, dry, hulled, 1 oz	7	4.2
Sunflower Seeds, dried, hulled, 1 oz	6	2
Tahini, 1 Tbsp, ½ oz	2.5	1.4
Granola & Food/Protein Bars		
Granola Bars, average, 1 bar, 2 oz	2	0.5
Atkins Advantage Bar	20	1
Balance Oasis Bars 1.76 oz	14	4.5
Bariatrix Proti-Bars, 1	15	3.6
Carb Sense Bar	30	2
Choice dm Bar, 1.23 oz	6	3.6
Dr Soy Protein Bars, 1.76 oz	11	18
Ensure Nutrition Energy Bar	9	3.6
Genisoy	14	4.5
Jenny Craig Bars, 1.97 oz	10	3.6
Met-Rx "Big 100", 100g	27	7.2
Planters Peanut Bar, 1.6 oz	7	0.7
Post Carb Well Bar	10	1
PowerBar, 1 bar, 2.3 oz	10	6.3
Slim-Fast Bar, 34g	8	2.7
Source One Bar, 2.2 oz	15	4.5
Twin Lab Protein Fuel, 3 oz	35	4.5
High Energy Bars, 2 oz	15	1.5

Nutritional & High Protein Drinks

	Pro	Iron
Atkins Shakes, 11 fl.oz can	20	**2.7**
Bariatrix Shakes, dry, 1 oz	15	**3.6**
Very High Protein, 1 pkt	35	**6.3**
Boost Ready To Drink, 8 oz can	15	**4.5**
Carnation Instant Breakfast, 10 oz	13	**4.5**
Curves Protein Drink, 2 scoops	15	**18**
Ensure High Protein, 8 oz can	12	**2.3**
GeniSoy Shake, 1 scoop, 35g	14	**3.6**
Kashi GoLean Shake (RTD), 11 oz can	15	**2.7**
Kindercal, 8 fl.oz	7	**2.5**
Met-Rx Protein Shake, 11 oz	35	**4.5**
Myoplex (EAS), Nutrition Shake, 1 pkt	42	**5.4**
Nature's Best, Protein Shake, 1 scoop	22	**3.6**
Optifast 800, made-up, 8 oz	14	**3.6**
Resource (Novartis) Standard, 8 fl.oz	9	**4.5**
Revival Soy, Plain, 58g pkt	20	**3**
Slim-Fast Shakes 325 ml can	10	**3.6**
Ultra Slim-Fast, 1 can	7	**6.3**
Usana Nutrimeal Mix, 2 scoops, 1½ oz	12	**6**
Walgreens Slim For Less, 11 oz can	10	**2.7**
Weider Muscle Builder, 2 scoops	17	**5**

Coffee, Tea, Soda

	Pro	Iron
Coffee, Coffee Substitutes, 1 cup	0	**0.1**
Tea (all types); Soft Drinks/Soda	0	**0**
Hot Chocolate, 6 fl.oz	2	**2.2**

Beer, Wine, Spirits

	Pro	Iron
Beer, 12 fl.oz	1	**0**
Wines, red/white, 1 glass	0	**0.4**
Spirits/Liquor	0	**0**

Fast-Foods/Burgers

For extra listings ~ see CalorieKing.com

	Pro	Iron
Pancakes: Average all outlets, 3	8	**2**
Shakes, Chocolate	12	**0.4**
Sundaes: Average all outlets	7	**0.3**
Arby's: Roast Beef Sandwich, reg.	21	**4**
Giant Roast Beef S/wich	32	**6**
Roast Chicken Club	27	**3**
Burger King: Whopper S/wich	30	**2.5**
Hamburger	17	**1.5**
Bacon Double Cheeseburger	35	**2.5**
BK Fish Sandwich	18	**2**
Carl's Jr: Famous Star Hamburger	24	**2**
Ranch Crispy Chicken	24	**2**
Super Star Hamburger	41	**3**
Charbroiled Chicken Club Sandwich	31	**2**

Fast Foods/Burgers (Cont)

	Pro	Iron
Domino's Pizza: Deep Dish (12"), 2 sl.		
Cheese, 2 slices	42	**4**
Pepperoni, Sausage, Ham	41	**4**
X-tra Cheese & Pepperoni	50	**4.5**
KFC: Original, Wing & Breast	51	**0.4**
3-Pce. Dinner, Original	72	**0.6**
Crispy Strips, 3	29	**0.4**
Original Recipe Sandwich	29	**1.5**
McDonald's: Big Mac	25	**4**
Cheeseburger	15	**3**
Chicken McNuggets (6)	15	**1**
Crispy Chicken Burger	22	**3**
Filet-O-Fish	15	**2**
Grilled Chicken Caesar Salad	29	**2**
Hamburger	12	**3**
Quarter Pounder w. Cheese	29	**5**
French Fries: Small, 2.4 oz	3	**0.4**
Large, 6 oz	8	**1**
Breakfast: Egg McMuffin	18	**3**
Bacon, Egg & Cheese McGriddles	19	**2**
Ham, Egg & Cheese Bagel	26	**4**
Sausage McMuffin w. Egg	20	**3**
Pizza Hut: *Per Medium, 2 slices*		
Pan Pizzas, average	26	**4**
Thin 'n Crispy, Supreme	22	**2**
Hand Tossed, Pepperoni	24	**3**
Personal Pan Pizza, Meat	35	**4**
Subway (6" Subs): Average	20	**2**
Meatball	25	**6**
Roast Chicken Breast	24	**3.5**
Steak & Cheese, 6"	23	**6**
Subway Club	22	**3.5**
Taco Bell: Bean Burrito	14	**3.5**
Beef Burrito Supreme	18	**3.5**
Tostado	10	**1.5**
Chicken/Steak Enchirito	16	**3**
Taco Supreme	10	**2**
Gordita Baja Beef	14	**2.5**
Chicken Quesadilla	28	**4**
Wendy's: Single Sandwich w. Everything	25	**3**
Big Bacon Classic Sandwich	33	**3**
Jr Hamburger Kid's Meal	15	**2**
Homestyle Chicken Sandwich	29	**4**

High Blood Pressure

Many American adults have hypertension (high blood pressure), and are unaware of it. It is generally symptomless, so **have your blood pressure checked annually** - particularly if it runs in the family.

Untreated hypertension overworks the heart, damages arteries and promotes atherosclerosis. This in turn greatly increases the risk of heart disease, stroke, blindness, kidney disease and impotence. The earlier hypertension is detected, the sooner it can be brought under control.

BLOOD PRESSURE CLASSIFICATIONS

National High Blood Pressure Educ. Prog. (2003)

	DIASTOLIC		SYSTOLIC
Normal	Below 80	and	**Below 120**
Prehypertension	80-89	or	**120-139**
Stage 1	90-99	or	**140-159**
Stage 2	100 or more	or	**160 or more**

Treating Hypertension

Prehypertension (in the chart above) means you don't have high blood pressure now but are likely to develop it in the future.

You can take steps to prevent it with healthy lifestyle habits: reducing sodium intake, eating adequate fruit and vegetables, losing weight if overweight, limiting alcohol to 2 drinks or less daily, quitting smoking, exercising regularly, and managing stress.

Stage 1 hypertension can often be treated with the above lifestyle changes.

Stage 2 hypertension usually requires drug therapy. However, salt restriction, abstaining from alcohol and the above lifestyle changes will improve the success of drug therapy, and enable smaller drug doses to be prescribed.

HYPERTENSION DAMAGES ARTERIES & PROMOTES ATHEROSCLEROSIS

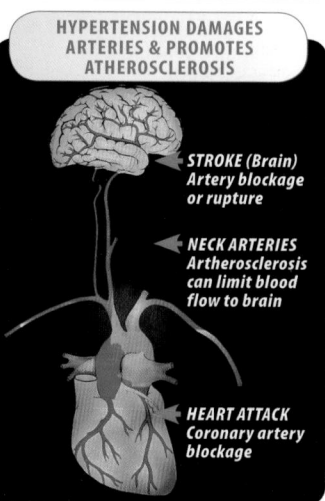

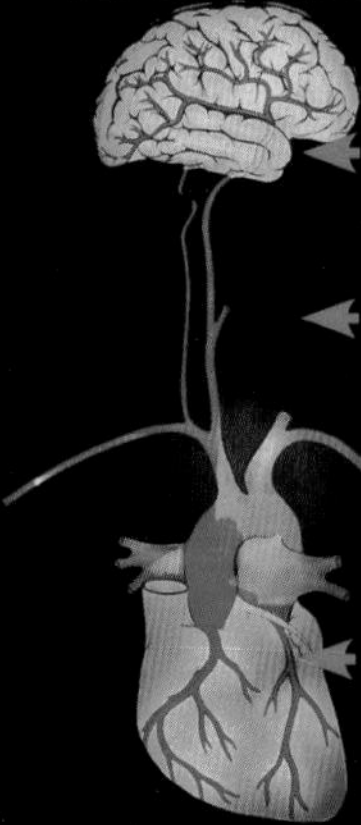

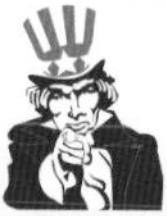

STROKE

KNOW THE WARNING SIGNS!

If you notice one or more of these signs, **call your doctor immediately**. They may be signalling a possible stroke or transient ischemic attack:

- **Sudden weakness** or numbness in your face, arm or leg on one side of your body.
- **Sudden dimness**, blurring or loss of vision, particularly in one eye.
- **Loss of speech**, or trouble talking or understanding speech.
- **Sudden severe headache** - 'a bolt out of the blue' - with no apparent cause.
- **Unexplained dizziness**, unsteadiness or a sudden fall, especially if accompanied by any of the other symptoms.

Salt & Sodium

- **Sodium is a mineral element** most commonly found in salt (sodium chloride). It also occurs naturally in much smaller amounts in animal and plant foods, and water - normally sufficient for our needs without having to add salt.
- **Sodium is required** for nerve and muscle function as well as to balance the amount of fluid in our tissues and blood.

  Sodium acts like a sponge to attract and hold fluids in body tissues.
- **Excess sodium** can cause water retention, and increase the risk of developing hypertension. Very high salt intake may also increase the risk of stomach cancer.
- **Too little sodium** may cause low blood pressure (hypotension), and decrease blood flow to the heart, brain and kidneys - especially during exercise. (A certain blood volume is required to sustain the blood pressure needed for adequate blood flow in the capillaries).

Salt-Sensitive Persons

- **Normally, our kidneys** excrete excess dietary sodium. The thirst we feel after a salty meal is the body calling for water to dilute the sodium, and enable the kidneys to flush out excess sodium.
- **However, 'salt - sensitive'** persons (up to 50% of adults) tend to retain excess sodium (above approximately 3000mg daily) instead of excreting it. Such persons are more likely to develop hypertension and would most benefit from sodium restriction. Assume you are susceptible if there is a family history of hypertension.
- **Although not everyone will benefit, all Americans are being asked to moderate their salt and sodium intake** as a public health measure - particularly that so many do not know whether or not they have hypertension; and also because we do not know just who is salt-sensitive.

Safe Sodium Levels

The American Heart Association recommends a **maximum sodium intake of 2400mg per day** for adults with normal blood pressure. However, people who consume less than 1500mg sodium have the lowest blood pressure levels.

Persons with hypertension and kidney ailments are usually restricted to as little as **1000mg sodium per day**. Your doctor will discuss the correct sodium level for you.

Persons engaged in prolonged strenuous work or exercise may lose sodium through heavy sweating - especially in hot, humid weather. Adequate salt (and fluids) is necessary to avoid dehydration. A little extra salt at mealtimes is usually sufficient to satisfy any extra need. Do not take salt tablets.

Finding Hidden Sodium

On average, **less than one third of our sodium intake comes from the salt shaker.** The rest is hidden in processed foods that have salt added during manufacture.

Sodium compounds added to food or medicinals can also contribute significant sodium.

Sodium bicarbonate in particular is widely used in antacid tablets and powders, and saline drink powders (such as Alka Seltzer). Sodium bicarbonate contains 27% sodium by weight. Each gram contributes 270mg sodium. Large amounts of sodium can be unwittingly consumed – up to 600mg per tablet.
(See Antacids ~ Page 294)

Other sodium compounds include mono-sodium glutamate (MSG), sodium ascorbate, sodium nitrite, and sodium citrate.

Alcohol Danger

Excessive alcohol intake contributes to hypertension. Susceptible persons should limit alcohol intake to 1-2 drinks per day.

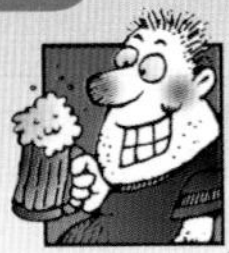

Salt Sodium Guide

Sodium accounts for only 40% of the weight of salt (sodium chloride). Examples:
1 gram (1000mg) Salt has 400mg Sodium
1 teaspoon (5g) Salt has 2000mg Sodium

Hints to Reduce Sodium

- **Watch the salt shaker.** Start with an easy 50% cut in sodium by using Lite Salt (*Morton*) or *Cardia* Salt. Then gradually cut back until you can leave the salt shaker off the table.
- **Taste your food before salting.** Use the pepper shaker (small holes) for more controlled sprinkling of salt.
- **Choose low sodium,** sodium free, and reduced sodium products in place of regular salted products.
- **Check labels for sodium levels.** The following sodium descriptors may appear on labels:
  Reduced Sodium: At least 75% less sodium than the original product.
  Low Sodium: 140 mg or less/serving.
  Very Low Sodium: 35mg or less/serving.
  Sodium Free: Less than 5mg per serving.
- **Use reduced-sodium breads,** butter and margarine. Regular varieties contain up to 2% salt. This is considered high in view of their significant contribution to our diet.
- **Go easy on condiments and sauces** such as tomato ketchup, mustard, soy sauce and spaghetti sauces, plus salad dressings. Use low sodium varieties.
- **Limit pizzas and salty fast-foods.** Check ***CalorieKing.com*** food database.
- **Avoid salty snack foods** such as potato chips, corn chips, salted nuts, pretzels and cheesy-flavored snacks. **Choose unsalted** popcorn, nuts or seeds. Eat more fruit.
- **Don't salt children's food** to your taste.
- **Limit or avoid antacids and saline powders with** sodium bicarbonate (such as *Alka-Seltzer*). They are high in sodium.

Foods High In Sodium

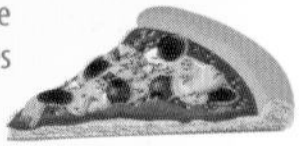

- Cheese, Butter, Margarine
- Pickles, Sauerkraut, Olives
- Condiments, Sauces
- Salad Dressings
- Canned vegetables/salads/beans
- Deli Salads (with dressing)
- Frozen/Packaged Meals/Entrees
- Soups: Canned/dry; bouillon cubes
- Meats: Ham, bacon, sausage, luncheon meats, smoked meats
- Canned Fish (in brine/salt)
- Sea Salt, Garlic/Celery Salt
- Snack Foods (potato chips, pretzels)
- Tomato Juice (Canned), V8 Vegetable Juice
- Fast Foods: Pizza, Burgers, Chicken
- *Alka-Seltzer* Antacid

Moderate Sodium

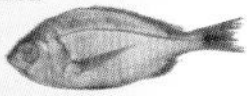

- Bread (Reduced Salt)
- Meat, Fish, Poultry - Unprocessed
- Milk, Yogurt, Soy Drinks, Eggs
- Peanut Butter
- Breakfast Cereals (less than 200mg/serving)
- Chocolate Candy, Fruit/Nut Bars
- *Reduced Sodium & Low Sodium* Products

Foods Low In Sodium

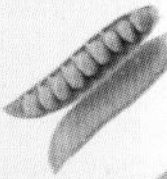

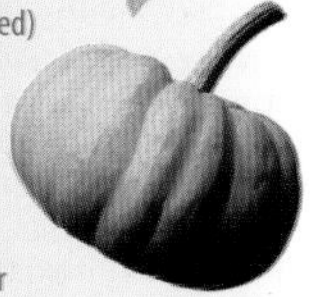

- Products labelled *Very Low Sodium*, or *Sodium Free*
- Fresh fruits and vegetables
- Canned and Dried Fruits
- Potatoes, Rice, Pasta
- Dried Beans & Lentils, Tofu
- Nuts & Seeds (unsalted)
- Corn & Popcorn (unsalted)
- Pepper, Spices, Herbs
- Jam, Honey, Syrup
- Candy, Gum
- Hard & Jelly Candy
- Coffee, Tea, Alcohol
- Fresh Fruit Juices, Water

> The American Heart Association recommends a sodium intake of **less than 2400mg/day**

Milk & Dairy Products

	Sodium
Milk: Whole/lowfat/skim, average	
1 cup, 8 fl.oz	120
Whole, low sodium, 1 cup	5
Choc Milk *(Hershey's)*, 1 cup	130
Soy Milk, 8 fl.oz	30
Buttermilk, cultured, 8 fl.oz	250
Dry/Powder, skim, ¼ cup, 1 oz	110
Yogurt, with fruit average, 8 oz	130
Cheese: Blue, 1 oz	330
Parmesan, 1 oz	450
Kraft Cheddar, 1 oz	180
Philadelphia Brand Cream Cheese	85
Process Cheese., average,1 oz	430
Swiss, 1 oz	40
Cottage Cheese, ½ cup, 4 oz	450
Ricotta Cheese, ½ cup, 4 oz	150

Icecream, Frozen Yogurt

Icecream, average,½ cup	50
Frozen Yogurt, ½ cup	50

Fats/Oils

Butter/Margarine:	
Regular, 2 Tbsp, 1 oz	230
Unsalted, reg., 2 Tbsp, 1 oz	5
Mayonnaise, aver., 2 Tbsp, 1 oz	160
Oils/Lard/Dripping	0
Cream, average, 1 Tbsp	6
Coffee-Mate: Powdered, 1 tsp	2
Liquid, 1 Tbsp	5

Eggs

Whole, 1 large	70
Omelet, 2 egg, plain	220
w. cheese	400
Egg Beaters (Fleischmann's), ¼ cup	80

Meats

Meat, average all types, cooked (Beef/Lamb/Veal/Pork), 4 oz	80
Corned Beef, cooked, 3 oz	800
Bacon, cooked, 2 slices, ½ oz	270
Ham, 3 oz	1100

Chicken & Turkey

Chicken/Turkey, cooked, unsalted, 4 oz	80
Stuffing Mixes, average., ½ cup	500

Sodium ~ Sodium (mg)

Sausages & Meats

	Sodium
Bologna, 1 oz	280
Frankfurter, 2 oz	640
Ham, chopped, ¾ oz slice	290
Liverwurst (Braunschweiger), 1 oz	320
Pepperoni, 5 slices, 1 oz	570
Salami, cooked, 1 oz	350
dry/hard, 1 oz	600
Sausage, 1 oz link	220
Pork, 2 oz patty	260
Turkey Roll, 1 oz	160

Fish:

Fresh Fish, average, plain	
Cooked, 4 oz (no bone)	60
Broiled w. butter, 4 oz	150
Breaded & fried, 4 oz	320
Fish fillets, batter-dipped 3 oz	350
Fish sticks, 1 oz stick	160
Gefilte Fish (w. broth), 1 pce, 1½ oz	220
Herring, pickled, 2 pces, 1 oz	260
Lobster, meat only, 4 oz	180
Oysters, fresh, 6 med., 3 oz	95
Salmon: Canned, 3 oz	460
No Salt Added, 3 oz	65
Smoked fish, average, 3 oz	650
Tuna: Canned, 3 oz	330
No Added Salt, 3 oz	40

Entrees & Meals

Frozen Meals, average	600-900
Lean Cuisine, average	700
Stouffer's, average	580
Dinners, average	900-1200
Side Dishes, average	400-600
Pizza, frozen, ¼ large, 6 oz	800-1200
Microwave Cup Meals	900-1200
Cup O'Noodles, average	1500

Fast-Foods & Restaurants

Cheeseburger	750
Chicken Dinner (3 piece)	2200
Chicken Nuggets w. Sauce	800
Fish/Chicken Sandwich	1000
French Fries, small, 2½ oz	150
Hamburger: Regular	500
Large with cheese	1100
Hot Dog (Frankfurter)	800
Pizza, 2 medium slices	1200
Shake, chocolate	250
Taco	400

Extra Listings ~ see CalorieKing.com

Sodium ~ Sodium (mg)

	Sodium
Soups: Condensed, 1 c., 8 oz	800-1000
Low Sodium	70
Chicken Noodle, 1 cup	900
Bouillon Cube, average	950
Cup-A-Soup: Average	850
Lite, average	450
Soup Mixes, average, 1 cup	900

Condiments, Sauces, Dressings

A-1 Sauce, 1 Tbsp	270
Barbecue Sauce, 1 Tbsp	130
Bragg Liquid Aminos, 1 tsp	220
Chili Sauce, 1 Tbsp	230
Ketchup: Tomato, 1 Tbsp	180
Low Sodium, 1 Tbsp	20
Mayonnaise, 1 Tbsp	80
Mustard, 1 tsp	70
Pizza Sauce, ½ cup	700
Salad Dressings, 2 Tbsp, 1 oz	160-400
Spaghetti Sauce, ½ cup	500
Soy Sauce: 1 Tbsp	900
Lite *(Kikkoman),* 1 Tbsp	600
Sweet & Sour, ½ cup	250
Tabasco, 1 tsp	25
Vinegar, Lemon Juice	0
Worcestershire, 1 Tbsp	200
Tomato: Sauce, 1 cup	1200
Paste/Puree (salted), ½ cup	1000
No Salt Added, ½ cup	25

Salt & Salt Substitutes

Table Salt: 1 teaspoon, 6g	2400
Single Serve package, 1 g	400
Cardia Salt, 1 teaspoon	1080
Lite Salt *(Morton)*, 1 teaspoon, 6g	1200
***Morton* Salt Substitute**	5
***No Salt* Salt Substitute,** 1 teaspoon	5
Garlic/Seasoned Salt 1 teaspoon, 4g	1300
Sea Salt, 1 teaspoon, 5g	2250

Seasonings, Herbs & Spices

Baking Powder, 1 tsp, 3g	340
Baking Soda (Sodium bicarb), 1 tsp, 3g	810
Accent (Flavor Enhancer), 1 tsp	600
Chili Powder, 1 tsp, 3g	25
Curry Powder	0
Lemon Pepper *(Lawry's)*, 1 tsp	340
Meat Tenderizer, 1 tsp, 5g	1750
MSG (Monosodium glutamate), 5g	500
Mrs Dash (Herb/Spice Blend), 1 tsp	0
Pepper, Mustard (dry), 1 tsp	1
Yeast, Nutritional, 1 Tbsp	10

Breakfast Cereals

Kellogg's:	Sodium
All-Bran, ⅓ cup, 1 oz	260
Oatbran Flakes, ¾ cup, 1 oz	220
Corn Flakes, 1 cup, 1 oz	290
Just Right, ½ cup, 1 oz	200
Mini Wheats Frosted, 1.8 oz	5
Health Valley Cereals, 1 serving	5
Quaker: Cap'n Crunch, ¾ cup, 1 oz	200
Crunchy Corn Bran, 1 cup, 1 oz	320
100% Natural Granola, ½ cup, 1 oz	15
Puffed Rice/Wheat, 2 cups, 1 oz	1
Total, 1 cup, 1 oz	140
Oatmeal: Regular, ¾ cup	1
Instant *(Quaker)*, ⅔ cup (1 pkt)	270

Breads, Bagels, Crackers

Bread: Average all types, 1 oz	140
Low Sodium, 1 oz	10
Bagels: Plain, 2 oz	200
Sara Lee, 3 oz	500
Biscuits, average, 1 oz	180
Bun/Roll, 1 medium, 1½ oz	200
Crackers: Saltine, 2 crackers	70
Low Salt (Premium), 2	45
Graham, 2 regular	50
Croissant, average, 2 oz	280
Rice Cakes, average	25
RyKrisp Crispbread, Sesame, 2	100

Cookies, Cakes, Desserts

Cookies: Average, 2-3 cookies, 1 oz	100
Mrs Fields', average, 2½ oz	180
Baked Custard, ½ cup	100
Brownie, ¼ oz piece	75
Cake, average, 3 oz piece	250
Cinnamon Sweet Roll, 2 oz	250
Danish, Apple	250
Donut, average	150
Muffins: 1 medium, 2 oz	150
Sara Lee, average, 2½ oz	300
Pancakes, 3 x 4"	360
Pie, average 1/6 of 9" pie	300
Pudding: Average, ½ cup	160
Jell-O (Mix), Instant, ½ cup	400
Waffles:	
Home-made, 7", 2½ oz	350
Frozen, average, 1¼ oz	260
Aunt Jemima, avg, 2½ oz	630

Fruit & Juices

	Sodium
Fresh Fruit, average all types, 1 serving	1
Dried/Canned Fruit, ½ cup	1
Fruit Juice: Fresh, sqz'd, 6 fl.oz	1
Commercial, aver., 6 fl.oz	20
Carrot Juice *(Ferraro's)*, 8 fl.oz	230
Tomato Juice *(Campbell's)*, 6 fl.oz	570
Low Sodium (No Salt Added)	20
V8 Vegetable *(Campbell's)*, 6 fl.oz	600
(No Salt Added), 6 fl.oz	45

Vegetables

Fresh/Frozen (No Salt Added): *Per ½ Cup*	
Asparagus, Bean Sprouts, Corn	3
Beets, Carrots, Celery, ½ cup	40
Broccoli, Cabbage, Cauliflower	10
Cucumber, Green Beans, Mushroom, Okra	3
Onions, Peas, Potato, Pumpkin, Squash	3
Peppers, Hot Chili, raw, each	3
Spinach, Turnips, ½ cup, ckd	40
Tomato, 1 medium, 5 oz	10
Canned: Asparagus, 4 spears	300
Beans, baked in tomato sauce	450
Beets, ½ cup, 3 oz	240
Corn Kernels, ½ cup, 3 oz	190
Creamed, ½ cup, 4½ oz	330
Mushrooms w. butter sce, 2oz	550
Peas, ½ cup, 3 oz	250
Sauerkraut, ½ cup, 4 oz	750

Pickles, Olives

Olives, pickled: Green, 1 large	90
Ripe/black, 1 large	40
Pickles: Bread & Butter, 4 sl., 1 oz	200
Dill, 1 pickle, 2½ oz	900
Sweet, 1 gherkin, ½ oz	130

Soybean Products

Miso (Soy Paste), ¼ c., 2½ oz	2500
Soybean Protein Isolate, 1 oz	280
Tempeh, ½ cup, 3 oz	5
Tofu, average, ½ cup, 4 oz	5

Jam, Honey, Syrups

Jam/Jelly, 1 Tbsp	2
Honey/Maple Syrup, 1 Tbsp	1
Log Cabin Syrup, 1 fl.oz	35
Lite, 1 fl.oz	90

Peanut Butter

Peanut Butter, regular, 1 Tbsp	70
Unsalted, 1 Tbsp	1

Snacks, Nuts

	Sodium
Cheese Balls/Curls, 1 oz	280
Corn/Tortilla Chips, average, 1 oz	220
Granola bars, average, 1 bar	80
Nuts: Plain, unsalted, 1 oz	1
Lightly salted, 1 oz	80
Salted or Honey Roasted, 1 oz	160
Popcorn: Plain (unsalted), 1 cup	1
Flavored, average, 1 cup	60
Salt added, 1 cup	180
Potato Chips: Plain, 1 oz	160
Flavored, average, 1 oz	250
Pretzels, regular, 3, 1 oz	450

Candy, Chocolate

Chocolate, milk, 1 oz	30
Carob Milk Bar, 1 oz	55
Fudge, chocolate, 1 oz	55
Candy Bars, average, 1½ oz	60
Hard Candy, Jelly Beans, 1 oz	10
Licorice, 1 oz	30

Beverages, Alcohol

Coffee (& Substitutes), Tea, 1 cup	1
Cocoa, dry, plain, 1 Tbsp	0
Mix, average, 1 envelope	120
Quik *(Nestle)*, 2 tsp	35
Soft Drinks, average, 8 fl.oz	20
Mineral Water, Perrier, 8 fl.oz	5
Gatorade Thirst Quencher, 8 fl.oz	110
Water: Average, 1 cup, 8 fl.oz	5
Drier regions, 1 cup	20+
Alcohol: Beer, average, 12 fl.oz	15
Wines, average, 4 fl.oz	10
Spirits (distilled), 1½ fl.oz	1

Antacids - Alka-Seltzer

	Sodium
Alka-Seltzer *(Per Tablet):*	
Alka-Seltzer P.M., 1 tablet	500
Original (Light Blue Box)	570
Extra Strength (Dark Blue Box)	590
Flavored Lemon/Lime & Cherry	500
Antacid (yellow Box)	310
Gelatine Capsule, 1	0
Alka-Mints, chewable	0
Bromo Seltzer, ¾ capful	760
Rolaids, All types	0
Tums, Regular/Extra Strength	0
Sodium Bicarbonate (27% sodium), 1g	270

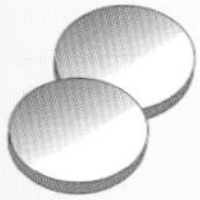

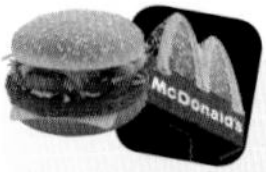

Fast-Food Restaurants Index
~ See Page 183 ~

FAST-FOOD INDEX
~ PAGE 183 ~

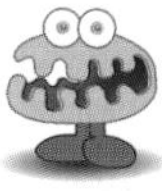

Index H - L

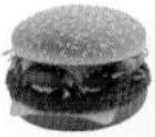

FAST-FOOD INDEX ~ PAGE 183 ~

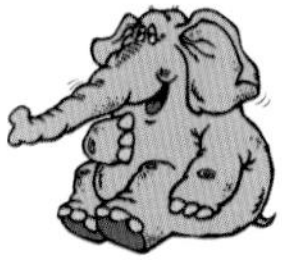

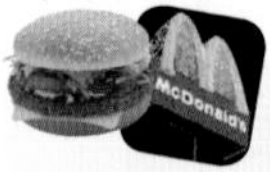

FAST-FOOD RESTAURANTS INDEX
~ SEE PAGE 183 ~

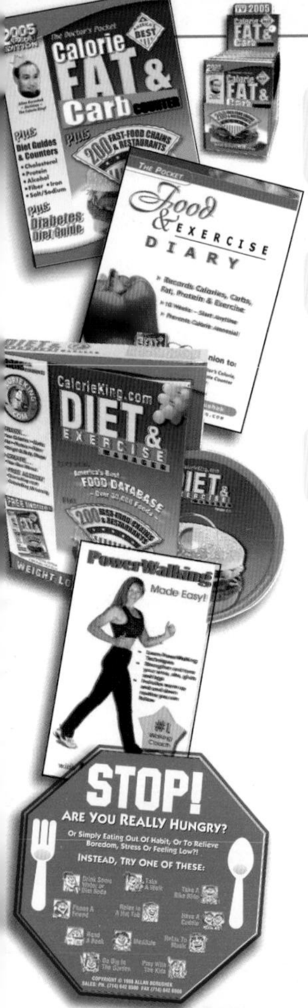

Mail Order *Service*

▶ **The Doctor's Pocket CALORIE, FAT & CARB COUNTER** **$7.00**

- **10-Book Display Box ($6.00 per book)** **$60.00**

(Special Quantity Discounts - Contact Publisher)

▶ **FOOD & EXERCISE DIARY (10 Weeks)** **$4.00**

▶ **DESKTOP DIET DIARY SOFTWARE** **$29.95**
Tracks your meals, snacks, exercise, weight and more!
Includes free access to CalorieKing.com University

▶ **FRIDGE POSTER** **$3.00**
STOP! ARE YOU REALLY HUNGRY?
(8″x 8″ size, with magnet) ~ See Page 55

▶ **POWERWALK VIDEO** **$19.00**
with Patti Joyce, America's Best Walking Coach
~ Fun, Motivational. Learn how to burn extra calories!

▶ **PEDOMETERS & WALKING PROGRAM**

- **Yamax (Clinical Calorie Model)** **$25.00**
  Measures steps, miles, calories
- **Omron Pedometer (Deluxe Clinical)** **$20.00**
  Measures steps, miles, calories,
  (Special Quantity Discounts)

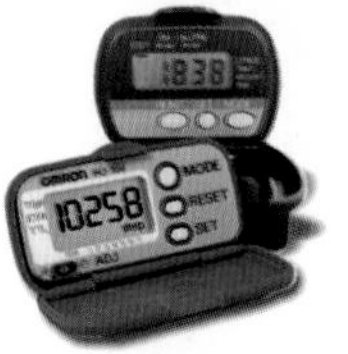

Shipping & Handling:

Add $3.00 for first item and
$1.00 for each extra item.
(In California, add 7¾% Sales Tax)

Phone (949) 642-8500

Online www.CalorieKing.com

OR Mail your order with payment to:

Family Health Publications
1001 West 17th St, Suite M
Costa Mesa, CA 92627

VISA · MasterCard · AMERICAN EXPRESS

SPECIAL QUANTITY DISCOUNTS
~ CONTACT PUBLISHER ~

Online ~ www.CalorieKing.com

Weight Control Tips

Eat Sensibly

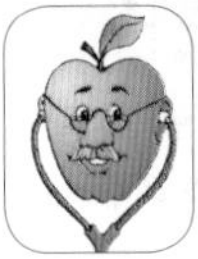

- Avoid fad diets. Eat 3 sensible meals daily with adequate fruit and vegetables.
- Limit portion size. Limit fats and high-fat foods, sugar, soda and alcohol. *(Sample Diet Plan ~ Page 11)*

Exercise Daily

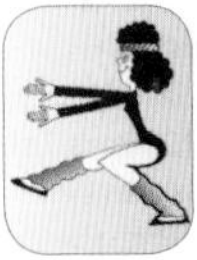

- Get active and exercise every day!
- Include muscle-strengthening exercises. You'll lose more fat and keep it off. You'll also feel and look better, and you can eat a little more! *(Exercise Guide ~ Page 12)*

Reshape Eating Behaviors

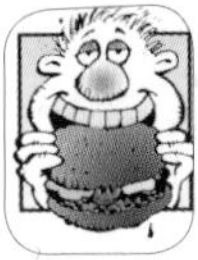

- Be aware of eating habits and behaviors that lead to overeating.
- Also focus on social and emotional situations that lead you to snack compulsively. *(Extra notes ~ Page 14)*

Keep a Food & Exercise Diary

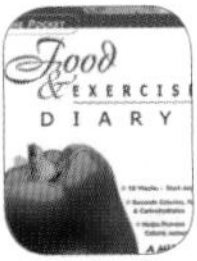

- A diary helps you see exactly what you eat and drink, and how much you exercise.
- An excellent motivator and proven weight loss aid. Keeps you honest!

Arrange Moral Support

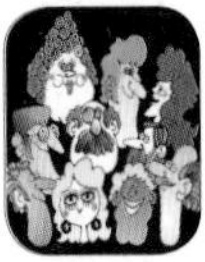

Gain the support of family and friends. Get extra professional help if required, from your doctor, dietitian, psychologist, exercise trainer, or slimming group. Beware of family saboteurs who discourage you from adopting a healthier lifestyle!

DOCTOR CHECK-UP

Ask your doctor to check your blood pressure, blood sugar and blood cholesterol levels.

HEALTHY WEIGHTS ~ MEN & WOMEN ~ (Over 18 Years)

Based on weights with least risk of disease or death from heart disease, diabetes, stroke and cancer.

Based on Body Mass Index of 20-35

BMI calculated as: $\frac{\text{Weight (kg)}}{\text{Height (m)}^2}$

Height (No Shoes) Ft Ins		Healthy Weight Range (Pounds)
4'7"	~	86-108
4'8"	~	88-110
4'9"	~	92-114
4'10"	~	97-121
4'11"	~	99-123
5'0"	~	101-127
5'1"	~	105-132
5'2"	~	110-136
5'3"	~	112-140
5'4"	~	114-145
5'5"	~	119-149
5'6"	~	123-156
5'7"	~	127-158
5'8"	~	129-162
5'9"	~	134-167
5'10"	~	138-173
5'11"	~	143-178
6'0"	~	145-182
6'1"	~	149-187
6'2"	~	156-193
6'3"	~	158-198
6'4"	~	162-202
6'5"	~	170-211
6'6"	~	172-215
6'7"	~	175-220

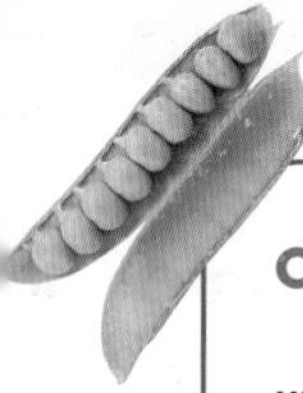

Contents

Calorie, Fat & Carbohydrate Counter

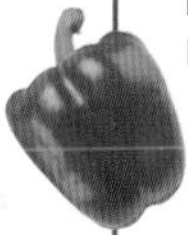

Diet Guides & Counters

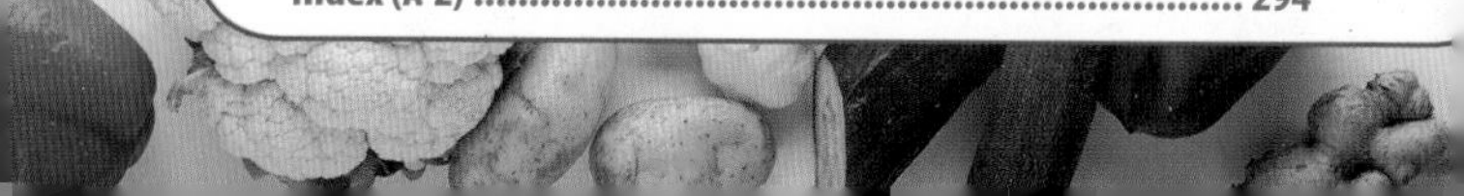